Complimentary Access

Your Personal AI Assistant

AF086158

Dr. Wise

Be Wise, Ask Dr. Wise!
You can search Anything, Anywhere, Anytime

- MCQs
- Short Notes
- Long Notes
- Images
- Flowcharts
- Explanations

Access the chatbot using the steps below
1. Scan QR and install App
2. Redemption Process:

New Users
- Click Redeem and enter redemption code
- Create Account and get access to online content

Existing Users
- Login with e-learning account credentials
- Redeem code inside more option

Redeem Code

*No return is acceptable if panel is scratched off

DOWNLOAD APP
Download on the App Store
GET IT ON Google Play

Essentials of Microbiology
(Organism-Based)

Apurba S Sastry MD (JIPMER) DNB MNAMS PDCR
*Officer In-charge, Hospital Infection Control and Prevention Unit (HICP)
Antimicrobial Stewardship Lead (Microbiology)
Additional Professor
Department of Microbiology
Jawaharlal Institute of Postgraduate Medical Education and Research (JIPMER)
Puducherry, India*

Sandhya Bhat (Gold medalist) MD DNB MNAMS PDCR
*Professor
Department of Microbiology
Pondicherry Institute of Medical Sciences (PIMS)
(A Unit of The Madras Medical Mission)
Puducherry, India*

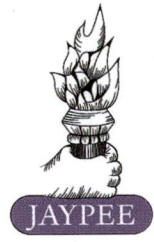

JAYPEE BROTHERS MEDICAL PUBLISHERS
The Health Sciences Publisher
New Delhi | London

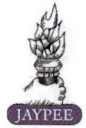

Jaypee Brothers Medical Publishers (P) Ltd

Headquarters

Jaypee Brothers Medical Publishers (P) Ltd
EMCA House, 23/23-B
Ansari Road, Daryaganj
New Delhi 110 002, India
Landline: +91-11-23272143, +91-11-23272703
+91-11-23282021, +91-11-23245672
Email: jaypee@jaypeebrothers.com

Corporate Office

Jaypee Brothers Medical Publishers (P) Ltd
4838/24, Ansari Road, Daryaganj
New Delhi 110 002, India
Phone: +91-11-43574357
Fax: +91-11-43574314
Email: jaypee@jaypeebrothers.com

Website: www.jaypeebrothers.com
Website: www.jaypeedigital.com

Overseas Office

J.P. Medical Ltd
83 Victoria Street, London
SW1H 0HW (UK)
Phone: +44 20 3170 8910
Fax: +44 (0)20 3008 6180
Email: info@jpmedpub.com

© 2025, Jaypee Brothers Medical Publishers

The views and opinions expressed in this book are solely those of the original contributor(s)/author(s) and do not necessarily represent those of editor(s) and Publisher of the book.

All rights reserved. No part of this publication may be reproduced, stored or transmitted in any form or by any means, electronic, mechanical, photocopying, recording or otherwise, without the prior permission in writing of the publishers.

All brand names and product names used in this book are trade names, service marks, trademarks or registered trademarks of their respective owners. The publisher is not associated with any product or vendor mentioned in this book.

Medical knowledge and practice change constantly. This book is designed to provide accurate, authoritative information about the subject matter in question. However, readers are advised to check the most current information available on procedures included and check information from the manufacturer of each product to be administered, to verify the recommended dose, formula, method and duration of administration, adverse effects and contraindications. It is the responsibility of the practitioner to take all appropriate safety precautions. Neither the publisher nor the author(s)/editor(s) assume any liability for any injury and/or damage to persons or property arising from or related to use of material in this book.

This book is sold on the understanding that the publisher is not engaged in providing professional medical services. If such advice or services are required, the services of a competent medical professional should be sought.

Every effort has been made where necessary to contact holders of copyright to obtain permission to reproduce copyright material. If any have been inadvertently overlooked, the publisher will be pleased to make the necessary arrangements at the first opportunity.

Inquiries for bulk sales may be solicited at: jaypee@jaypeebrothers.com

Essentials of Microbiology (Organism-Based)

First Edition: **2025**

ISBN: 978-93-5696-848-6

Printed at: Samrat Offset Pvt. Ltd.

Dedicated to

Our Beloved Parents

Family Members

And, above all, the Almighty

Golden Rules of Goal Setting

Dear Students

Here are some important tips which will help you in setting your goals in studies:

1. **Set Goals That Motivate You:** This means making sure that they are important to you, and that there is value in achieving them
2. **Set SMART Goals**
   - Specific: Your goal must be clear and well defined, not vague or generalized
   - Measurable: Goals must have measurable objectives
   - Attainable: Make sure that your goals are achievable and within your limit
   - Relevant: Will take you to the direction you want your life and career to go
   - Time Bound: You must know when you have the deadline and can celebrate success
3. **Set Goals in Writing:** Written commitment in presence of your close people (parents, close friends) will always push and remind you whenever you tend to deviate from your goal
4. **Make an Action Plan:** Do not focus only on the outcome, but make planning of all small steps that collectively take to the outcome. This is especially important if your goal is big and demanding, or long-term
5. **Monitor Yourself:** Compliance to the action plan should be monitored at least weekly (for one month goal) or monthly (for a yearly goal), depending upon your goal size.

Remember

"Success is not final; failure is not fatal: It is the courage to continue that counts." —*Winston S Churchill*

"There are two types of people who will tell you that you cannot make a difference in this world: those who are afraid to try and those who are afraid you will succeed." —*Ray Goforth*

Preface

It gives us immense pleasure to announce the release of *Essentials of Microbiology (Organism-Based)*. The excitement reaches its height as our efforts of the last three months have come to an end. The idea of scripting an organism-based book on Microbiology came to our mind as we received numerous requests from the Microbiology faculty and paramedical students across the country to write a Microbiology book with an organism-based approach that can cater to several courses such as BScMLT (Bachelor's Degree in Medical Lab Technology) and other Allied Health Science Courses, BPT (Bachelor of Physiotherapy) and AYUSH courses—BAMS (Bachelor of Ayurvedic Medicine and Surgery), BHMS (Bachelor of Homeopathic Medicine and Surgery), BUMS (Bachelor of Unani Medicine and Surgery), BNYS (Bachelor of Naturopathy and Yoga Science) and BSMS (Bachelor of Siddha Medicine and Surgery). The existing books on these subjects are discouraging with suboptimal matter and do not cover the syllabus properly. Keeping all the above-mentioned aspects in mind, we have drafted this textbook with a unique approach to suit the needs of students of India—both in their examination and in clinical/laboratory practice.

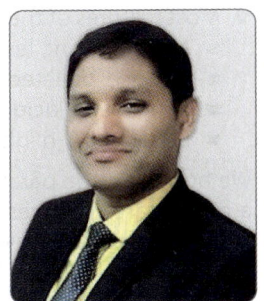

Apurba S Sastry

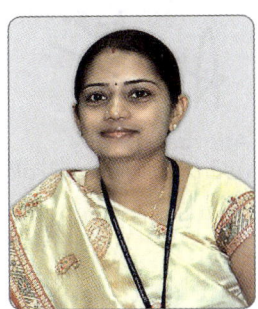

Sandhya Bhat

- ❖ **Section 1:** *General Microbiology* section is meticulously structured with the inclusion of general bacteriology, which is further reorganized into several sub-chapters.
- ❖ **Section 2:** *Immunology* section covers topics such as immunity, antigen, antibody, complement, antigen-antibody reactions, components of the immune system, immune response, hypersensitivity reactions, autoimmunity, immunodeficiency disorders, immunoprophylaxis, national immunization schedule, and immunohematology.
- ❖ **Section 3:** *Hospital Infection Control* section comprises topics such as healthcare-associated infections (HAI), standard precautions including hand hygiene and PPE, transmission-based precautions, major HAI types, HAI surveillance, infection control committee, sterilization and disinfection (including CSSD), biomedical waste management (BMW), needle stick injury, environmental surveillance, and antimicrobial stewardship.
- ❖ **Section 4:** *Systematic Bacteriology* section covers topics such as gram-positive cocci (*Staphylococcus*, *Streptococcus*, Pneumococcus, *Enterococcus*), and gram-negative cocci (meningococcus and gonococcus), gram-positive bacilli (*Corynebacterium* and *Bacillus*), anaerobes (including non-sporing anaerobes), mycobacteria (*Mycobacterium tuberculosis*, NTM, and *M. leprae*), gram-negative bacilli (Enterobacterales, Vibrio, non-fermenters, fastidious bacteria, miscellaneous gram-negative bacteria), Spirochetes, Rickettsiae, Chlamydiae, and *Mycoplasma*.
- ❖ **Section 5:** *Virology* section covers topics such as DNA viruses like Herpes and others, and RNA viruses such as Myxoviruses, rubella virus, coronaviruses, arboviruses, rabies virus, poliovirus, HIV, hepatitis viruses, Ebola virus, viral gastroenteritis, oncogenic viruses, and others. COVID-19, the most catastrophic disease of today's date has been addressed as a completely new chapter covering in detail.
- ❖ **Section 6:** *Parasitology* section covers topics such as Amoebae, flagellates (*Giardia, Trichomonas, Leishmania*, and *Trypanosoma*), malaria parasite (*Plasmodium*), coccidian parasites, cestodes, trematodes, nematodes (intestinal and tissue), and ectoparasites.
- ❖ **Section 7:** *Mycology* section covers topics such as superficial mycoses, subcutaneous mycoses, systemic (deep) mycoses, and opportunistic fungal infections.
- ❖ **Section 8:** *Applied Microbiology* section comprises topics on various infective syndromes such as bloodstream infection, meningitis, UTI, diarrhea, respiratory infection, and others. A separate chapter on *Specimen Collection* has been incorporated (under Section 8) covering in-depth various aspects of appropriate specimen collection—correct technique, adequate volume, and at the correct time (before the start of antimicrobials).

Preface

- ❖ **Annexures** incorporated at the end cover relevant topics such as laboratory-acquired infections and laboratory safety, quality control in Microbiology, and practical Microbiology. The Annexure on Practical Microbiology enlists the common practical exercises required for the above-mentioned courses and also gives information regarding the chapters and page numbers where these exercises have been discussed in detail in various sections.
- ❖ Most features of the author's popular MBBS book have been maintained in this book:
  - More content, less pages—saves student's time
  - Concise, bulleted format, and to-the-point text—easy-to-read during the examination
  - Simple and lucid language—makes the understanding easy
  - Separate highlight boxes—for important topics and treatment boxes for quick review.

We hope that the paramedical students will relish reading this book and find it useful. We also hope that we have made a good start in addressing the varied needs of paramedical students and faculty teaching microbiology with a single comprehensive book. We will be glad to receive your valuable feedback, which will enable us to improve further.

Apurba S Sastry
apurbasastrymicrobiology@gmail.com

Sandhya Bhat
sandhyabhatk@gmail.com

Acknowledgments

The release of *Essentials of Microbiology (Organism-Based)* would not have been possible without our close association with many people. We take this opportunity to extend our sincere gratitude and appreciation to all those who made this book possible.

Hearty acknowledgments to our teachers, departmental staff, family members, and others, for their blessings and support.

- We are extremely thankful to Director, JIPMER, Puducherry, and Director-Principal, Pondicherry Institute of Medical Sciences (PIMS), Puducherry to encourage for writing books.
- **Faculty, residents and postgraduates** of Department of Microbiology, JIPMER, Puducherry and Pondicherry Institute of Medical Sciences (PIMS), Puducherry for their inputs during the manuscript preparation.
- **For providing photographs**—We are extremely thankful to all people/institutes/companies who have agreed to provide valuable photographs.
- **Microbiology faculty from various institutes**—Dr Anand B Janagond, Dr Deepashree R, Dr Ketan Priyadarshi, and Dr Sarumathi for their inputs during the manuscript preparation.

As you know, human errors are inevitable; and no book is immune to them. We would request all the readers to provide any errata found and also valuable inputs. If any reader wishes to share feedback, suggestions, updates, and errata, please feel free to mail us at *apurbasastrymicrobiology@gmail.com*. As a token of gratitude, the reader will be acknowledged in the subsequent edition of the book.

Special Acknowledgments to My Publisher

Jaypee Brothers Medical Publishers (P) Ltd, New Delhi, India

- Shri Jitendar P Vij (Group Chairman)
- Mr Ankit Vij (Managing Director)
- Mr MS Mani (Group President)
- Dr Madhu Choudhary (Director–Educational Publishing): She has been a great support throughout the manuscript preparation
- Ms Pooja Bhandari [Director–Production (Books and Journals)]
- Ms Seema Dogra (Cover Visualizer)
- Mr Aditya Tayal (Editorial Manager–Content Strategy): Extremely dynamic, have lot of patience and available 24x7 to address to our queries
- **Development team:** Mr Deep Kumar (Typesetter), Mr Nitin Bhardwaj (Graphic Designer) and Ms Neelam Kakriya (Proofreader). These guys are simply outstanding in their work. The way Nitin Bhardwaj does the designing of photographs is extraordinary. It is a treat for us to work with all of them. These guys are extremely workaholic and have a very good team spirit. We salute them, for their professionalism.
- **Marketing heads from various zones:** Mr Narendra Shekhawat (Vice President–Sales), Mr Venugopal V (South Head), Mr Rishi Sharma (North Region Head), CS Gawde (Western Head) and Sandip Gupta (Eastern Head).
- **Branch managers and sales manager from various branches:** Bengaluru branch (Ravi Kumar, A Palani, E Venkatesh), Chennai branch [Maran A (Adoption Head for South), Dharani Kumar P, RK Dharani, Dharanidaran], Kochi branch (Sujeesh VS, Diffin Robin, Arun Kumar), Hyderabad branch (Parimal Guha Neogy, Marthanda Sarma, Rajesh Malothu, Hamza Ali), Mumbai branch (Sameer S Mulla), Nagpur branch (Rajesh Shrivas), Ahmedabad branch (Ms Priyanka Kansara, Dinesh Waghade), Delhi branch (Sujatha Puri) and Kolkata branch (Sanjoy Chakraborthy).

Lastly, we would like to keep in record that without the support of our son (Master Adarsh), and parents (of both Dr Sandhya and Dr Apurba), it would have been impossible to continue the spirit on, during the journey of the current edition.

Apurba S Sastry
Sandhya Bhat

Contents

Section 1: General Microbiology — 1

1. Introduction and History — 3
2. Microscopy — 6
3. General Bacteriology
   - 3.1 Morphology and Physiology of Bacteria — 11
   - 3.2 Laboratory Diagnosis of Bacterial Infections — 19
   - 3.3 Bacterial Genetics — 40
   - 3.4 Antimicrobial Agents and Antimicrobial Resistance — 45
   - 3.5 Bacterial Pathogenesis — 49
4. Normal Microbial Flora — 52
5. Epidemiology of Infectious Diseases — 54

Section 2: Immunology — 57

6. Immunity (Innate and Acquired) — 59
7. Antigen, Antibody and Complement — 63
8. Antigen–Antibody Reaction — 71
9. Components of Immune System: Organs, Cells and Products — 81
10. Immune Responses: Cell-mediated and Antibody-mediated — 86
11. Hypersensitivity Reactions — 91
12. Autoimmunity, Immunodeficiency Disorders, Transplant and Tumor Immunology — 94
13. Immunoprophylaxis and Immunization Schedule — 99
14. Immunohematology — 104

Section 3: Hospital Infection Control — 107

15. Healthcare-associated Infections — 109
16. Sterilization and Disinfection — 118
17. Biomedical Waste Management — 130
18. Needle Stick Injury (Occupational Exposure) — 135
19. Environmental Surveillance (Bacteriology of Water, Air, Surface, and Food) — 139
20. Antimicrobial Stewardship — 143

Section 4: Systematic Bacteriology — 147

Gram-positive Cocci
21. *Staphylococcus* — 149
22. *Streptococcus*, Pneumococcus and *Enterococcus* — 153

Gram-negative Cocci
23. *Neisseria*: Meningococcus and Gonococcus — 158

Gram-positive Bacilli
24. *Corynebacterium* — 161
25. *Bacillus* — 165
26. Anaerobes: *Clostridium* and Non-sporing Anaerobes — 168
27. Mycobacteria: *M. tuberculosis*, Nontuberculous Mycobacteria and *M. leprae* — 172
28. Miscellaneous Gram-positive Bacilli (Actinomycetes and *Listeria*) — 178

Gram-negative Bacilli
29. Enterobacterales (*Escherichia coli, Klebsiella, Shigella, Salmonella* and Others) — 181
30. *Vibrio* — 189
31. *Pseudomonas, Acinetobacter* and Other Nonfermenters — 192

32.	Fastidious Gram-negative Bacilli: *Haemophilus, Brucella* and *Bordetella*	196
33.	Miscellaneous Gram-negative Bacilli: *Campylobacter, Helicobacter, Legionella, Pasteurella*, Agents of Bacterial Vaginosis, Rat-bite Fever	200
34.	Spirochetes: *Treponema, Borrelia* and *Leptospira*	*203*
35.	Rickettsiae, Chlamydiae and *Mycoplasma*	207

Section 5: Virology — 211

36.	General Virology	213
37.	Herpesviruses	219
38.	Other DNA Viruses (including Bacteriophage)	224
39.	Myxoviruses and Rubella Virus	227
40.	Coronaviruses	233
41.	Arboviruses	236
42.	Rabies Virus	241
43.	Picornaviruses (Poliovirus, Coxsackievirus and Rhinovirus)	244
44.	HIV/AIDS	248
45.	Hepatitis Viruses	254
46.	Miscellaneous RNA Viruses	260

Section 6: Parasitology — 265

47.	General Parasitology	267
48.	Amoebae (*Entamoeba* and Free-living Amoebae)	273
49.	Intestinal and Genital Flagellates: *Giardia* and *Trichomonas*	278
50.	Hemoflagellates: *Leishmania* and *Trypanosoma*	282
51.	Malaria Parasite and *Babesia*	286
52.	Opportunistic Coccidian Parasites and Others	292
53.	Cestodes: *Taenia, Echinococcus, Hymenolepis, Diphyllobothrium* and Others	297
54.	Trematodes: *Schistosoma*, Hepatic Flukes, *Fasciolopsis*, and *Paragonimus*	303
55.	Intestinal Nematodes: *Trichuris, Enterobius, Ascaris*, Hookworm, and *Strongyloides*	308
56.	Tissue Nematodes: Filarial Nematodes, *Dracunculus*, and *Trichinella*	316
57.	Medical Entomolgy (Ectoparasites)	321

Section 7: Mycology — 327

58.	Medical Mycology	329

Section 8: Applied Microbiology — 343

59.	Bloodstream Infections	345
60.	Meningitis	348
61.	Urinary Tract Infection	351
62.	Diarrheal Diseases	354
63.	Respiratory Tract Infections	357
64.	Miscellaneous Infective Syndromes	360
65.	Specimen Collection and Transport	365

Annexures — 371

1.	Laboratory-acquired Infections and Laboratory Safety	373
2.	Quality Control in Microbiology	375
3.	Practical Microbiology	378

Index — *379*

SECTION 1

General Microbiology

SECTION OUTLINE

1. Introduction and History
2. Microscopy
3. General Bacteriology
    - 3.1 Morphology and Physiology of Bacteria
    - 3.2 Laboratory Diagnosis of Bacterial Infections
    - 3.3 Bacterial Genetics
    - 3.4 Antimicrobial Agents and Antimicrobial Resistance
    - 3.5 Bacterial Pathogenesis
4. Normal Microbial Flora
5. Epidemiology of Infectious Diseases

Introduction and History

CHAPTER 1

CHAPTER PREVIEW
- Clinical Microbiology
- Classification of Microorganisms
- History

CLINICAL MICROBIOLOGY

Medical microbiology is a branch of medicine that deals with the study of microorganisms and their role in human health and diseases. It is also concerned with the diagnosis, treatment, and prevention of various infectious diseases. The branches of medical microbiology are as follows:

- **General microbiology:** It deals with the study of general properties of microorganisms—taxonomy, morphology, pathogenesis, laboratory diagnosis, and treatment for their effective killing
- **Immunology:** It deals with the study of the immune system, immunological mechanisms of infectious diseases and various immunological methods for diagnosis of infectious diseases
- **Hospital infection control:** It deals with the study of various control measures to prevent the transmission of healthcare associated infections
- **Systemic microbiology:** Microorganisms infect various organ systems of our body. Four kinds of microorganisms cause infectious disease: bacteria, fungi, parasites, and viruses
  1. *Bacteriology:* The study of bacteria
  2. *Virology:* The study of viruses
  3. *Mycology:* The study of fungi
  4. *Parasitology:* The study of parasites; it has two arms
     i. Protozoology: The study of protozoa
     ii. Helminthology: The study of helminths.

CLASSIFICATION OF MICROORGANISMS

Microorganisms are grouped under both prokaryotes and eukaryotes.
- Bacteria are placed under prokaryotes. They have a primitive nucleus, and other properties of a prokaryotic cell **(Table 1.1)**
- Whereas fungi and parasites (protozoa and helminths) belong to eukaryotes; having a well-defined nucleus and various eukaryotic cellular organelles

Table 1.1: Characteristics of prokaryotes and eukaryotes.

Characteristics		Prokaryotes	Eukaryotes
Microorganisms		Bacteria	Fungi, parasites
Nucleus		Diffuse	Well defined
	Nuclear membrane	Absent	Present
	Nucleolus	Absent	Present
	Ribonucleoprotein	Absent	Present
	Cell division	Binary fission	Mitosis, meiosis
	Chromosome	One, circular	Many, linear
Extrachromosomal DNA		Found in plasmid	Found in mitochondria
Cell membrane		Does not contain sterols except in *Mycoplasma*	Contain sterols
Cellular organelles like mitochondria, etc.		Absent (except ribosome)	Present
Ribosome		70S	80S
Site of respiration		Mesosome	Mitochondria

(S: Svedberg unit)

- Viruses are neither considered as prokaryotes nor eukaryotes because they lack the characteristics of living things, except the ability to replicate.

HISTORY

The existence of microorganisms was hypothesized for many centuries before their actual discovery. The teaching of Mahavira (Jainism, 6th century BC) and the postulation of Varo and Columella (who named the invisible organisms as '*Animalia minuta*') were some of those attempts. The eminent personalities in the field of Microbiology and their important contributions have been described below.

Antonie Philips van Leeuwenhoek (1676)

He was the first scientist who observed bacteria and other microorganisms, using a single-lens microscope constructed by him and he named those small organisms as *'Little animalcules'* **(Fig. 1.1A)**.

Louis Pasteur

Microbiology developed as a scientific discipline from the era of Louis Pasteur (1822–1895). He is also known as **'father of microbiology'**. He was a professor of chemistry in France. His studies on fermentation led him to take interest to work in microbiology **(Fig. 1.1B)**. His contributions to microbiology are as follows:

- He had proposed the **principles of fermentation** for preservation of food
- He introduced the **sterilization techniques** and developed steam sterilizer, hot air oven and autoclave
- He described the method of **pasteurization of milk**
- He had also contributed for the vaccine development against several diseases, such as anthrax, fowl cholera and rabies
- He disproved the theory of spontaneous generation of disease and postulated the **'germ theory of disease'**. He stated that disease cannot be caused by bad air or vapor, but it is produced by the microorganisms present in air
- **Liquid media concept:** He used nutrient broth to grow microorganisms
- He was the founder of the Pasteur Institute, Paris.

Joseph Lister

Joseph Lister (1867) is considered to be the **'father of antiseptic surgery'**. He had observed that postoperative infections were greatly reduced by using disinfectants such as diluted carbolic acid during surgery to sterilize the instruments and to clean the wounds.

Robert Koch

Robert Koch provided remarkable contributions to the field of microbiology. He was a German general practitioner (1843–1910) **(Fig. 1.1C)**. His contributions are as follows:

- He introduced **solid media** for the culture of bacteria. Eilshemius Hesse, the wife of, one of the Koch's assistants had suggested the use of **agar** as solidifying agents
- He also introduced methods for isolation of bacteria in **pure culture**
- He described **hanging drop** method for testing motility
- He **discovered bacteria** such as the anthrax bacilli, tubercle bacilli and cholera bacilli
- He introduced staining techniques by using aniline dye
- **Koch's postulates:** Robert Koch had postulated that a microorganism can be accepted as the causative agent of an infectious disease only if four criteria are fulfilled. These criteria are as follows:
  1. The microorganism should be constantly associated with the lesions of the disease
  2. It should be possible to isolate the organism in pure culture from the lesions of the disease
  3. The same disease must result when the isolated microorganism is inoculated into a suitable laboratory animal
  4. It should be possible to re-isolate the organism in pure culture from the lesions produced in the experimental animals.

Exceptions to Koch's postulates: There are some bacteria that do not satisfy one or more of the four criteria of Koch's postulates. Those organisms are: *Mycobacterium leprae* and *Treponema pallidum*. They cannot be grown in vitro; however, they can be maintained in experimental animals.

Other Important Contributors

- **Paul Ehrlich (1854–1915):** He is known as **'father of chemotherapy'**. He was also the first to report the *acid-fast nature* of tubercle bacillus. He was the founder and first director of what is known now as the Paul Ehrlich Institute, Germany **(Fig. 1.1D)**
- **Edward Jenner (1796):** He developed the first vaccine of the world, the smallpox vaccine. He used the cowpox virus (*Variolae vaccinae*) to immunize children against smallpox from which the term **'vaccine'** has been derived. The same principles are even used today for developing vaccines
- **Ignaz Semmelweis (1846):** He introduced the importance of hand hygiene in healthcare facilities. He

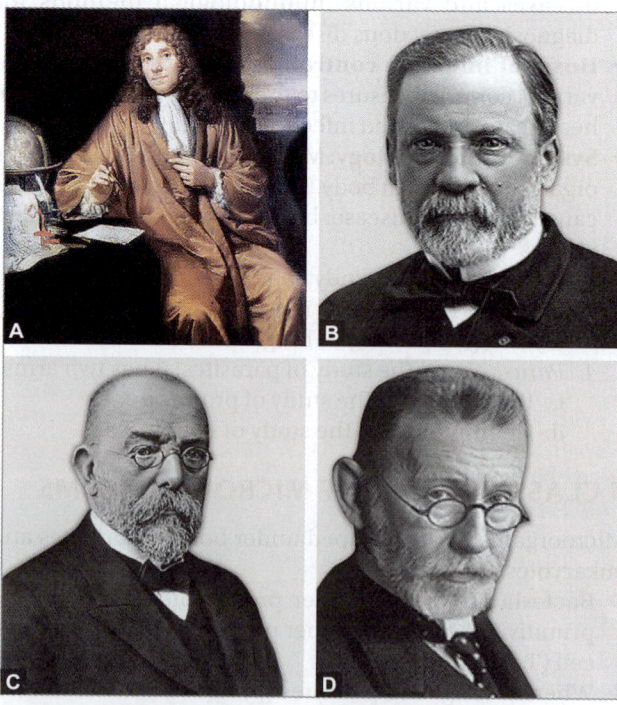

Figs. 1.1A to D: Eminent microbiologists: **A.** Antonie van Leeuwenhoek; **B.** Louis Pasteur; **C.** Robert Koch; **D.** Paul Ehrlich.
Source: Wikipedia (with permission).

CHAPTER 1 ◆ Introduction and History

proposed that improper hand hygiene practice during delivery led to the transmission of infection causing outbreak of puerperal fever
- **Hans Christian Gram (1884):** He developed a method of staining bacteria which was named as 'Gram stain' to make them more visible and differentiable under a microscope
- **Ernst Ruska:** He was the founder of electron microscope (1931)
- **Alexander Fleming (1929):** He discovered the most commonly used antibiotic substance of the last century, i.e. penicillin
- **Barbara McClintock:** She described the mobile genetic elements in bacteria called transposons
- **Walter Gilbert and Frederick Sanger** were the first to develop (1977) the method of DNA sequencing
- **Karry B Mullis:** Discovered polymerase chain reaction (PCR) and was awarded Noble Prize in 1993.

Discovery of Microorganisms

Several microorganisms were discovered by the scientists **(Table 1.2)**. The names of some of the bacteria have been coined in the honor of the scientists who discovered them **(Table 1.3)**.

Nobel Laureates

A number of scientists in medicine or physiology have been awarded Nobel Prizes for their contributions in microbiology **(Table 1.4)**.

Table 1.2: Discovery of important microorganisms.	
Discoverer	Organism
Ogston	*Staphylococcus aureus*
Neisser	*Neisseria gonorrhoeae*
Loeffler	*Corynebacterium diphtheriae*
Bruce	*Brucella melitensis*
Hansen	*Mycobacterium leprae*
Schaudinn and Hoffman	*Treponema pallidum*
d'Herelle	Bacteriophages
WH Welch	*Clostridium perfringens*
Anthony Epstein and Yvonne Barr	Epstein-Barr virus

Table 1.3: Bacteria named after the discoverers.	
Common name	Scientific name
Kleb-Loeffler bacillus	*Corynebacterium diphtheriae*
Pfeiffer's bacillus	*Haemophilus influenzae*
Whitmore's bacillus	*Burkholderia pseudomallei*
Eaton's agent	*Mycoplasma pneumoniae*
Gaffky-Eberth bacillus	*Salmonella* Typhi

Table 1.4: Nobel laureates in medicine or physiology for their contributions in microbiology.		
Nobel laureate	Year	Research done
Sir Ronald Ross	1902	Life cycle of malarial parasite in mosquitoes
Robert Koch	1905	Discovery of the causative agent of tuberculosis
Charles LA Laveran	1907	Discovery of malarial parasite in unstained preparation of blood
Sir Alexander Fleming	1945	Discovery of penicillin
J Lederberg and EL Tatum	1958	Discovery of conjugation in bacteria
Watson and Crick	1962	Discovered double helix structure of DNA
BS Blumberg	1976	Discovered Australia antigen (HBsAg)
Barbara McClintoch	1983	Discovered mobile genetic elements (transposon)
Kary B Mullis	1993	Invented polymerase chain reaction
Stanley B Prusiner	1997	Described Prions
Luc Montagnier and Barre-Sinoussi	2008	Discovery of human immunodeficiency virus (HIV)
William C Campbell and S Omura	2015	For discovering ivermectin for the treatment of roundworm infections
Youyou Tu	2015	For discovering artemisinin, a novel drug used for malaria

EXPECTED QUESTIONS

I. Write short notes on:
 1. Contributions of Louis Pasteur to Microbiology.
 2. Koch's postulates.

II. Multiple Choice Questions (MCQs):
 1. Who has introduced the sterilization techniques?
    a. Louis Pasteur   b. Edward Jenner
    c. Robert Koch   d. Paul Ehrlich

 2. Who is considered to be the 'father of antiseptic surgery'?
    a. Edward Jenner
    b. Robert Koch
    c. Alexander Fleming
    d. Joseph Lister

Answers
1. a   2. d

CHAPTER 2

Microscopy

CHAPTER PREVIEW

- Micrometry
- Bright-field or Light Microscope
- Dark Field Microscope
- Phase Contrast Microscope
- Fluorescence Microscope
- Electron Microscope

■ INTRODUCTION

Microorganisms are extremely small. The size of the bacteria, fungi and parasites is expressed in micrometers (1 μm = 10^{-3} mm) whereas viruses are measured in nanometers (1 nm = 10^{-3} μm).

Most bacteria, parasites and fungi can be observed by light microscope, whereas viruses need an electron microscope. Therefore, it is important to understand the principle and the functioning of each microscope.

Microscopy refers to the use of a specialized instrument—called 'microscope' to view objects and areas of objects that cannot be seen with the naked eye (objects that are not within the resolution range of the normal eye). There are various types of microscopes that are used in diagnostic Microbiology.

- Bright-field or light microscope
- Dark field (or dark ground) microscope
- Phase contrast microscope
- Fluorescence microscope
- Electron microscope.

Properties of a Microscope

A good microscope should have at least three properties:
1. **Good resolution:** Resolution or resolving power refers to the ability to produce separate images of closely placed objects so that they can be distinguished as two separate entities. The resolution power of:
   - Unaided human eye is about 0.2 mm (200 μm)
   - Light microscope is about 0.2 μm
   - Electron microscope is about 0.5 nm.

   Resolution depends on **refractive index** of the medium. Oil has a higher refractive index than air; hence, use of oil enhances the resolution power of a microscope.
2. **Good contrast:** This can further be improved by staining the specimen. When the stains bind to the cells, the contrast is increased
3. **Good magnification:** This is achieved by use of convex lenses.

■ MICROMETRY

Micrometry refers to the measurement of dimensions of the microorganisms under a microscope by using micrometers. There are two micrometers, namely (1) ocular micrometer and (2) stage micrometer **(Figs. 2.1A and B)**.

- ❖ **Ocular micrometer** is a circular glass disk that fits into the eyepiece of the microscope. It has 100 equally spaced divisions (marked as 0–10, at every 10 division interval) **(Fig. 2.1A)**
- ❖ The **stage micrometer** is clipped to the stage of the microscope. In the center of the stage micrometer, a known 1 mm distance is divided into 10 divisions (0.1 mm); each one is further divided into 10 graduations of 0.01 mm or 10 μm each
- ❖ **Calibration:** The graduations on both micrometers are superimposed on each other. Then the graduations on the ocular microscope are calibrated against the standard graduations on the stage micrometer as given below **(Fig. 2.1A):**

> **Calibration factor** for one division on ocular micrometer (in μm) =
>
> $$\frac{\text{Known distance between two lines on stage micrometer, i.e., 100 μm}}{\text{Number of divisions on ocular micrometer that lies between two lines of stage micrometer}}$$
>
> Therefore in the above example **(Fig. 2.1)**, one division of ocular micrometer (i.e., calibration factor) measures to 100/37 = 2.7 μm.
>
> Hence, size of the bacteria = The number of divisions of ocular micrometer it corresponds to × 2.7 μm

- ❖ **Measurement:** After calibration, the ocular micrometer is used to measure the size of various microbes, such as length, breadth, and diameter. First, count the number of divisions occupied in ocular micrometer by the organism. Then, multiply this number by the calculated calibration factor. This value indicates the size of the organism **(Fig. 2.1B)**.

CHAPTER 2 ◆ Microscopy

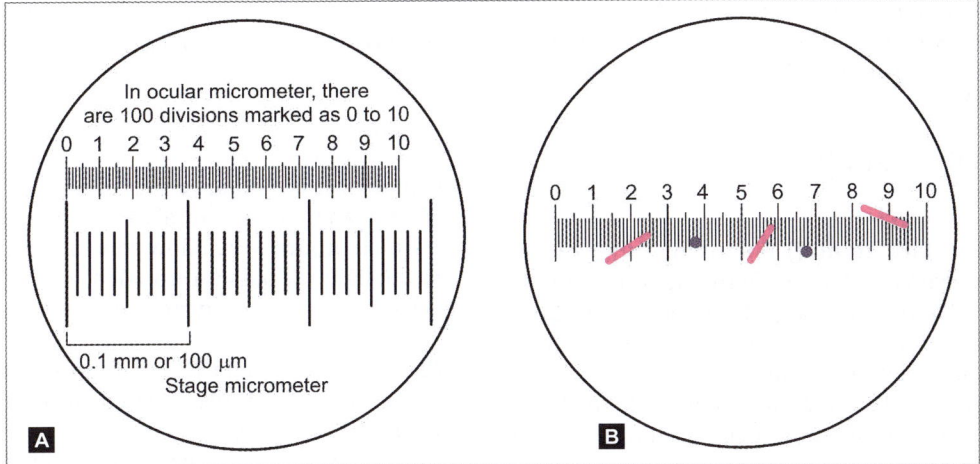

Figs. 2.1A and B: (A) Principle of micrometry [The divisions of ocular micrometer are superimposed on graduations of stage micrometer. Distance between two graduations of stage micrometer equals to 37 divisions of ocular micrometer. Therefore, one division of ocular micrometer (i.e., calibration factor) measures to 100/37 = 2.7 μm]; (B) Stage micrometer is removed. Slide containing bacteria is focused. Size of the bacteria is determined by number of divisions of ocular micrometer it corresponds × 2.7 μm.

■ BRIGHT-FIELD OR LIGHT MICROSCOPE

The bright-field or light microscope forms a dark image against a brighter background, hence the name.

Structure

The parts of a bright-field microscope are divided into three groups **(Fig. 2.2)**:

Mechanical Parts

- ❖ **Base:** It holds various parts of the microscope, such as the light source, the fine and coarse adjustment knobs
- ❖ **C-shaped arm:** It holds the microscope, and it connects the ocular lens to the objective lens
- ❖ **Mechanical stage:** The arm bears a stage with stage clips to hold the slides and the stage control knobs to move the slide during viewing. It has an aperture at the center that permits light to reach the object from the bottom.

Magnifying Parts

- ❖ **Ocular lens:** The arm contains an eyepiece that bears an ocular lens of 10x magnification power. Microscopes with two eye pieces are called as binocular microscopes. Ocular lens has a magnification power of 10x.
- ❖ **Objective lens:** The arm also contains a revolving nose piece that bears three to four objectives with lenses of differing magnifying power (4x, 10x, 40x and 100x).
- ❖ The total magnification of a field is the product of the magnification of the objective lens and ocular lens:
  - Scanning field (40x)
  - Low power field (100x)
  - High power field (400x) and
  - Oil immersion field (1000x).

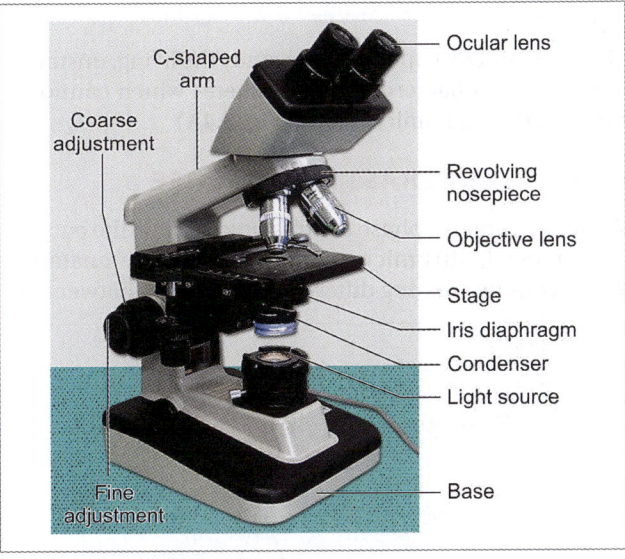

Fig. 2.2: Bright-field microscope.
Source: Nikon Alphaphot (*with permission*).

Illuminating Parts

- ❖ **Condenser:** It is mounted beneath the stage which focuses a cone of light on the slide
- ❖ **Iris diaphragm:** It controls the light that passes through the condenser
- ❖ **Light source:** It may be a mirror or an electric bulb
- ❖ **Fine and coarse adjustment knobs:** They sharpen the image.

Working Principle

The rays emitted from the light source pass through the iris diaphragm and fall on the specimen. The light rays passing through the specimen are gathered by the objective and a magnified image is formed. This image is further magnified by the ocular lens to produce the final magnified virtual image **(Fig. 2.3)**.

■ DARK FIELD MICROSCOPE

Principle

In dark field (or dark ground) microscope, the object appears bright against a dark background. This is made possible by use of a special dark field condenser **(Fig. 2.3)**.
- ❖ The dark field condenser has a central opaque area that blocks light from entering the objective lens directly and has a peripheral annular hollow area which allows the light to pass through and focus on the specimen obliquely
- ❖ Only the light which is reflected by the specimen enters the objective lens whereas the unreflected light does not enter the objective. As a result, the specimen is brightly illuminated; but the background appears dark.

Applications

Dark field microscope is used to study the living, unstained cells and thin bacteria like spirochetes which cannot be visualized by light microscopy **(Fig. 2.4A)**.

■ PHASE CONTRAST MICROSCOPE

As per its name, in phase contrast microscope the contrast is enhanced. This microscope visualizes the unstained living cells by creating difference in contrast between the cells and water. It converts slight differences in refractive index and cell density into easily detectable variations in light intensity.

Principle

The condenser is similar to that of dark field microscope, consists of an opaque central area with a thin transparent ring, which produces a hollow cone of light.
- ❖ As the light ray passes through a cell, gets retarded due to variations in density and refractive index within the specimen
- ❖ The undeviated light passing through the phase ring (a special optical disk located in the objective) gets advanced in wavelength
- ❖ The deviated and undeviated waves will cancel each other when they come together to form an image **(Fig. 2.5)**
- ❖ The background, formed by undeviated light, is bright, while the unstained object appears dark and well-defined **(Fig. 2.4B)**.

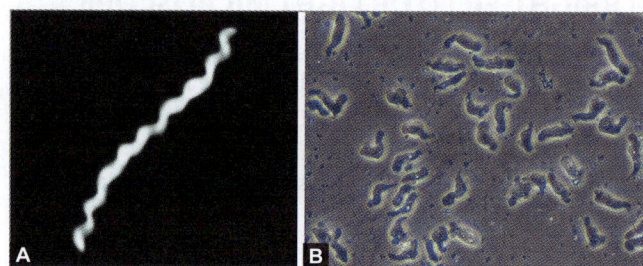

Figs. 2.4A and B: A. Dark ground microscopic picture demonstrating spirally coiled bacteria (spirochete); **B.** Phase-contrast microscopic picture demonstrating *Naegleria fowleri* trophozoites (free-living amoeba).

Source: **A.** Public Health Image Library, ID# 2043; Centers for Disease Control and Prevention (CDC), Atlanta (*with permission*); **B.** Centers for Disease Control and Prevention (CDC), Atlanta (*with permission*).

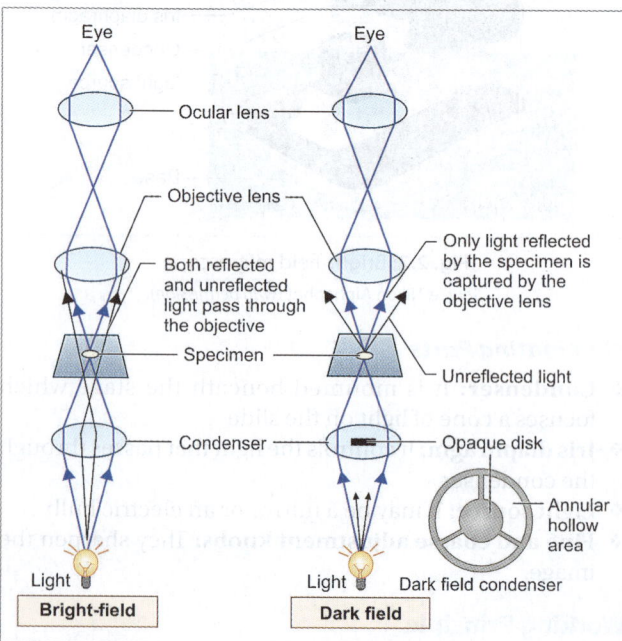

Fig. 2.3: Light pathways of bright-field and dark field microscopes.

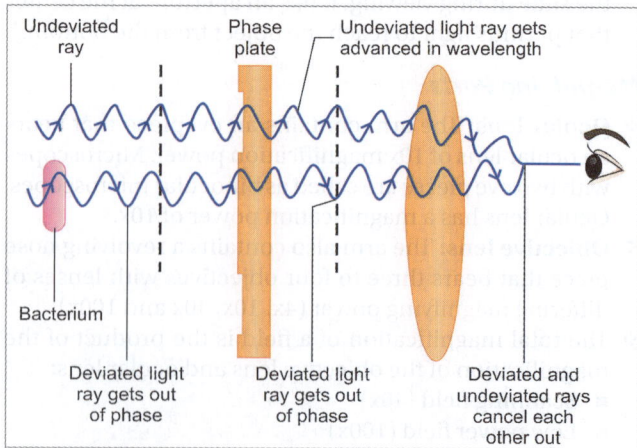

Fig. 2.5: Principle of phase contrast microscope.

Applications

Phase contrast microscopy is especially useful for studying:
- Microbial motility
- Determining the shape of living cells, and
- Detecting microbial internal cellular components, such as the cell membrane, nuclei, endospores and inclusion bodies; which become clearly visible because they have refractive indices markedly different from that of water.

■ FLUORESCENCE MICROSCOPE

The "fluorescence microscope" refers to any microscope that uses fluorescence property to generate an image.

Principle

When fluorescent dyes are exposed to ultraviolet (UV) rays, they become excited and are said to fluoresce, i.e. they convert this invisible, short wavelength rays into light of longer wavelengths (i.e. visible light) **(Fig. 2.6A)**.
- The source of light may be a mercury lamp which emits rays that pass through an excitation filter
- The excitation filter is so designed that it allows only short wavelength UV light (about 400 nm, called as the exciting wavelength of light) to pass through; blocking all other long wavelength rays
- The exciting rays then get reflected by a dichromatic mirror in such a way that they fall on the specimen which is previously stained by fluorescent dye and focused under the microscope
- The fluorescent dye absorbs the exciting rays of short wavelength, gets activated and in turn emits rays of higher wavelength
- A barrier filter positioned after the objective lenses removes any remaining ultraviolet light, which could otherwise damage the viewer's eyes, or blue and violet light, which would reduce the image's contrast.

Applications

- **Autofluorescence:** Certain microbes directly fluoresce when placed under UV lamp, e.g. *Cyclospora* (a protozoan parasite)
- **Microbes coated with fluorescent dye:** Certain microbes fluoresce when they are stained non-specifically by fluorochrome dyes
  - Acridine orange dye for the detection malaria parasites and filarial nematodes
  - Auramine phenol is used for the detection of tubercle bacilli **(Fig. 2.6B)**.
- **Immunofluorescence:** It uses fluorescent dye tagged immunoglobulins to detect cell surface antigens or antibodies bound to cell surface antigens (described in detail in **Chapter 8**).

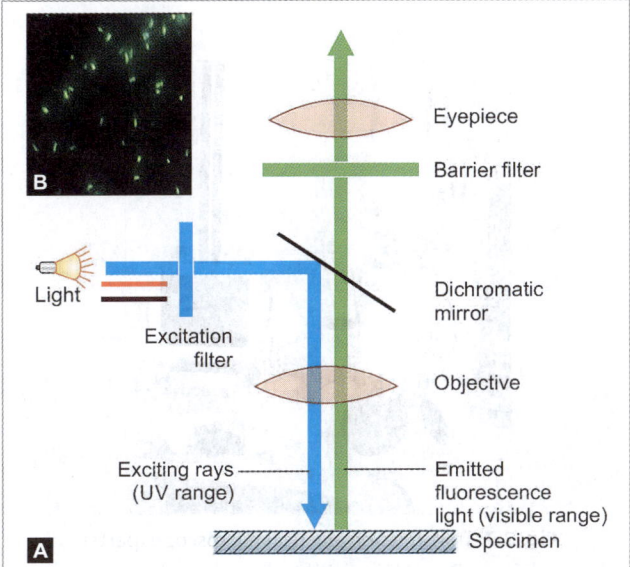

Figs. 2.6A and B: A. Principle of fluorescence microscope; **B.** Tubercle bacilli seen under fluorescence microscope.
Source: Department of Microbiology, JIPMER, Puducherry (*with permission*).

■ ELECTRON MICROSCOPE

An electron microscope (EM) uses accelerated electrons as a source of illumination. Because the wavelength of electrons can be up to 100,000 times shorter than that of visible light photons, the EM has a much better resolving power than a light microscope; hence, it can reveal the details of flagella, fimbriae and intracellular structures of a cell. It was invented by German physicist **Ernst Ruska** in 1931. Differences between light microscope and EM are listed in **Table 2.1**. Electron microscopes are of two types:
1. Transmission electron microscope (TEM, most common type) **(Fig. 2.7)**
2. Scanning electron microscope (SEM).

Table 2.1: Differences between light microscope and electron microscope.

Features	Light microscope	Electron microscope
Highest practical magnification	About 1,000–1,500	Over 100,000
Best resolution	0.2 µm	0.5 nm
Radiation source	Visible light	Electron beam
Medium of travel	Air	High vacuum
Specimen mount	Glass slide	Copper grid
Type of lens	Glass	Electromagnet

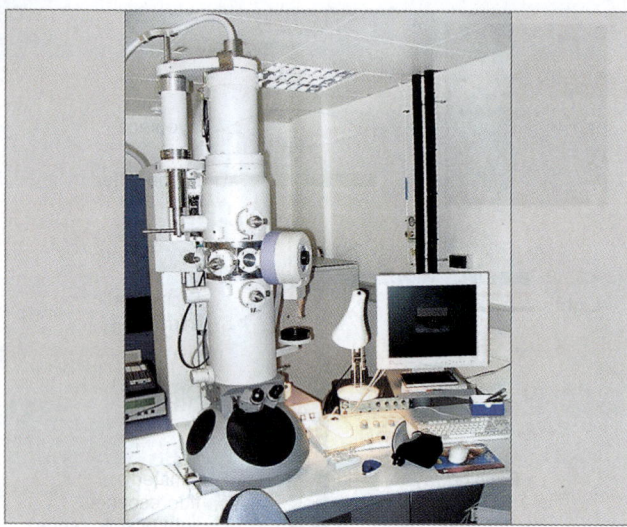

Fig. 2.7: Transmission electron microscope (parts).
Source: David J Morgan/Wikipedia (*with permission*).

Transmission Electron Microscope

Specimen Preparation

The specimen to be viewed under EM should be able to maintain its structure when it is bombarded with electrons. Hence, only very thin specimens (20-100 nm thickness) are suitable for EM. However, bacterial cells are thicker than this; hence, they need to be sliced into thin layers using an ultramicrotome knife.

Electron Pathway

Electrons are generated by electron gun, which travel in high speed. The electrons are then made to travel in a path of vacuum to avoid deflection by collision with air molecules.

- Electrons pass through a magnetic condenser and then bombard on the thin sliced specimen mounted on the copper slide
- The specimen scatters electrons passing through it, and then the electron beam is focused by magnetic lenses to form an enlarged, visible image of the specimen on a fluorescent screen.

Applications of Electron Microscope

The most important use of EM in diagnostic microbiology is detection of viruses. It can detect viruses either—(i) directly from the clinical specimens (e.g., rotavirus from stool) or (ii) from tissue cultures.

Scanning Electron Microscope

Scanning electron microscope (SEM) has been used to examine the surfaces of microorganisms in great detail. It has a resolution of 7 nm or less. The SEM differs from TEM, in producing an image from electrons emitted by an object's surface rather than from transmitted electrons.

EXPECTED QUESTIONS

I. **Write short notes on:**
  1. Principle and uses of dark field microscope.
  2. Principle and uses of fluorescence microscope.

II. **Multiple Choice Questions (MCQs):**
  1. Unaided human eye has a resolution power of:
     a. 0.2 mm b. 0.2 μm
     c. 0.2 nm d. 0.5 nm
  2. Which of the following microscopes, the object appears bright against a dark background?
     a. Simple light microscope
     b. Dark ground microscope
     c. Compound light microscope
     d. Electron microscope
  3. **Highest useful magnification available in light microscope is____.**
     a. 100X
     b. 400X
     c. 1000X
     d. 2000X

Answers
1. a   2. b   3. c

General Bacteriology: Morphology and Physiology of Bacteria

CHAPTER 3.1

CHAPTER PREVIEW
- Medically Important Bacteria
- Bacterial Taxonomy
- Morphology of Bacteria
- Physiology of Bacteria

■ MEDICALLY IMPORTANT BACTERIA

Based on Gram stain, the bacteria can be grouped into gram-positive cocci, gram-negative cocci, and gram-positive bacilli, gram-negative bacilli and miscellaneous bacteria (that do not take up/poorly take up Gram stain) **(Table 3.1.1)**.

■ BACTERIAL TAXONOMY

Bacterial taxonomy comprises of three separate but interrelated important areas.

1. **Classification:** It refers to hierarchy based arrangement of bacteria into taxonomic groups on the basis of similarities or differences in their biochemical, physiological, genetic, and morphological properties.
   - The most recent taxonomic classification of bacteria is based on **Cavalier and Smith's six** kingdoms classification (1998).
   - Kingdom **Bacteria** is divided in decreasing order of hierarchy into phylum/division, class, order, suborder, family, tribe, genus and species.
2. **Nomenclature:** It refers to the naming of taxa according to their characteristics, by following the international rules. Bacterial nomenclature follows the modern system of binomial nomenclature.
   - Scientific names for taxonomic levels above genus are always capitalized but not italicized; for example, Phylum Proteobacteria
   - In binomial nomenclature system, the scientific name of bacteria comprises of a genus name (starts with a capital letter) and species name. Both genus and species should be written in italic, e.g. *Staphylococcus aureus*
3. **Identification:** It refers to the practical use of a classification scheme such as: (1) Identification of an unknown taxon by comparing with a defined and named taxon, (2) To isolate and identify the causative agent of a disease.

Table 3.1.1: Medically important bacteria.

Gram-positive cocci
• *Staphylococcus*—e.g. *S. aureus* • *Streptococcus*—e.g. β-hemolytic streptococci, and pneumococcus • *Enterococcus*—e.g. *E. faecalis, E. faecium*
Gram-negative cocci
Neisseria—e.g. meningococcus and gonococcus
Gram-positive bacilli
• *Corynebacterium*—e.g. *C. diphtheriae* • *Bacillus*—e.g. *B. anthracis* • *Mycobacterium*—e.g. *M. tuberculosis, M. leprae* • Miscellaneous gram-positive bacilli—*Listeria, Actinomycetes* and *Nocardia*
Gram-negative bacilli
• Enterobacterales—e.g. *Escherichia coli, Klebsiella, Proteus, Shigella, Salmonella, Yersinia* • Non-fermenting gram-negative bacilli—e.g. *Pseudomonas, Acinetobacter, Burkholderia* • *Vibrio*—e.g. *Vibrio cholerae* • Fastidious gram-negative bacilli—*Haemophilus, Bordetella, Brucella* • Miscellaneous gram-negative bacilli—*Campylobacter, Helicobacter, Legionella*, etc.
Anaerobic bacterial infections
• Sporing anaerobes—*Clostridium* • Non-sporing anaerobes—*Bacteroides*
Miscellaneous bacteria
• Spirochetes—*Treponema, Borrelia, Leptospira* • Rickettsiae, chlamydiae and *Mycoplasma*

■ MORPHOLOGY OF BACTERIA

Shape of Bacteria

Depending on their shape, bacteria are classified into:
- ❖ Cocci (singular coccus, from; kokkos, meaning berry) are oval or spherical cells, and
- ❖ Bacilli or rods (singular bacillus, meaning rod-shaped).

Cocci are arranged in groups (clusters), pairs, or chains. Similarly, bacilli can be arranged in chains, pairs, and some bacilli are curved, comma-shaped, or cuneiform-shaped (**Fig. 3.1.1 and Table 3.1.2**).

Based on Gram staining property, both cocci and bacilli are further classified into (**Fig. 3.1.1 and Table 3.1.2**):
* Gram-positive cocci
* Gram-negative cocci
* Gram-positive bacilli
* Gram-negative bacilli.

Miscellaneous group: However, some bacteria are weakly Gram stained and hence need special stains for their demonstration, such as:
* Spirochetes (*Treponema* and *Leptospira*)—thin spirally coiled bacilli
* *Mycoplasma* (cell wall deficient free-living bacteria)
* Rickettsiae and chlamydiae are obligate intracellular bacteria.

Bacterial Cell Anatomy

Bacterial cell anatomy comprises the following structures (**Fig. 3.1.2**):
* The **outer layer** or the envelope of a bacterial cell consists of—(1) a rigid cell wall and (2) an underlying plasma membrane
* The **cytoplasm** contains cytoplasmic inclusions (mesosomes, ribosomes, inclusion granules, vacuoles) and a diffuse nucleoid containing a single circular chromosome

Table 3.1.2: Classification of bacteria depending on their morphology and Gram staining property.

Bacteria	Example
Gram-positive cocci arranged in	
Cluster	Staphylococcus
Short chain	Streptococcus
Long chain	Viridans streptococci
Pairs, lanceolate shaped	Pneumococcus
Pairs or in short chain	Enterococcus
Gram-negative cocci arranged in	
Pairs, lens-shaped	Meningococcus
Pairs, kidney-shaped	Gonococcus
Gram-positive bacilli arranged in	
Chain (bamboo stick appearance)	*Bacillus anthracis*
Chinese letter or cuneiform pattern	*Corynebacterium diphtheriae*
Branched and filamentous form	*Actinomyces, Nocardia*
Gram-negative bacilli arranged in	
Pleomorphic (various shapes—cocci, coccobacilli, bacilli, etc.)	*Haemophilus, Proteus*
Coccobacilli	*Acinetobacter*
Comma shaped	*Vibrio cholerae*
Others	
Spirally coiled, flexible	Spirochetes
Bacteria that lack cell wall	*Mycoplasma*

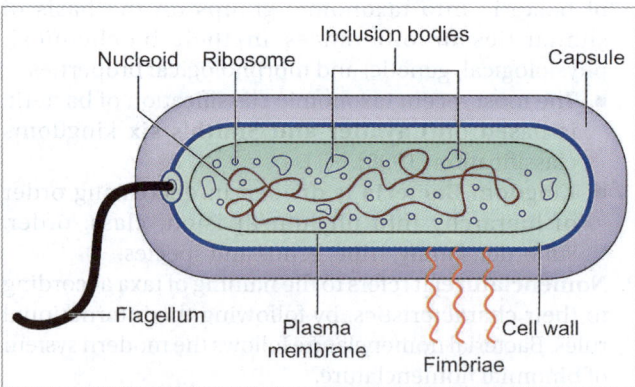

Fig. 3.1.2: Structure of bacterial cell.

* Some bacteria may possess additional **cell wall appendages** such as capsule, flagella and fimbriae.

Bacterial Cell Wall

The cell wall is a tough and rigid structure, surrounding the bacterium. It is 10–25 nm in thickness.

The cell wall has the following functions:
* It protects the cell against osmotic lysis
* It confers rigidity upon bacteria due to the presence of a peptidoglycan layer in the cell wall

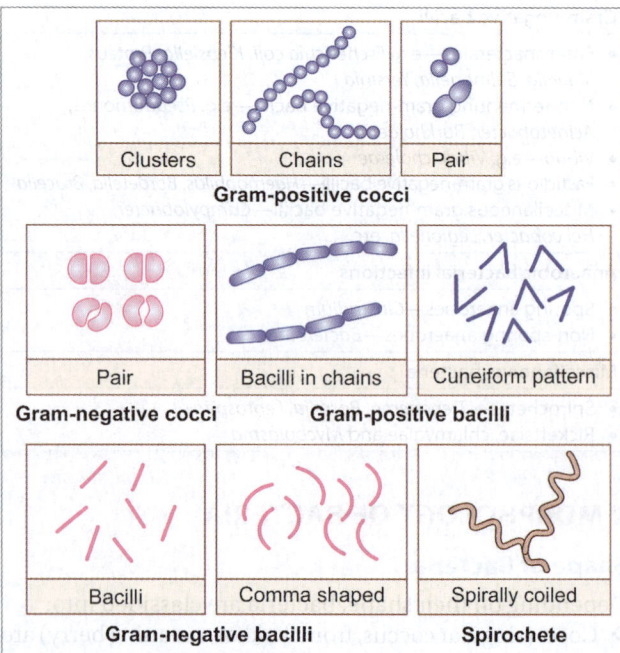

Fig. 3.1.1: Different morphology of bacteria and Gram staining property.

- It is the site of action of several antibiotics
- **Virulence factors:** Bacterial cell wall contains certain virulence factors (e.g. endotoxin), which contribute to their pathogenicity
- **Immunity:** Antibody raised against specific cell wall antigens (e.g. antibody to LPS) may provide immunity against some bacterial infections.

Gram-positive Cell wall

The cell wall of gram-positive bacteria is simpler than that of gram-negative bacteria **(Table 3.1.3)**, made up of the following structure.
- **Peptidoglycan:** It is made up of layers of mucopeptide chains. It is much thicker (50–100 layers thick, 16–80 nm) than the gram-negative cell wall **(Fig. 3.1.3)**
- **Teichoic acid:** Gram-positive cell wall contains a significant amount of teichoic acid; which is absent in gram-negative bacteria. It constitutes major surface antigens of gram-positive bacteria.

Gram-negative Cell wall

The gram-negative cell wall is thinner and more complex than the gram-positive cell wall, comprising of the following components **(Fig. 3.1.4 and Table 3.1.3)**.

Table 3.1.3: Differences between gram-positive and gram-negative cell wall.		
Characters	Gram-positive cell wall	Gram-negative cell wall
Peptidoglycan layer	Thicker (16–80 nm)	Thinner (2 nm)
Lipid content	Nil or scanty (2–5%)	Present (15–20%)
Lipopolysaccharide	Absent	Present **(endotoxin)**
Teichoic acid	Present	Absent

- **Peptidoglycan layer:** It is very thin (2 nm) compared to that of the gram-positive cell wall, made up of 1–2 layers of mucopeptide chain
- **Outer membrane:** This is a phospholipid layer that lies outside the thin peptidoglycan layer. It serves as a protective barrier to the cell. Outer membrane proteins (OMP) or porin proteins help in the transport of smaller molecules and also they are target sites for many antibiotics
- **Lipopolysaccharide (LPS):** This layer is unique to gram-negative bacteria, which is absent in gram-positives. It consists of three parts as:
  1. *Lipid A or the endotoxin*: It is an important virulence factor for gram-negative bacteria
  2. *Core polysaccharide*: It projects from lipid A region
  3. *O side chain*: O antigens are used for serotyping for bacteria and they also induce antibody formation.
- **Periplasmic space:** It is the space between the inner cell membrane and outer membrane. It encompasses the peptidoglycan layer.

Cell Membrane

The plasma membrane is essential for the survival of the bacteria. It is 5–10 nm thick, and composed of bilayered phospholipid in which several proteins are embedded **(Figs. 3.1.2 to 3.1.4)**. The plasma membrane serves important functions in the bacterial cell such as:
- It is a **semipermeable membrane** that acts as an osmotic barrier; selectively allows particular ions, nutrients into the cell, and also helps in waste excretion
- It acts as the site for a variety of crucial metabolic processes such as respiration, synthesis of lipids and cell wall, etc.

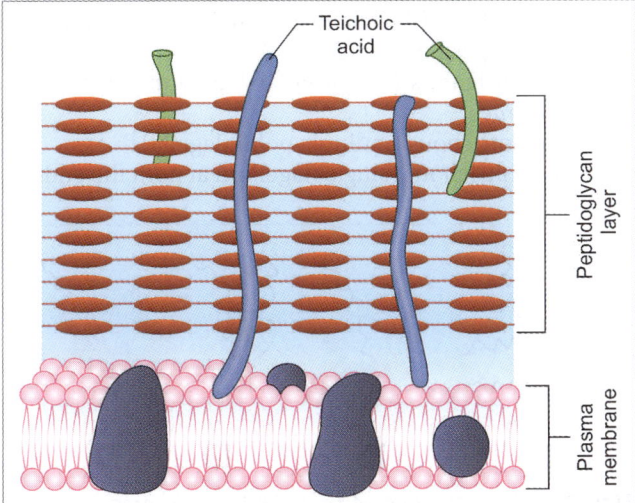

Fig. 3.1.3: Structure of gram-positive cell wall.

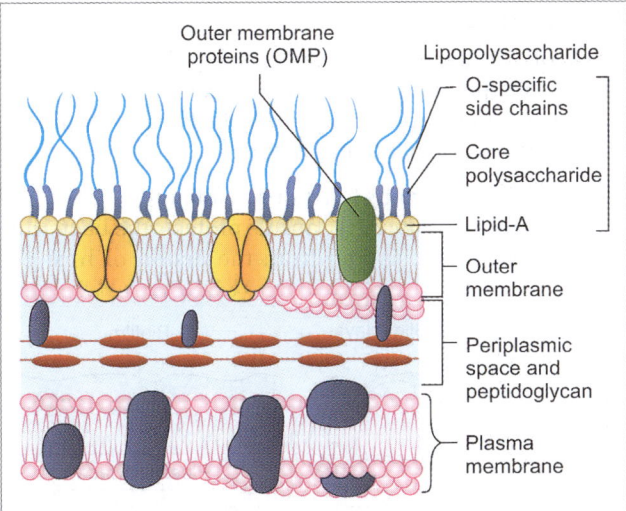

Fig. 3.1.4: Gram-negative cell wall.

Cytoplasmic Matrix

Bacterial cytoplasm is mainly composed of water and is packed with the following structures:

- ❖ **Ribosomes:** They are the sites for protein synthesis; composed of rRNA and ribosomal proteins. Ribosomes are integrated with the mRNA and at this site, the genetic codons of the mRNA are translated into peptide sequences
- ❖ **Intracytoplasmic inclusions:** They are the storage sites of nutrients/energy present in some bacteria. They are formed by the bacteria under nutritional deficiency conditions. For examples, include glycogen granules and metachromatic granules
- ❖ **Mesosomes:** They are invaginations of the plasma membrane. They possess respiratory enzymes and are involved in bacterial respiration; are analogous to the mitochondria of eukaryotes
- ❖ **Nucleoid:** Bacteria do not have a true nucleus, but the genetic material is located in an irregularly shaped region called the nucleoid. There is no nuclear membrane or nucleolus
    - Bacteria possess a single haploid chromosome, comprising circular double-stranded DNA
    - Bacterial DNA divides by simple binary fission
    - Bacteria also possess extrachromosomal DNA called **plasmids**.

Cell Wall Appendages

Capsule and Slime Layer

Some bacteria possess a layer of amorphous viscid material lying outside the cell wall called **capsule**. When the capsule is in the form of unorganized loose material, it is called a **slime layer (Fig. 3.1.5)**.

Function/Uses

Most of the bacterial capsules are polysaccharide in nature—e.g. pneumococcus, meningococcus, *Haemophilus influenzae, Klebsiella pneumoniae*. In *Bacillus anthracis*, the capsule is polypeptide in nature.

The capsule has various functions as follows:
- ❖ **Bacterial virulence:** (i) Capsule protects the bacterium from phagocytosis and from the action of host cell lysozymes. (ii) It also helps in biofilm formation. Biofilm is an extracellular polysaccharide layer, which helps in bacterial adhesion to foreign body surfaces and thereby promotes diseases such as prosthetic valve endocarditis and catheter-associated urinary tract infections, etc.
- ❖ **Identification:** Capsular antigens can be used for the identification and typing of bacteria
- ❖ **Used as vaccine:** Capsular antigens of a few bacteria are used for vaccine preparation; e.g. pneumococcus, meningococcus, and *Haemophilus influenzae* serotype-b.

Demonstration of Capsule

Capsule can be detected by various methods as follows:
- ❖ **Negative staining** by India ink and nigrosin stain: Capsule appears as a clear refractile halo around the bacteria against a black background
- ❖ **M'Fadyean capsule stain:** It is used for demonstration of the capsule of *Bacillus anthracis* by using polychrome methylene blue stain
- ❖ **Quellung reaction** for demonstrating capsule in *Streptococcus pneumoniae* by adding capsular antisera mixed with methylene blue
- ❖ **Latex agglutination test:** Capsular antigens can be detected in the sample (e.g. CSF) by latex agglutination test by using specific anticapsular antibodies coated on latex particles. This is available for pneumococcus, *Haemophilus influenzae* and meningococcus.

Flagella

Flagella are thread-like appendages, protruding from the cell wall. They measure 5–20 µm in length and 0.01–0.02 µm in thickness.
- ❖ **Arrangement:** There are various patterns of arrangement of flagella with respect to the bacterial surface **(Figs. 3.1.6A to D)**:
    - Peritrichous (flagella distributed over the entire cell surface), e.g. *Escherichia coli*
    - Monotrichous (single polar flagellum), e.g. *Vibrio cholerae*
    - Lophotrichous (multiple polar flagella)
    - Amphitrichous (single flagellum at both the ends).

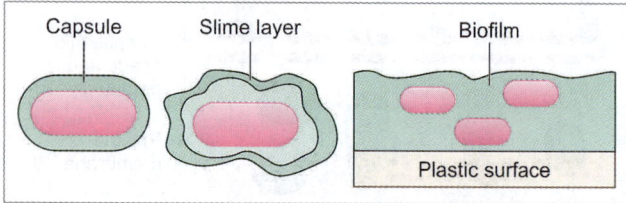

Fig. 3.1.5: Capsule, slime layer and biofilm.

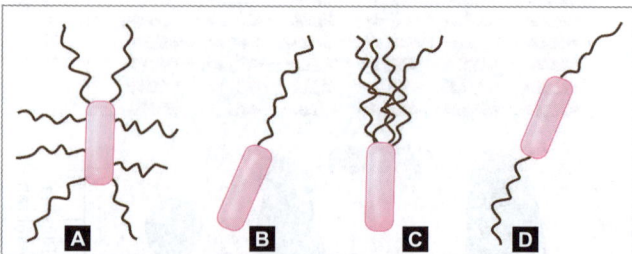

Figs. 3.1.6A to D: Types of bacterial flagellar arrangement: **A.** Peritrichous; **B.** Monotrichous; **C.** Lophotrichous; **D.** Amphitrichous.

- ❖ **Ultrastructure of flagella:** Flagellum is composed of three parts—(i) filament, (ii) basal body, and (iii) hook
- ❖ **Bacterial motility:** Flagella confer motility to the bacteria (organ of locomotion). Bacteria can produce characteristic type of motility which helps in their identification **(Table 3.1.4)**
- ❖ **Detection of flagella:** Flagella can be demonstrated by:
  - Direct demonstration by electron microscopy
  - Indirect means by demonstrating the motility by hanging drop method, dark ground or phase contrast microscopy.

Fimbriae or Pili

Fimbriae or pili are short, fine, hair-like appendages, smaller to flagella, but numerous in number. According to the functions, pili are of two types **(Fig. 3.1.7A)**.
1. **Common pili or fimbriae:** They help in **bacterial adhesion** to epithelial surfaces helping in colonization. They are present in gram-negative and some gram-positive bacteria
2. **Sex pili:** They help in bacterial conjugation by forming a conjugation tube through which the bacterial gene transfer takes place. They are only found in gram-negative bacteria.

Table 3.1.4: Types of motility shown by different bacteria.	
Types of motility	**Bacteria**
Tumbling motility	*Listeria*
Gliding motility	*Mycoplasma*
Stately motility	*Clostridium*
Darting motility	*Vibrio cholerae*
Swarming on agar plate	*Proteus*
Corkscrew motility	Spirochetes

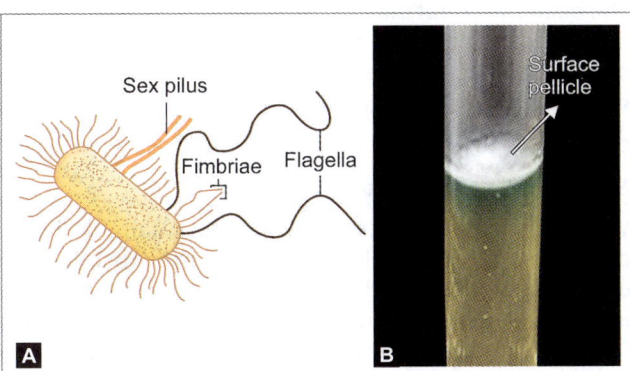

Figs. 3.1.7A and B: A. Differentiation between fimbriae, sex pilus and flagella; **B.** Surface pellicle (arrow showing).

Source: Department of Microbiology, JIPMER (*with permission*).

Detection of fimbriae: Fimbriae can be detected either directly by electron microscope, or indirectly through the formation of the **surface pellicle**. It is a thin layer formed at the surface of liquid culture **(Fig. 3.1.7B)**.

L Form (Cell Wall Deficient Forms)

They are the cell wall deficient bacteria, discovered by E Klieneberger. She named it as L form after its place of discovery, i.e. Lister Institute, London (1935).
- ❖ When bacteria lose cell wall, they become spherical irrespective of their original shape. This may occur spontaneously or after exposure to lysozyme or cell wall-acting antibiotics such as penicillin
- ❖ L forms play a role in the persistence of pyelonephritis and other chronic infections
- ❖ Some bacteria like *Mycoplasma* lack cell wall permanently and has been suggested that they may represent stable L form.

Bacterial Spores

Spores are highly resistant resting stage of the bacteria formed in unfavorable environmental conditions as a result of the depletion of exogenous nutrients.

Structure

The bacterial spore comprises several layers. From the innermost to the outermost, the layers are—core, cortex, coat, and exosporium **(Fig. 3.1.8)**.
- ❖ The core is the innermost part containing the DNA material and is walled off from the cortex by an inner membrane and the germ cell wall
- ❖ Cortex and the coat layers lie external to the core and are separated from each other by an outer membrane
- ❖ The outermost layer is called the exosporium.

Sporulation

Sporulation refers to the process of formation of spores from the vegetative stage of bacteria. Sporulation

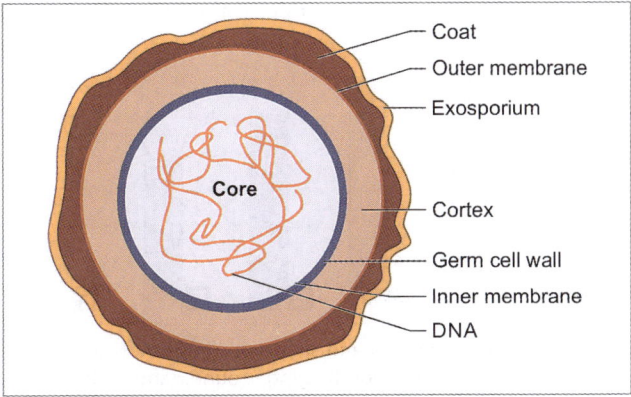

Fig. 3.1.8: Structure of bacterial spore.

commences when growth ceases due to a lack of nutrients. The mature spore formed is extremely resistant to heat and disinfectant.

Germination

It is the transformation of dormant spores into active vegetative cells when grown in a nutrient-rich medium.

Shape and Position of Spores

For a given species, the position, shape, and relative size of the spore are constant.
- **Position:** Spores may be central, subterminal, or terminal (**Figs. 3.1.9A to F**)
- **Shape:** They may be oval or spherical
- **Width:** The diameter of the spore may be the same or less than the width of bacteria (non-bulging spore—e.g. as in *Bacillus*), or may be wider than the bacillary body producing a bulge in the cell (bulging spore, e.g. as in *Clostridium*).

Sporicidal Agents

Spores are resistant to most of the routinely used disinfectants. Only limited agents called sterilants are capable of killing the spores, e.g. autoclave, ethylene oxide sterilizer, etc. (*refer* **Chapter 16**).

Demonstration of Spores

- **Gram staining:** Spores appear as unstained refractile bodies within the cells
- **Modified Ziehl–Neelsen staining:** Spores are weakly acid-fast and appear red color when ZN staining is performed using 0.25–0.5% sulfuric acid as a decolorizer
- **Schaeffer–Fulton stain:** It is a special staining technique to demonstrate spores.

Applications

Spores of certain bacteria are employed as indicators of proper sterilization. Absence of the spores (inability to grow) after autoclaving or processing in hot air oven indicates proper sterilization.
- Spores of *Geobacillus stearothermophilus* are used as sterilization control for autoclave and plasma sterilizer
- Spores of *Bacillus atrophaeus* are used as sterilization control for hot air oven and ethylene oxide sterilizer.

■ PHYSIOLOGY OF BACTERIA

Bacterial Growth and Nutrition

Water constitutes about 80% of the total bacterial cell. The minimum nutritional requirements essential for the growth of bacteria include sources of carbon, nitrogen, hydrogen, oxygen, and small amounts of inorganic salts such as sulfur, phosphorus, and sodium, etc.

Some fastidious bacteria require additional growth factors called **bacterial vitamins**, which need to be added to the culture medium for their growth, e.g.—*Haemophilus influenzae* requires niacin.

Bacterial Cell Division

Bacteria divide by **binary fission**. The nuclear division precedes cytoplasmic division and then the two daughter cells get separated. In a few bacteria, the daughter cells may remain partially attached even after cell division; so that the bacterial cells are arranged in pairs or chains (e.g. streptococci) or clusters (e.g. staphylococci).

Rate of Multiplication in Bacteria

Generation time is the time required for a bacterium to give rise to two daughter cells under optimum conditions. The generation time for most of the important pathogenic bacteria (e.g. *Escherichia coli*) is 20 minutes. In *Mycobacterium tuberculosis*, it is about 10–15 hours and for *Mycobacterium leprae*, it is about 12–13 days.

Bacterial Count

The bacterial count may be expressed in terms of the total count and viable count. **The total count** indicates the total number of bacteria (live or dead) in the specimen. **Viable count** measures the number of living (viable) cells in the given specimen.

Bacterial Growth Curve

When a bacterium is inoculated into a suitable liquid culture medium and incubated, its growth follows a definite course. When the bacterial count of such culture is determined at different intervals and plotted in relation to time, a **bacterial growth curve** is obtained comprising of four phases (**Table 3.1.5 and Fig. 3.1.10**).
1. **Lag phase:** It is the period between inoculation and the beginning of the multiplication of bacteria. After inoculating into a culture medium, bacteria do not start

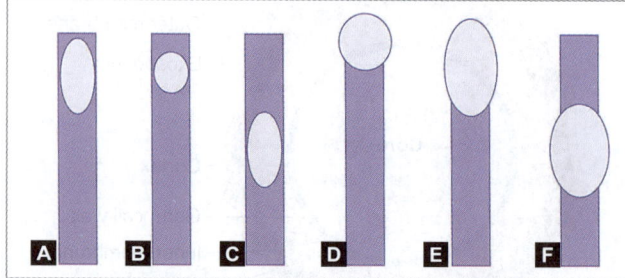

Figs. 3.1.9A to F: Position and shape of spores: **A.** Non-bulging, oval and terminal; **B.** Non-bulging, round, and subterminal; **C.** Non-bulging, oval and central; **D.** Bulging, round and terminal; **E.** Bulging, oval and terminal; **F.** Bulging, oval, and central.

CHAPTER 3.1 ❖ General Bacteriology: Morphology and Physiology of Bacteria

Table 3.1.5: Various phases of bacterial growth curve.				
	Lag	Log	Stationary	Decline
Bacteria divide	No	Yes	Yes	No
Bacterial death	No	No	Yes	Yes
Total count	Flat	Raises	Raises	Flat
Viable count	Flat	Raises	Flat	Falls
Special features	Accumulation of enzymes and metabolites Attains a maximum size	Uniformly stained Metabolically active Small size	Gram variable **Produce:** Granules, spores, exotoxin, bacteriocin	**Produce:** Involution forms

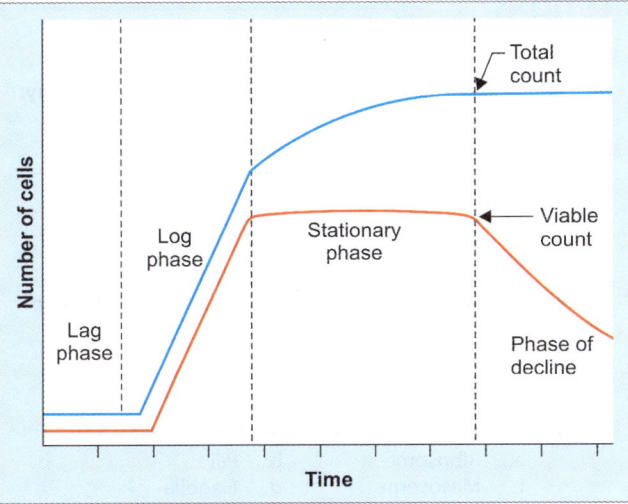

Fig. 3.1.10: Bacterial growth curve.

multiplying immediately but take some time to build up enzymes and metabolites
- Bacteria increase in size due to the accumulation of enzymes and metabolites
- Bacteria reach their maximum size at the end of the lag phase.
2. **Log phase:** In this phase bacteria divide exponentially so that the growth curve takes a shape of a straight line. At this stage, the bacterium is:
   - Smaller in size and biochemically active
   - Uniformly stained: It is the best time to perform the Gram stain.
3. **Stationary phase:** After the log phase, the bacterial growth ceases almost completely due to exhaustion of nutrients, accumulation of toxic products, and autolytic enzymes
   - The number of progeny cells formed is just enough to replace the number of cells that die
   - Hence, the number of viable cells remains stationary as there is almost a balance between the dying cells and the newly formed cells. But the total count keeps rising. In this phase:
     ♦ Bacterium becomes gram-variable
     ♦ More storage granules are formed
     ♦ Sporulation occurs in this phase
     ♦ Bacteria produce exotoxins, antibiotics, and bacteriocins.
4. **Decline phase:** Gradually, the bacteria stop dividing completely; while the cell death continues due to exhaustion of nutrients, and accumulation of toxic products. Involution forms are seen in this phase. There is a decline in the viable count but not in total count.

Factors Affecting Growth of Bacteria

Several environmental factors affect the growth of the bacteria.

Oxygen

Based on their oxygen requirements bacteria are classified as:
- ❖ **Obligate aerobes:** They can grow only in the presence of oxygen (e.g. *Pseudomonas, Mycobacterium tuberculosis, Bacillus*)
- ❖ **Facultative anaerobes:** They are aerobes that can also grow anaerobically (e.g. most of the pathogenic bacteria, e.g. *Escherichia coli, Staphylococcus aureus*, etc.)
- ❖ **Microaerophilic bacteria:** They can grow in the presence of low oxygen tension, i.e. 5–10% of oxygen (e.g. *Campylobacter* and *Helicobacter*)
- ❖ **Obligate anaerobes:** These bacteria can grow only in absence of oxygen, as oxygen is lethal to them (e.g. *Clostridium tetani*).

Temperature

Most of the pathogenic bacteria grow optimally at 37°C (i.e. human body temperature). However, the optimal temperature range varies with different bacterial species.
- ❖ **Psychrophiles**—grow best at temperatures below 20°C, e.g. *Pseudomonas*
- ❖ **Mesophiles**—grow within a temperature range 25°C and 40°C, e.g. most of the pathogenic bacteria
- ❖ **Thermophiles**—these bacteria grow at a high-temperature range of 55°C–80°C, e.g. *Geobacillus stearothermophilus*.

Other Important Factors Affecting Growth of Bacteria

- **Carbon dioxide:** Organisms that require higher amounts of carbon dioxide (5–10%) for growth are called *capnophilic bacteria*. Examples include *Brucella abortus*, *Streptococcus pneumoniae*, etc.
- **pH:** Most pathogenic bacteria grow between pH 7.2–and pH 7.6. Very few bacteria (e.g. lactobacilli) can grow at acidic pH and *Vibrio cholerae* are capable of growing at alkaline pH
- **Light:** Bacteria (except phototrophs) grow well in darkness. Photochromogenic mycobacteria produce pigments only on exposure to light
- **Moisture and desiccation:** Moisture is an essential requirement for the growth of bacteria because 80% of the bacterial cell consists of water. Some organisms like *Treponema pallidum* and *N. gonorrhoeae* die quickly after drying, while *M. tuberculosis* and *S. aureus* may survive drying for several weeks.

Metabolism of Pathogenic Bacteria

The bacterial metabolism is dependent on whether they are aerobic or anaerobic.
- Aerobic bacteria utilize glucose by oxidation by Krebs cycle
- Anaerobes utilize glucose by fermentation via three pathways:
  1. Glycolysis (Embden–Meyerhof–Parnas pathway): Glucose is converted to pyruvate; seen in most of the bacteria
  2. Entner–Doudoroff (ED) pathway: Seen in *Pseudomonas*
  3. Pentose phosphate pathway.

EXPECTED QUESTIONS

I. **Write an essay on:**
   1. Describe in detail the structure and function of the cell wall of gram-negative bacilli with the help of a diagram.

II. **Write short notes on:**
   1. Bacterial capsule.
   2. Bacterial growth curve.
   3. List the differences between cell wall of gram-positive bacteria and gram-negative bacteria.

III. **Multiple Choice Questions (MCQs):**
   1. The cuneiform arrangement is characteristic of:
      a. *Staphylococcus*
      b. *Streptococcus*
      c. *Corynebacterium diphtheriae*
      d. *Bacillus anthracis*
   2. A bacterial capsule can be best demonstrated by:
      a. Gram staining
      b. Acid-fast staining
      c. Negative staining
      d. Albert staining
   3. The bacterial structure involved in motility is:
      a. Ribosome   b. Pili
      c. Mesosome   d. Flagella
   4. Lipopolysaccharide is a component of cell wall of:
      a. Gram-positive bacteria
      b. Gram-negative bacteria
      c. Virus
      d. Fungi
   5. Bacterial structure involved in respiration is:
      a. Ribosome   b. Pili
      c. Mesosome   d. Flagella

Answers
1. c   2. c   3. d   4. b   5. c

General Bacteriology: Laboratory Diagnosis of Bacterial Infections

CHAPTER 3.2

CHAPTER PREVIEW
- Specimen Collection
- Direct Detection
- Culture, Identification and AST
  - Culture Media
- Culture Methods
- Culture Identification
- Antimicrobial Susceptibility Test
- Serology
- Molecular Methods
- Microbial Typing

INTRODUCTION

Laboratory diagnosis of bacterial infections comprises of several steps—specimen collection, direct detection, culture, identification and antimicrobial susceptibility test, serology and molecular methods (refer box).

LABORATORY DIAGNOSIS — Bacterial infections

1. **Specimen collection**
2. **Direct detection**
   - Microscopy: Gram stain, acid-fast stain, Albert stain, histopathological staining, dark ground, phase-contrast and fluorescence microscopy
   - Antigen detection from clinical specimen
   - Molecular diagnosis: Detecting bacterial DNA or RNA from clinical specimen
3. **Culture**
   - Culture media
   - Culture methods
   - Colony morphology, smear and motility testing
4. **Identification**
   - Biochemical identification
   - Automated identification methods
5. **Antimicrobial susceptibility testing**
6. **Serology**—Antigen and antibody detection
7. **Molecular methods**
8. **Typing methods**

SPECIMEN COLLECTION

Specimen collection depends upon the type of underlying infections **(Table 3.2.1)**.

General Principles

The following general principles should be followed while collecting the specimen:

- ❖ **Standard precautions** should be followed for collecting and handling all specimens (**Chapter 15** for details)
- ❖ **Before antibiotics start:** Whenever possible, culture specimens should be collected prior to administration of any antimicrobial agents
- ❖ **Contamination** with indigenous flora should be avoided, especially when collecting urine and blood culture specimens
- ❖ **Swabs** are though convenient but considered inferior to tissue, aspirate and body fluids
- ❖ **Container:** Specimens should be collected in sterile, tightly sealed, leak proof, wide-mouth, screw-capped containers
- ❖ **Labeling:** All specimens must be appropriately labelled with name, age, gender, treating physician, diagnosis, antibiotic history, type of specimen, and desired investigation name
- ❖ **Rejection:** Specimens grossly contaminated or compromised or improperly labeled may be rejected
- ❖ If **anaerobic culture** is requested, proper anaerobic collection containers with media should be used
- ❖ Specimen should not be sent in container containing **formalin** for microbiological analysis.

Specimen Transport

The specimens should reach the laboratory for further processing as soon as possible after the collection. If required appropriate transport media should be used (discussed subsequently in this chapter).

For most of the specimens, transport time should not exceed **two hours**. However, there are some exceptions.

- ❖ Specimens that require an **immediate transport** (<15 minutes)—such as CSF and body fluids, ocular

Table 3.2.1: Types of infections and various specimens collected.	
Type of infections	Specimens collected
Bloodstream infection, sepsis, endocarditis	Paired blood culture specimens • Collected aseptically by two-step disinfection of skin; first with alcohol followed by chlorhexidine • 8–10 mL of blood (for adults) collected in blood culture bottles
Infectious diseases requiring serology	• Blood (2 mL/investigation) • Collected by minimal asepsis (one-step skin disinfection with alcohol) • Collected in vacutainer
Diarrheal diseases	Stool (mucus flakes), rectal swab
Meningitis	Cerebrospinal fluid (CSF)
Infections of other sterile body area	Sterile body fluids; e.g. pleural fluid, synovial fluid, peritoneal fluid
Skin and soft tissue infections	Pus or exudate, wound swabs, aspirates from abscess and tissue bits
Anaerobic infections	Aspirates, tissue specimens, blood and sterile body fluids, bone marrow (swabs, sputum not satisfactory)
Upper respiratory tract infections	Throat swab with membrane over the tonsil, nasopharyngeal swab, per-nasal swab
Lower respiratory tract infections	Sputum, endotracheal aspirate, bronchoalveolar lavage (BAL), protected specimen brush (PSB) and lung biopsy
Pulmonary tuberculosis	• Sputum—early morning and spot • Collected in well-ventilated area • Gastric aspirate for infants
Urinary tract infections	• Midstream urine • Suprapubic aspirated urine • Catheterized patient—collected from the catheter tube, after clamping distally and disinfecting; not from urobag
Genital infections	• Urethral swab, cervical swab—for urethritis • Exudate from genital ulcers
Eye infections	• Conjunctival swabs • Corneal scrapings • Aqueous or vitreous fluid
Ear infections	• Swabs from outer ear • Aspirate from inner ear

specimens, tissue specimens, suprapubic aspirate and bone specimen

- **Urine (midstream)** added with preservative (boric acid) is acceptable up to 24 hours, otherwise should be transported within 2 hours
- **Stool culture:** Stool specimen should be transported within 1 hour, but with transport medium (Cary-Blair medium) up to 24 hours is acceptable
- **Rectal swabs**—up to 24 hours is acceptable
- **For anaerobic culture:** Specimens should be put into Robertson's cooked meat broth or any specialized anaerobic transport system and transported immediately to the laboratory.

Specimen Storage before Processing

Most specimens can be stored **at room temperature** immediately after receipt, for **up to 24 hours**. However, there are some exceptions.

- **Blood cultures**—should be incubated at 37°C immediately upon receipt
- **Sterile body fluids, bone, vitreous fluid, suprapubic aspirate**—should be immediately plated upon receipt and incubated at 37°C
- **Corneal scraping**—should be immediately plated at bed-side on to blood agar and chocolate agar
- **Stool culture**—can be stored up to 72 hours at 4°C
- **Urine** (midstream and from the catheter), **lower respiratory** tract specimen, **gastric biopsy** (for *Helicobacter pylori*)—can be stored up to 24 hours at 4°C.

DIRECT DETECTION

Direct detection of bacteria in the clinical specimen plays a very important role in early institution of antimicrobial therapy. These methods include microscopic demonstration of bacteria—staining techniques and other methods such as detection of antigen or nucleic acid in the clinical specimen.

STAINING TECHNIQUES

Structural details of bacteria cannot be seen under a light microscope due to lack of contrast. Hence, it is necessary to use staining methods to produce color contrast and thereby increase the visibility. Before staining, the smears are fixed so that they will not be displaced during the staining process. Fixation also protects the internal structures of cells in a fixed position. It is done by two methods.

1. **Heat fixation:** It is done by gently flame heating an air-dried film, used for bacterial smears
2. **Methanol fixation:** Used for blood smears.

Common staining techniques used in diagnostic bacteriology include:

- **Simple stain:** Basic dyes, such as methylene blue or basic fuchsin are used as simple stains. They provide the color contrast, but impart the same color to all the bacteria in a smear
- **Negative staining:** A drop of bacterial suspension is mixed with dyes, such as India ink or nigrosin. The background gets stained black whereas unstained bacterial/yeast capsule stand out in contrast. This is very useful in the demonstration of bacterial/yeast capsules which do not take up simple stains

- ❖ **Impregnation methods:** Bacterial cells and structures that are too thin to be seen under the light microscope, are thickened by impregnation of silver salts on their surface to make them visible, e.g. for demonstration of spirochetes and bacterial flagella (by Leifson staining technique)
- ❖ **Differential stains:** Here, two stains are used which impart different colors to different bacteria or bacterial structures, which help in differentiating bacteria. The most commonly employed differential stains are:
    - **Gram stain:** It differentiates bacteria into gram-positive and gram-negative groups.
    - **Acid-fast stain:** It differentiates bacteria into acid-fast and non acid-fast groups.
- ❖ **Special stains:** These staining techniques are useful to identify various bacterial structures of importance. Examples include—(1) Albert staining (to demonstrate metachromatic granules), (2) Spore staining (e.g. Schaeffer–Fulton stain).

Gram Stain

This staining technique was originally developed by Hans Christian Gram (1884).

Procedure (Fig. 3.2.1)

- ❖ **Fixation:** The smear made on a slide from bacterial culture or specimen is air-dried and then heat-fixed
- ❖ **Step 1 (Primary stain):** The smear is stained with pararosaniline dyes such as crystal violet (or gentian violet or methyl violet) for one minute. Then the slide is rinsed with water. Crystal violet stains all the bacteria violet in color (irrespective of whether they are gram-positive or gram-negative)
- ❖ **Step 2 (Mordant):** Gram's iodine (dilute solution of iodine) is poured over the slide for one minute. Then the slide is rinsed with water. Gram's iodine acts as a mordant, binds to the dye to form bigger dye-iodine complexes in the cytoplasm
- ❖ **Step 3 (Decolorization):** Next step is pouring of few drops of decolorizer to the smear, e.g. acetone (for 2–3 sec) or ethyl alcohol (20–30 sec) or acetone alcohol (for 10 sec). Slide is immediately rinsed with water. Decolorizer removes the primary stain from gram-negative bacteria while the gram-positive bacteria retain the primary stain

    > *Note:* **Decolorization** is the most crucial step of Gram staining. If the decolorizer is poured for more time, even gram-positive bacteria lose color (**over decolorization**) and if poured for less time, the gram-negative bacteria do not lose the color of primary stain properly (**under decolorization**).

- ❖ **Step 4 (Counterstain):** Secondary stains such as safranin or dilute carbol fuchsin is added for 30 seconds.

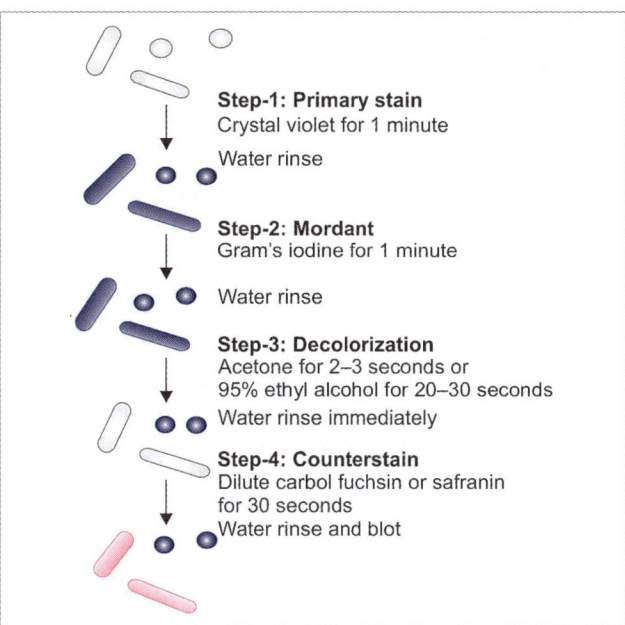

Fig. 3.2.1: Principle and procedure of Gram staining.

It imparts pink or red color to the gram-negative bacteria. Alternatively, neutral red may also be used as counterstain, especially for gonococci. The slide is rinsed in tap water, dried, and then examined under oil immersion objective.

Interpretation of Gram Stain

Smear is examined under oil immersion objective (Fig. 3.2.2A).
- ❖ Gram-positive bacteria resist decolorization and retain the color of primary stain, i.e. violet
- ❖ Gram-negative bacteria are decolorized and, therefore, take counterstain and appear pink.

Principle of Gram Staining

Though the exact mechanism is not understood, the following theories have been put forward.
- ❖ **pH theory:** Cytoplasm of gram-positive bacteria is more acidic, hence, can retain the basic dye (e.g. crystal violet) for longer time. **Iodine** serves as mordant, i.e. it combines with the primary stain to form a dye-iodine complex which gets retained inside the cell
- ❖ **Cell wall theory:** This is believed to be the most important postulate to describe the mechanism of Gram stain
    - Gram-positive cell wall has a thick peptidoglycan layer (50–100 layers thick), with tight cross linkages
    - The peptidoglycan itself is not stained; instead, it seems to act as a permeability barrier preventing loss of crystal violet. Large dye-iodine complexes are not able to penetrate this tightened peptidoglycan layer in a gram-positive bacteria

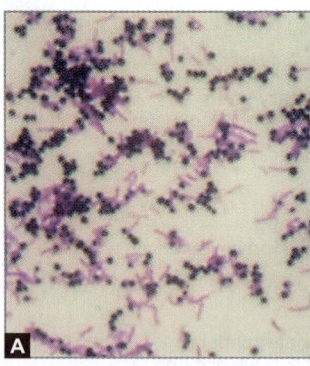 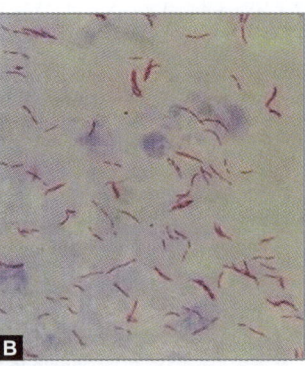

Figs. 3.2.2A and B: A. Gram staining demonstrating violet-colored gram-positive cocci in clusters and pink colored gram-negative bacilli in scattered arrangement; **B.** Acid-fast staining shows long slender straight or slightly curved beaded red acid-fast bacilli.

Source: A. Department of Microbiology, Pondicherry Institute of Medical Sciences, Puducherry; B. Department of Microbiology, JIPMER, Puducherry (*with permission*).

- Gram-negative cell wall is more permeable thus allowing the outflow of crystal violet easily. This is attributed to:
    - The thin peptidoglycan layer in gram-negative cell wall which is not tightly cross linked
    - Presence of lipopolysaccharide layer in the cell wall of gram-negative bacteria, which gets disrupted easily by the decolorizer; forming larger pores, that allow the dye-iodine complexes to escape from the cytoplasm
- **Magnesium ribonucleate theory:** It is present in the cell membrane of gram-positive bacteria but not in gram-negative bacteria and helps to retain the primary dye.

> **Uses of Gram Stain**
> - **To differentiate bacteria into gram-positive and gram-negative**
> - **For identification:** Gram staining from bacterial culture gives an idea to put the corresponding biochemical tests for further identification of bacteria
> - **To start empirical treatment:** Gram stain from the specimen gives a preliminary clue about the bacteria present so that the empirical treatment can be started
> - **Anaerobic organisms,** such as *Clostridium* do not grow in routine culture. Therefore, organisms detected in Gram stain, but aerobic culture-negative gives a preliminary clue to perform an anaerobic culture of the specimen
> - **Yeasts:** In addition to stain the bacteria, Gram stain is useful for staining certain fungi such as *Candida* and *Cryptococcus* (appear gram-positive)
> - **Quality of specimen:** Gram stain helps in screening the quality of the **sputum specimen** before processing it for culture. Presence of more pus cells and less epithelial cells indicates good quality specimen.

Acid-fast Stain

The acid-fast stain was discovered by Paul Ehrlich and subsequently modified by Ziehl and Neelsen. This staining is done to identify acid-fast organisms, such as *Mycobacterium tuberculosis* and others. Acid-fastness is due to presence of mycolic acid in the cell wall.

Ziehl-Neelsen Technique (Hot Method)

Smear Preparation

Smear measuring 2 × 3 cm in size is prepared in a new clean grease free scratch free slide from the yellow purulent portion of the sputum.

- The smear should neither be too thick nor too thin. When placed over a printed matter, the print should be readable through the smear
- Smear preparation should be done near a flame, as six inches around the flame is considered sterile zone (as heat coagulates the aerosols raised during the smear preparation).

Heat Fixation

The smear is air dried and then heat fixed by passing over the flame 3–5 times for 3–4 seconds each time. Coagulation of the proteinaceous material in the sputum will facilitate fixing of the smear.

Procedure

Step 1 (Primary stain)
Smear is poured with strong carbol fuchsin (1%) for 5 minutes. Intermittent heating is done by flaming the underneath of the slide until the vapor rises. Heating helps in better penetration of the stain.

- Care must be taken to ensure that the smear does not dry out, to prevent drying more solution of stain is added to the slide and the slide reheated
- Rinse the slide with tap water, until all free carbol fuchsin stain is washed away. At this point, the smear on the slide looks red in color.

Step 2 (Decolorization)
It is done by pouring 25% sulfuric acid over the slide and allowing it to stand for 2–4 minutes. The slide is gently rinsed with tap water and tilted to drain off the water.

- A properly decolorized slide appears colorless or light pink. If the slide is still red, sulfuric acid is reapplied for 1–3 minutes and then rinsed gently with tap water.

Step 3 (Counter staining)
0.1% methylene blue is poured onto the slide and left for 30 seconds. Then the slide is rinsed gently with tap water and allowed to dry.

- The slide is examined under the light microscope using low power objective (10×) to select a suitable area and then examined under oil immersion field (100×)

- Contaminated materials/used slide should be discarded in a jar containing 5% phenol.

Interpretation

Mycobacterium tuberculosis appears as long slender, straight or slightly curved and sometimes beaded, red colored acid-fast bacillus. Other non-acid fast organisms present in the smear and the background take up the counter stain and appear blue **(Fig. 3.2.2B)**.

Modifications of Acid-Fast Staining

Hot method (Ziehl–Neelsen technique) was widely used before. Now various **cold methods** are used, where the intermittent heating is not required. Examples include:
- **Kinyoun's method:** First step, flood Kinyoun's carbolfuchsin over the smear for 5 minutes; second step, decolorize with acid alcohol for 3 minutes and third step, counterstain with methylene blue for 4 minutes (*refer* **Chapter 27**)
- **Gabbet's method:** It is a two-step method—first, flood the smear with basic fuchsin-phenol stain for 10 minutes and then counterstain with Gabbet's methylene blue (containing sulfuric acid) for 2 minutes.

Higher is the content of mycolic acid in the cell wall, more is the acid-fastness; hence higher percentage of sulfuric acid is required for decolorization **(Table 3.2.2)**.

Albert Stain

Albert stain is used to demonstrate the metachromatic granules of *Corynebacterium diphtheriae*.

Procedure

- After heat fixing, the smear is covered with Albert I stain for 5 minutes, then the excess stain is drained out
- Albert II (iodine solution) is added for 1 minute
- Slide is washed with water, blotted dry and examined under oil immersion field.

Composition

Composition of Albert stain includes:

Table 3.2.2: Acid-fast organisms/structures and percentage of sulfuric acid suitable for staining.	
Acid-fast organisms/structures	**Sulfuric acid (%) needed for decolorization**
Mycobacterium tuberculosis	25%
Mycobacterium leprae	5%
Nocardia	1%
Acid-fast parasites such as Cryptosporidium, Cyclospora, Cystoisospora	0.5%
Bacterial spore	0.25–0.5%

- **Albert I:** Comprises of toluidine blue, malachite green, glacial acetic acid, alcohol (95% ethanol), and distilled water
- **Albert II:** Contains iodine in potassium iodide.

Interpretation

Corynebacterium diphtheriae appears as green colored bacilli arranged in Chinese letter or cuneiform pattern, with bluish black metachromatic granules at polar ends (*refer* **Fig. 24.1C, Chapter 24**). These can be differentiated from diphtheroids which do not show granules and are arranged in palisade pattern. However, certain bacteria, such as *Corynebacterium xerosis* and *Gardnerella vaginalis* also possess metachromatic granules.

Other Microscopic Techniques

Other microscopic techniques include:
- **Dark-ground and phase-contrast microscopy**—for demonstration of spirochetes in genital specimens
- **Hanging drop preparation** for stool specimen (see below highlight box).

> **Hanging drop preparation**
> Hanging drop preparation is one of the most commonly used method to demonstrate bacterial motility. The procedure is explained in **Figure 3.2.3**. After the drop is prepared on a coverslip and kept over the cavity slide, the edge of the drop is focused.
> ❑ The edge is focused because (i) it provides better contrast at the edge, (ii) aerobic bacteria usually migrate toward the edge to get more oxygen
> ❑ Hanging drop may give some clue about the identification, especially when a typical pattern of motility is observed (e.g. darting motility as for *Vibrio cholerae* in the stool specimen).

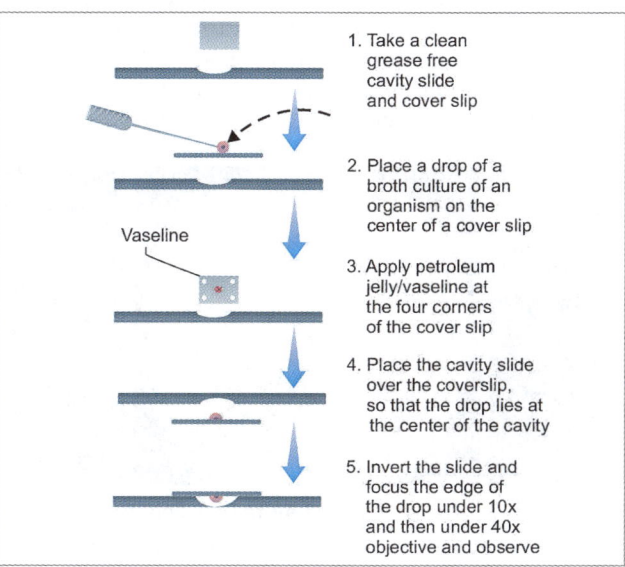

Fig. 3.2.3: Hanging drop method (procedure).

CULTURE, IDENTIFICATION AND AST

Culture is the most common diagnostic method used for detection of bacterial infections. Specimens are inoculated on to various culture media and incubated. The colonies grown are subjected to identification and antimicrobial susceptibility test (AST).

■ CULTURE MEDIA

A microbiological culture medium is a liquid or solid substance that contains nutrients to support the growth, and survival of microorganisms.

Constituents of Culture Media

The important constituents of culture media are water, electrolytes, peptone (a complex mixture of partially digested proteins), agar, meat extract and yeast extract.
- ❖ **Agar** is used for solidifying the culture medium.
  - It is prepared from the cell wall of seaweeds and available commercially in powder form
  - It is used as 1–2% for solid medium, 0.5% for semisolid agar and 6% to inhibit *Proteus* swarming.
- ❖ In addition, **blood** (e.g. 5% sheep blood) or **serum** may be added to provide extra nutrition to fastidious bacteria.

Types of Culture Media

Bacteriological culture media can be classified in two ways.
A. Based on consistency, culture media are grouped into—liquid (or broth), semisolid and solid media.
B. Based on the method of growth detection, culture media are classified as:
1. **Conventional culture media:** Here, the bacterial growth is detected manually by visual inspection of turbidity or colony morphology. They are of various types such as—simple/basal media, enriched media, enrichment broth, selective media, differential media, transport media and anaerobic media, etc.
2. **Automated culture media:** They are mainly available for blood and sterile body fluid culture. The growth is detected automatically by the equipment.

Conventional Culture Media

Simple/Basal Media

They contain minimum ingredients that support the growth of non-fastidious bacteria. Examples include—
- ❖ **Peptone water:** It contains peptone (1%) + NaCl (0.5%) + water **(Fig. 3.2.4A)**
- ❖ **Nutrient broth:** It is made up of peptone water + meat extract (1%).
- ❖ **Nutrient agar:** It is made up of nutrient broth + 2% agar **(Fig. 3.2.4B)**
- ❖ **Semisolid medium:** It is prepared by reducing the concentration of agar to 0.2–0.5%.

> **Uses of Basal Media**
> The basal media are used for:
> ❑ Testing the non-fastidiousness of bacteria
> ❑ They serve as the base for the preparation of many other media
> ❑ Nutrient broth is used for studying the bacterial growth curve
> ❑ Nutrient agar is the preferred medium for:
>   ➢ Performing the biochemical tests, such as oxidase, catalase and slide agglutination test, etc.
>   ➢ To study the colony morphology
>   ➢ Pigment demonstration.

Enriched Media

When a basal medium is added with additional nutrients, such as blood, serum or egg, it is called enriched medium. In addition to non-fastidious organisms, they also support the growth of fastidious nutritionally exacting bacteria. Examples include:
- ❖ **Blood agar:** It is prepared by adding 5–10% of sheep blood to the molten nutrient agar at 45°C **(Fig. 3.2.4C)**. It is the most widely used medium in diagnostic bacteriology.

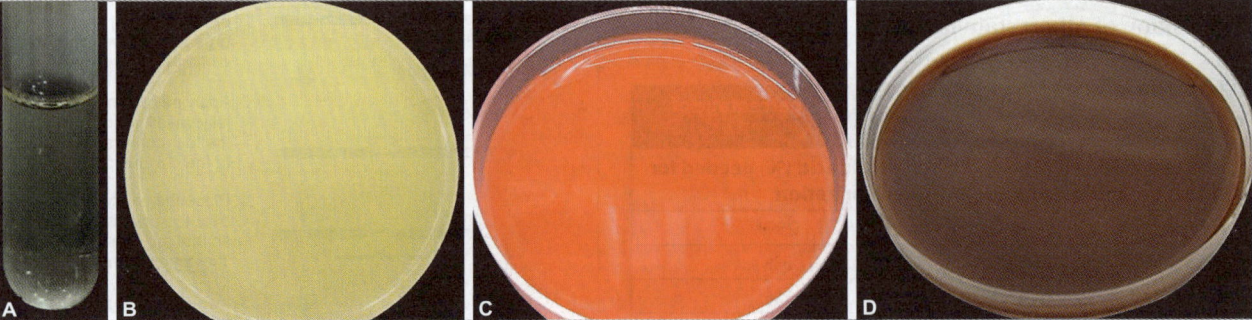

Figs. 3.2.4A to D: A. Peptone water; **B.** Nutrient agar; **C.** Blood agar; **D.** Chocolate agar.
Source: A to D. Department of Microbiology, JIPMER, Puducherry (*with permission*).

Blood agar also tests the hemolytic property of the bacteria, which may be either: (1) partial or α (green) hemolysis and (2) complete or β-hemolysis (described subsequently in this chapter)

- **Chocolate agar:** It is the heated blood agar, prepared by adding 5–10% of sheep blood to the molten nutrient agar at 70°C, so that the RBCs will be lysed and the content of RBCs will be released, changing the color of the medium to brown **(Fig. 3.2.4D)**. It is more nutritious than blood agar, and even supports certain highly fastidious bacteria, such as *Haemophilus influenzae* that does not grow on blood agar
- **Loeffler's serum slope:** It contains serum. It is used for isolation of *Corynebacterium diphtheriae*
- **Blood culture media:** They are used for isolating microorganisms from blood. They are available either as conventional or automated blood culture media (described later in this chapter).

Enrichment Broth

They are the liquid media added with some inhibitory agents which selectively allow certain organism to grow and inhibit others. This is important for isolation of the pathogens from clinical specimens which also contain normal flora (e.g. stool and sputum specimen). Examples for enrichment broth include:
- Gram-negative broth—Used for isolation of *Shigella*
- Selenite F broth—Used for isolation of *Shigella*
- Alkaline peptone water (APW)—Used for *Vibrio cholerae*.

Selective Media

They are solid media containing inhibitory substances that inhibit the normal flora present in the specimen and allow the pathogens to grow.
- **Lowenstein–Jensen (LJ) medium:** It is used for isolation of *Mycobacterium tuberculosis* **(Fig. 3.2.5A)**
- **Thiosulfate citrate bile salt sucrose (TCBS) agar:** It is used for isolation of *Vibrio* species **(Fig. 3.2.5B)**
- **DCA (deoxycholate citrate agar) and XLD (xylose lysine deoxycholate) agar:** They are used for the isolation of enteric pathogens, such as *Salmonella* and *Shigella* from stool **(Figs. 3.2.6A and B)**
- **Potassium tellurite agar (PTA):** It is used for isolation of *Corynebacterium diphtheriae*.

Transport Media

They are used for the transport of the clinical specimens suspected to contain delicate organism or when delay is expected while transporting the specimens from the site of collection to the laboratory **(Table 3.2.3)**. Bacteria do not multiply in the transport media, they only remain viable.

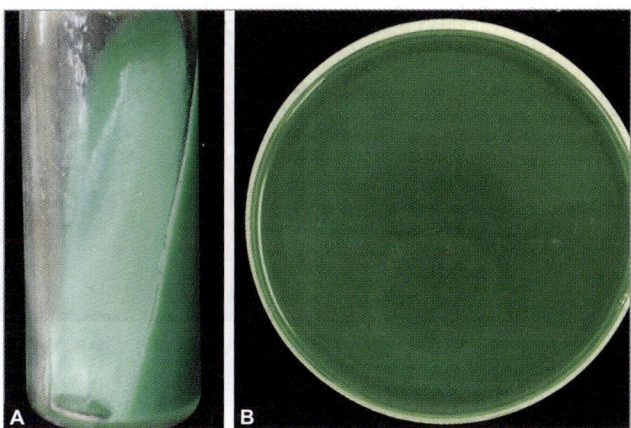

Figs. 3.2.5A and B: A. Lowenstein–Jensen medium; **B.** TCBS agar.
Source: Department of Microbiology, JIPMER, Puducherry (with permission).

Table 3.2.3: Transport media used for common bacteria.

Organism	Transport media
Neisseria	Amies medium and Stuart's medium
Vibrio cholerae	• VR (Venkatraman-Ramakrishnan) medium • Autoclaved sea water • Cary-Blair medium
Shigella, Salmonella	• Buffered glycerol saline • Cary-Blair medium

Differential Media

These media differentiate between two groups of bacteria by using an indicator, which changes the color of the colonies of a particular group of bacteria but not the other group.
- **MacConkey agar:** It is a differential and low selective medium, commonly used for the isolation of enteric gram-negative bacteria **(Fig. 3.2.6C)**
  - It differentiates organisms into LF or lactose fermenters (produce pink colored colonies, e.g. *Escherichia coli*) and NLF or non-lactose fermenters (produce colorless colonies, e.g. *Shigella*)
  - **Composition:** It contains peptone, lactose, agar, neutral red (indicator) and taurocholate
  - Most laboratories use combination of blood agar and MacConkey agar for routine bacterial culture.
- **CLED agar (cysteine lactose electrolyte-deficient agar):** This is another differential medium similar to MacConkey agar, capable of differentiating between LF and NLF. It is used as an alternative to combination of blood agar and MacConkey agar, for the processing of urine specimens **(Fig. 3.2.6D)**.

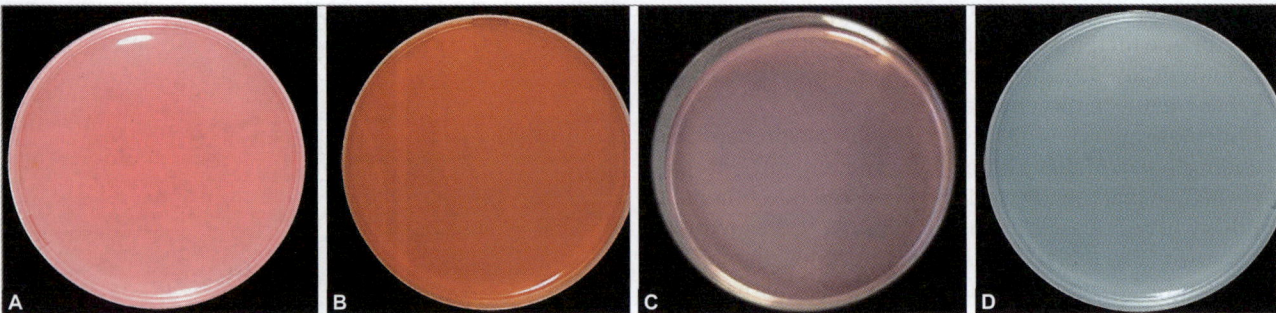

Figs. 3.2.6A to D: A. DCA; **B.** XLD agar; **C.** MacConkey agar; **D.** CLED agar.
Source: Department of Microbiology, JIPMER, Puducherry (*with permission*).

Anaerobic Culture Media

Anaerobic media contain reducing substances which take-up oxygen and create lower redox potential and thus permit the growth of obligate anaerobes, such as *Clostridium*. Examples are as follows:

- **Robertson's cooked meat (RCM) broth:** It contains chopped meat particles (beef heart), which provide glutathione (a sulfhydryl group containing reducing substance) and unsaturated fatty acids. It is the most widely used anaerobic culture medium **(Fig. 3.2.7A)**. It is also used for maintenance of stock cultures
- **Other anaerobic media** include:
  - Thioglycollate broth **(Fig. 3.2.7B)**
  - Anaerobic blood agar
  - Egg yolk agar
  - Phenyl ethyl agar
  - *Bacteroides* bile esculin agar (BBE agar).

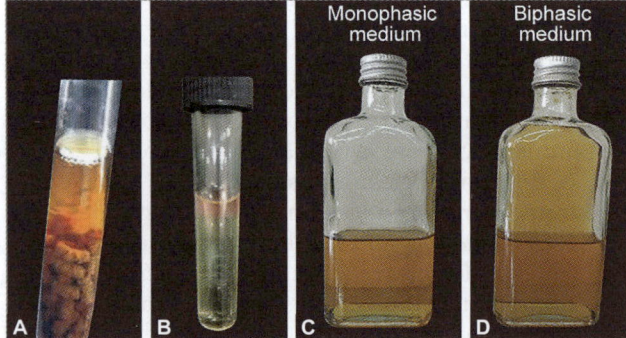

Figs. 3.2.7A to D: A. Robertson's cooked meat medium; **B.** Thioglycollate broth; **C.** Brain-heart infusion broth; **D.** Biphasic medium (Brain-heart infusion broth/agar).
Source: A, C and D. Department of Microbiology, JIPMER, Puducherry; B. Department of Microbiology, Pondicherry Institute of Medical Sciences, Puducherry (*with permission*).

Blood Culture Media

Recovery of bacteria from blood is difficult as they are usually present in lesser quantity in the blood and many of the blood pathogens are fastidious. Therefore, enriched media are used for isolating microorganisms from blood. Blood culture media are available either as conventional or automated media.

Conventional Blood Culture Media

The conventional blood culture media are of two types:
1. **Monophasic medium:** It contains brain-heart infusion (BHI) broth **(Fig. 3.2.7C)**
2. **Biphasic medium:** It has a liquid phase containing BHI broth and a solid agar slope made up of BHI agar **(Fig. 3.2.7D)**.

The recovery of organisms in the blood is enhanced by mixing the blood in the broth periodically. If any growth occurs, it can be detected by manual subcultures onto solid media, performed periodically for 1 week.

Automated Blood Culture Techniques

Automated blood culture (ABC) systems have been in use for two decades. Examples include BacT/ALERT **(Fig. 3.2.8A)**, and BACTEC systems. Following inoculation, the ABC bottles are loaded inside the automated culture instrument.

- **Medium:** Automated blood culture bottles **(Fig. 3.2.8B)** contain:
  - Tryptic soy broth and/or brain heart infusion broth (as enriched media) added with
  - Polymeric resin beads which adsorb and neutralize the antimicrobials present in the blood specimen.
- **Advantages:** ABC systems offer continuous periodic monitoring (once in every 10 minutes). Hence, it gives a higher yield of positive cultures from clinical specimens

CHAPTER 3.2 ◆ General Bacteriology: Laboratory Diagnosis of Bacterial Infections

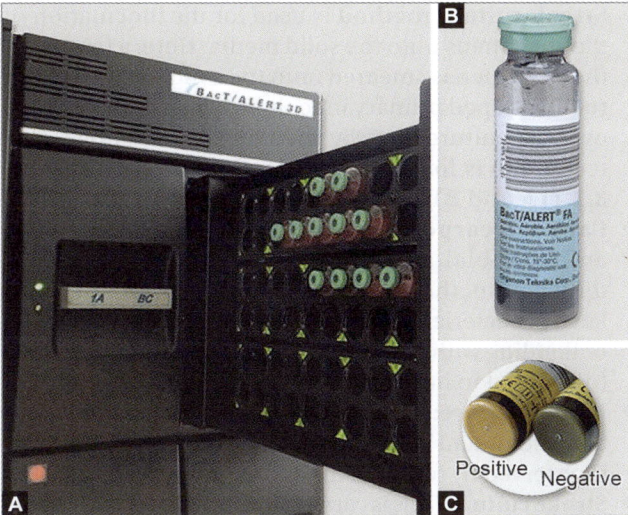

Figs. 3.2.8A to C: A. BacT/ALERT automated blood culture system; **B.** BacT/ALERT blood culture bottle; **C.** BacT/ALERT bottle showing colorimetric detection of positive blood culture.
Source: Department of Microbiology, JIPMER, Puducherry (*with permission*).

Table 3.2.4: Selection of media for various specimen types.

Specimens	Recommended culture media
Exudate specimens*	Blood agar plus MacConkey agar
Sterile body fluids	Blood agar, plus MacConkey agar, plus chocolate agar or Automated blood culture bottles
Blood	Blood culture bottles (Conventional or automated)
Urine	Blood agar plus MacConkey agar CLED agar can be used alternatively
Stool	Selenite-F broth plus MacConkey agar plus DCA and/or XLD agar (if cholera is suspected- add TCBS agar)
Respiratory specimens	Blood agar, plus MacConkey agar, plus chocolate agar (if diphtheria is suspected - add LSS and PTA)

*Exudate specimens include pus, wound swab, aspirates, and tissue bits.
(CLED, cysteine lactose electrolyte deficient agar; DCA, deoxycholate citrate agar; XLD, xylose lysine deoxycholate; TCBS, thiosulfate-citrate-bile salts-sucrose agar; LSS, Loeffler serum slope; PTA, potassium tellurite agar)

in less time. They are less labor intensive, as fully-automated
❖ **Disadvantages:** (i) High cost of the instrument and culture bottles and (ii) inability to observe the colony morphology, as liquid medium is used.

■ CULTURE METHODS

Culture methods involve inoculating the specimen on to appropriate culture media, followed by incubating the culture plates in appropriate conditions.

Selection of Media

The first step of a culture investigation is selection of appropriate media, which in turn depends up on the type of specimen to be processed. In general, combination of blood agar and MacConkey agar is commonly used for processing of most specimens. However, there are few specimens for which additional or alternative media are used **(Table 3.2.4)**.

Inoculation of the Specimens

Inoculation of the specimens onto the culture media is carried out with the help of bacteriological loops made up of platinum or nichrome wire **(Fig. 3.2.9A)**.

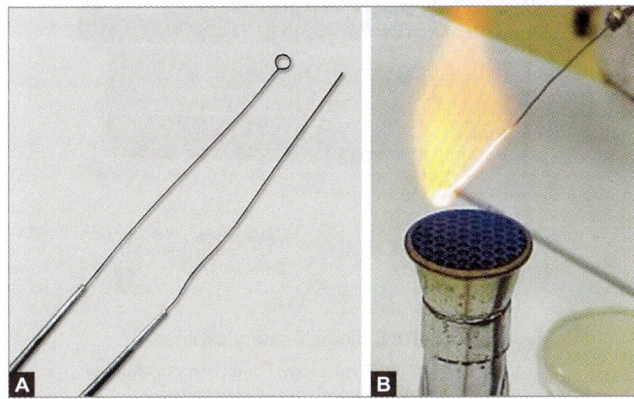

Figs. 3.2.9A and B: A. Bacteriological loop and straight wire; **B.** Flaming the loop (red hot).
Source: A. Department of Microbiology, JIPMER, Puducherry (*with permission*).

❖ The inoculating loop is first heated in the Bunsen flame by making it red hot **(Fig. 3.2.9B)** and then made cool waiting for 10 seconds
❖ The entire process of bacteriological culture method should be carried out in a biological safety cabinet and wearing appropriate personal protective equipment such as gloves, laboratory coat or gown and mask (for respiratory specimens).

> **Biosafety Cabinet (BSC)**
> It is an enclosed, ventilated laboratory work station, used to protect the laboratory personnel while working with potential infectious clinical specimens.
> - They are specially designed in a way that the air is blown into the cabinet away from the worker and then exhausted outside through a duct lined with HEPA filters **(Fig. 3.2.10)**
> - There are various types of BSCs, depending upon air velocity and percentage of air recirculated. Most of the microbiology laboratories require Class 2A BSC. A higher class of BSCs may be required for certain high-risk pathogens.

Inoculation Methods

Common inoculation methods are streak culture, liquid culture and lawn culture.

- **Streak culture method** is used for the inoculation of the specimens onto the solid media. Here, a loopful of the specimen is smeared onto the solid media to form round-shaped primary inoculum, which is then spread over the culture plate by streaking parallel lines. This technique is followed to get isolated colonies **(Figs. 3.2.11A and B)**
- **Lawn or carpet culture:** It is useful to carry out antimicrobial susceptibility testing (AST) by disk diffusion method **(Fig. 3.2.11C)**. Here, the uniform lawn of bacterial growth is obtained by either swabbing or flooding with a bacterial broth onto the culture plate (discussed in detail subsequently in this chapter)
- **Liquid culture:** It is used for culture of the blood and body fluids and also for water analysis. Bacterial growth is observed by turbidity in the medium
- **Stroke culture:** This is carried out on agar slopes or slants by streaking the straight wire in a zigzag fashion. It is used for biochemical test such as urease test.

Incubatory Conditions

Most of the pathogenic bacteria are aerobes or facultative anaerobes; grow best at 37°C, i.e. body temperature of human beings. Therefore, the inoculated culture plates are incubated at 37°C aerobically overnight in an incubator.

> **Bacteriological Incubator**
> It is an equipment used to incubate the culture plates, biochemical tests and AST plates **(Fig. 3.2.12)**. The incubator maintains optimal temperature. Some incubators are specially designed to maintain other conditions, such as humidity and CO_2.

Other Incubatory Conditions

The incubatory conditions may vary depending upon the bacteria to be isolated.

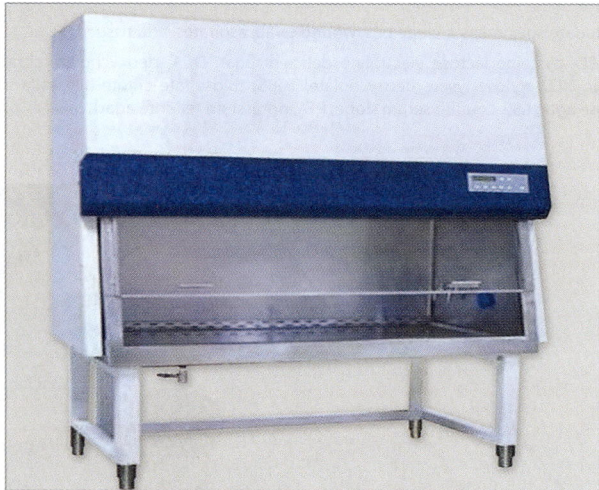

Fig. 3.2.10: Biological safety cabinet.
Source: Department of Microbiology, Pondicherry Institute of Medical Sciences, Puducherry (*with permission*).

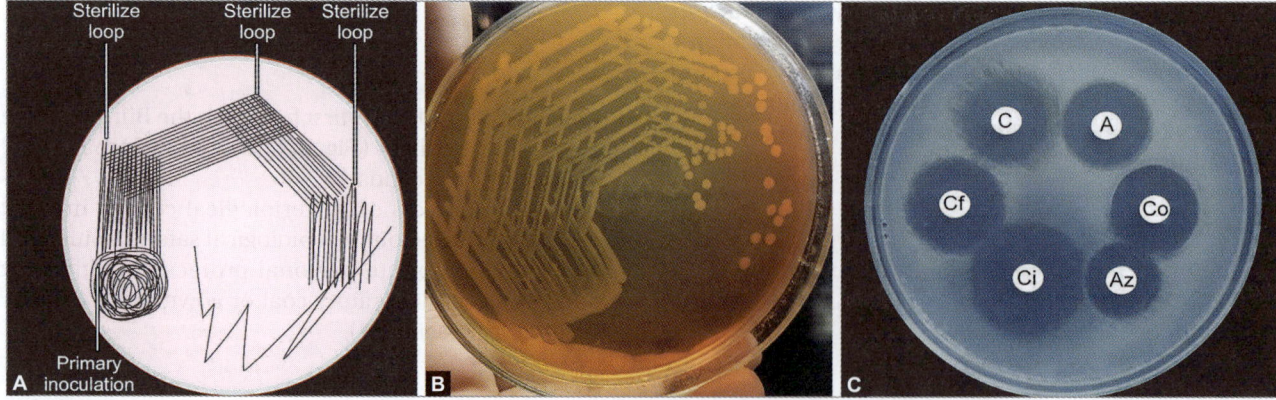

Figs. 3.2.11A to C: A. Streak culture (schematic representation); **B.** Isolated colonies grown by following streak culture; **C.** Lawn culture of a bacterial isolate to perform the antimicrobial susceptibility testing.
Source: Department of Microbiology, JIPMER, Puducherry (*with permission*).

CHAPTER 3.2 ◆ General Bacteriology: Laboratory Diagnosis of Bacterial Infections

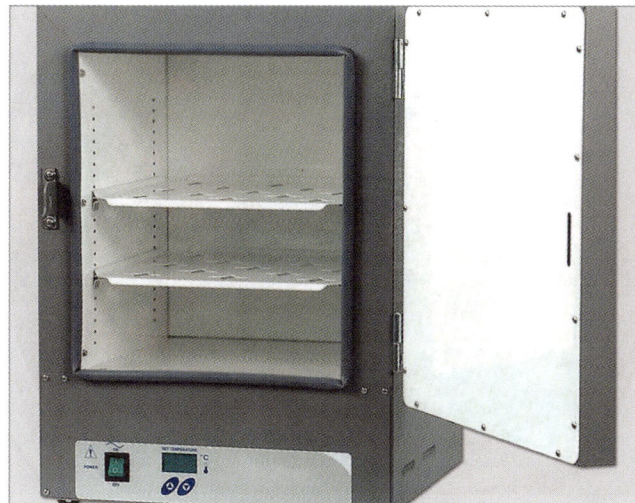

Fig. 3.2.12: Bacteriological incubator.
Source: Department of Microbiology, JIPMER, Puducherry (*with permission*).

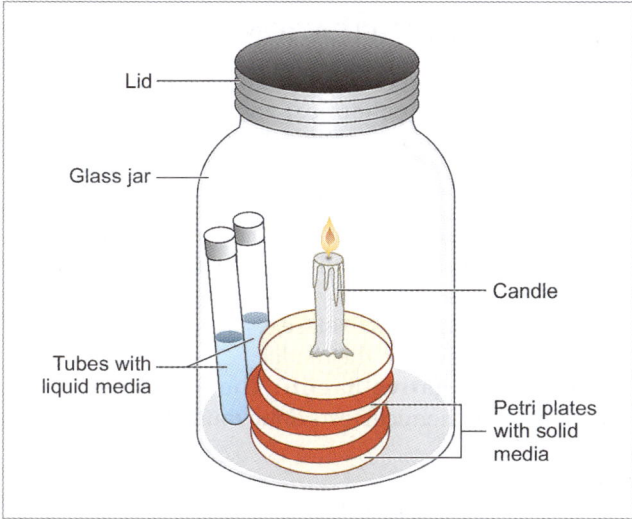

Fig. 3.2.13: Candle jar.

- **For capnophilic bacteria** candle jar is used. Here, inoculated media are placed inside a jar, along with a lighted candle and then jar is sealed. This provides an atmosphere of approximately 3–5% CO_2 **(Fig. 3.2.13)**. This is useful for capnophilic bacteria, such as *Brucella*, *Streptococcus*, pneumococcus and gonococcus
- **For microaerophilic bacteria,** such as *Campylobacter* and *Helicobacter* require 5% oxygen for optimum growth
- **For obligate anaerobes,** anaerobic culture methods are used (see below).

Anaerobic Culture Methods

Obligate anaerobic bacteria can grow only in the absence of oxygen. The following are the methods used to create anaerobiosis.
- **Evacuation and replacement method** by using:
  - *McIntosh and Filde's anaerobic jar* **(Fig. 3.2.14A)**: It was the most popular method in the past
  - *Anoxomat* **(Fig. 3.2.14B)**: It automatically evacuates air and replaces it with hydrogen gas from a cylinder. It is easier to use and highly effective for creating anaerobiosis.
- **Absorption of oxygen by chemical methods:** *GasPak system* works on this principle **(Fig. 3.2.15)**. It is the most commonly used method for anaerobiosis. Here, the oxygen is removed by chemical reactions
- **Anaerobic glove box** and **anaerobic work station** for easy processing, incubation and examination of the specimens, without exposure to oxygen
- **Reducing agents** such as glucose, thioglycollate, and cooked meat pieces can be used to reduce oxygen in culture media. Robertson cooked meat broth **(RCM)** is commonly used; which uses chopped meat particles as reducing agent **(Fig. 3.2.7A)**.

Indicator of anaerobiosis: The effectiveness of anaerobiosis can be checked by:
- **Chemical indicator:** Reduced methylene blue remains colorless in anaerobic conditions, but turns blue on exposure to oxygen
- **Biological indicator** using obligate aerobe such as *Pseudomonas*: The absence of its growth indicates that complete anaerobiosis has been achieved.

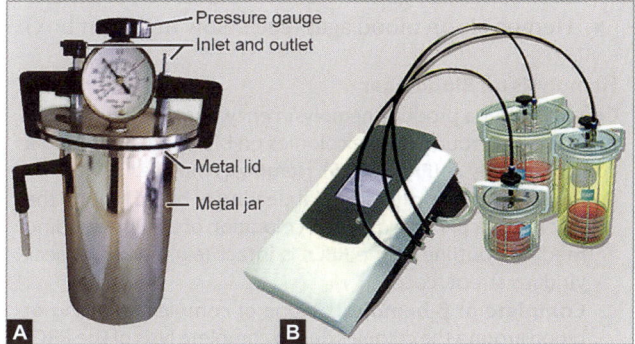

Figs. 3.2.14A and B: A. McIntosh and Filde's anaerobic jar; **B.** Anoxomat anaerobic system.
Source: A. Department of Microbiology, Pondicherry Institute of Medical Sciences, Puducherry; B. Department of Microbiology, JIPMER, Puducherry (*with permission*).

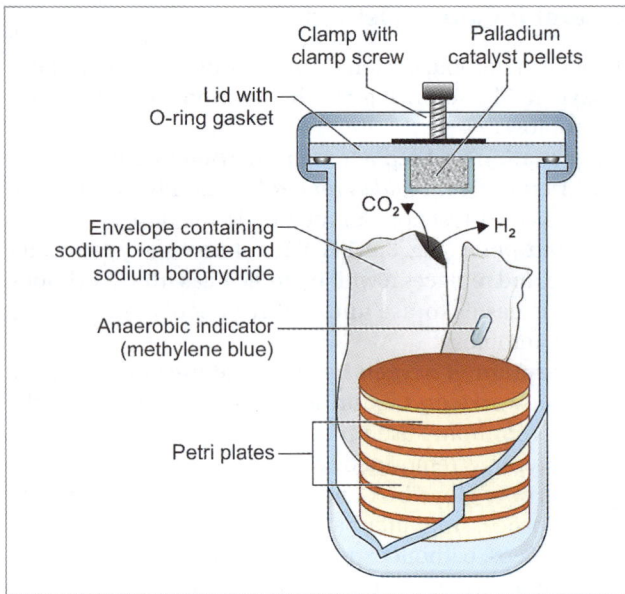

Fig. 3.2.15: GaSPak anaerobic system.

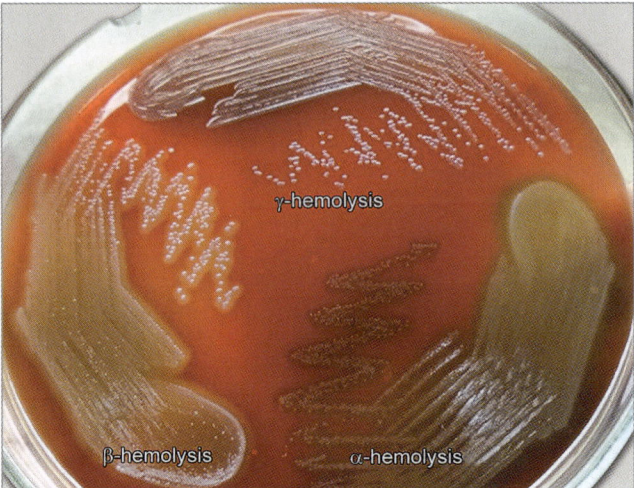

Fig. 3.2.16: Hemolysis on blood agar.
Source: Department of Microbiology, Pondicherry Institute of Medical Sciences, Puducherry (*with permission*).

Colony Morphology

After overnight incubation, the culture media are removed from the incubator and examined under bright illumination.
- The appearance of the bacterial colony on the culture medium helps in their preliminary identification.
- The colony characteristics that help in the preliminary identification are—
  - Size, shape, consistency (e.g. dry, moist or mucoid)
  - Color (e.g. pink or pale colony on MacConkey agar)
  - Pigment production: e.g. blue-green pigments by *Pseudomonas*, golden-yellow colonies by *S. aureus*
  - Hemolysis on blood agar (see below highlight box).

> **Hemolysis on Blood Agar**
> Certain bacteria produce hemolysin enzymes that lyse the red blood cells surrounding the colonies on blood agar, forming a zone of hemolysis **(Fig. 3.2.16)**. Hemolysis may be:
> - **Partial or α-hemolysis:** Partial clearing of blood around the colonies occurs with green discoloration of the surrounding medium; outline of the RBCs is intact (e.g. pneumococci, viridans streptococci)
> - **Complete or β-hemolysis:** Zone of complete clearing of blood around the colonies due to complete lysis of the RBCs (e.g. *Staphylococcus aureus* and *Streptococcus pyogenes*)
> - **No hemolysis (γ-hemolysis, a misnomer):** There is no color change surrounding the colony (e.g. *Enterococcus*)

Culture Smear and Motility Testing

The colonies grown on the culture media are subjected to Gram staining and motility testing by hanging drop method.

■ CULTURE IDENTIFICATION

Identification of bacteria from culture is made either by conventional biochemical tests or by automated identification systems.

Biochemical Identification

Based on the type of colony morphology and Gram staining appearance observed in culture smear, the appropriate biochemical tests are employed.
1. **Initially,** catalase and oxidase tests are done on all types of colonies grown on the media
2. **For gram-negative bacilli:** The following are the common biochemical tests done routinely, abbreviated as 'ICUT':
   - Indole test
   - Citrate utilization test
   - Urea hydrolysis test
   - Triple sugar iron test (TSI).
3. **For gram-positive cocci:** The useful biochemical tests are as follows:
   - Coagulase test (for *Staphylococcus aureus*)
   - CAMP (Christie-Atkins-Munch-Petersen) test for group B *Streptococcus*
   - Bile esculin hydrolysis test (for *Enterococcus*)
   - Heat tolerance test (for *Enterococcus*)
   - Inulin fermentation (for pneumococcus) and
   - Bile solubility test (for pneumococcus)
   - Antimicrobial susceptibility tests done for bacterial identification are as follows:
     - Optochin susceptibility test—done to differentiate pneumococcus (sensitive) from viridans streptococci (resistant)

- Bacitracin susceptibility test—done to differentiate group A (sensitive) from group B (resistant) *Streptococcus*.

Some of the important biochemical tests are described below. Coagulase test and other biochemical reactions for gram-positive cocci are described in the respective chapters.

Catalase Test

When a colony of any catalase producing bacteria is mixed with a drop of hydrogen peroxide (3% H_2O_2) placed on a slide, effervescence or bubbles appear due to breakdown of H_2O_2 by catalase to produce oxygen **(Fig. 3.2.17)**.
- Catalase test is primarily used to differentiate between *Staphylococcus* (catalase positive) from *Streptococcus* (catalase negative)
- It is also positive for members of the families Enterobacteriaceae, Vibrionaceae, Pseudomonadaceae, etc.

Oxidase Test

It detects the presence of cytochrome oxidase enzyme in bacteria, which catalyzes the oxidation of reduced cytochrome by atmospheric oxygen.
- When a filter paper strip or disk, soaked in oxidase reagent is smeared with a bacterial colony producing cytochrome oxidase enzyme, the smeared area turns deep purple within 10 seconds due to oxidation of the dye to form a purple colored compound indophenol blue
- Interpretation **(Fig. 3.2.18A)** and examples:
  - **Oxidase positive (deep purple):** Examples include *Pseudomonas*, *Vibrio*, *Neisseria*, *Bacillus*, *Haemophilus*, etc.
  - **Oxidase negative (no color change):** Examples include; members of family Enterobacteriaceae, *Acinetobacter*, etc.

Indole Test

It detects the ability of certain bacteria to produce an enzyme tryptophanase that breaks down amino acid tryptophan present in the medium into indole.
- When Kovac's reagent is added to an overnight incubated broth of a bacterial colony, it complexes with indole to produce a cherry red color ring near the surface of the medium
- ❖ **Indole positive (Fig. 3.2.18B):** A red colored ring is formed near the surface of the broth. Examples include *Escherichia coli, Proteus vulgaris, Vibrio cholerae*, etc.
- ❖ **Indole negative (Fig. 3.2.18B):** Yellow colored ring is formed near the surface of the broth, e.g. *Klebsiella pneumoniae, Proteus mirabilis, Pseudomonas, Salmonella*, etc.

Citrate Utilization Test

It detects the ability of a few bacteria to utilize citrate as the sole source of carbon for their growth, with production of alkaline metabolic products. Test is performed on Simmon's citrate medium. Citrate utilizing bacteria produce growth and a color change, i.e. original green color changes to blue **(Fig. 3.2.19A)**.
- ❖ Citrate test is positive for *Klebsiella pneumoniae, Citrobacter, Enterobacter*, etc.
- ❖ The test is negative for *Escherichia coli, Shigella*, etc.

Urea Hydrolysis Test

Urease producing bacteria can split urea present in the medium to produce ammonia that makes the medium alkaline.
- ❖ Test is done on Christensen's urea medium, which contains phenol red indicator that changes to pink color in alkaline medium **(Fig. 3.2.19B)**
- ❖ **Urease test is positive** for *Klebsiella pneumoniae, Proteus* species, *Helicobacter pylori, Brucella*, etc.
- ❖ **Urease test is negative** for *Escherichia coli, Shigella, Salmonella*, etc.

Triple Sugar Iron (TSI) Agar Test

TSI is a very important medium employed widely for identification of gram-negative bacteria. TSI medium contains three sugars—glucose, sucrose and lactose in

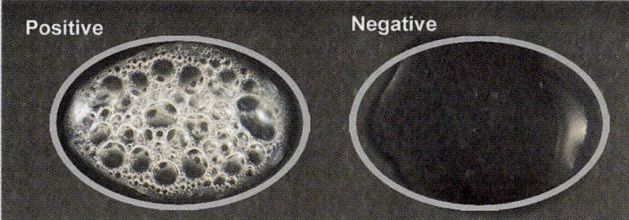

Fig. 3.2.17: Catalase test.
Source: Department of Microbiology, JIPMER, Puducherry (*with permission*).

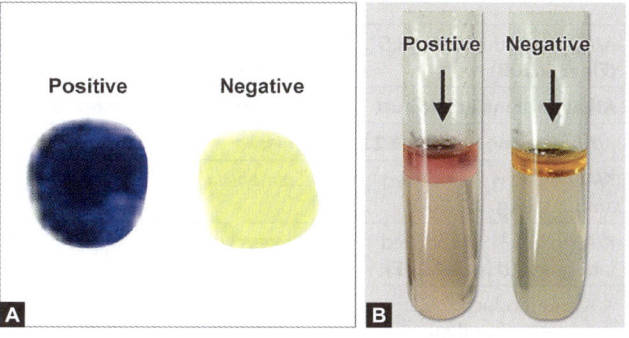

Figs 3.2.18A and B: A. Oxidase test; **B.** Indole test.
Source: Department of Microbiology, Pondicherry Institute of Medical Sciences, Puducherry (*with permission*).

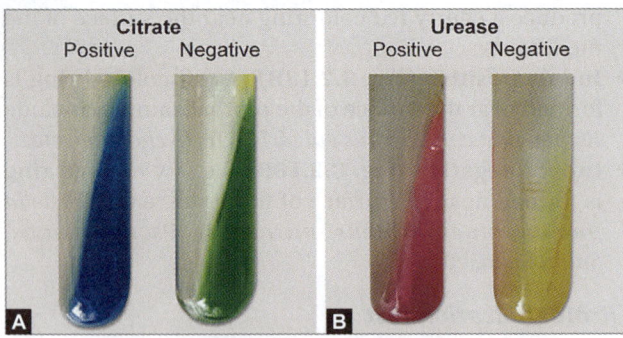

Figs. 3.2.19A and B: A. Citrate utilization test; **B.** Urea hydrolysis test.

Source: Department of Microbiology, Pondicherry Institute of Medical Sciences, Puducherry (*with permission*).

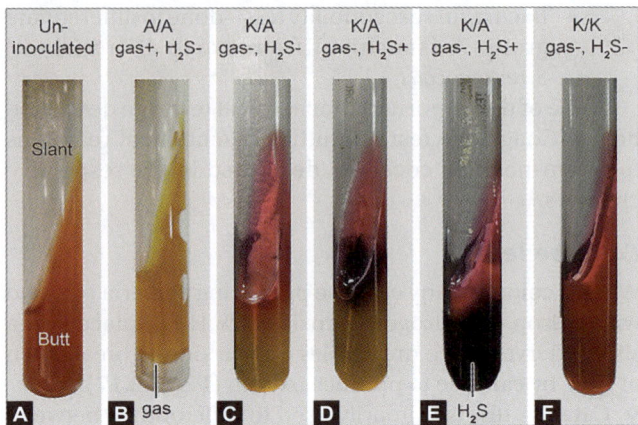

Figs 3.2.20A to F: Triple sugar iron test.

Source: Department of Microbiology, JIPMER, Puducherry (*with permission*).

the ratio of 1:10:10 parts. Uninoculated TSI medium is red in color; has a slant and a butt **(Fig. 3.2.20A)**. After inoculation, the medium is incubated at 37°C for 18–24 hours.

Interpretation

TSI detects three properties of bacteria, which includes fermentation of sugars to produce acid and/or gas and production of H_2S **(Figs. 3.2.20B to F and Table 3.2.5)**.

❖ **Acid production:** If acid is produced, the medium is turned yellow from red. Accordingly the organisms are categorized into three groups:
1. **Nonfermenters:** They do not ferment any sugars, hence the medium (both slant and butt) remain red, producing Alkaline slant/Alkaline butt (K/K) reaction **(Fig. 3.2.20F)**; e.g. *Pseudomonas* and *Acinetobacter*
2. **Glucose only fermenters:** They ferment only glucose and produce little acid only at the butt, whereas the slant remains alkaline giving rise to Alkaline slant/Acidic butt (K/A) reaction **(Fig. 3.2.20C)**; e.g. *Salmonella* and *Shigella*
3. **≥2 sugars fermenters:** They ferment glucose and also ferment lactose and/or sucrose to produce large amount of acid so that the medium (both slant and butt) change to yellow giving rise to Acidic slant/Acidic butt (A/A) reaction **(Fig. 3.2.20B)**; e.g., *E. coli* and *Klebsiella*.

❖ **Gas production:** If gas is produced, the medium is lifted up or broken with cracks **(Fig. 3.2.20B)**; e.g., *E. coli* and *Klebsiella*

❖ **H_2S production:** If H_2S is produced, the medium changes color to black **(Figs. 3.2.20D and E)**; e.g., *Salmonella* Typhi and *Proteus vulgaris*.

Automated Systems for Bacterial Identification

Automated identification systems are revolutionary in diagnostic microbiology.
❖ They have several advantages—(i) produce faster results, (ii) can identify a wide range of organisms with accuracy, which are otherwise difficult to identify (e.g. anaerobes) through conventional biochemical tests
❖ Examples of automated systems used for bacterial identification are—
- **MALDI–TOF:** Matrix-assisted laser desorption ionization time-of-flight
- **VITEK 2 system** and **Phoenix** automated identification and AST system.

> **MALDI-TOF MS**
> MALDI-TOF MS technology (Matrix Assisted Laser Desorption Ionization Time-of-Flight Mass Spectrometry) has revolutionized the identification of organisms in clinical microbiology laboratories

Table 3.2.5: Various reactions in TSI with examples.	
Reactions in TSI	**Examples**
Acidic slant/acidic butt	**≥2 sugars fermented** (1) glucose, (2) lactose or/and sucrose
A/A, gas produced, no H_2S **(Fig. 3.2.20B)**	*Escherichia coli* *Klebsiella pneumoniae*
Alkaline slant/acidic butt	**Only glucose-fermenter group**
K/A, no gas, no H_2S **(Fig. 3.2.20C)**	*Shigella*
K/A, no gas, H_2S produced (small amount) **(Fig. 3.2.20D)**	*Salmonella* Typhi
K/A, no gas, H_2S produced (abundant) **(Fig. 3.2.20E)**	*Proteus vulgaris*
K/A, gas produced, H_2S produced (abundant)	*Salmonella* Paratyphi B
K/A, gas produced, no H_2S	*Salmonella* Paratyphi A
Alkaline slant/alkaline butt	**Non-fermenters group**
K/K, no gas, no H_2S **(Fig. 3.2.20F)**	*Pseudomonas, Acinetobacter*

Contd...

Contd...

> - **Principle:** It identifies the organism based on the pattern of ribosomal proteins present.
>   - The colony is mixed with a **matrix** solution on a slide, then the slide is loaded into the system and subjected to laser beam.
>   - The **laser** causes **desorption** and **ionization** of bacterial ribosomal proteins, generating singly protonated ions
>   - The ions then travel in a flight tube, with a speed according to their mass to charge (m/z) ratio.
>   - Based on the **time-of-flight** of the ions, a characteristic spectrum is generated which is unique to a species as it represents the conserved ribosomal proteins.
> - **Applications:** (i) It can accurately identify bacteria, fungi, and mycobacteria etc; (ii) turnaround time of few minutes, and (iii) it can also be used to identify organism directly from positively flagged blood culture bottles.

VITEK 2 Automated System

VITEK 2 is the most widely used automated system in India for identification and AST of bacteria and yeast. Principle of VITEK for identification is discussed below, VITEK for AST is discussed later in this chapter.
- The identification card contains several wells, each well contains a test substrate that measures specific metabolic activity, which is then detected by colorimetry.
- The identification of the organism is made based on the reactions produced by all the wells.
- Separate ID cards are available for gram-negative, gram-positive bacteria, fastidious bacteria and yeasts **(Fig. 3.2.21)**.
- The result of identification is usually available within 4–6 hours.

■ ANTIMICROBIAL SUSCEPTIBILITY TEST

Antimicrobial susceptibility test (AST) is the most important investigation carried out by a Microbiology laboratory.

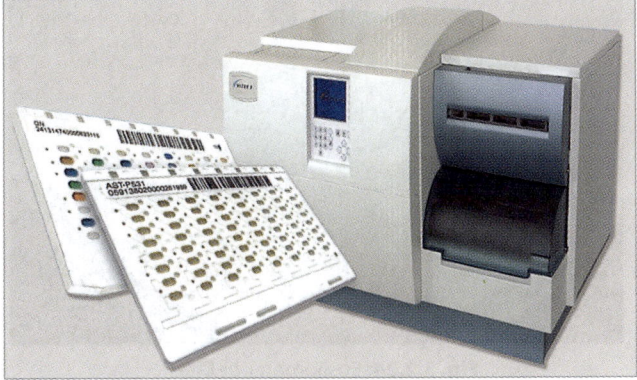

Fig. 3.2.21: VITEK 2 system with its panels (reagent cards) for identification and antimicrobial susceptibility test.
Source: Department of Microbiology, JIPMER, Puducherry (*with permission*).

- Bacteria exhibit great strain variations in susceptibility to antimicrobial agents. Therefore, AST plays a vital role to guide the clinician for tailoring the empirical antibiotic therapy to pathogen-directed therapy
- AST is performed only for pathogenic bacteria isolated from the specimen, and not for the commensal bacteria. For example, *E. coli* isolated from urine specimen should be subjected to AST, whereas *E. coli* isolated from stool is a commensal; hence, AST is not performed.

Classification of AST Methods

AST methods are classified into phenotypic and genotypic methods.
- The phenotypic methods are further grouped into—
  - Disk Diffusion Method, e.g. Kirby–Bauer's disk diffusion (DD) test
  - Dilution tests: Broth dilution and agar dilution methods
  - Epsilometer or E-test
  - Automated AST, e.g. Vitek, Phoenix and Microscan systems.
- Genotypic methods such as PCR detecting drug-resistant genes (e.g. *mecA* gene for *S. aureus*).

Disk Diffusion Method

Kirby–Bauer's disk diffusion (DD) test is the most widely used AST method. They are suitable for rapidly growing pathogenic bacteria.
- **Procedure:** Mueller–Hinton agar (MHA) is the medium used for DD test.
  - Bacterial colony suspension (of 0.5 McFarland turbidity) is prepared in saline and then inoculated onto MHA by spreading (lawn culture) with sterile swabs.
  - Antimicrobial disks are then placed on the surface of MHA plate. Then the plates are incubated at 37°C for 16–18 hours and then interpreted.
- **Interpretation:** Susceptibility to the drug is determined by the zone of inhibition of bacterial growth around the disk, measured by using a Vernier caliper **(Fig. 3.2.23)**. The interpretation of zone size into sensitive, intermediate or resistant is based on the standard zone size interpretation chart, provided by standard guidelines, e.g. Clinical and Laboratory Standards Institute (CLSI) **(Fig. 3.2.22 and Table 3.2.6)**.

Direct Disk Diffusion Test

The direct DD (or direct susceptibility test, i.e. DST) is indicated when results are required urgently and for the specimens that are expected to contain single pathogen (for positively-flagged blood culture bottle, sterile body fluids or urine).

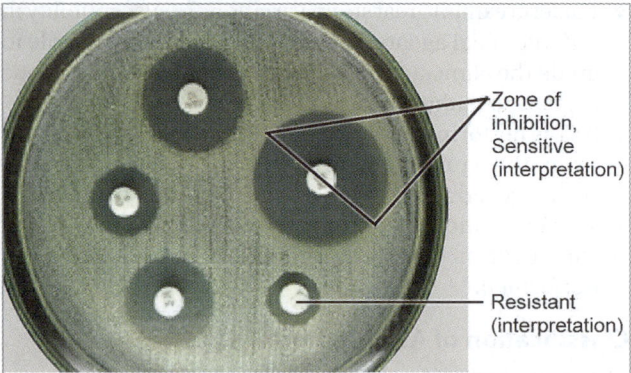

Fig. 3.2.22: Kirby–Bauer disk diffusion method.
Source: Department of Microbiology, Pondicherry Institute of Medical sciences, Puducherry (*with permission*).

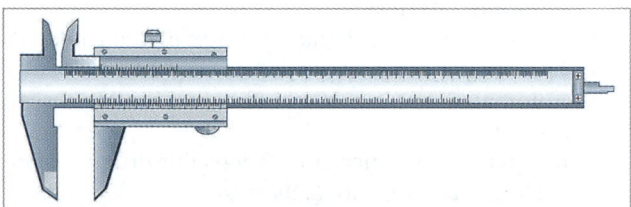

Fig. 3.2.23: Vernier caliper.

Table 3.2.6: Commonly used disk concentrations and interpretation of disk diffusion test (as per CLSI 2024 guideline).

Breakpoints for Enterobacterales				
Antimicrobial agents	Disk strength (µg)	Zone diameter break points (mm)		
		S	I	R
Ceftriaxone	30	≥23	20–22	≤19
Ciprofloxacin	5	≥26	22–25	≤21
Piperacillin-tazobactam*	100/10	≥25	21–24	≤20
Amikacin	30	≥17	15–16	≤14
Meropenem	10	≥23	20–22	≤19

(CLSI, Clinical and Laboratory Standards Institute; S, Sensitive; I, Intermediate; R, Resistant)

*For piperacillin-tazobactam, susceptible dose dependent breakpoint is applicable instead of intermediate breakpoint.

- Here, the specimen is directly inoculated uniformly on to the surface of an agar plate and the antibiotic disks are applied
- The results of the direct-DD test should always be verified by performing AST from the colony subsequently
- This test is of no use when mixed growth is suspected in the specimen, e.g. pus, stool, sputum, etc.

Dilution Tests

Here, the inoculum of the test organism is added to serial dilutions of antimicrobial agent in presence of a suitable medium. After overnight incubation, it is examined to determine the MIC.

- **MIC (minimum inhibitory concentration):** It is the lowest concentration of the drug that will inhibit the visible growth of an organism
- **Types:** Based on the platform where the test is performed, there are various types of dilution methods.
  - *Broth dilution:* It uses Mueller-Hinton broth. It can be performed using tube (broth macrodilution) or microtiter plate (broth microdilution)
  - *Agar dilution:* It is performed on Mueller-Hinton agar.

Epsilometer or E-test

E-test is an absorbent strip that contains predefined gradient of antibiotic concentrations along its length.
- It is a MIC-based method, that uses the principles of both dilution and diffusion of the drug into the medium
- E-strip is applied to a lawn inoculum of a bacterium. Following incubation of the test organism, an elliptical zone of inhibition is produced surrounding the strip
- The antibiotic concentration at which the ellipse edge intersects the strip, is taken as MIC value **(Fig. 3.2.24)**.

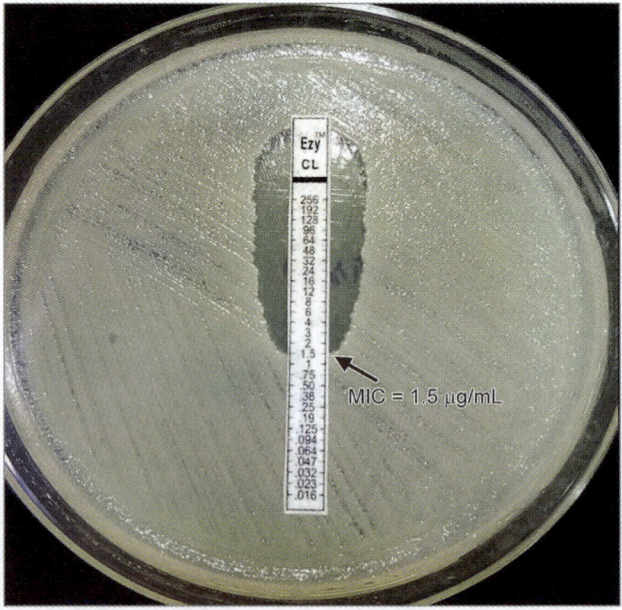

Fig. 3.2.24: Epsilometer or E-test.
Source: Department of Microbiology, Pondicherry Institute of Medical Sciences, Puducherry (*with permission*).

Automated Antimicrobial Susceptibility Tests

Most systems are computer assisted and have sophisticated softwares to analyze the growth rates and determine the antibiotic susceptibility report. Several automated systems are available now, such as:
- **VITEK 2** identification and antimicrobial sensitivity system (bioMérieux, **Fig. 3.2.21**)
- **Phoenix System** (Becton Dickinson)
- **MicroScan Walk Away** system.

VITEK 2 Automated System for AST

VITEK 2 is the most widely used automated AST system in India; can perform AST of bacteria and yeasts; whereas other automated AST systems can perform AST of bacteria only, not for yeasts.
- **Principle:** It works on the principle of on microbroth dilution
- **AST card:** The wells present in the VITEK AST card contain doubling dilution of antimicrobial agents. The organism suspension (of 0.5 McFarland turbidity) is added to these wells **(Fig. 3.2.21)**
- **Growth detection:** The cards are incubated in the system at 35.5 ±1°C. The reading is taken once in every 15 minutes by the optical system of the equipment. Presence of any turbidity in a well indicates the organism has grown in that antibiotic well
- **MIC:** The MIC is determined as the highest dilution of the antimicrobial agent which inhibits the growth of organism and there is no turbidity in the well
- **Time:** The results are available within 8–10 hours for gram-negative bacilli and 16–18 hours for gram-positive cocci.

Role of MIC-based Methods

The clinical microbiology laboratory should perform a MIC-based method whenever possible. This is because the MIC-based methods are much superior to disk diffusion test for a number of reasons.
- **For confirming the AST results** obtained by disk diffusion tests, as they are more reliable and accurate than the latter
- AST of bacteria for which disk diffusion test is not standardized should only be performed by MIC testing (e.g. Vancomycin for *S. aureus*).

Interpretation of AST

The result of AST (whether disk diffusion or MIC based methods) is always expressed in four interpretative categories.
- **Susceptible (S):** Indicates that the antibiotic is clinically effective when used in standard therapeutic dose
- **Intermediate (I):** Indicates that the antibiotic is not clinically effective when used in standard dose; but may be active when used in increased dose. Antibiotics reported as 'I' should be avoided for treatment if alternative agents are available
- **Susceptible dose dependent (SDD):** Indicates that the antibiotic will be clinically active only if given in increased dose. This category is available only for few agents such as cefepime for Enterobacteriaceae
- **Resistant (R):** Indicates that the antibiotic is NOT clinically effective when used in either standard dose or increased dose; and therefore should not be included in the treatment regimen.

Choice of Antibiotics to be included in Panel

It is neither possible nor desirable to test the susceptibility against all the drugs. The panel of the drugs to be tested against an isolate depends upon various factors:
- **Clinically indicated:** Include only those antibiotics for testing which are clinically indicated for the suspected infective syndrome
- **Organism isolated**, for which the AST is going to be performed, and its **local resistance pattern** (as per hospital antibiogram)
- **Intrinsic resistance:** The antibiotics to which the isolate is intrinsically resistant must be excluded from testing
- **Locally available** antibiotic at the hospital
- **Site of action:** Only those antibiotics should be tested which are active in the site. For example, antibiotics such as clindamycin, macrolide and chloramphenicol are excluded from testing for urine isolates.

■ SEROLOGY

The serological tests play an important role in the diagnosis of various bacterial infections. These include detection of either antigen or antibody in the serum of the patient, by various immunological assays—precipitation, agglutination, ELISA, and rapid test. The detail of these methods is discussed in **Chapter 8**. The important serological tests used for diagnosis of bacterial infections include:
- Widal test for enteric fever
- Standard agglutination test for brucellosis
- Microscopic agglutination test and rapid diagnostic test for leptospirosis
- Weil-Felix test for rickettsial infections
- VDRL (venereal disease research laboratory) test and RPR (rapid plasma reagin) test for syphilis
- ELISA is available for various bacterial diseases such as chlamydial infections, brucellosis, *Mycoplasma* pneumonia, leptospirosis and rickettsial infections, etc.

■ MOLECULAR METHODS

Molecular methods are broadly grouped into amplification based and non-amplification based methods.

Nucleic acid amplification techniques (NAATs) have been increasingly used in diagnostic microbiology. Various NAATs used are:
- ❖ Polymerase chain reaction (PCR)
- ❖ Real-time polymerase chain reaction (rt-PCR)
- ❖ Loop mediated isothermal amplification (LAMP)
- ❖ Automated PCR such as Biofire FilmArray
- ❖ Automated real-time PCR such as cartridge based nucleic acid amplification test (CBNAAT): Used for tuberculosis, described in **Chapter 27**.

Non-amplification molecular methods include DNA hybridization method, e.g. line probe assay.

Polymerase Chain Reaction (PCR)

PCR is a technology in molecular biology used to amplify a single or few copies of a piece of DNA to generate millions of copies of DNA. It was developed by Kary B Mullis (1983) for which he and Michael Smith were awarded the Nobel Prize in Chemistry in 1993.

> **Principle of PCR**
> PCR involves three basic steps.
> 1. **DNA extraction from the organism:** This involves lysis of the organisms and release of the DNA which may be done by various methods—boiling, adding enzymes (e.g. lysozyme, proteinase K), etc. DNA extraction kits are also available commercially
> 2. **Amplification of extracted DNA:** This is carried out in a special PCR machine called thermocycler **(Fig. 3.2.25A)**. The extracted DNA is subjected to repeated cycles (30–35 numbers) of amplification which takes about 3–4 hours. Each amplification cycle has three steps **(Fig. 3.2.26)**.
>
> Contd...

> Contd...
> - ➢ **Denaturation at 95°C:** This involves separation of the dsDNA into two separate single strands
> - ➢ **Primer annealing (55°C):** Primer is a short oligonucleotide complementary to a small sequence of the target DNA. It anneals to the complementary site on the target ssDNA
> - ➢ **Extension of the primer (72°C):** This step is catalyzed by Taq Polymerase enzyme which keeps on adding the free nucleotides to the growing end of the primer. Taq Polymerase is a special type of DNA polymerase (isolated from the plant bacterium *Thermus aquaticus*), capable of withstanding the high temperature of PCR reaction.
> 3. **Gel electrophoresis of amplified product:** The amplified DNA is electrophoretically migrated according to their molecular size by performing agarose gel electrophoresis **(Fig. 3.2.25B)**. The amplified DNA forms clear band, which can be visualized under ultraviolet (UV) light **(Fig. 3.2.25C)**.

Applications of PCR

PCR is now a common and often indispensable technique used in medical diagnostics and research laboratories for a variety of applications. It has the following advantages compared to the conventional culture methods:
- ❖ **More sensitive:** It can amplify very few copies of a specific DNA, so it is more sensitive
- ❖ **More specific:** Use of primers targeting specific DNA sequence of the organism makes the PCR assays highly specific
- ❖ PCR can be done to amplify the DNA of the organism: (1) either directly from the sample, or (2) to confirm the organism grown in culture
- ❖ PCR can also detect the organisms that are highly fastidious or noncultivable by conventional culture methods

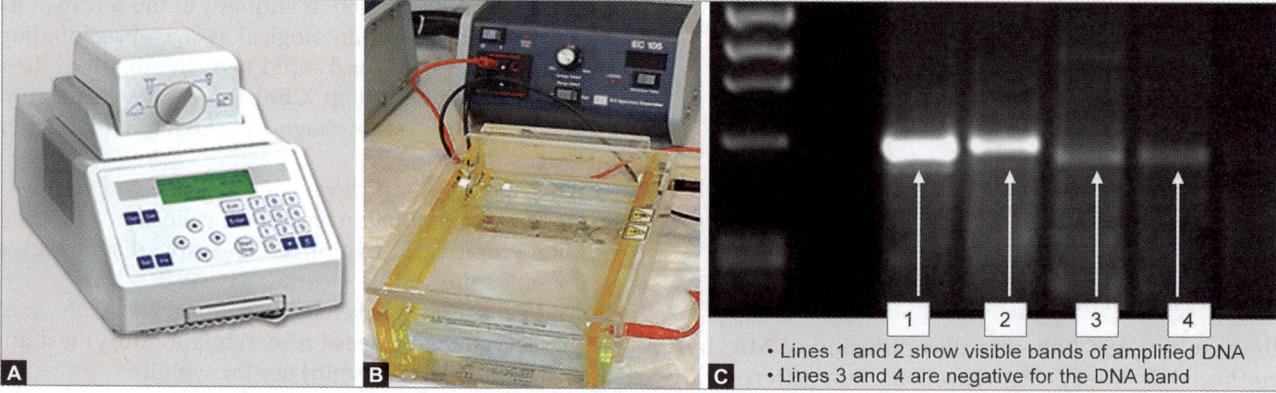

Figs. 3.2.25A to C: **A.** Thermocycler machine (Eppendorf); **B.** Gel electrophoresis of amplified product; **C.** Visualization of amplified DNA under UV light.

Source: Department of Microbiology, JIPMER, Puducherry (with permission).

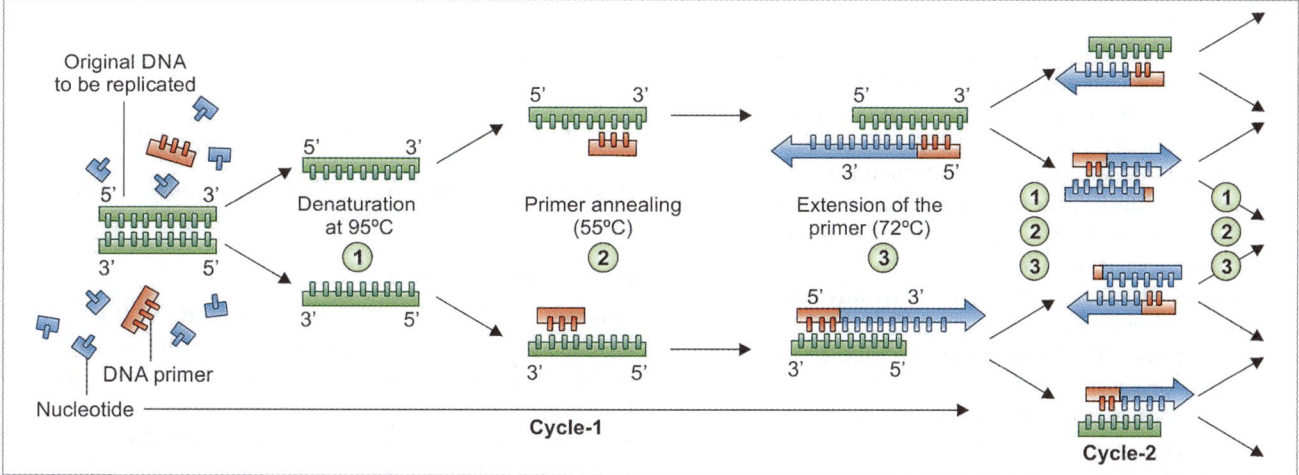

Fig. 3.2.26: Polymerase chain reaction cycle—3 basic steps of amplification.

- PCR can be used to detect the genes in the organism responsible for drug resistance (e.g. *mec* A gene detection in *Staphylococcus aureus*)
- Detects genetic diseases, such as sickle cell anemia, phenylketonuria, and muscular dystrophy.

Disadvantages of PCR

Conventional PCR detects only the DNA, but not the RNA (latter can be detected by reverse transcriptase PCR).

- **Qualitative, not quantitative:** Conventional PCR can only detect the presence or absence of DNA. It cannot quantitate the amount of DNA of the organism present in the sample. This is possible by real time PCR
- **Viability:** PCR cannot differentiate between viable or nonviable organisms. It only detects the presence of DNA in the sample which may be extracted from viable or nonviable organism
- **False-positive amplification:** It may occur due to contamination with environmental DNA. Hence, strict asepsis should be maintained in the PCR laboratory
- **False-negative:** The PCR inhibitors present in some specimens, such as blood, feces, etc. may inhibit the amplification of target DNA.

Modifications of PCR

1. **Reverse transcriptase PCR (RT-PCR):** Conventional PCR amplifies only the DNA. For amplifying RNA, RT-PCR is done
   - After RNA extraction, the first step is addition of reverse transcriptase enzyme that coverts RNA into DNA. Then, the amplification of DNA and gel documentation steps are similar to that described for conventional PCR
   - It is extremely useful for detection of RNA viruses or 16S rRNA genes of the organisms.
2. **Nested PCR:** It is modification of PCR, where two rounds of PCR amplification are carried out by using two primers that are targeted against two different DNA sequences of same organism
   - The amplified products of the first round PCR is subjected to another round of amplification using a second primer which targets the same organism but a different DNA sequence
   - More sensitive: Double round of amplification yields high quantity of DNA
   - More specific: Use of two primers targeting two regions of DNA of the same organisms makes the test more specific
   - Application: Nested PCR is used for detection of *Mycobacterium tuberculosis* (targeting IS6110 gene) in samples

   Disadvantage: There is more chance of contamination of the PCR tubes, which may lead to false-positive results.
3. **Multiplex PCR:** It uses more than one primer which can detect many DNA sequences of several organisms in one reaction
   - Syndromic approach: Multiplex PCR is useful for the diagnosis of the infectious diseases that are caused by more than one organism
   - For example, for the etiological diagnosis of pyogenic meningitis, different primers targeting the common agents of pyogenic meningitis, such as pneumococcus, meningococcus and *H. influenzae* can be added simultaneously in the same reaction tube
   - Contamination issues: There is a risk of the reaction tubes being contaminated with environmental DNA.

Real-time PCR (rt-PCR)

It is based on PCR technology, which is used to amplify and simultaneously detect or quantify a targeted DNA molecule on a real-time basis. Reverse transcriptase real-time PCR formats can detect and quantify RNA molecules of the test organism in the sample on a real-time basis.

It uses a different thermocycler than the conventional PCR. It is very expensive, 5-10 times more than the cost of conventional PCR **(Fig. 3.2.27)**.

Advantages: Real-time PCR has many advantages over a conventional PCR, such as:

- ❖ **Quantitative:** Real-time PCR can quantitate the DNA or RNA present in the specimen; hence can be used for monitoring the disease progression in response to treatment, e.g. viral load monitoring in HIV or hepatitis B viral infection
- ❖ **Takes less time:** In rt-PCR, the amplification can be visualized simultaneously during the process of amplification unlike the conventional PCR where there is an extra-step of gel electrophoresis to detect the amplicons
- ❖ **Contamination rate** is extremely less
- ❖ **Sensitivity and specificity** of rt-PCR assays are much more than the conventional PCR.

Detection of amplification products of real-time PCR is carried out by using a variety of fluorogenic molecules which may be either nonspecific or specific.

- ❖ **Nonspecific methods:** They use SYBR green dye that stains any nucleic acid nonspecifically
- ❖ **Specific methods:** They use fluorescent labeled oligonucleotide probe which binds (i.e. hybridizes) only to a particular region of amplified nucleic acid. Three types of hybridization probes are commonly used:
  - TaqMan or hydrolysis probe
  - Molecular beacon
  - Fluorescence resonance energy transfer (FRET) probe.

Post-amplification melting curve analysis is used for quantitation of the nucleic acid load.

Nucleic Acid Probes

Nucleic acid probes are radiolabeled or fluorescent labelled pieces of single stranded DNA or RNA, which can be used for the detection of homologous nucleic acid by hybridization.

- ❖ Hybridization is the technique in which two single strands of nucleic acid come together to form a stable double stranded molecule
- ❖ There are two types of nucleic acid probes—DNA probes (hybridizes with DNA) and RNA probes (hybridizes with RNA)
- ❖ Nucleic acid probes are used to detect the specific nucleic acid from:
  1. Clinical samples directly *or*
  2. Following amplification of small quantity nucleic acid present in the clinical sample (e.g. in real time PCR) *or*
  3. From culture isolates.
- ❖ **Line probe assay** is a classic example of molecular test that uses nucleic acid probe technology. It is used for diagnosis of tuberculosis.

■ MICROBIAL TYPING

Microbial typing refers to characterization of an organism beyond its species level.

Applications: Microbial typing is an important tool for hospital microbiologists and epidemiologists. It helps to: (i) Investigate outbreaks, (ii) Determine the source and routes of infections, (iii) Differentiate between recurrence and infection with new strain and (iv) Evaluate the effectiveness of control measures.

Classification: Typing methods are broadly classified as phenotypic and genotypic methods.

- ❖ **Phenotypic Methods**
  - *Biotyping:* It is based on biochemical properties of organisms. It is used for Vibrio cholerae O1, which is classified into two biotypes—(1) Classical, and (2) El Tor.
  - *Antibiogram typing:* It classifies organisms based on their resistance pattern to different antimicrobials.
  - *Serotyping:* It is a typing method based on antigenic property of the organism. Examples include—

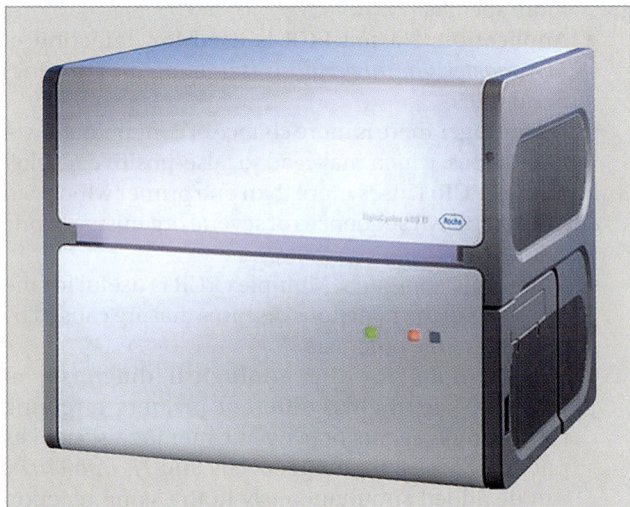

Fig. 3.2.27: Real-time PCR.
Source: Department of Microbiology, JIPMER, Puducherry (*with permission*).

CHAPTER 3.2 ❖ General Bacteriology: Laboratory Diagnosis of Bacterial Infections

(1) *Streptococcus* (Lancefield grouping, based on carbohydrate antigen) and (ii) serotyping of *Shigella*, *Salmonella* and *Vibrio cholerae* based on somatic antigen.

❖ **Genotypic Methods** include—(i) Restricted Fragment Length Polymorphism (RFLP), (ii) Pulse Field Gel Electrophoresis (PFGE) and (iii) Sequencing-based methods such as nucleotide sequencing and whole genome sequencing.

EXPECTED QUESTIONS

I. **Write short notes on:**
   1. Gram staining.
   2. Selective media.
   3. Anaerobic culture methods.
   4. Automations in Microbiology.
   5. Polymerase chain reaction.
   6. Real-time PCR.

II. **Multiple Choice Questions (MCQs):**
   1. **Recommended transport medium for stool specimen suspected to contain *Vibrio cholerae* is:**
      a. Buffered glycerol saline medium
      b. Venkatraman-Ramakrishnan medium
      c. Nutrient broth
      d. Blood agar
   2. **Which is an enriched medium?**
      a. Selenite F broth   b. Peptone water
      c. MacConkey agar   d. Chocolate agar
   3. **Agar concentration required to prepare nutrient agar is:**
      a. 2%   b. 6%
      c. 0.25%   d. 0.5%
   4. **Robertson cooked meat broth is an example of:**
      a. Enriched media   b. Enrichment media
      c. Anaerobic media   d. Nutrient media
   5. **Blood culture bottle contains:**
      a. BHI broth   b. Peptone water broth
      c. Selenite F broth   d. Alkaline peptone water
   6. **The three components of PCR involves all, *except*:**
      a. DNA extraction   b. Amplification
      c. Gel documentation d. Blotting

Answers
1. b   2. d   3. a   4. c   5. a   6. d

General Bacteriology: Bacterial Genetics

CHAPTER 3.3

CHAPTER PREVIEW
- Principles of Bacterial Genetics
- Mutation
- Horizontal Gene Transfer
  - Transformation
- Transduction
- Lysogenic Conversion
- Conjugation
- Transposition
- Gene Transfer by Artificial Methods (Genetic Engineering)

PRINCIPLES OF BACTERIAL GENETICS

Bacterial DNA is present in the chromosome as well as in extrachromosomal genetic material as a plasmid.
- **Chromosome:** Bacteria possess a single haploid chromosome, comprising of coiled circular double-stranded DNA. Bacteria do not have a true nucleus; but the genetic material is located in an irregularly-shaped region called the nucleoid
- **Plasmids:** They are the extrachromosomal double-stranded circular DNA molecules that exist in a free state in the cytoplasm of bacteria and also found in some yeasts
  - Plasmids are not essential for life
  - They are capable of replicating independently
  - Sometimes, they may integrate with chromosomal DNA of bacteria and such plasmids are called as episomes
  - **Functions of plasmids** include—(i) *Fertility or F-plasmids* code for the expression of sex pili that help in bacterial conjugation, (ii) *Resistance (R) plasmids* contain genes that code for resistance to various antibiotics and (iii) *Virulence plasmids* code for certain virulence factors and toxins that help in bacterial pathogenesis.

GENE TRANSFER IN BACTERIA

Bacteria undergo genetic variation and acquire new gene through a mechanism called mutation. Following which, the newly acquired genes are transferred either vertically to their offsprings during cell division or horizontally to other bacteria in the surrounding.

MUTATION

A mutation is a random, undirected heritable variation caused by a change in the nucleotide sequence of the genome of the cell.

- The frequency of mutation ranges from 10^{-2} to 10^{-10} per bacterium per division
- Mutations can be spontaneous or induced by physical [e.g. ultraviolet (UV) radiations] or chemical agents (e.g. alkylating agents, and 5-bromouracil)
- Mutation is best appreciated when it involves a function, which can be readily observed by experimental methods. For example, *E. coli* mutant that loses its ability to ferment lactose can be readily detected on MacConkey agar (produce non-lactose fermenting colonies).

HORIZONTAL GENE TRANSFER

Horizontal gene transfer occurs in bacteria by several methods, such as:
- Transformation (uptake of naked DNA)
- Transduction (through bacteriophage)
- Lysogenic conversion
- Conjugation (plasmid mediated via conjugation tube).

TRANSFORMATION

When bacteria die, the cell wall gets lysed and the DNA fragmented are released to the surrounding environment
- Transformation is a natural process of random uptake of free DNA fragment from the surrounding medium by a bacterial cells and incorporation of this DNA fragment into its chromosome in a heritable form
- Natural transformation has been studied in certain bacteria such as *Streptococcus, Bacillus, Haemophilus, Neisseria, Pseudomonas*, etc.
- **Griffith experiment:** It was an experiment performed by Griffith (1928) on mice using pneumococci and provided direct evidence of transformation.
  - Griffith found that mice died when they were injected with a mixture of live noncapsulated pneumococci

and heat killed capsulated pneumococci strains. However, neither of which separately proved fatal to mice **(Fig. 3.3.1)**
- He stated that the live noncapsulated strains were transformed into the capsulated strains due to transfer of the capsular genes released from the lysis of the killed capsulated strains.

TRANSDUCTION

Transduction is defined as the transfer of a portion of DNA from one bacterium to another by a bacteriophage.

Mechanism of Transduction

Bacteriophage (or phage) is a virus that infects and multiplies inside the bacterium.
- During the transmission of phage from one bacterium to other, a part of the host DNA may accidentally get incorporated into the phage and then gets transferred to the recipient bacterium.
- This leads to acquisition of new characters by the recipient bacterium coded by the donor DNA.

Life Cycles of Phage

After entering into a new bacterium, the phage can perform two types of life cycle.
- **Lytic or virulent cycle:** The phage multiplies in host cytoplasm, produces a large number of progeny phages, which subsequently are released causing lysis and death of the host cell
- **Lysogenic or temperate cycle:** Here, the phage DNA remains integrated with the bacterial chromosome as the prophage, and multiplies synchronously with bacterial DNA. The phage DNA when transferring to a new bacterium gets disintegrated from the parent bacterial chromosome and in the process, may take up a few bacterial genes.

Types of Transduction

Transduction is of two types, either generalized or restricted.
- **Generalized transduction** involves transfer of any part of the donor bacterial genome into the recipient bacteria. It usually occurs due to defective assembly during lytic cycle of virulent phages.
  - Packaging errors may happen occasionally due to defective assembly of the daughter phages. Instead of their own DNA, a part of host DNA may accidentally be incorporated into the daughter bacteriophages
  - The resulting bacteriophage often injects the donor DNA into another bacterial cell but does not initiate a lytic cycle as the original phage DNA is lost **(Fig. 3.3.2)**.
- **Restricted or specialized transduction:** It is capable of transducing only a particular genetic segment of the bacterial chromosome that is present adjacent to the phage DNA. It occurs as a result of defect in the disintegration of the lysogenic phage DNA from the bacterial chromosome.
  - When a lysogenic bacteriophage is integrated with the bacterial chromosome, leaves the host chromosome, portions of the bacterial chromosome present adjacent to the phage DNA may get wrongly excised along with it
  - Such transducing phages carrying a part of bacterial DNA in addition to their DNA, when infect another bacterium, the transfer of the donor DNA takes place.

Role of Transduction

- Transduction may be a mechanism for the transfer of bacterial genes coding for drug resistance; for example, plasmid coded penicillin resistance in staphylococci.
- It has also been proposed as a method of genetic engineering in the treatment of some inborn metabolic defects.

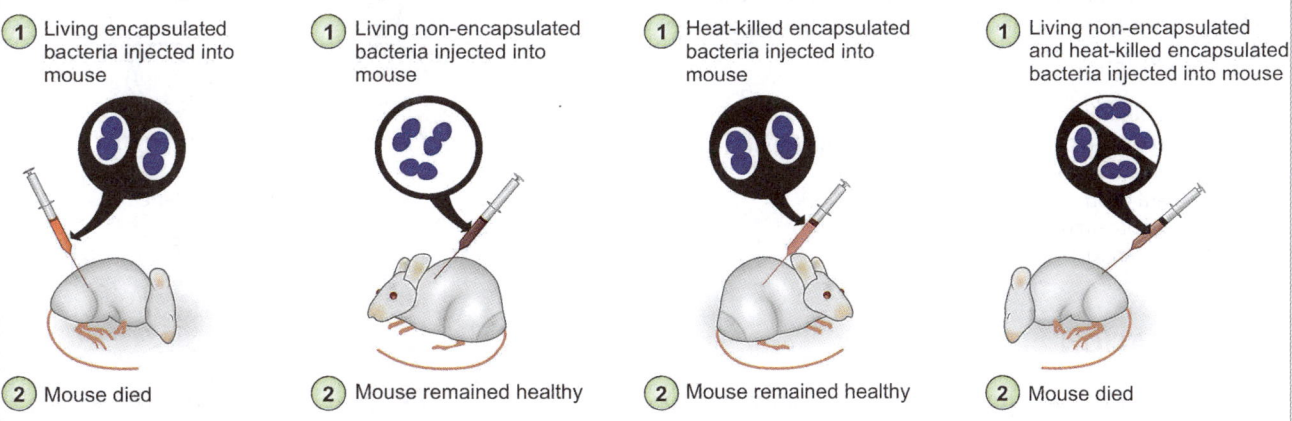

Fig. 3.3.1: Griffith experiment demonstrating transformation.

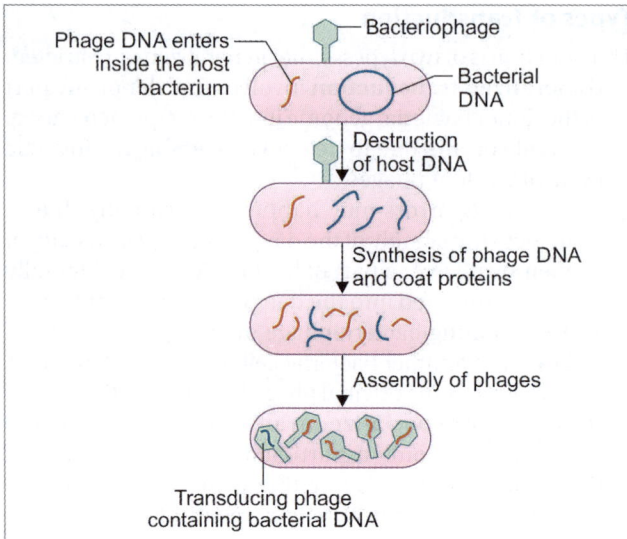

Fig. 3.3.2: Generalized transduction.

■ LYSOGENIC CONVERSION

Here, the phage DNA which is integrated into the host bacterial chromosome (during the lysogenic cycle), itself codes for several virulence factors such as toxins. When such bacteriophage infects a new host, the virulence genes also get transferred.

❖ The prophage acts as an additional chromosomal element which encodes for new characters and is transferred to the daughter cells. This process is known as lysogeny or lysogenic conversion

❖ **Imparts toxigenicity to the bacteria:** Phage DNA may be responsible for bacterial virulence by coding for their toxin production. For example, in *Corynebacterium diphtheriae*, the diphtheria toxin is coded by a lysogenic phage DNA which is integrated with the bacterial chromosome. Elimination of the phage from a toxigenic strain renders the bacterium nontoxigenic.

> **Phage Coded Toxins**
> Bacterial toxins that are coded by lysogenic phages include:
> ❑ Diphtheria toxin
> ❑ Cholera toxin
> ❑ Verocytotoxin of *E. coli*
> ❑ Botulinum toxin C and D

■ CONJUGATION

Conjugation refers to the transfer of genetic material from one bacterium (donor or male) to another bacterium (recipient or female) by mating or contact with each other and forming the conjugation tube.

F^+ X F^- Mating

The F^+ cell (also called as the donor or the male bacterium) contains a plasmid called F factor or fertility factor. The bacteria lacking the F factor are called as recipient or female bacteria or F^- cells.

❖ F factor is a conjugative plasmid; carries genes that encode for the formation of sex pilus (that helps in conjugation) and self plasmid transfer
❖ The F pilus brings the donor and nearby recipient cells close to each other and form a conjugation tube that bridges between the donor and recipient cells **(Fig. 3.3.3)**
❖ During conjugation, the plasmid DNA replicates by the rolling-circle mechanism, and a copy moves to the recipient bacterium through the conjugation tube. Then, in the recipient, the entered strand is copied to produce complete F factor with ds DNA

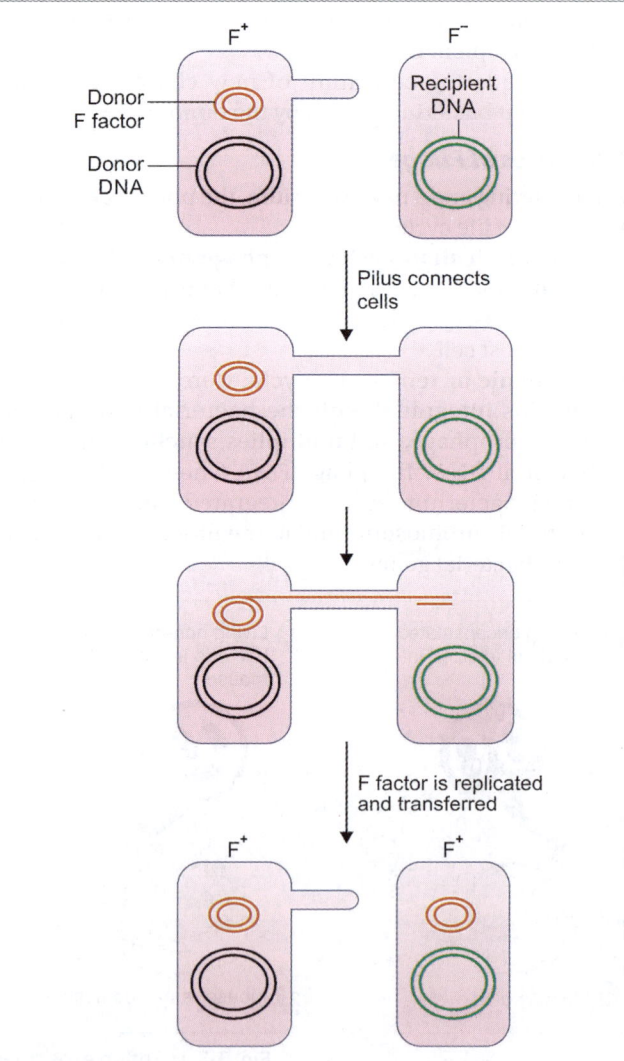

Fig. 3.3.3: Bacterial conjugation (F^+ X F^- mating).

- As a result, the recipient (F⁻) becomes (F⁺) cell and can in turn conjugate with other (F⁻) cells.

HFR Conjugation

F factor being a plasmid, it may integrate with bacterial chromosome and behave as episome.
- Such donor cells are able to transfer chromosomal DNA to recipient cells with high frequency in comparison to F⁺ cells, therefore, named as Hfr cells (high frequency of recombination)
- During conjugation of Hfr cell with an F⁻ cell, only few chromosomal genes along with a part of the F factor get transferred. Connection between the cells usually breaks before the whole genome is transferred
- As the entire F factor does not get transferred, hence following conjugation, F⁻ recipient cells do not become F⁺ cells.

Role of Conjugation

- Conjugation plays an important role in the transfer of plasmids coding for antibacterial drug resistance [resistance transfer factor (RTF)] and bacteriocin production [Colicinogenic (Col) factor.
- Conjugation is the most common mechanism of transfer of plasmids coding for multiple drug resistance among bacteria. Several drug resistance genes can be transferred together along with the F factor, which is the main reason for the emergence of **multi-drug resistance** in bacteria.

Mutational and transferrable drug resistance have been discussed in **Chapter 3.4**.

■ TRANSPOSITION

Transposons are the bacterial genes that are capable of intracellular transfer between chromosome to chromosome, plasmid to plasmid, and chromosome to plasmid or vice versa and the process of such intracellular transfer of transposons is called as transposition. As transposons move around the genome in a cut-and-paste manner, they are also called **jumping genes** or **mobile genetic elements**.
- Unlike plasmids, transposons are not self-replicating and are dependent on chromosomal or plasmid DNA for replication
- Transposons were first discovered in the 1940s by Barbara McClintock for which she won the Nobel Prize in 1983
- **Types of transposons include**—(i) insertion sequence transposon (simplest form) and (ii) composite transposon (larger and carry additional genes coding for antibiotic resistance or toxin production).

GENE TRANSFER BY ARTIFICIAL METHODS

■ GENETIC ENGINEERING

Genetic engineering refers to deliberate modification of an organism's genetic information by directly altering its nucleic acid genome. Genetic engineering is accomplished by a precise mechanism known as recombinant DNA technology.

The gene coding for any desired protein is isolated from an organism, and then inserted into suitable vector, which is then cloned in such a way that it can be expressed in the formation of specific (desired) protein.

Recombinant DNA Technology

The procedure of recombinant DNA technology involves the following steps:
1. **Treatment with restriction enzyme:** The DNA from the microorganism is extracted and then is cleaved by enzymes called restriction endonucleases to produce a mixture of DNA fragments
2. **Southern blot:** The fragment containing the desired gene is isolated from the mixture of DNA fragments. This is done by:
   - DNA fragments are electrophoretically separated by subjecting to agar gel electrophoresis
   - The separated DNA fragments are transferred from the gel to a nitrocellulose membrane
   - The DNA fragment containing the desired gene is detected adding a specific DNA probe, complementary to the gene of interest
   - The band containing the desired gene is isolated by DNA extraction and then, is subjected to electrophoresis in a different gel.
3. **Recombination with a vector:** The isolated DNA fragment is annealed with a vector by DNA ligase enzyme
4. **Introduction of the vector into bacteria:** The vector is introduced into bacteria usually by transformation and rarely by transduction
5. **Cloning:** Culture of the bacteria containing the desired gene followed by expression of the gene products, yields a large quantity of desired protein.

Applications of Genetic Engineering

- **Production of vaccines,** e.g., subunit vaccines for hepatitis B and papillomavirus
- **Production of antigens used in diagnostic kits:** Used for specific antibody detection (e.g. ELISA)
- **Production of proteins used in therapy:** These include interferons, interleukin-2, tumor necrosis factor, etc.
- **Gene therapy:** Genetic diseases can be cured by replacing the defective gene by introducing the normal gene into the patient.

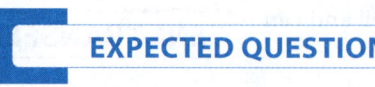

EXPECTED QUESTIONS

I. Write essay on:
1. Name various methods of horizontal gene transfer. Discuss in detail about mechanism of conjugation.

II. Write short notes on:
1. Transformation.
2. Transposition.
3. Transduction.
4. Genetic engineering.

III. Multiple Choice Questions (MCQs):
1. Mechanism of direct transfer of free DNA:
    a. Transformation
    b. Conjugation
    c. Transduction
    d. Transposition
2. Phage mediated transfer of DNA from one bacterium to another bacterium is known as:
    a. Transformation
    b. Transduction
    c. Transmission
    d. Conjugation
3. NOT a method of horizontal gene transfer is:
    a. Conjugation
    b. Mutation
    c. Transformation
    d. Transduction
4. Sometimes, the plasmid may integrate with chromosomal DNA of bacteria and such plasmids are called as:
    a. Episomes
    b. Transfer factors
    c. Vectors
    d. Cosmids
5. The Griffith experiment on mice using pneumococci strains provide the direct evidence of:
    a. Transformation
    b. Transduction
    c. Conjugation
    d. Transposition

Answers
1. a   2. b   3. b   4. a   5. a

General Bacteriology: Antimicrobial Agents and Antimicrobial Resistance

CHAPTER 3.4

CHAPTER PREVIEW

- Antimicrobial Agents
- Antimicrobial Resistance

■ ANTIMICROBIAL AGENTS

Antimicrobials are the agents that kill or inhibit the growth of microorganisms. They can be classified in various ways:

1. According to microorganisms against which they are used—antibacterial, antifungal, antiparasitic, antiviral agents. Only antibacterial agents are discussed in this chapter
2. According to their ability to kill (ends with suffix cidal) or inhibit (ends with suffix static) the microorganism, e.g. bactericidal and bacteriostatic
3. According to the chemical structure and mechanism of action—the antimicrobial agents can be further divided into many classes, as described in **Table 3.4.1**.

■ ANTIMICROBIAL RESISTANCE

Antimicrobial resistance refers to the development of resistance to an antimicrobial agent by a microorganism. It can be of two types—intrinsic and acquired resistance.

Intrinsic Resistance

It refers to the innate ability of a bacterium to resist a class of antimicrobial agents due to its inherent structural or functional characteristics.

- ❖ This imposes negligible threat as it is a defined pattern of resistance and is non-transferable. However, the clinicians must be aware to exclude these antibiotics from therapy
- ❖ Some of the important examples include—
  - Gram-negative bacteria are resistant to vancomycin
  - Gram-positive bacteria are resistant to colistin
  - Aerobic bacteria are resistant to metronidazole
  - *Klebsiella pneumoniae* are resistant to ampicillin and ticarcillin
  - *Proteus* species are resistant to ampicillin, first and second-generation cephalosporins, tetracyclines, nitrofurantoin, and polymyxins
  - *Pseudomonas aeruginosa* is resistant to ampicillin, ceftriaxone, amoxicillin-clavulanate, ampicillin-sulbactam, ertapenem, tetracyclines, tigecycline, co-trimoxazole, and chloramphenicol
  - *Acinetobacter baumannii* is resistant to ampicillin, amoxicillin, amoxicillin-clavulanate, ertapenem, aztreonam, chloramphenicol, and fosfomycin

Acquired Resistance

This refers to the emergence of resistance in bacteria that are ordinarily susceptible to antimicrobial agents, by acquiring the genes coding for resistance. Most of the antimicrobial resistance shown by bacteria belongs to this category.

The emergence of resistance is a major problem worldwide in antimicrobial therapy. Infections caused by resistant microorganisms often fail to respond to the standard treatment, resulting in prolonged illness, higher healthcare expenditures, and a greater risk of death.

- ❖ Overuse and misuse of antimicrobial agents is the single most important cause of the development of acquired resistance
- ❖ The evolution of resistant strains is a natural phenomenon, which can occur among bacteria especially when an antibiotic is an overuse
- ❖ The use of a particular antibiotic poses selective pressure in a population of bacteria which in turn promotes resistant bacteria to thrive and the susceptible bacteria to die off **(Fig. 3.4.1)**
- ❖ Thus the resistant bacterial populations flourish in areas of high antimicrobial use, where they enjoy a selective advantage over susceptible populations
- ❖ The resistant strains then spread in the environment and transfer the genes coding for resistance to other unrelated bacteria.

Table 3.4.1: Antimicrobial agents—classification and indication.		
Class/mechanism	Drugs	Spectrum of activity
A. Inhibit Cell Wall Synthesis		
β-lactam antibiotics: Binds to penicillin-binding protein, thereby blocking peptidoglycan cross-linking		
Penicillins — Penicillin	Penicillin G, Procaine penicillin G, Benzathine penicillin G	*Streptococcus*, pneumococcus, meningococcus, gonococcus, *Corynebacterium diphtheriae, Clostridium perfringens,* and *Treponema pallidum*
Penicillins — Penicillinase-resistant-penicillins	Cloxacillin, dicloxacillin, nafcillin, oxacillin, and methicillin	**Same as penicillin** *plus* Penicillinase producing *Staphylococcus aureus*
Penicillins — Aminopenicillins (extended-spectrum)	Ampicillin, amoxicillin	**Same as penicillin** *plus Enterococcus faecalis, Escherichia coli, Salmonella* and *Shigella*
Penicillins — Ureidopenicillins and carboxypenicillins	Ticarcillin, piperacillin, carbenicillin	**Same as aminopenicillins** *plus Pseudomonas aeruginosa*
Cephalosporin — 1st generation	Cefazolin, cephalexin	*Staphylococcus aureus, Escherichia coli,* and *Klebsiella*
Cephalosporin — 2nd generation	Cefuroxime, cefoxitin	Same as 1st generation *plus* gram-negative activity and anaerobic activity (cefoxitin)
Cephalosporin — 3rd generation	Ceftriaxone, cefotaxime; Ceftazidime, cefoperazone	*Escherichia coli* and *Klebsiella*; *Pseudomonas* (ceftazidime); Pneumococci, meningococci (ceftriaxone)
Cephalosporin — 4th generation	Cefepime, cefpirome	Good activity against gram-positive and negative bacteria including *Pseudomonas*
Cephalosporin — 5th generation	Ceftobiprole, ceftaroline	Same as 3rd generation and MRSA
β-lactam + β-lactamase inhibitors	Amoxicillin-clavulanate*, Cefoperazone-sulbactam, Piperacillin-tazobactam*, Ceftazidime-avibactam	Same as the spectrum of the respective β-lactam drug plus active against β-lactamase producing bacteria. *Have excellent anaerobic coverage
Carbapenems	Imipenem, meropenem, doripenem	Broadest range of activity against most bacteria, which include gram-positive cocci, Enterobacterales, *Pseudomonas, Listeria*, and anaerobes
Monobactam	Aztreonam	Gram-negative rods
Other cell wall inhibitors		
Glycopeptides	Vancomycin, teicoplanin	Active against most gram-positive bacteria including MRSA (drug of choice), and for *Clostridioides difficile*
Fosfomycin	Fosfomycin	Active against *Escherichia coli, Enterococcus*, etc.
B. Protein Synthesis Inhibition		
Binds and inhibits 30S ribosomal subunit		
Aminoglycosides	Gentamicin, amikacin, tobramycin	Enterobacterales, *Pseudomonas, Acinetobacter, Enterococcus*: Gentamicin *plus* cell wall active agent given
Tetracyclines	Tetracycline, doxycycline, minocycline	Rickettsiae, Chlamydiae, *Mycoplasma, Vibrio cholerae*; Minocycline: *Acinetobacter, Burkholderia*
Glycylglycines	Tigecycline	*Acinetobacter, Enterococcus, Staphylococcus*
Binds and inhibits 50S ribosomal subunit		
Chloramphenicol	Chloramphenicol	*Haemophilus influenzae*, anaerobic infection
Macrolides	Erythromycin, azithromycin	*Streptococcus, Haemophilus influenzae, Mycoplasma*
Lincosamides	Clindamycin	*S. aureus*, streptococci, anaerobic infection
Oxazolidinones	Linezolid	Resistant gram-positives like MRSA and VRE infections
Streptogramins	Quinupristin-dalfopristin	MRSA and VRE infections
Mupirocin	Mupirocin	Topical ointment—skin infections, nasal carriers of MRSA

Contd...

Contd...

Class/mechanism	Drugs	Spectrum of activity
C. Nucleic Acid Synthesis Inhibitors		
DNA synthesis inhibitors		
Fluoroquinolones	Inhibit DNA gyrase and topoisomerase IV, thus inhibiting DNA synthesis	
1st generation	Norfloxacin, ciprofloxacin, ofloxacin	Enterobacterales
2nd generation	Levofloxacin, moxifloxacin, sparfloxacin	Others: *Haemophilus, Pseudomonas*
Nitroimidazoles (damage DNA)	Metronidazole, tinidazole	Anaerobic organisms, also active against protozoa: *Entamoeba, Giardia* and *Trichomonas*
Nitrofuran	Nitrofurantoin	Urinary tract infection *(E. coli, Klebsiella)*
RNA synthesis inhibitors		
Rifamycins	Rifampicin	Mycobacteria *(M. tuberculosis, M. leprae,* etc.)
D. Mycolic Acid Synthesis Inhibitors		
Isonicotinic acid hydrazide	Isoniazid (INH)	*M. tuberculosis*
E. Folic Acid Synthesis Inhibitors		
Bacteriostatic: Competitively inhibit enzymes involved in two steps of folic acid synthesis		
Antifolates (Sulfonamides and trimethoprim)	• Sulfadiazine • Cotrimoxazole (Trimethoprim + sulfamethoxazole)	**Sulfadiazine:** Used topically in burn wound surface **Cotrimoxazole** is indicated for: UTI pathogens (*E. coli, Klebsiella,* etc.) *Toxoplasma gondii, Pneumocystis jirovecii*
F. Antimicrobial Agents that Act on the Cell Membrane		
Lipopeptides	Daptomycin	Gram-positive bacteria including VRE and MRSA
Polymyxins	Polymyxin B and colistin	Multidrug-resistant gram-negative bacterial infections

(MRSA, methicillin-resistant *Staphylococcus aureus*; VRE, vancomycin-resistant *Enterococcus*)

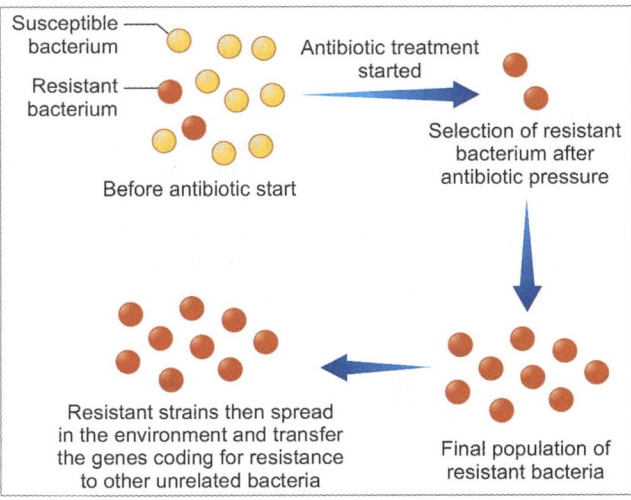

Fig. 3.4.1: Mechanism of development of acquired resistance.

Other factors favoring the spread of antimicrobial resistance include—
- Poor infection control practices in hospitals, e.g. poor hand hygiene practices can facilitate the transmission of resistant strains
- Inadequate sanitary conditions
- Irrational use of antibiotics by doctors, not following antimicrobial susceptibility report
- Uncontrolled sale of antibiotics over the counters without prescription.

Mutational and Transferable Drug Resistance

In presence of selective antibiotic pressure, bacteria acquire new genes (i.e. acquired resistance) mainly by two broad methods.

Mutational Resistance

Resistance can develop due to mutation of the resident genes.
- It is typically seen in *Mycobacterium tuberculosis*, developing resistance to antitubercular drugs
- Mutational drug resistance differs from transferable drug resistance in many ways **(Table 3.4.2)**
- Usually, it is a low-level resistance, developed to one drug at a time; which can be overcome by using a combination of different classes of drugs
- That is why multidrug therapy is used in tuberculosis using 4–5 different classes of drugs, such as isoniazid, rifampicin, pyrazinamide, ethambutol, and streptomycin.

Transferrable Drug Resistance

In contrast, transferrable drug resistance is plasmid coded and usually transferred by conjugation or rarely by transduction, or transformation (explained in **Chapter 3.3**).

Table 3.4.2: Mutational vs transferable drug resistance.	
Mutational drug resistance	**Transferable drug resistance**
Resistance to one drug at a time	Multiple drugs resistance at the same time
Low-degree resistance	High-degree resistance
Resistance can be overcome by a combination of drugs	Cannot be overcome by drug combinations
Virulence of resistance mutants may be lowered	Virulence not decreased
Resistance is not transferable to other organisms	Resistance is transferable to other organisms
Spread to off-springs by vertical spread only	Spread by: Horizontal spread (conjugation, or rarely by transduction/transformation)

❖ The resistance coded plasmid (called R plasmid) can carry multiple genes, each coding for resistance to one class of antibiotic
❖ Thus, it results in a high degree of resistance to multiple drugs, which cannot be overcome by using combination of drugs.

Mechanism of Antimicrobial Resistance

Bacteria develop antimicrobial resistance through several mechanisms.

Decreased Permeability across the Cell Wall

Certain bacteria modify their cell membrane porin channels; either in their frequency, size, or selectivity; thereby preventing the antimicrobial agents from entering the cell. This resistance mechanism has been observed in many gram-negative bacteria, such as *Pseudomonas*, *Enterobacter*, and *Klebsiella* species against drugs, such as imipenem, aminoglycosides, and quinolones.

Efflux Pumps

Certain bacteria possess efflux pumps that mediate expulsion of the drug(s) from the cell, soon after their entry; thereby preventing the intracellular accumulation of drugs. This strategy has been observed in:
❖ *Escherichia coli* and other Enterobacterales against tetracyclines, chloramphenicol
❖ *Staphylococcus aureus* and *Streptococcus pneumoniae* against fluoroquinolones.

By Enzymatic Inactivation

Certain bacteria can inactivate the antimicrobial agents by producing various enzymes, such as:
❖ **β-lactamase** enzyme production: It breaks down the β-lactam rings, thereby inactivating the β-lactam antibiotics. There are various types of β-lactamase enzymes
  ▪ Gram-positive bacteria produce: Penicillinase
  ▪ Gram-negative bacteria produce enzymes such as extended-spectrum β-lactamase (ESBL), AmpC β-lactamase, and carbapenemases.
❖ **Aminoglycoside modifying enzymes** can be produced by both gram-negative and gram-positive bacteria—they destroy the structure of aminoglycosides.

By Modifying the Target Sites

Modification in the target sites of antimicrobial agents (which are within the bacteria) is a very important mechanism. It is observed in:
❖ **MRSA (Methicillin-resistant *Staphylococcus aureus*):** In these strains, the target site of penicillin, i.e. penicillin-binding protein (PBP) gets altered to PBP-2a. The altered PBP, coded by a chromosomally coded gene *mecA*, does not sufficiently bind to β-lactam antibiotics and therefore prevents them from inhibiting the cell wall synthesis
❖ **Vancomycin resistance in enterococci (VRE):** These strains have a change in the target site of vancomycin (i.e. D-alanyl-D-alanine side chain of peptidoglycan).

 EXPECTED QUESTIONS

I. Write short notes on:
  1. Mechanism of antibiotic resistance.
  2. Mutational and transferable drug resistance.
II. Multiple Choice Questions (MCQs):
  1. MRSA is mediated by:
     a. Plasmid   b. *mecA* gene
     c. Transposons   d. None
  2. All of the following antimicrobial agents act on the cell wall, *except*:
     a. Imipenem   b. Penicillin
     c. Polymyxins   d. Vancomycin
  3. All of the following are true regarding transferrable drug resistance, *except*:
     a. Multiple drugs resistance at the same time
     b. Virulence not decreased
     c. Low-degree resistance
     d. Cannot be overcome by drug combinations

Answers
1. b   2. c   3. c

Bacterial Pathogenesis

CHAPTER 3.5

CHAPTER PREVIEW
- Mechanism of Bacterial Pathogenesis

■ MECHANISM OF BACTERIAL PATHOGENESIS

The ability of bacteria to produce disease or tissue injury is referred to as 'pathogenesis'. While the term 'virulence' is used more specifically to describe the relative degree of pathogenesis (tissue damage), which may vary between different strains of the same organism. The virulence of a strain may undergo spontaneous or induced variation.

- **Exaltation:** Enhancement of virulence is known as exaltation, which can be induced experimentally by serial passage into susceptible hosts
- **Attenuation:** It refers to the reduction of virulence, which can be achieved by passage through unfavorable hosts, repeated cultures in artificial media, etc.

Pathogenesis involves several steps such as—transmission of the organism, infective dose, adhesion, invasion, intracellular survival, and expression of several virulence factors (like toxins and enzymes, etc.).

Route of Transmission

The route of transmission of infection plays a crucial role in the pathogenesis of certain bacteria. This difference is probably related to the modes by which different bacteria can initiate tissue damage and establish themselves **(Table 3.5.1)**.

Infective Dose

The infective dose of the bacteria is referred to as the minimum inoculum size that is capable of initiating an infection.

- **Low infective dose:** Certain organisms require a relatively small inoculum to initiate infection
  - *Shigella*: Very low (as low as 10 bacilli)
  - *Campylobacter jejuni* (500 bacilli).
- **Large infective dose:** In contrast, bacteria with a high infective dose can initiate the infection only when the inoculum size exceeds a particular critical size
  - *Salmonella* (10^2–10^5 bacilli)
  - *Vibrio cholerae* (10^6–10^8 bacilli).

The infective dose varies depending upon the factors, such as:

- **Virulence of the organism:** Higher the virulence, the lower is the infective dose
- Host's age and overall immune status
- The ability of the organism to resist gastric acidity: *Shigella* can survive gastric acidity, even a low infective dose can initiate the infection. In contrast, *Vibrio* is extremely acid labile, hence requiring a heavy inoculum to bypass the gastric barrier.

Adhesion

Adhesion of the bacteria to body surfaces is the initial event in the pathogenesis of the disease. It is mediated by specialized molecules called adhesins that bind to specific host cell receptors.

- **Fimbriae or pili:** They are the most important adhesins present in some bacteria. They directly bind to the sugar residues on host cells
- **Other adhesins:** Apart from pili, there are other adhesins found in certain bacteria, such as M protein (*Streptococcus pyogenes*), lipoteichoic acid (gram-positive cocci), etc.

Table 3.5.1: Mode of transmission of bacterial infections.	
Transmission	**Bacterial agents/diseases**
Contact	Multi-drug resistant organisms in hospitals such as *S. aureus, E. coli, Klebsiella*, etc.
Droplet	Meningococcus, *C. diphtheriae* Pneumococcus
Aerosol	*M. tuberculosis*
Ingestion	*Salmonella* and *Shigella* *Vibrio* and diarrheagenic *E. coli*
Vector-borne	Rickettsiae and *Borrelia*
Sexual	Gonococcus, *Chlamydia trachomatis* *Treponema pallidum*
Vertical	*Treponema pallidum*
Birth canal	Listeria, *Streptococcus agalactiae*

❖ **Biofilm formation:** It is another mechanism by which certain bacteria mediate strong adherence to certain structures, such as catheters, prosthetic implants, and heart valves. Biofilm is a group of bacterial cells which stick to each other on a surface and are embedded within a layer of a self-produced matrix of the glycocalyx.

Invasion

Invasion refers to the entry of bacteria into host cells, leading to its spread within the host tissues.
- ❖ Highly invasive pathogens produce spreading or generalized lesions (e.g. streptococcal infections)
- ❖ While less invasive pathogens cause localized lesions (e.g. staphylococcal abscess).

Important virulence factors that help in invasion include:
- ❖ Virulence marker antigen or invasion plasmid antigens in *Shigella*
- ❖ **Enzymes:** The invasion of bacteria is enhanced by many enzymes such as hyaluronidase, collagenase, streptokinase, IgA proteases.

Intracellular Survival

Some organisms survive in the intracellular environment. They are grouped into obligate and facultative intracellular organisms **(Table 3.5.2)**. Various bacterial strategies that inhibit phagocytosis are:
- ❖ The bacterial capsule prevents the phagocyte from adhering to the bacterium. Examples of capsulated bacteria—*Neisseria meningitidis*, *Haemophilus influenzae* and *Streptococcus pneumoniae*
- ❖ Inhibition of phagolysosome fusion by *Mycobacterium tuberculosis*
- ❖ Resistance to lysosomal enzymes by *Coxiella* species and *Mycobacterium leprae*.

Toxins

Endotoxins

Endotoxins are the lipid A portion of lipopolysaccharide (LPS).
- ❖ They are present as an integral part of the cell wall of gram-negative bacteria
- ❖ They are released from the bacterial surface by lysis of the bacteria
- ❖ They are responsible for various biological effects in the host such as—macrophage activation, platelet activation, activation of complement and coagulation pathway leading to disseminated intravascular coagulation (DIC) and septic shock and possibly death.

Exotoxins

They are heat-labile proteins; secreted by certain species of both gram-positive and gram-negative bacteria (examples are given in **Table 3.5.3**).
- ❖ **High potency:** Exotoxins are highly potent even in minute amounts
- ❖ **Used for vaccine:** Exotoxins can be converted into toxoids by treatment with formaldehyde
- ❖ **Specific action:** They are highly specific for a particular tissue, e.g. tetanus toxin for CNS.

Exotoxins differ from endotoxins in several ways **(Table 3.5.4)**.

Table 3.5.2: Intracellular bacteria.

Facultative intracellular bacteria	Obligate intracellular
Salmonella typhi, *Brucella*	*Mycobacterium leprae*
Legionella, *Listeria*	*Rickettsia*
Neisseria meningitidis	*Chlamydia*
Mycobacterium tuberculosis	*Coxiella burnetii*

Table 3.5.3: Bacterial exotoxins.

Organisms	Toxins (Exotoxins)
Staphylococcus aureus	Exfoliative toxin Enterotoxin Toxic shock syndrome toxin
Streptococcus pyogenes	Pyrogenic exotoxin
Corynebacterium diphtheriae	Diphtheria toxin
Bacillus anthracis	Anthrax toxin
Clostridium tetani	Tetanus toxin
Clostridium botulinum	Botulinum toxin
Diarrheagenic *E. coli*	Heat labile toxin Heat stable toxin Verocytotoxin
Shigella	Shiga toxin
Vibrio cholerae	Cholera toxin
Pseudomonas	Exotoxin-A

Table 3.5.4: Differences between bacterial endotoxins and exotoxins.

Endotoxins	Exotoxins
Lipopolysaccharides in nature	Proteins in nature
Part of the cell wall of gram-negative bacteria	Secreted both by gram-positive and gram-negative bacteria
Produce nonspecific action (fever, shock, etc.)	Specific action on particular tissues
Less potent	More potent
Poorly antigenic	Highly antigenic
No effective vaccine is available using endotoxin	Toxoid forms are used as a vaccine, e.g. tetanus toxoid

CHAPTER 3.5 ◆ Bacterial Pathogenesis

EXPECTED QUESTIONS

I. **Write short notes on:**
   1. Mechanisms of bacterial pathogenesis.
   2. Differences between endotoxins and exotoxins.

II. **Multiple Choice Questions (MCQs):**
   1. **The chemical nature of endotoxin is:**
      a. Protein
      b. Lipopolysaccharide
      c. Carbohydrate
      d. None
   2. **The following are exotoxins, *except*:**
      a. Botulinum toxin
      b. Anthrax toxin
      c. Diphtheria toxin
      d. Lipid A portion of LPS
   3. **Obligate intracellular bacteria are all, *except*:**
      a. *M. leprae*   b. *Rickettsia*
      c. *Chlamydia*   d. *M. tuberculosis*
   4. **The following bacteria require large infective dose, *except*:**
      a. *Escherichia coli*
      b. *Shigella*
      c. *Salmonella*
      d. *Vibrio cholerae*
   5. **Bacteria transmitted by droplet route include all, *except*:**
      a. Meningococcus
      b. *Mycobacterium tuberculosis*
      c. Pneumococcus
      d. *Corynebacterium diphtheriae*
   6. **Capsule prevents phagocytosis all of the following bacteria, *except*:**
      a. *Neisseria meningitidis*
      b. *Streptococcus pneumoniae*
      c. *Haemophilus influenzae*
      d. *Staphylococcus aureus*
   7. **True about exotoxin is:**
      a. Chemically lipopolysaccharide
      b. Neutralizing antibodies ineffective
      c. Can be fatal in small doses
      d. Nonspecific effects

Answers
1. b   2. d   3. d   4. b   5. b   6. d   7. c

General Bacteriology: Normal Microbial Flora

CHAPTER 4

CHAPTER PREVIEW
- Microbiology of Normal Flora

MICROBIOLOGY OF NORMAL FLORA

Normal microbial flora refers to the diverse group of microbial populations that every human being harbors on skin and mucous membranes. They do not cause harm; rather they have a beneficiary effect on the host.

- Humans acquire the normal flora soon after the birth and then continue to harbor it until death
- In humans, the normal flora is located in various sites such as the gastrointestinal tract (GIT), respiratory tract, genitourinary tract, and skin
- Most of the normal flora predominantly contain bacteria and to a less extent some fungi and parasites
- GIT is the predominant site of normal flora, where the most common flora is *Bacteroides fragilis* (anaerobic flora). Among aerobes, *Escherichia coli* is the most common.

The microbiological profile of the normal flora in various sites of the human body is given in **Table 4.1**.

Role of Normal Flora

Various microorganisms present as the normal flora have a different relationship with the host. They may have a beneficiary effect on the host, or may be harmful to the host.

Beneficial Effects

The normal microbial flora has several beneficial effects on the host:
- **Prevent colonization of pathogen:** By competing for attachment sites or essential nutrients
- **Synthesize vitamin:** Human enteric bacteria secrete several vitamins such as vitamin K and B complex (e.g. vitamin B12) in excess
- **Waste produced antagonizes other bacteria:** Normal flora may inhibit or kill other nonindigenous organisms by producing a variety of waste substances such as—fatty acids, peroxides, lactic acid, etc.

Table 4.1: Common normal flora of human host.

Anatomical site	Organisms as normal flora
Oral cavity	Nonsporing anaerobes Viridans streptococci, Yeast
Nasopharynx	Nonsporing anaerobes Streptococci, *Neisseria* (non-pathogenic) *Staphylococcus epidermidis*
Gastrointestinal tract	Nonsporing anaerobes (e.g. *Bacteroides fragilis*) Enterobacteriaceae and other gram-negative rods Enterococci *Candida* species Commensal *Entamoeba* species*
Vagina	Nonsporing anaerobes Diphtheroids *Lactobacillus* *Streptococcus agalactiae* *Candida*
Skin	Nonsporing anaerobes *Staphylococcus epidermidis* Diphtheroids, *Micrococcus*

*Parasites as a part of normal flora

- **Immune stimulation:** Normal microbiota being foreign to the host stimulates the host's immune system.

Disturbed Normal Flora Promote Infection

When the composition of normal flora is disturbed, it facilitates pathogenic organisms to enter and cause disease. Several mechanisms by which the normal flora is disturbed are as follows:
- **Injudicious use of broad-spectrum antimicrobial agent:** It may completely suppress the normal flora thus permitting the pathogen to take the upper hand and cause infection
- **Host factors** such as immune suppression, reduced peristalsis may promote the pathogen to grow

CHAPTER 4 ◆ General Bacteriology: Normal Microbial Flora

❖ **Physical destruction** of the normal flora by irradiations, chemicals, burns, etc.

Harmful Effects

Members of the normal flora may cause various endogenous disease.
❖ When the host immunity is lowered, *or*
❖ If they enter the wrong site or tissue—then even the resident flora can produce disease **(Table 4.2)**.

Probiotics

The term "Probiotics" is defined as the live microorganisms (part of normal flora) that, when administered in adequate amounts, confer a health benefit to the host.
❖ They are extremely useful in the conditions where the normal intestinal flora is suppressed
❖ Probiotics are commercially available in the form of capsules or sachets, consisting of a mixture of some important beneficiary bacteria and yeast of human intestinal flora such as *Bifidobacterium*, *Lactobacillus*, etc.
❖ Probiotics are found to have a beneficiary role in treating the following conditions:
  ▪ Gastroenteritis due to any cause
  ▪ Antibiotic-associated diarrhea
  ▪ Lactose intolerance
  ▪ Irritable bowel syndrome and colitis
  ▪ Necrotizing enterocolitis
  ▪ *Helicobacter pylori* infection.

Table 4.2: Diseases produced by normal flora.

Diseases	Anatomical site from which the flora is transferred
Urinary tract infection	Intestinal flora such as *Escherichia coli*, *Klebsiella*
Endocarditis	Oral flora (Viridans streptococci)
Dental caries	Oral flora
Peritonitis	Intestinal flora

EXPECTED QUESTIONS

I. **Write short notes on:**
  1. Resident flora and transient flora.
  2. Beneficial effects of the normal flora.

II. **Multiple Choice Questions (MCQs):**
  1. The most common commensal in human intestine is:
     a. *Bacteroides fragilis*
     b. *Escherichia coli*
     c. *Klebsiella pneumoniae*
     d. *Lactobacillus*
  2. Which of the following is not a commensal in human female genital tract?
     a. *Lactobacillus* species
     b. *Streptococcus agalactiae*
     c. *Neisseria* (non-pathogenic species)
     d. *Trichomonas vaginalis*
  3. **All of the following are diseases produced by normal flora, *except*:**
     a. Urinary tract infection by intestinal flora
     b. Endocarditis viridans streptococci
     c. Bacterial dysentery by *Shigella*
     d. Dental caries and periodontal disease by oral flora

Answers
1. a   2. d   3. c

Epidemiology of Infectious Diseases

CHAPTER 5

CHAPTER PREVIEW
- Infection and Related-terminologies
- Epidemiological Patterns
- Eradication and Elimination
- Epidemiological Determinants of Disease Causation

The epidemiology branch of infectious disease deals with the distribution and determinants of infection-related health states in specified populations, and their application to control the disease.

INFECTION AND RELATED-TERMINOLOGIES

Following the entry of the microorganism into the body, it may lead to either infection or colonization; both the terms need to be distinguished.
- ❖ **Infection:** It is a process in which a pathogenic organism enters, establishes itself, multiplies, and invades the normal anatomical barrier of the host resulting in disease
- ❖ **Colonization:** Here, the pathogenic organism enters, multiplies but does not invade, and neither causes disease nor elicits a specific immune response
    - Colonizers are different from normal flora
    - They have pathogenic potential and may invade and cause disease in another host or the same host later.
- ❖ **Healthcare-associated infection (HAIs):** Defined as the new infections acquired in a healthcare facility (HCF) by a patient after 48 hours of admission, which was neither present nor incubating at the time of admission (*refer* **Chapter 15**).
- ❖ **Community-associated infections:** Refers to the infections which developed in the community or within 48 hours of admission to a healthcare facility.

EPIDEMIOLOGICAL PATTERNS

The spread of communicable diseases in the community may occur in several epidemiological patterns—outbreak, epidemic, pandemic, hyperendemic and sporadic.
- ❖ **Outbreak** is a sudden rise in the number of cases in a limited geographic area; e.g. Nipah virus encephalitis outbreak in Kerala in 2018, resulting in 18 cases with 16 deaths.
- ❖ **Epidemic:** If the infection occurs at a much higher rate than usual in a particular geographical area, it is known as an epidemic. It usually affects a large number of people within a community, population, or region. Example includes—SARS-CoV epidemic in China in 2003.
- ❖ **Pandemic:** An infection that spreads rapidly to large areas of the world is known as a pandemic. Example includes—COVID-19 pandemic in 2020 affecting >200 countries.
- ❖ **Endemic:** When a disease occurs at a persistent, usually low level in a certain geographical area, it is called an endemic. India is endemic to several diseases such as typhoid fever, cholera, malaria, etc.
- ❖ **Sporadic:** Infections occur at irregular intervals or only in a few places; scattered or isolated. For example, several sporadic cases of cholera occur in India every year.

ERADICATION AND ELIMINATION

Eradication, elimination, and control of an infectious disease are related terminologies with distinct differences.

Eradication

It refers to the complete and permanent worldwide reduction to 'zero new cases' of the disease through deliberate efforts. If a disease has been eradicated, no further control measures are required. Example includes—Smallpox was the only disease to be eradicated from the whole world (in 1980).

Elimination

It refers to the 'reduction to zero' (or a very low defined target rate) of new cases in a defined geographical area. The diseases which attained elimination in India include neonatal tetanus and leprosy.

CHAPTER 5 ◆ Epidemiology of Infectious Diseases

Control

It refers to the reduction of disease incidence, prevalence, morbidity, or mortality to a locally acceptable level as a result of deliberate efforts.

EPIDEMIOLOGICAL DETERMINANTS OF DISEASE CAUSATION

The **Epidemiological Triad** depicts the causation of infectious disease. The triad consists of an external **agent**, a susceptible **host**, and an **environment** that brings the host and agent together.

Agent Factors

It refers to the infectious microorganisms such as a virus, bacterium, parasite, or fungus that are responsible for the causation of the disease. A variety of agent-related factors influence whether the exposure to an organism will result in disease **(Table 5.1)**.

- ❖ **Organism's pathogenicity:** It refers to the ability of the organism to cause disease.
- ❖ **Infective dose:** It is the minimum inoculum size that is capable of initiating an infection.
  - **Low infective dose:** For example, *Shigella, Cryptosporidium parvum* and *Giardia*.
  - **Large infective dose:** For example, *Salmonella, Vibrio cholerae*.
- ❖ **Source and reservoir:** The starting point for the occurrence of an infectious disease is known as a source or/and reservoir of infection. Human sources may be either cases or carriers.

Table 5.1: Epidemiological determinants of disease causation.
Agent
• Organism's pathogenicity
• Infective dose
• Source and reservoir: Human or animal
• Mode of transmission: Contact, inhalation, ingestion, vector-borne, vertical transmission
• Infectivity or communicability
Host
• Age, gender, and race
• Underlying disease, pregnancy, etc.
• Underlying immune status and nutritional status
• Occupational status
• Personal practices: Hygiene and sexual practices
• Genetic make-up
Environment
• Seasonality
• Resistance to disinfectants
• Soil, moisture, rainfall

- **Cases or patients:** They are the persons in a given population identified as having a particular disease
- **Carrier:** It refers to the persons who harbor the infectious agent in the absence of any clinical symptoms and shed the organism from the body via contact, air, or secretions.

❖ **Mode of transmission:** Microorganisms may be transmitted from the reservoir or source to a susceptible host in different ways. Mode of transmission of common diseases/agents are:
- **Contact (direct/indirect):** Common cold, skin infections
- **Inhalation (droplet/aerosol transmission):** Measles, SARS-CoV, tuberculosis
- **Ingestion:** Cholera, enteric fever
- **Inoculation (by animal bite):** Rabies
- **Vector borne:** Malaria parasites, dengue
- **Transplacental transmission:** The pathogens causing congenital infections are abbreviated as 'TORCH': **T**oxoplasma gondii, **O**thers (*Treponema pallidum*, varicella-zoster virus), **R**ubella virus, **C**ytomegalovirus and **H**erpes simplex virus.

❖ **Infectivity or communicability:** It refers to the ability of an infectious agent to transmit from one person to another. A **period of communicability** is the time during which an infectious agent may be transferred directly or indirectly from an infected person to another person. Examples include:
- **Measles:** From -4 to +4 days of onset of rash
- **COVID-19:** From -2 to +10 days of onset of symptoms.

Host Factors

Host refers to the human who can get the disease. A variety of factors intrinsic to the host, sometimes called risk factors, can influence an individual's exposure, susceptibility, or response to a causative agent.

- ❖ **Age:** Most viral infections are common at extremes of age, i.e. childhood and old age
- ❖ **Gender:** Males have a greater exposure risk to infections transmitted in work environments and females are at higher risk of acquiring sexually transmitted infections such as HIV and gonorrhea
- ❖ **Pregnancy:** Certain agents can cause transplacental infections during pregnancy (e.g. CMV, rubella)
- ❖ **Host immune status:** Low immunity predisposes to many infections, such as CMV
- ❖ **Prior immunity:** Prior immunity to the agent due to vaccination or past infection can protect the individual from further infection. Some viral infections such as smallpox, chickenpox, measles, mumps, and rubella provide lifelong immunity

- **Nutritional status:** Malnutrition lowers the host immunity and thus predisposes to many viral infections, e.g. measles
- **Underlying comorbid disease:** People with diabetes, immunodeficiency disorders, or receiving steroid therapy are more prone to acquire various infections
- **Occupational status:** Sometimes, infectious diseases are more common in certain occupations; for example, zoonotic diseases such as anthrax are common among butchers, abattoirs, and farmers
- **Sexual practices:** People with multiple sex partners, men who have sex with men are more prone to develop various sexually-transmitted infections such as HIV
- **Hygiene:** Poor hygiene, poor sanitation, over crowding, etc. predispose to several diseases such as acute diarrheal illness and typhoid fever
- **Genetic makeup:** Certain individuals are more prone to develop some microbial infections. This depends on the genetic makeup of the individual.

Environmental Factors

Environmental factors play an important role in disease causation.

- **Seasonality:** Many diseases are common in winters such as influenza and meningococcal meningitis; whereas vector-borne diseases such as malaria, dengue are more common in the rainy season
- **Disinfectants:** The organisms which are more resistant to the action of disinfectant can survive in the environment for longer. This is particularly important in the hospital environment where the multidrug-resistant organisms such as *Pseudomonas, Acinetobacter* and *Klebsiella,* etc. are widely prevalent
- **Soil:** Damp, sandy, or friable soil with vegetation is suitable for certain soil-transmitted helminths such as hookworm, *Ascaris,* and *Trichuris* than clay soil
- **Moisture:** Moisture is necessary for the survival of most microbes as dryness is rapidly fatal.

EXPECTED QUESTIONS

I. **Write short notes on:**
   1. Epidemiological patterns.
   2. Epidemiological determinants of disease causation.

II. **Multiple Choice Questions (MCQs):**
   1. If the infection occurs at a much higher rate than usual in a particular geographical area, it is known as:
      a. Epidemic
      b. Pandemic
      c. Outbreak
      d. Sporadic
   2. Organisms with low infective dose include all, *except*:
      a. *Shigella*
      b. *Cryptosporidium parvum*
      c. *Giardia*
      d. *Vibrio cholerae*
   3. Healthcare associated infection is defined as new infection acquired in a healthcare facility which was neither present nor incubating at the time of admission, within:
      a. 24 hours
      b. 48 hours
      c. 36 hours
      d. 72 hours
   4. The complete and permanent worldwide reduction to zero new cases of the disease through deliberate efforts is known as:
      a. Reduction
      b. Elimination
      c. Eradication
      d. Control

Answers
1. a   2. d   3. b   4. c

SECTION 2: Immunology

SECTION OUTLINE

6. Immunity (Innate and Acquired)
7. Antigen, Antibody and Complements
8. Antigen–Antibody Reaction
9. Components of Immune System: Organs, Cells and Products
10. Immune Responses: Cell-mediated and Antibody-mediated
11. Hypersensitivity Reactions
12. Autoimmunity, Immunodeficiency Disorders, Transplant and Tumor Immunology
13. Immunoprophylaxis and Immunization Schedule
14. Immunohematology

Immunity (Innate and Acquired)

CHAPTER 6

CHAPTER PREVIEW
- Innate Immunity
- Acquired or Adaptive Immunity
- Active Immunity
- Passive Immunity
- Other Types of Immunity

The term "immunity" is defined as the resistance offered by the host against microorganism(s) or any foreign substance(s). Immunity can be broadly classified into two types:
1. Innate immunity—present right from birth
2. Acquired/adaptive immunity—acquired during the course of life.

INNATE IMMUNITY

Innate immunity is the inborn resistance against infections that an individual possesses right from birth, due to his genetic or constitutional makeup.

Innate immunity has certain unique properties by which it can be differentiated from acquired immunity (**Table 6.1**).

- **Acts in minutes:** Innate immunity is the **first line of host defense** against infections; occurs immediately after the microbial entry
- **Prior microbial exposure is not required:** Innate immunity is independent of prior exposure to the microbes; presents even before the first entry of the microorganism
- **Non-specific:** Cells of innate immunity are non-specific in their action; can be directed against any microbial antigen(s)
- **No memory:** Innate immunity does not have a memory component. Response to a repeat infection is identical to the primary response.

Mechanism of Innate Immunity

Following exposure to microorganisms, several mediators of innate immunity are recruited to the site of infection. The first step that takes place is **attachment,** which involves binding the surface molecules of organisms to the receptors on the cells of innate immunity (e.g. toll-like receptors).

Components of Innate Immunity

There are several mediators of innate immunity.
- **Anatomical barriers:** Such as skin and mucosal surfaces have a spectrum of antimicrobial activities
  - Mechanically prevents entry of microbes
  - Mucosa produces mucus which entraps microbes
  - Cilia present in the lower respiratory tract propel the microbes outside.
- **Physiological barriers** are also capable of inhibiting certain microbes; examples include:
  - Normal body temperature
  - Gastric acidity
  - Secretory products of mucosa such as saliva, tears, trypsin and bile salts, etc.
- **Host immune cells:** Several immune cells such as phagocytes, NK cells, mast cells, and dendritic cells play a crucial role in innate immunity
  - *Phagocytes* such as neutrophils, and macrophages are the main components of innate immunity. They are rapidly recruited to the site of infection and mediate phagocytosis (i.e. engulfment of microbes and subsequent microbial killing)
  - *Natural killer (NK) cells:* They are a class of lymphocytes that kill intracellular pathogens, virus-infected cells, and tumor cells
  - *Mast cells:* They are present in the epithelial lining of respiratory and other mucosa and are capable of killing the microbes by releasing several inflammatory mediators
  - *Dendritic cells:* They respond to microbes by producing numerous cytokines that initiate inflammation.
- **Complement pathways:** Alternative and mannose-binding pathways are the chief mediators of innate immunity
- **Inflammatory response:** Inflammation is defined as the biological response of vascular tissues to harmful stimuli, such as microorganisms or other foreign substances. The

major events that take place during an inflammatory response following a microbial entry are as follows:
- Vasodilation due to release of vasoactive substances from the damaged tissues
- Leakage of plasma proteins through blood vessels
- Recruitment of phagocytes (e.g. neutrophils) to the site of inflammation
- Engulfment of microbes and dead material by the phagocytes
- Destruction of the microbes

❖ **Normal resident flora** lining the intestinal, respiratory, and genital tract can compete with the pathogens for nutrition. They also produce antibacterial substances

❖ **Cytokines:** In response to the microbial antigens, dendritic cells, macrophages, and other cells secrete several cytokines that mediate many of the cellular reactions of innate immunity such as:
- Tumor necrosis factor-α (TNF-α)
- Interleukin-1 (IL-1), IL-6, IL-8, IL-12 and IL-16
- Interferons (IFN-α, β)

❖ **Acute phase reactant proteins (APRs):** They are the proteins synthesized by liver at a steady concentration, but their synthesis increases exponentially during acute inflammatory conditions. Examples of APR include: C-reactive protein, serum amyloid A, complement proteins, coagulation protein, and mannose-binding protein.

Table 6.1: Differences between innate and acquired immunity.

Properties	Innate immunity	Acquired/Adaptive immunity
Resistance to infection that an individual	Possesses right from birth	Acquires during his lifetime
Duration	The immune response occurs in minutes	The immune response occurs in days
Prior exposure to the antigen	Not required	Required
Immunological memory	Absent	Present
Host cell receptors	Non-specific, e.g. toll-like receptor	Specific, e.g. T cell receptors and B cell immunoglobulin receptors
Important components of innate immunity	• Anatomical and physiological barriers • Host immune cells: Phagocytes, NK cells, mast cells, dendritic cells, etc. • Complement pathways—alternative and mannose-binding pathways • Normal resident flora	T cell B cell Classical complement pathway

> **C-Reactive Protein (CRP)**
> It is one of the most common markers of acute inflammation, used in most diagnostic laboratories.
> ❑ The level of CRP rises in acute inflammatory conditions including bacterial infection
> ❑ **Marked increase** of CRP (>10 mg/dL): It occurs in conditions such as acute bacterial infections, major trauma and systemic vasculitis.
> ❑ Following an injury or inflammation, the CRP level starts increasing by 6 hr, doubles every 8 hr, reaches its peak by 48 hr.
> ❑ CRP is so named because it precipitates with the C-carbohydrate antigen of pneumococcus. However, it is not an antibody against the C-antigen of pneumococcus; it is non-specific, can be raised in any inflammatory conditions
> ❑ It can be detected by latex agglutination test using latex particles coated with anti-CRP antibodies. Detection limit of CRP by latex agglutination test is 0.6 mg/dL.

The differences between innate and acquired immunity are depicted in **Table 6.1**.

■ ACQUIRED IMMUNITY

Acquired immunity is defined as the resistance against the infecting foreign substance that an individual acquires or adapts during the course of his life.

❖ **Mediators: T cells and B cells** are the chief mediators of acquired immunity. Other mediators include:
- Classical complement pathway
- Antigen-presenting cells
- Cytokines (IL-2, IL-4, IL-5).

❖ **The response occurs in days:** Acquired immunity involves activation of T and B cells against the microbial antigens; which takes several days to weeks to develop, following the microbial entry

❖ **Requires prior microbial exposure:** Acquired immunity develops only after exposure to the microbes

❖ **Specific:** Acquired immunity is highly specific; directed against specific antigens of the microbes

❖ **Memory present:** Acquired immunity does have a memory component. A proportion of T and B cells become memory cells following primary contact with the microbe, which play an important role when the microbe is encountered subsequently

❖ **Host cell receptors** of acquired immunity are specific for a particular microbial antigen. Examples include T cell receptors and B cell immunoglobulin receptors.

Types of acquired immunity: Acquired immunity can be classified in two ways:

CHAPTER 6 ◆ Immunity (Innate and Acquired)

1. Active and passive immunity
2. Artificial and natural immunity.

Active Immunity

Active immunity is the resistance developed by an individual towards an antigenic stimulus.
- ❖ Here, the host's immune system is actively involved against the antigenic stimulus; leading to the activation of T and B cells, and the production of specific antibodies
- ❖ Active immunity may be induced naturally or artificially
  - **Natural active immunity** occurs following exposure to microbial infection (e.g. measles virus infection)
  - **Artificial active immunity** develops following exposure to an immunogen by vaccination (e.g. measles vaccine). Vaccines are discussed in detail in **Chapter 13**.
- ❖ As the host's immune apparatus is actively involved, active immunity often fails to develop when the host is immunocompromised
- ❖ Active immunity **develops slower**; as there is an initial **lag phase**, required for activation of the T and B cells
- ❖ **Long-lasting:** Active immunity usually lasts for longer periods, but the duration varies depending on the type of pathogen.

Types of immune response in active immunity are of two types: Primary immune response and secondary immune response.

Primary Immune Response

It occurs when the antigenic exposure occurs for the first time. The following events take place:
- ❖ **Latent or lag period:** Active immunity develops only after a latent period following the antigenic exposure, which corresponds to the time required for the host's immune apparatus to become active
- ❖ **Effector cells:** Majority of activated T and B cells against the antigenic stimulus become effector T and B cells
- ❖ **Memory cells:** A minor proportion of stimulated T and B cells become memory cells, which are the key cells for secondary immune response
- ❖ **Antibody surge:** Effector B cells (plasma cells) produce antibodies (mainly IgM type). Antibodies appear in the serum in slow and sluggish manner; reach peak, maintain the level for a while and then fall down.

Secondary Immune Response

It occurs when the same antigenic exposure occurs subsequently. The events which take place are as follows:
- ❖ **Latent period** is either absent or of short duration. This is because memory cells become active soon after the antigenic exposure
- ❖ **Negative phase:** At the onset of secondary immune response, there may be a negative phase during which the antibody level may become lower than it was before the antigenic stimulus. This is because the exposed antigen combines with the pre-existing antibody and thus the antibody level in serum falls down
- ❖ **Antibody surge:** Secondary antibody response is prompt, powerful, long-lasting and mainly of IgG type. Hence, it is said that, the booster doses of vaccines are more effective than the first dose.

Passive Immunity

Passive immunity is defined as the resistance that is transferred passively to a host in a "readymade" form without the active participation of the host's immune system.
- ❖ Passive immunity can also be induced naturally or artificially
  - **Natural passive immunity** involves the IgG antibody transfer from mother to fetus across the placenta
  - **Artificial passive immunity** develops following the readymade transfer of commercially prepared immunoglobulin (e.g. Rabies immunoglobulin).
- ❖ Passive immunity plays a very important role in:
  - Immunodeficient individuals (as the host's immune apparatus is not effective), and
  - Post-exposure prophylaxis; when an immediate effect is warranted.
- ❖ Passive immunity **develops faster**; there is no lag phase
- ❖ There is no **immunological memory** as the memory cells are not involved
- ❖ **Booster doses are not effective:** As the memory component is absent, the effect produced following subsequent immunoglobulin administration is the same as the effect produced after the primary dose.

The differences between active and passive immunity are listed in **Table 6.2**.

■ OTHER TYPES OF IMMUNITY

Local (or Mucosal) Immunity

Local or mucosal immunity is the immune response that is active at the mucosal surfaces such as intestinal or respiratory or genitourinary mucosa.
- ❖ It is mediated by a type of IgA antibody called secretory IgA, which prevents the entry of microbes at the local site itself
- ❖ Local immunity can only be induced by natural infection or by live vaccination, e.g. live oral polio vaccine (but not by killed vaccines).

Table 6.2: Differences between active and passive immunity.

Properties	Active immunity	Passive immunity
Mechanism	Produced actively by host immune system	Immunoglobulins received passively
Induced by	• Infection (natural) • Vaccination (artificial)	• Mother to fetus IgG transfer (natural) • Readymade antibody transfer (artificial)
Duration	Long-lasting	Short-lasting
Lag period	Present	No lag period
Memory	Present	No memory
Booster doses	Useful	Less effective
In Immunodeficient individuals	Not useful	Useful
Post-exposure prophylaxis	Less useful	Useful

Herd Immunity

Herd immunity is defined as the overall immunity of a community (or herd) toward a pathogen.

❖ It plays a vital role in preventing epidemic diseases
❖ If herd immunity is good, that means a large population of the community is immune to a pathogen. Hence, epidemics are less likely to occur and eradication of the disease may be possible

❖ Herd immunity develops following effective vaccination against some diseases like:
  ▪ Diphtheria and pertussis vaccine
  ▪ Measles, mumps, and rubella (MMR) vaccine
  ▪ Polio (oral polio vaccine)
  ▪ Smallpox vaccine.

EXPECTED QUESTIONS

I. Write an essay on:
1. Define immunity. Describe in detail about the properties and mediators of innate immunity.

II. Write short notes on:
1. Herd immunity.
2. Differences between innate and acquired immunity.
3. Differences between active and passive immunity.

III. Multiple Choice Questions (MCQs):
1. Which is not a mediator of innate immunity?
   a. T cells
   b. NK cell
   c. Phagocytes
   d. Neutrophil
2. Which of the following about innate immunity is wrong?
   a. The immune response occurs in minutes
   b. Non-specific
   c. It is first line of defense
   d. Need prior contact with the antigen
3. Which of the following about active immunity is correct?
   a. No lag phase
   b. Booster doses are useful
   c. Useful in immunodeficient people
   d. No memory cells
4. The type of immunity that develops after infection is:
   a. Artificial immunity
   b. Acquired immunity
   c. Passive immunity
   d. Combined immunity
5. The immunity develops after the vaccination is an example for:
   a. Natural active immunity
   b. Artificial active immunity
   c. Natural passive immunity
   d. Artificial passive immunity

Answers
1. a   2. d   3. b   4. b   5. b

Antigen, Antibody and Complement

CHAPTER 7

CHAPTER PREVIEW
- Antigen
- Antibody
- Complement

ANTIGEN

Antigen (Ag) is defined as any substance that satisfies two distinct immunologic properties—immunogenicity and antigenicity.
1. **Immunogenicity:** It is the ability of an antigen to induce an immune response in the body
2. **Antigenicity (immunological reactivity):** It is the ability of an antigen to combine specifically with antibodies.

The substance that satisfies the first property, i.e. immunogenicity (inducing a specific immune response) is more appropriately called **"immunogen"** rather than using the word "antigen".

Hapten
Haptens are low molecular weight molecules that **lack immunogenicity** (cannot induce an immune response) but **retain antigenicity or immunological reactivity** (i.e. can bind to their specific antibody or T cell receptor). Haptens can become immunogenic when combined with a larger protein molecule called a **carrier**.

Epitope
Epitope or antigenic determinant is the smallest unit of an antigen that is capable of reacting with the specific site of an antibody. The specific site of an antibody that reacts with the corresponding epitope of an antigen is called **paratope**.

Antigen Host Relationship
Based on the antigen-host relationship, antigens can be grouped into two types:
1. **Self or autoantigens:** They belong to the host itself; hence they are not immunogenic. Host's immune system does not react to its own antigen, which is due to exhibiting a mechanism called **immunological tolerance** (*refer* Chapter 12).
2. **Non-self or foreign antigens:** They are immunogenic and are of three types:
   i. **Alloantigens** are species specific. Tissues of all individuals in a species contain species-specific antigens
   ii. **Isoantigens** are types of antigens that are present only in subsets of a species, e.g. blood group antigens and histocompatibility antigens.
   iii. **Heteroantigens:** Antigens belonging to two different species are called heteroantigens. A **heterophile antigen** is a type of heteroantigen that exists in unrelated species; but they share epitopes with each other. So, antibody produced against antigen of one species can react with the other and vice versa. Heterophile antigens can be used in various serological tests. Examples include—Weil-Felix reaction (for typhus fever), Paul-Bunnell test (for infectious mononucleosis), etc.

Factors Influencing Immunogenicity of Ag
There are various factors that influence the immunogenicity of an antigen.
- **Size of the antigen:** Larger is the size more potent is the molecule as an immunogen
- **Chemical nature of the antigen:** Proteins are stronger immunogens than carbohydrates or lipids
- **Susceptibility of antigen to tissue enzymes:** Only substances that are susceptible to the action of tissue enzymes are immunogenic
- **Structural complexity:** Polymers made up of at least two or more amino acids are immunogenic
- **Foreignness to the host:** Higher is the phylogenetic distance between the antigen and the host; more is the immunogenicity
- **Genetic factor:** Different individuals of a given species show different types of immune responses towards the same antigen due to genetic differences

- **Optimal dose of antigen:** An antigen is immunologically active only in the optimal dose range. A too little dose or too large dose fails to elicit an immune response
- **Route of antigen administration:** In general, the immune response is better induced following the parenteral administration of an antigen
- **Sometimes, repeated doses of antigens** may be required to generate an adequate immune response.

> **Adjuvant**
>
> The term "adjuvant" refers to any substance that enhances the immunogenicity of an antigen. They are usually added to vaccines to increase the immunogenicity of the vaccine antigen.
>
> ***Examples of Adjuvants***
> - **Alum** (aluminum hydroxide or phosphate)
> - **Lipopolysaccharide** (LPS) fraction of *Bordetella pertussis* is an excellent adjuvant for diphtheria and tetanus toxoids. This explains the reason for using combined immunization for diphtheria, pertussis and tetanus in the form of DPT vaccine.
>
> ***Mechanism of Adjuvant Action:*** Adjuvants act through the following steps:
> - Delaying the release of antigen
> - By activating phagocytosis
> - By activating helper T (T_H) cells.

Biological Classes of Antigens

Different biological classes of antigens are:
- **T-dependent (TD) antigens:** Most of the normal antigens are T cell dependent, they are processed and presented by antigen-presenting cells (APCs) to T cells which lead to T cell activation. The activated T cells secrete cytokines that in turn stimulate the B cells to produce antibodies.
- **T-independent (TI) antigens:** There are a few antigens such as **bacterial capsule, flagella** and **LPS** (lipopolysaccharide) that do not need the help of T cells and APCs. They directly bind to immunoglobulin receptors present on B cells and stimulate B cells polyclonally. It leads to increased secretion of non-specific antibodies.
- **Superantigens:** They can activate T cells directly without being processed by antigen-presenting cells (APCs).
  - Non-specific activation of T cells leads to a massive release of cytokines known as "cytokine storm," which include inflammatory mediators such as interferon-γ, IL-1, IL-6, TNF-α, and TNF-β. Various products of microorganisms act as superantigens.
  - Examples include—Staphylococcal toxic shock syndrome toxin-1 (TSST-1) and exfoliative toxin, streptococcal pyrogenic exotoxin (SPE)-A and C, etc.

ANTIBODY

Antibody or immunoglobulin is a specialized glycoprotein, produced from activated B cells (plasma cells) in response to an antigen, and is capable of combining with the antigen that triggered its production.
- Immunoglobulin (Ig) constitutes 20–25% of total serum proteins
- There are five classes of Ig recognized—IgG, IgA, IgM, IgD, and IgE.

Structure of Antibody

An antibody molecule is a 'Y-shaped' heterodimer, composed of four polypeptide chains **(Fig. 7.1)**—two light (L) chains and two heavy (H) chains.
- **Bonds:** All four H and L chains are bound to each other by disulfide bonds, and by noncovalent interactions
- **Ends:** The chains have two ends—an amino-terminal end (NH_3) and a carboxyl-terminal end (COOH)
- **H chain classes:** There are five classes of H chains. Each Ig has one type of H class. The five classes of Igs (IgG, IgA, IgM, IgD, and IgE) are classified based on the type of H chains they possess **(Table 7.1)**.
- **L chains** are of two types—kappa (κ) and lambda (λ), named after Korngold and Lipari who originally described them. In humans, 60% of the light chains are kappa and 40% are lambda type. Both the light chains of an antibody molecule are of same type, either κ or λ, but never both.

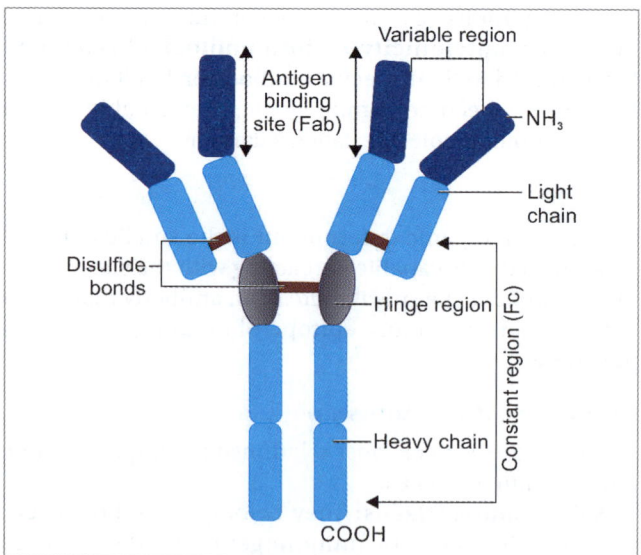

Fig. 7.1: General structure of an antibody.

CHAPTER 7 ◆ Antigen, Antibody and Complement

Table 7.1: Type of heavy chain in each immunoglobulin class.

Immunoglobulin class	Heavy chain type
IgG	γ (gamma)
IgA	α (alpha)
IgM	μ (mu)
IgD	δ (delta)
IgE	ε (epsilon)

Variable and Constant Regions

Each H and L chain comprises two regions—variable and constant region.
1. **Variable region:** Contains a variable sequence of amino acids. It is the antigen-binding region of an antibody
    - It comprises a hypervariable region called paratope, which makes actual contact with the epitope of the antigen
    - Antibodies produced against various antigens differ from each other in the amino acid sequences of the variable region.
2. **Constant region (Fc):** It constitutes the remaining part of an Ig molecule other than that of the variable region
    - The amino acid sequence of the Fc region shows a uniform pattern
    - The Fc region of antibody mediates various effector functions such as binding to the complements, and various other cell types such as phagocytes, lymphocytes, mast cells, NK cells, eosinophils, etc. **(Fig. 7.2)**
    - These cells bear Fc receptors (FcR) that bind to the Fc region of immunoglobulins.

Functions of Immunoglobulins

- ❖ **Antigen binding (by Fab region):** Binding to the antigen is the primary function of an antibody, which can result in protection of the host. The Fab fragment bears the variable region and is involved with the interaction with the antigen

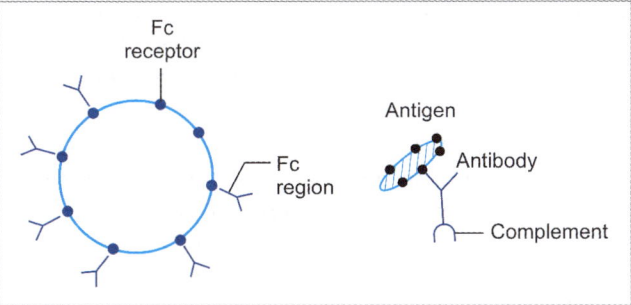

Fig. 7.2: Function of the constant region (Fc) of antibody.

- ❖ **Effector functions (by Fc region):** A variety of secondary "effector functions" are produced; mediated by Fc region of the antibody. These effector functions include:
    - Fixation of complement: Antibody coating the target cell binds to complement through its Fc receptor which leads to complement mediated lysis of the target cell
    - Binding to various cells: Phagocytes, lymphocytes, platelets, mast cells, NK cell, eosinophils and basophils bear Fc receptors (FcR) that bind to Fc region of immunoglobulins. This binding can activate the cells to perform some biological functions.

Immunoglobulin Classes

There are five classes of immunoglobulins.

Immunoglobulin G (IgG)

It constitutes about 70–80% of total Ig in the body. It mediates various functions.
- ❖ IgG can **cross the placenta**; hence providing immunity to the fetus and newborn
- ❖ **Complement fixing:** Fc region of IgG can bind to complement factors; thus activating the classical pathway of the complement system
- ❖ **Phagocytosis:** IgG bind to Fc receptors present on phagocytes (macrophages, neutrophils) and enhances the phagocytosis (opsonization) of antigen bound to them
- ❖ It mediates precipitation and neutralization reactions
- ❖ IgG is raised after a long time following infection and represents chronic or past infection (recovery).

Immunoglobulin M (IgM)

Among all Ig, IgM has the highest molecular weight. It is present only in the intravascular compartment, not in body fluids or secretions. It exists either in monomeric form with 2 valencies or pentameric form (5 Ig joined together by a J chain) with a valency of 10 **(Fig. 7.3A)**. IgM mediates various functions.
- ❖ **Acute infection:** IgM is the first antibody to be produced following an infection; represents acute or recent infection. It is also called a primary immune response antibody
- ❖ **Complement fixing:** It is the most potent activator of the classical complement pathway
- ❖ It is also present on B cell surface in monomeric form and serves as **B cell receptor** for antigen binding
- ❖ It acts as an **opsonin**; binds to an antigen which is then easily recognized and removed (opsonization)
- ❖ **Fetal immunity:** It is the first antibody to be synthesized in fetal life; thus provides immunity to the fetus

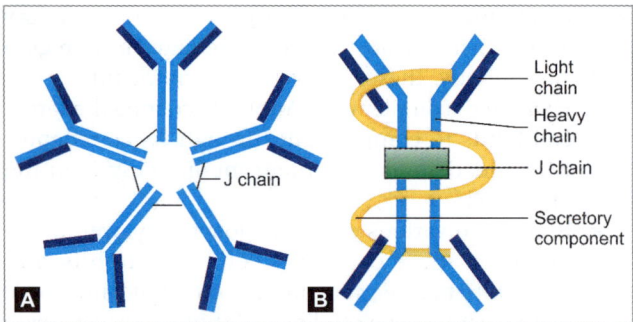

Figs. 7.3A and B: A. Pentameric IgM; **B.** Dimeric IgA.

- Protection against **intravascular organisms**: IgM being intravascular, is responsible for protection against blood invasion by microorganisms
- IgM mediates **agglutination** reaction.

Immunoglobulin A (IgA)

IgA is the second most abundant class of Ig next to IgG, constituting about 10–15% of total serum Ig. IgA exists as two isotypes such as IgA1 and IgA2. It exists in both monomeric and dimeric forms.
- **Serum IgA:** IgA in serum is predominantly in monomeric form
- **Secretory IgA:** It is dimeric in nature, with a valency of four; the two IgA monomeric units are joined by **J chain** (Fig. 7.3B)
    - *Location:* Secretory IgA is the predominant antibody found in body secretions like milk, saliva, tears, intestinal and respiratory tract mucosal secretions
    - *Function:* The secretory IgA mediates **local or mucosal immunity**; protects against pathogens by cross-linking the antigens and preventing their entry through the mucosal surfaces.

Immunoglobulin E (IgE)

Among all Ig, IgE is having the lowest serum concentration. It is also the only heat-labile antibody.
- IgE is highly potent and mediates **type I hypersensitivity** reactions by binding to the mast cells (*refer* **Chapter 11**)
- IgE is elevated in **helminthic infections**.

Immunoglobulin D (IgD)

IgD is found as membrane Ig on the surface of B cells and acts as a B cell receptor along with IgM.

Monoclonal Antibody

Monoclonal antibodies (mAb) are defined as the antibodies derived from a single clone of plasma cell; all having the same antigen specificity, i.e. produced against a single epitope of an antigen.

- **Production:** Monoclonal antibodies are produced by a method called as hybridoma technique
    - In the hybridoma technique, antibody-forming mouse splenic B cells are fused with myeloma cells (cancerous plasma cells) to produce hybridoma cells
    - These hybridoma cells can grow and survive long producing the desired antibody.
- **Uses:** mAb has various uses such as:
    - *Diagnostic reagents:* The antigen detection kits employ various mAb tagged with detection molecules, such as an enzyme, which detects the specific antigens in the clinical specimens by using various formats like ELISA, rapid tests, etc.
    - *Passive immunity:* For post-exposure prophylaxis against various infections, mAb targeting specific antigens of infecting organisms can be administered. Examples include—immunoglobulins against hepatitis B, rabies, and tetanus
    - *Therapeutic use:* Monoclonal antibodies are used in the treatment of various inflammatory conditions, allergic diseases, and cancers.

COMPLEMENT

The term 'complement' (C) represents a group of proteins normally found in the serum in an inactive form, but when activated they augment the immune responses. They constitute about 5% of normal serum proteins.

Complements have the following general properties:
- **Bind to Fc region of antibody:** The binding of complement to an antibody is described by various terms as, **fixing** or **consumption**
- **Role of antigen:** The classical pathway of complements do not bind to free antibodies but they can only fix those antibodies which are bound with antigens
- **Species nonspecific:** Complements from one species can react with antibodies from other species, though the efficiency decreases with an increase in taxonomic distance
- **Heat labile:** Complements get denatured by heating the serum at 56°C for 30 minutes. Such serum with lost complement activity is called **inactivated serum**.

Complement Components

The complement system comprises of about 30 serum proteins grouped into complement components, the properdin system and the regulatory proteins.
- **Components:** There are nine components; C1 to C9. C1 has three subunits—C1q, C1r and C1s. The properdin system and the regulatory proteins are named by letter symbols, e.g. factor-B.

CHAPTER 7 ◆ Antigen, Antibody and Complement

- ❖ **Synthesis:** The liver is the major site for the synthesis of complement proteins.
- ❖ **Complement activation:** All the complement proteins are synthesized in an inactive form and are activated by proteolysis. Complements have two unequal fragments (large and small fragments). During proteolysis, the smaller fragment is removed exposing the active site of the larger fragment, which participates in the cascade reaction of complement pathway.
- ❖ **Cascade reaction:** The fragments of complements interact in a definite sequential manner with a cascade-like effect, which leads to the formation of the complex. Such complex having enzymatic activity is designated by putting a bar over the number or symbol (e.g. $\overline{CbBb}$).

Complement Pathways

There are three pathways of complement activation:
1. **Classical pathway:** This is an antibody dependent pathway. Pathway is triggered by the antigen–antibody complex formation
2. **Alternative pathway:** This is an antibody independent pathway, triggered by the antigen directly
3. **Lectin pathway:** This is a recently described pathway. It resembles classical pathway, but it is antibody independent.

Stages of complement activation

There are four main stages in the activation of any of the complement pathways.
1. Initiation of the pathway
2. Formation of C3 convertase
3. Formation of C5 convertase
4. Formation of membrane attack complex (MAC).

All the three pathways **(Fig. 7.5)** differ from each other in their initiation till formation of C3 convertase. Then, the remaining stages are identical in all the pathways.

Classical Pathway

Classical pathway **(Fig. 7.5)** is antibody dependent. Decreasing order of ability of antibodies to fix complement is—IgM (most potent) > IgG3 > IgG1 > IgG2. The classical pathway begins with activation of C1 and binding to antigen–antibody complex.

Initiation

The first step is the binding of C1 to the antigen–antibody complex.
- ❖ The first binding portion of C1 is C1q, which reacts with the Fc portion of IgM or IgG bound to antigen
- ❖ Effective activation of classical pathway begins only when C1q is attached to the Fc portion of antibody by at least two of its globular binding sites
- ❖ C1q binds in presence of calcium ions, which in turn activates sequentially C1r followed by C1s.

Formation of C3 Convertase

Activated $\overline{C1s}$ acts as an esterase (C1s esterase), which can cleave C4 to produce C4a (an anaphylatoxin), and C4b which binds to C1 and participates further in complement cascade.
- ❖ $\overline{C14b}$ in the presence of magnesium ions cleaves C2 into C2a, which remains linked to complement complex, and C2b (has kinin like activity), which is released outside
- ❖ $\overline{C14b2a}$ is referred to as C3 convertase of the classical pathway.

Formation of C5 Convertase

C3 convertase hydrolyses many C3 molecules into two fragments: C3a (an anaphylatoxin) and C3b which remains attached to $\overline{C14b2a}$ to form $\overline{C14b2a3b}$ complex, which acts as C5 convertase of classical pathway.

Formation of Membrane Attack Complex

This phase begins with C5 convertase cleaving C5 into C5a (an anaphylatoxin, released into the medium) and C5b, which continues with the cascade.
- ❖ $\overline{C5b}$ is extremely labile, and gets stabilized by binding soon with C6 and C7 to form $\overline{C5b67}$ followed by addition of C8
- ❖ The hydrophobic regions on C7 and C8 help in penetration into the target cell membrane
- ❖ This inserted membrane complex ($\overline{C5b678}$) has a catalytic property to bind to C9 molecule
- ❖ Penetration of C9 causes the formation of channels or pores on the target cell membrane
- ❖ Because $\overline{C5b6789}$ destroys the target cell by attacking the cell membrane; it is called membrane attack complex (MAC) and the process of cytolysis is referred to as complement-mediated cytotoxicity **(Figs. 7.4 and 7.5)**.

Alternative Pathway

Alternative pathway **(Fig. 7.5)** is independent of antibody; hence is considered as a part of innate immunity. Unlike the classical pathway which involves all complement components from C1 to C9; in alternative pathway three

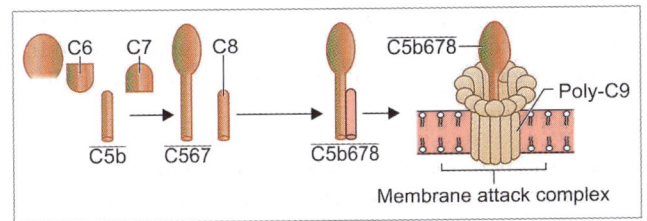

Fig. 7.4: Formation of membrane attack complex.

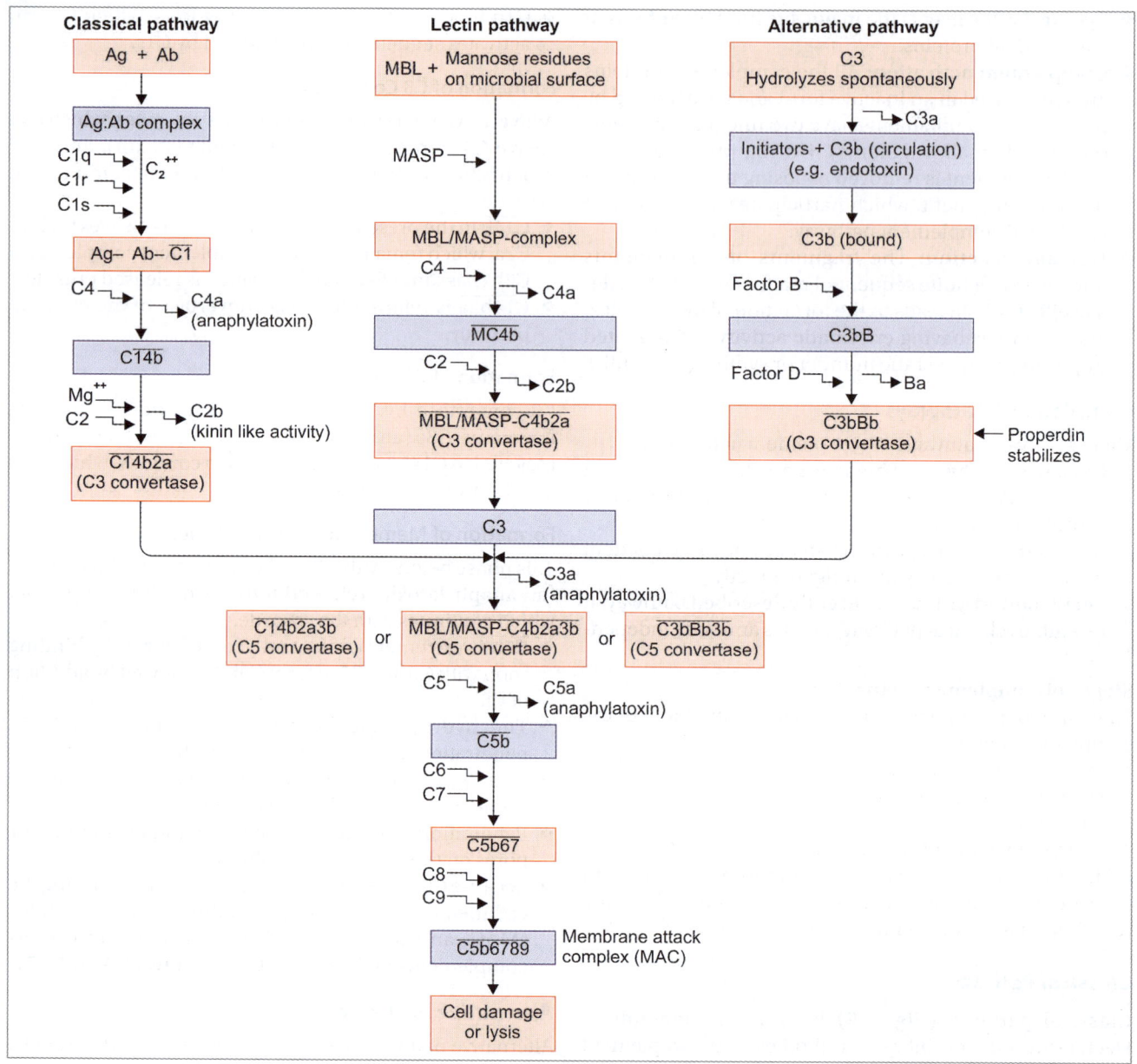

Fig. 7.5: The complement pathways.
(MBL, mannose binding lectins; MASP, MBL-associated serine protease)

complement components C1, C4 and C2 are not involved. Instead, it requires three other complement proteins present in serum named factor B, factor D and properdin.

Initiation

The alternative complement cascade is initiated by various cell surface constituents that are foreign to the host, e.g. bacterial endotoxin, teichoic acid from gram-positive bacteria, fungal cells, cobra venom factor, etc.

The first complement component to be involved in the alternative pathway is free C3 in the serum. C3 hydrolyzes spontaneously, to generate:
* C3a which diffuses out and
* C3b fragment which attaches to foreign cell surface antigen.

Formation of C3 Convertase

* In the next step, **Factor B** binds to C3b coated foreign cells

- **Factor D**, another alternative pathway complement factor, acts on factor B, and cleaves it into Ba (diffuses out) and Bb (remains attached)
- $\overline{C3bBb}$ is also called C3 convertase of alternative pathway
- $\overline{C3bBb}$ has a very short half-life of 5 minutes. If it is stabilized by another complement protein called properdin its half-life is increased to 30 minutes.

The remaining two stages, i.e. formation of C5 convertase and formation of membrane attack complex are identical to that of classical pathway.

Lectin Pathway

Lectin pathway is another complement pathway of innate immunity that works independent of antibody.
- It is mediated through lectin proteins of the host that interact with mannose residues present on microbial surface
- Lectin pathway involves all complement components used for classical pathways except C1 (i.e. from C2 to C9); instead of C1, host lectin protein called mannose binding lectins mediate the first 'initiation' stage (see **Fig. 7.5**)
- After binding of mannose binding lectins (MBL) to microbial surface, another host protein called MBL-associated serine protease (MASP) gets complexed with MBL (acute phase reactant protein, similar to C1q in structure)
- The remaining three stages are similar to the classical pathway.
- The MBL–MASP complex cleaves C4 which in turn splits C2 and the MBL/MASP-C4b2a act as C3 convertase.

Effector Functions of Complement

The membrane attack complex (MAC) and other complement by-products produced during the activation of complement pathways augment the immune response in many ways; which are collectively called as the effector functions of complement products. The functions are as follows:
- **Target cell lysis by MAC:** As already explained, bacteria, enveloped viruses, damaged cells, tumor cells, etc. are killed by complement-mediated cell lysis
- **Inflammatory response:** The complement byproducts such as C3a, C4a, and C5a induce mast cell degranulation leading to vasoconstriction, and increased vascular permeability
- **Opsonization:** Some complement byproducts (C3b and C4b) act as major opsonins and facilitate phagocytosis
- Complement helps in removing the immune complexes from blood
- **Viral neutralization:** Complements play a crucial role in the neutralization of viruses.

Evasion of Complement System by Microorganisms

In order to escape from the complement mediated effector mechanisms, microorganisms can develop various counter mechanisms to evade the complement system as follows:
- Thick peptidoglycan cell wall of gram-positive bacteria (*Staphylococcus, Streptococcus*) and polysaccharide side chain of gram-negative bacteria (*Escherichia coli, Salmonella*) can prevent membrane attack complex (MAC) insertion
- Elastases produced by *Pseudomonas* destroy C3a and C5a
- Bacterial capsule forms a physical barrier between C3b and CR1 interaction, e.g. *Streptococcus pneumoniae*.

Complement Deficiencies

Complement deficiency associated diseases fall into two categories; diseases associated with—(1) complement protein deficiencies and (2) complement regulator protein deficiencies **(Table 7.2)**.

Table 7.2: Complement deficiency diseases.		
Complement deficiencies	**Pathway(s) involved**	**Disease/pathology**
Complement protein deficiencies		
C1, C2, C3, C4	C1, C2, C4—classical pathway C3—common deficiency	Systemic lupus erythematosus (SLE), glomerulonephritis and pyogenic infections
Properdin, Factor D	Alternative pathway	*Neisseria* and pyogenic infection
Membrane attack complex (C5-C9)	Common deficiency	Disseminated *Neisseria* infection
Complement regulatory protein deficiencies		
C1 esterase inhibitor	Overactive classical pathway	Hereditary angioneurotic edema

EXPECTED QUESTIONS

I. Write essays on:
1. Define antibody. Describe in detail the structure and functions of various types of antibodies.
2. What is complement? Explain in detail about classical complement pathway. List various effector functions of complement.

II. Write short notes on:
1. Monoclonal antibodies and their applications.
2. The structure and function of IgG antibody.
3. The structure and function of IgA.
4. The structure and function of IgM.
5. Adjuvants.
6. Alternative complement pathway.

III. Multiple Choice Questions (MCQs):
1. Which antibody crosses the placenta?
   a. IgA b. IgG
   c. IgE d. IgM
2. What is the total vacancies of IgM?
   a. 10 b. 5
   c. 2 d. 1
3. Which antibody is elevated in acute infection?
   a. IgA b. IgG
   c. IgE d. IgM
4. Which antibody mediates mucosal immunity?
   a. IgA b. IgG
   c. IgE d. IgM
5. Endotoxin acts by:
   a. Classical pathway
   b. Lectin pathway
   c. Alternative pathway
   d. None
6. 70-80% total antibody is constituted by:
   a. IgA b. IgE
   c. IgG d. IgM
7. The most potent activator of classical complement pathway is:
   a. IgA b. IgM
   c. IgG d. IgE
8. Complement mediated cell lysis is done by:
   a. Anaphylatoxins
   b. Activation of apoptosis
   c. Membrane attack complex
   d. Inhibition of protein synthesis
9. Which part of the bacteria is most antigenic?
   a. Protein
   b. Carbohydrate
   c. Lipid
   d. Nucleic acid
10. The smallest determinant of antigenicity is called:
    a. Antigen b. Immunogen
    c. Epitope d. Paratope

Answers
1. b 2. a 3. d 4. a 5. c 6. c 7. b 8. c 9. a 10. c

Antigen–Antibody Reaction

CHAPTER 8

CHAPTER PREVIEW
- General Properties
- Conventional Immunoassays
  - Precipitation Reaction
  - Agglutination Reaction
- Newer Techniques
  - ELISA
  - Enzyme-linked Fluorescent Assay
  - Immunofluorescence Assay
- Chemiluminescence Immunoassay
- Western Blot
- Rapid Tests

The antigen (Ag)-antibody (Ab) reaction refers to the binding of antigen and antibody with each other specifically and in an observable manner.

GENERAL PROPERTIES OF ANTIGEN–ANTIBODY REACTIONS

Antigen (Ag)–antibody (Ab) reactions are characterized by the following general properties:
- **Specific:** Ag-Ab reaction involves specific interaction between the epitope of an antigen with the corresponding paratope of its homologous antibody
- **Noncovalent interactions:** The union of antigen and antibody requires the formation of a large number of noncovalent interactions between them
- **Immunoassays:** Because Ag-Ab reactions are specific and observable, they are extensively used in laboratories for the diagnosis of infectious diseases. Such assays are called immunoassays:
  - *Antigen detection assays:* Detect antigens in the patient's sample by employing a specific antibody
  - *Antibody detection assays:* Detect antibodies in a patient's sample by employing a specific antigen.
- **Serological tests:** Immunoassays can be developed for the detection of antigens or antibodies in various clinical specimens, the most common being serum specimen. The immunoassays that are designed specifically for testing on serum specimens are called serological tests
- **Titer:** The exact amount of antibody in serum can be estimated by serial dilution of the patient's serum and mixing each dilution of the serum with a known quantity of antigen. The measurement of antibodies is expressed in terms of titer
  - The antibody titer of serum is the highest dilution that shows an observable reaction with the antigen
- Antigen titer can also be similarly measured in the sera by testing the series of diluted sera against a known quantity of antibodies.

Lattice Hypothesis

When the sera-containing antibody is serially diluted (in normal saline), the antibody level gradually decreases.
- ❖ When a fixed quantity of antigen is added to such a set of test tubes containing serially diluted sera, then it is observed that the Ag-Ab reaction occurs at its best only in the middle test tubes where the amount of antigen and antibody are equivalent to each other (*zone of equivalence*)
- ❖ The Ag-Ab reaction is weak or fails to occur when the number of antigens and antibodies are not proportionate to each other **(Figs. 8.1A to C)**
  - In the earlier test tubes, *antibodies are excess*, hence the Ag-Ab reaction does not occur. This is called as **prozone phenomenon**

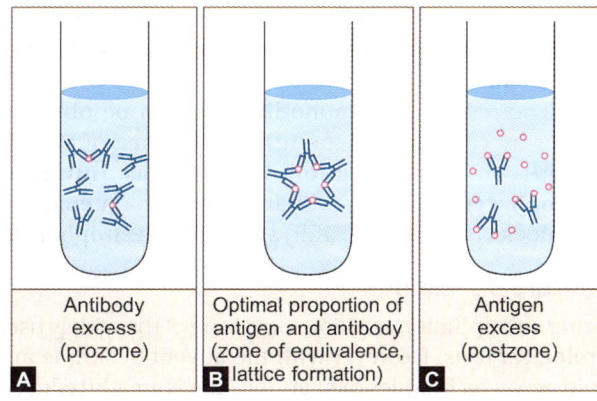

Figs. 8.1A to C: A. Prozone; **B.** Zone of equivalence; **C.** Postzone.

SECTION 2 ❖ Immunology

Table 8.1: Types of antigen–antibody reactions.

Conventional techniques	
• Precipitation reaction	• Complement fixation test
• Agglutination reaction	• Neutralization test
Newer techniques	
• Enzyme-linked immunosorbent assay (ELISA)	
• Enzyme-linked fluorescent assay (ELFA)	
• Immunofluorescence assay (IFA)	
• Chemiluminescence-linked immunoassay (CLIA)	
• Immunohistochemistry	

• Rapid tests
  ➤ Lateral flow assay (Immunochromatographic test)
  ➤ Flow through assay	

• Western blot	

■ In the later test tubes, *antigen* is *excess*, hence the Ag-Ab reaction fails to occur. This is called as **postzone phenomenon**.

TYPES OF ANTIGEN–ANTIBODY REACTIONS

The antigen–antibody reactions used in diagnostic laboratories are based on various techniques which are broadly classified as conventional techniques and newer techniques **(Table 8.1)**.

CONVENTIONAL IMMUNOASSAYS

■ PRECIPITATION REACTION

Definition

When a **soluble antigen** reacts with its antibody in the presence of optimal temperature, pH and electrolytes (NaCl), it leads to formation of the antigen–antibody complex in the form of:
❖ **Insoluble precipitation band** when gel or agar containing medium is used (called immunodiffusion) or
❖ **Insoluble floccules** when liquid medium is used (called flocculation test).

Note: The results of immunodiffusion can be obtained quicker by carrying out the test in presence of electric current. This modification is called as **immuno-electrophoresis**. It has two variants such as countercurrent immunoelectrophoresis (CIEP) and rocket electrophoresis.

Clinical Applications

Earlier, precipitation reactions were one of the widely used serological tests. However with the advent of simple and rapid newer techniques their application is greatly reduced. There are only limited situations where precipitation reaction is still in use; discussed below.

Slide Flocculation Test (for Syphilis)

It is used for serodiagnosis of syphilis, a sexually transmitted disease caused by *Treponema pallidum*.
❖ **Procedure:** When a drop of antigen is mixed with a drop of patient's serum (containing antibody) on a slide, then the precipitates formed remain suspended as floccules
❖ **Examples** include VDRL (Venereal Disease Research Laboratory) and RPR (Rapid Plasma Reagin) tests. Refer highlight box given below.

> **Venereal Disease Research Laboratory (VDRL)**
> This test was named after Venereal Disease Research Laboratory (VDRL), New York, where the test was developed. It works on the principle of precipitation (slide flocculation) test.
> ❑ **Procedure:** 50 μL of patient's serum (heat inactivated) is mixed with a drop of VDRL antigen on a concave slide, which is then mixed by rotating the slide for 4 minutes **(Figs. 8.2A and B)**
> ❑ **Result:** Positive test (i.e. reactive) is indicated by formation of medium to large clumps of antigen anti-body complexes; visualized by focusing the slide under microscope (10x)
> ❑ **CSF antibodies:** VDRL test can also be performed on CSF specimen to detect antibodies
> ❑ **Uses:** VDRL test is cheaper and preferred as a screening test for laboratory with higher sample load and for batch testing (e.g. antenatal screening) and also to monitor treatment response.

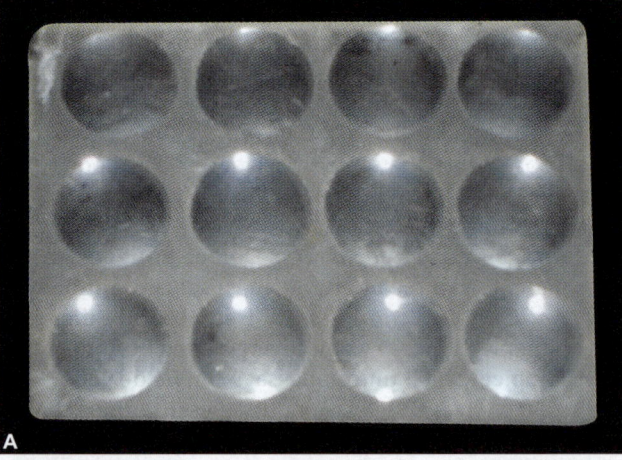

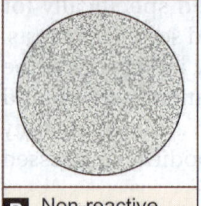
Non-reactive

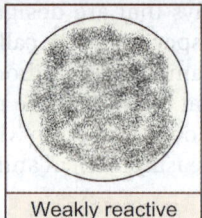
Weakly reactive

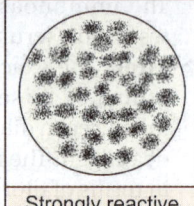
Strongly reactive

Figs. 8.2A and B: A. VDRL slide; **B.** VDRL test results.
Source: Department of Microbiology, JIPMER, Puducherry (*with permission*).

Rapid Plasma Reagin (RPR)
RPR is another slide flocculation test using disposable plastic cards having clearly defined circles. It is similar to VDRL test with some differences such as:
- RPR antigen has a prolonged shelf-life, therefore it is preferred to test individual sample (less sample load); whereas VDRL is preferred when samples are tested in batches (large sample load)
- Results can be read in naked eyes, without the need of a microscope, as the clumps formed are bigger in size
- It can only be used for detecting antibodies in blood; not in CSF
- It is more expensive than VDRL.

Elek's Gel Precipitation Test (Detecting Diphtheria Toxin)

The *Corynebacterium diphtheriae* strain isolated is streaked on to a medium containing a filter paper soaked with diphtheria antitoxin (*refer* **Chapter 24** for detail).
- If the strain is toxigenic, it produces the toxin, which diffuses in the agar, meets with the antitoxin and produces arrow-shaped precipitation band (*refer* **Fig. 24.3**)
- This test can also be used to know the relatedness between the strains isolated during an outbreak.

AGGLUTINATION REACTION

Definition
When a **particulate** or **insoluble** antigen is mixed with its antibody in the presence of electrolytes at a suitable temperature and pH, the particles are clumped or agglutinated.
- **Advantage:** Agglutination is more sensitive than precipitation test and the clumps are better visualized and interpreted as compared to bands or floccules
- **Applications:** Agglutination reactions are classified as direct, indirect (passive) and reverse passive agglutination reactions. All these agglutination tests are performed either on a slide, or in tube or in card or sometimes in microtiter plates.

Direct Agglutination Test
Here, the antigen directly agglutinates with the antibody.

Slide Agglutination
It is usually performed to confirm the identification and serotyping of bacterial colonies grown in culture. It is also the method used for blood grouping and cross matching.

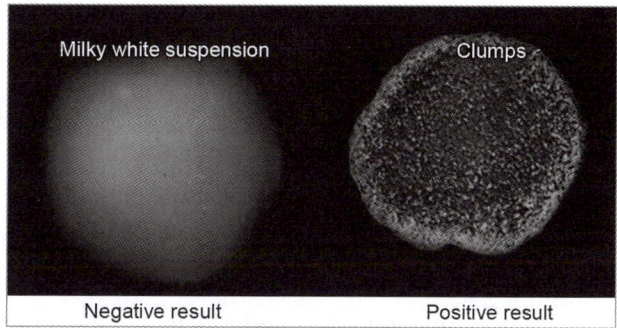

Fig. 8.3: Slide agglutination test.
Source: Department of Microbiology, JIPMER, Puducherry (*with permission*).

Bacterial colony is mixed with a drop of saline on a slide to form a uniform smooth milky white suspension
↓
To this, a drop of the antiserum (serum containing appropriate antibody) is added and the slide is shaken thoroughly (manually or by rotator) for few seconds
↓
A positive result is indicated by visible clumping with clearing of the suspension **(Fig. 8.3)**
or
If the milky white suspension remains unchanged, indicates a negative result **(Fig. 8.3)**

Tube Agglutination
This is a quantitative test done for estimating antibody in serum. The **antibody titer** can be estimated as the highest dilution of the serum which produces a visible agglutination.

A fixed volume of a particulate antigen suspension is added to an equal volume of serial dilutions of a serum sample (containing appropriate antibody) in test tubes
↓
Positive test indicates agglutination (clump formation at the bottom of the tube with clearing of the supernatant)
or
Negative test indicates agglutination has not occurred (Ag suspension forms button at the bottom of the tube)

Tube agglutination is routinely used for the serological diagnosis of various diseases, such as:
- Typhoid fever (Widal test): It detects antibodies against both H (flagellar) and O (somatic) antigens of *Salmonella* Typhi (explained in **Chapter 29**)
  - H antigen–antibody clumps appear as loose fluffy clumps

- O antigen–antibody clumps appear as chalky white granular dense deposits.
- ❖ Acute brucellosis (Standard agglutination test)
- ❖ Coombs antiglobulin test (explained later in this chapter)
- ❖ Heterophile agglutination tests:
  - Typhus fever (Weil-Felix reaction)
  - Infectious mononucleosis (Paul-Bunnell test)
  - *Mycoplasma* pneumonia (Cold agglutination test).

Microscopic Agglutination

Here, the agglutination test is performed on a microtiter plate and the result is read under a microscope. The classical example is microscopic agglutination test (MAT) done for leptospirosis.

Indirect or Passive Agglutination Test (for Antibody Detection)

As agglutination test is more sensitive and better interpreted than precipitation test, attempt has been made to convert a precipitation reaction into an agglutination reaction. This is possible by coating the soluble antigen on the surface of a carrier molecule (e.g. RBC, latex or bentonite), so that the antibody binds to the coated antigen and agglutination takes place on the surface of the carrier molecule.

Indirect Hemagglutination Test (IHA)

It is a passive agglutination test where RBCs are used as carrier molecules. IHA was used widely in the past, but is less popular at present.

Latex Agglutination Test (LAT) for Antibody Detection

Here, polystyrene latex particles (0.8–1 μm in diameter) are used as carrier molecules which are capable of adsorbing several types of antigens. For better interpretation of result, the test is performed on a black color card.
- ❖ Drop of patient's serum (containing antibody) is added to a drop of latex solution coated with the antigen and the card is rotated for uniform mixing
- ❖ Positive result is indicated by formation of visible clumps (Fig. 8.4). LAT is one of the most widely used tests at present as it is very simple and rapid
- ❖ It is used for detection of ASO (antistreptolysin O antibody).

Reverse Passive Agglutination Test (for Antigen Detection)

In this test, the antibody is coated on a carrier molecule which detects antigen in the patient's serum.
- ❖ **Reverse passive hemagglutination assay (RPHA):** Here, the RBCs are used as carrier molecules. RPHA was used in the past for detection of hepatitis B surface antigen (HBsAg); now obsolete
- ❖ **Latex agglutination test for antigen detection:** It is used widely for detection of CRP (C reactive protein),

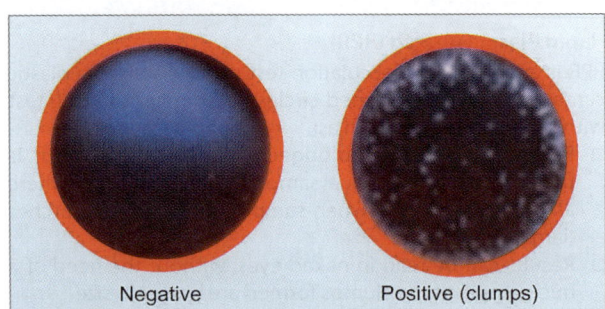

Fig. 8.4: Passive (latex) agglutination test.
Source: Department of Microbiology, JIPMER, Puducherry (*with permission*).

RA (rheumatoid arthritis factor), capsular antigen detection in CSF (for pneumococcus, meningococcus and *Cryptococcus*) and streptococcal grouping
- ❖ **Coagglutination test:** Here, *Staphylococcus aureus* (protein A) acts as carrier molecule. This test was used in the past to detect antigen from clinical specimens; now obsolete.

Hemagglutination Test

It refers to the agglutination tests that use RBCs as source of antigen. Hemagglutination tests are of two types: direct (described below) and indirect (or IHA, obsolete now).

Direct Hemagglutination Test

Serum antibodies directly agglutinate with surface antigens of RBCs to produce a matt. Examples include:
- ❖ **Paul-Bunnell test:** It employs sheep RBCs as antigens to detect Epstein-Barr virus antibodies in serum. The test is performed in tubes
- ❖ **Cold agglutination test:** It uses human RBCs as antigens to detect *Mycoplasma* antibodies in serum. Test is performed in tubes
- ❖ **Blood grouping** (ABO and Rh grouping)
- ❖ **Coombs test** or **antiglobulin test:** It is performed to diagnose Rh incompatibility by detecting Rh antibody from mother's and baby's serum.

Technical Issues in Agglutination Reactions

Two main problems pertaining to agglutination are prozone phenomenon and blocking antibody; both can cause false-negative agglutination test.
- ❖ **Prozone phenomenon:** Serum containing excess antibodies may fail to agglutinate with its antigen. This can be obviated by serial dilution of the serum and testing the antigen with each dilution of the serum sample
- ❖ **Blocking antibodies:** They are incomplete IgG antibodies. When they bind to antigens, they themselves cannot produce a visible agglutination. Such blocking antibodies may be detected by performing the test in hypertonic (4%) saline or more reliably by adding antiglobulin or Coombs reagent.

COMPLEMENT FIXATION TEST

Complement fixation test (CFT) detects the antibodies in patient's serum that are capable of fixing with complements. It was once very popular, now is almost obsolete.

Applications

- CFT was widely used for detection of complement fixing antibodies in *Rickettsia, Chlamydia, Mycoplasma* infections and some viral infections, such as arboviral infections
- Complements are also used for various other serological tests such as: *Treponema pallidum* immobilization test for syphilis and Sabin-Feldman dye test for *Toxoplasma*.

NEUTRALIZATION TEST

Neutralization tests are also less commonly used in modern days. Various examples are as follows:

- **Viral neutralization test:** It detects the presence of neutralizing antibody in patient's serum. When the serum is mixed with a live viral suspension and poured onto a cell line, specific serum antibody neutralizes the surface antigen, making the virus unable to infect a cell line
- **Plaque inhibition test:** This is done for bacteriophages
- **Toxin–antitoxin neutralization test:** Example includes—**Nagler's reaction** used for detection of α-toxin of *Clostridium perfringens*
- **Hemagglutination inhibition (HAI) test:** Antibodies in patient's sera can agglutinate with the hemagglutinin antigens present on the surfaces of some viruses. This test was used in the past for the diagnosis of various viral diseases, e.g. influenza.

NEWER TECHNIQUES

The newer techniques use a detector molecule to label antibody or antigen which in turn detects the corresponding antigen or the antibody in the sample by producing a visible effect **(Table 8.2)**.

ENZYME-LINKED IMMUNOSORBENT ASSAY

Enzyme-linked immunosorbent assay (ELISA) is an immunoassay that detects either antigen or antibodies in the specimen, by using enzyme–substrate–chromogen system for detection.

Principle of ELISA

ELISA is so named because of its two components:
- **Immunosorbent:** Here, an absorbing material is used (e.g. polystyrene, polyvinyl) that specifically absorbs the antigen or antibody present in serum
- **Enzyme** is used to label one of the components of immunoassay (i.e. antigen or antibody).

Substrate-chromogen system: A substrate-chromogen system is added at the final step of ELISA.
- The enzyme reacts with the substrate, which in turn activates the chromogen to produce a color
- The classical example is, horseradish peroxidase used as enzyme which reacts with its substrate (hydrogen peroxide), that in turn activates the chromogen (tetramethyl benzidine) to produce a color
- The color change is detected by spectrophotometry in an ELISA reader. Intensity of the color is directly proportional to the amount of the detection molecule (Ag or Ab) present in test serum.

> (Ag-Ab complex)-enzyme + substrate → activates the chromogen → color change → detected by spectrophotometry (ELISA reader, **Fig. 8.5A**)

Procedure of ELISA

ELISA is performed on a microtiter plate containing 96 wells **(Fig. 8.6)**, made up of polystyrene, polyvinyl or polycarbonate material.
- ELISA kits are commercially available; contain all necessary reagents (such as enzyme conjugate, dilution buffer, substrate/chromogen, etc.)

Table 8.2: Immunoassays and the types of molecule used for labeling.			
Abbreviation	Immunoassay method	Molecules used for labeling	Type of visible effect
ELISA	Enzyme-linked immunosorbent assay	Enzyme-substrate-chromogen complex	Color change is detected by spectrophotometer
ELFA	Enzyme-linked fluorescent assay	Enzyme-substrate	Fluorometric detection
IFA	Immunofluorescence assay	Fluorescent dye	Emits light, detected by fluorescence microscope
CLIA	Chemiluminescence-linked immunoassay	Chemiluminescent compounds	Emits light, detected by luminometer
IHC	Immunohistochemistry	Enzyme or fluorescent dye	Color change (naked eye) or fluorescence microscope
WB	Western blot	Enzyme	Color band (naked eye)
Rapid tests	Immunochromatographic test	Colloidal gold or silver	Color band (naked eye)
	Flow-through assay	Protein A conjugate	Color band (naked eye)

Note: Radioimmunoassay (RIA) is used for quantitative detection of hormones, drugs or microbial antigens. Because of the radiohazard associated, its use is reduced.

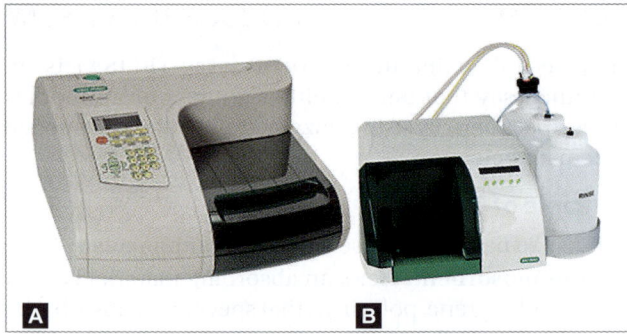

Figs. 8.5A and B: A. ELISA reader (Biorad); **B.** ELISA washer.
Source: Biorad Pvt. Ltd (*with permission*).

- The procedure involves a series of steps done sequentially. At each step, a reagent is being added, and then incubated, followed by washing of the wells [manually or by an automated ELISA washer **(Fig. 8.5B)**].

Types of ELISA

There are several types of ELISA, which differ from each other in their principles.

Direct ELISA

It is used for detection of antigen in test serum. Here, the primary antibody (targeted against the serum antigen) is labeled with the enzyme.
- **Step 1:** Wells of microtiter plate are empty, not precoated with Ag or Ab
- **Step 2:** Test serum (containing antigen) is added into the wells. Antigen becomes attached to the solid phase by passive adsorption
- **Step 3:** After washing, the enzyme-labeled primary antibodies (raised in rabbits) are added
- **Step 4:** After washing, a substrate–chromogen system is added and color is measured.

> Well + Ag (test serum) + primary Ab-Enzyme + substrate-chromogen → Color change **(Fig. 8.7A)**

Indirect ELISA

It is used for detection of antibody or less commonly antigen in serum. It differs from the direct ELISA in that the secondary antibody is labeled with enzyme instead of primary antibody. The secondary antibody is an anti-species antibody, e.g. anti-human Ig (an antibody targeted to Fc region of any human Ig). Indirect ELISA for antibody detection is described below **(Fig. 8.7B)**.
- **Step 1:** The solid phase of the wells of microtiter plates are precoated with the Ag
- **Step 2:** Test serum (containing primary Ab specific to the Ag) is added to the wells. Ab gets attached to the Ag coated on the well

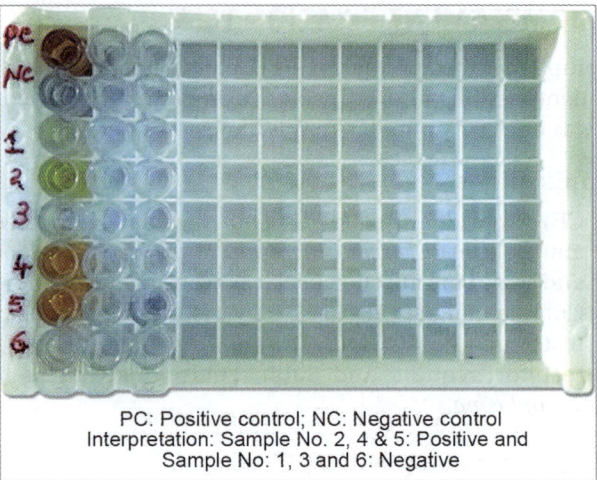

PC: Positive control; NC: Negative control
Interpretation: Sample No. 2, 4 & 5: Positive and Sample No: 1, 3 and 6: Negative

Fig. 8.6: ELISA for HBsAg.
Source: Department of Microbiology, Pondicherry Institute of Medical Sciences, Puducherry (*with permission*).

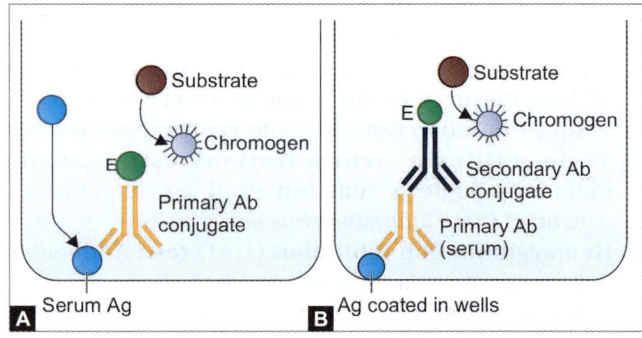

Figs. 8.7A and B: A. Direct ELISA (for antigen detection); **B.** Indirect ELISA (for antibody detection).

- **Step 3:** After washing, enzyme-labeled secondary Ab (anti-human immunoglobulin) is added
- **Step 4:** After washing, a substrate-chromogen system is added and color is developed.

> Wells are coated with Ag + primary Ab (test serum) + secondary Ab-enzyme + substrate-chromogen → development of color **(Fig. 8.7B)**

Sandwich ELISA

It detects the antigen in test serum. It is so named because the antigen gets sandwiched between a capture antibody and a detector antibody **(Fig. 8.8A)**.

> Wells precoated with capture Ab + Ag (test serum) + primary (detector) Ab-enzyme + substrate–chromogen → color **(Fig. 8.8A)**

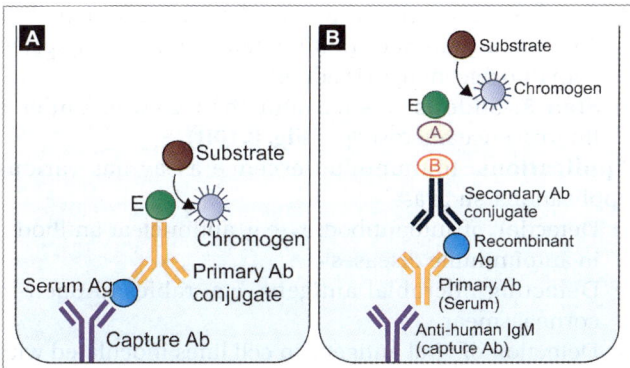

Figs. 8.8A and B: A. Sandwich ELISA (for antigen detection); **B.** IgM antibody capture (MAC) ELISA.

IgM Antibody Capture (MAC) ELISA

This is an enzymatically amplified sandwich-type immunoassay. This format of ELISA is widely used for dengue, Japanese encephalitis and West Nile virus, scrub typhus, leptospirosis, toxoplasmosis, etc. **(Fig. 8.8B).**
- It is based on capturing primary IgM Ab (in test serum) on a microtiter plate pre-coated with anti-human-IgM Ab, followed by addition of recombinant antigen (e.g. dengue antigen)
- Subsequently, enzyme labeled secondary antibody specific for the antigen is added, followed by addition of substrate-chromogen system
- The use of avidin-biotin system helps in amplifying the signal generated between enzyme-antibody complex, thus increases the sensitivity of the assay.

> Wells coated with capture anti-IgM Ab + IgM Ab (test serum) + recombinant antigen + secondary Ab-biotin +avidin-enzyme + substrate–chromogen → color **(Fig. 8.8B)**

Advantages of ELISA

ELISA is the method of choice for detection of antigens/antibodies in serum in modern days, especially in big laboratories as large number of samples can be tested together using the 96 well microtiter plate.
- It is economical, takes 2–3 hours for performing the assay
- ELISA has a high sensitivity; that is why, it is commonly used for performing screening test at blood banks and tertiary care sites
- Its specificity used to be low. But now, with use of more purified recombinant and synthetic antigens, and monoclonal antibodies, ELISA has become more specific.

Disadvantages of ELISA
- In small laboratories having less sample load, ELISA is less preferred than rapid tests
- It takes more time (2–3 hours) compared to rapid tests which take 10–20 minutes
- It needs expensive equipment such as ELISA washer and reader.

Applications of ELISA

ELISA can be used both for antigen and antibody detection.
- ELISA used for antigen detection: Hepatitis B [hepatitis B surface antigen (HBsAg) and precore antigen (HBeAg)], NS1 antigen for dengue, etc.
- ELISA can also be used for antibody detection against hepatitis B, hepatitis C, HIV, dengue, EBV, HSV, etc.

ENZYME-LINKED FLUORESCENT ASSAY (ELFA)

It is an modification of ELISA, differs from ELISA in two ways: (i) automated system, all steps are performed by the instrument itself, (ii) Ag-Ab-enzyme complex is detected by fluorometric method. VIDAS and miniVIDAS (bioMérieux) are commercially available systems based on ELFA technology **(Fig. 8.9)**.
- **Advantages:** It has many advantages over ELISA: (i) an automated system, (ii) easy to perform and user friendly, (iii) less contamination chance, (iv) gives quantitative results and (v) more sensitive and specific
- **Disadvantages:** (i) Expensive, (ii) can run only 12–30 number of tests of a single parameter at a time, (iii) limited number of parameters can be tested at the same time
- **Use:** It can be used to detect numerous parameters
  - *Infectious diseases:* Markers of hepatitis viruses and HIV (Ag and Ab), Ab to TORCH infection, dengue, SARS-CoV-2, and antigen of rotavirus, etc.
  - *Other uses:* Biomarkers (e.g. procalcitonin), hormones, tumor markers and screening for allergy.

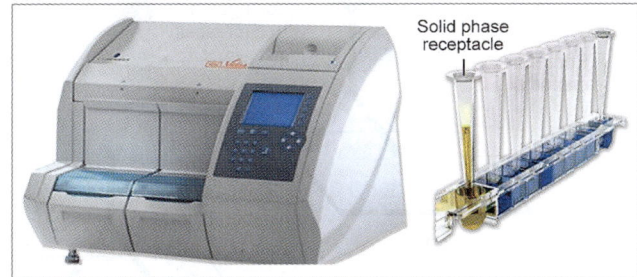

Fig. 8.9: miniVIDAS system and reagent strip (first well is solid phase receptacle coated with Ag or Ab and other wells contain various reagents).

Source: Department of Microbiology, JIPMER, Puducherry (*with permission*).

IMMUNOFLUORESCENCE ASSAY (IFA)

It is a technique similar to ELISA, but differs by some important features:
- Fluorescent dye is used instead of enzyme for labeling of antibody
- It detects cell surface antigens. It is also used to detect antibodies bound to cell surface antigens, unlike ELISA which detects free antigen or antibody.

Principle

Fluorescence refers to absorbing high energy-shorter wavelength ultraviolet light rays by the fluorescent compounds and in turn emitting visible light rays with a low energy-longer wavelength.
- The fluorescent dye is used to conjugate the antibody and such labeled antibody can be used to detect the antigens or antigen–antibody complexes on the cell surface
- The fluorescent compounds commonly used is fluorescein isothiocyanate (FITC).

Types

Direct Immunofluorescence Assay

- **Step 1:** Sample containing cells carrying surface antigens is smeared on a slide
- **Step 2:** Primary antibody specific to the antigen, tagged with fluorescent dye is added
- **Step 3:** Slide is washed to remove the unbound antibodies and then viewed under a fluorescence microscope **(Fig. 8.10A)**.

Indirect Immunofluorescence Assay

This detects antibodies in sample. Slides smeared with cells carrying known antigens are commercially available.
- **Step 1:** Test serum containing primary antibody is added to the slide
- **Step 2:** Slide is washed to remove the unbound antibodies. A secondary antibody (antihuman antibody conjugated with fluorescent dye) is added
- **Step 3:** Slide is washed and then viewed under a fluorescence microscope **(Fig. 8.10B)**.

Applications: Immunofluorescence assay has various applications, such as:
- Detection of autoantibodies (e.g. antinuclear antibody) in autoimmune diseases
- Detecting microbial antigens, e.g. rabies antigen in corneal smear
- Detection of viral antigens in cell lines inoculated with the specimens.

Flow Cytometry

Flow cytometry is a laser-based technology that quantitatively analyses and separates the cells as they pass through the laser beam. Flow cytometry can be used to analyze multiple parameters of cells (e.g. leukocytes) such as cell counting, cell sorting, analysis of size, shape, granularity, DNA or RNA content of a cell, etc. It is useful for estimation of CD4 T cell count in HIV infected patients.

CHEMILUMINESCENCE IMMUNOASSAY (CLIA)

Chemiluminescence refers to the emission of light (luminescence), as a result of a chemical reaction. The principle of CLIA is similar to that of ELISA; however, the chromogenic substance is replaced by chemiluminescent compounds (e.g. luminol and acridinium ester) that generate light during a chemical reaction (luxogenic). The light (photons) can be detected by a photomultiplier, also called as luminometer **(Fig. 8.11)**.

(Ag-Ab complex)-enzyme (e.g. HRP) + chemiluminescent substrate (e.g. luminol and acridinium ester) → product + light (photons) → detected by luminometer or photomultiplier.

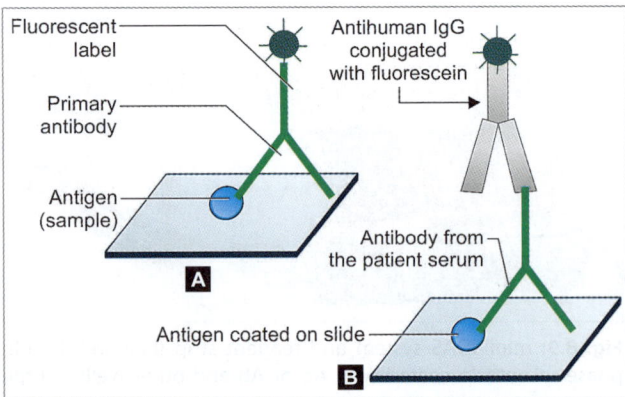

Figs. 8.10A and B: Immunofluorescence assay: **A.** Direct; **B.** Indirect.

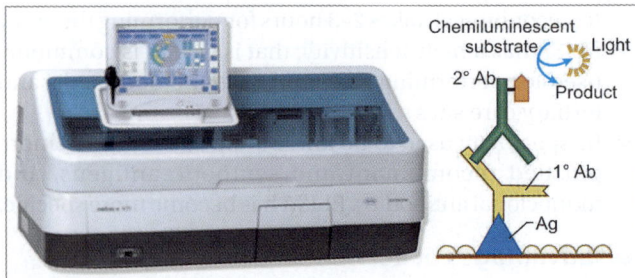

Fig. 8.11: Chemiluminescence system (CLIA) and its principle.
Source: Department of Microbiology, JIPMER, Puducherry (*with permission*).

Advantages of CLIA

CLIA claims to be 10 times more sensitive than ELISA.
* CLIA can be further modified by using an enhancer that potentiates the chemical reaction.
* Most samples have no 'background' signal, i.e. luminol compounds do not themselves emit light
* Measurement of chemiluminescence is not a ratio unlike the measurement of fluorescence (IFA) and or color (ELISA)
* Individual specimens can be tested.

Applications

CLIA has limited applications in diagnostic microbiology compared to ELISA. Currently, it is available for detection of antigens or antibodies against various infections such as hepatitis viruses, HIV, TORCH infections and biomarkers such as procalcitonin.

WESTERN BLOT

Western blot detects specific proteins (antibodies) in a sample containing a mixture of antibodies each targeted against different antigens of the same microbe.
* **Procedure:** It has three steps: (i) separation of antigen mixture into individual antigen fragments by *gel electrophoresis* according to their molecular weight, (ii) transfer of antigen fragments onto a *nitrocellulose membrane*, (iii) detection of individual antibodies in serum against each antigenic fragments by *enzyme immunoassay*
* **Advantages:** Western blot has excellent specificity. Hence, it is often used as a supplementary test to confirm the result of ELISA or other immunoassays having higher sensitivity.
* **Applications:** Western blot formats are available to detect antibodies in various diseases such as HIV, cysticercosis, hydatid disease, etc.

RAPID TESTS

Rapid tests are revolutionary in the diagnosis of infectious diseases. They are very simple to perform (one step method), rapid (takes 10–20 minutes), require minimal training, do not need any sophisticated instruments.
* These tests are also called **point-of-care** (POC) tests; as they can be performed independent of laboratory equipment and deliver instant results
* Two principles of rapid tests are available—lateral flow assay and flow through assay
* Both the formats are available for the diagnosis of various diseases such as malaria, hepatitis B, hepatitis C, HIV, leptospirosis, *Helicobacter pylori*, syphilis, etc.

Immunochromatographic Test (Lateral Flow Assay)

Immunochromatographic test (ICT) is based on lateral flow technique. It is widely used in diagnostic laboratories because of its simplicity, low-cost and rapidity. It can be used for both antigen and antibody detection in sample. Principle of antigen detection method is described below.

Principle of ICT (Antigen Detection)

The test system consists of a nitrocellulose membrane (NCM) and an absorbent pad. Two formats are available: cassette or strip **(Figs. 8.12A and B)**. The NCM is coated at two places in the form of lines—a test line, coated with monoclonal antibody targeted against the test antigen and a control line, coated with anti-species immunoglobulin. Specific Ab against the target Ag labelled with chromogenic marker (specific Ab tagged with *colloidal gold* or *silver*, a visually detectable marker) is infiltrated in the absorbent pad lining the sample window.
* The sample (serum) containing the test antigen is added to sample well; it reacts with antibody labeled with chromogenic marker (*colloidal gold* or *silver*, a visually detectable marker)
* Both 'Ag-specific Ab-colloidal gold complex' as well as the 'free colloidal gold labeled Ab' move laterally along the nitrocellulose membrane
* **Test band:** At the test line, the Ag-labeled Ab complex is immobilized by binding to the monoclonal Ab in the test line to form a colored band **(Fig. 8.12)**
* **Control band:** The free colloidal gold labeled Ab can move further and binds to the anti-human Ig to form a color control band. If the control band is not formed, then the test is considered invalid irrespective of whether the test band is formed or not **(Fig. 8.12)**.

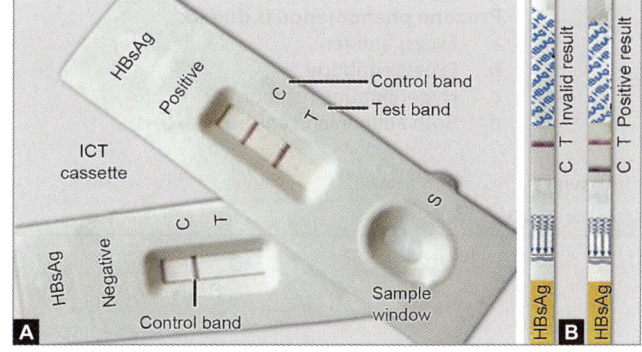

Figs. 8.12A and B: ICT for HBsAg detection:
A. Cassette format; **B.** Strip format.
Source: Department of Microbiology, Pondicherry Institute of Medical sciences, Puducherry (*with permission*).

Flow-through Assay

Flow-through tests are another type of rapid diagnostic assays which differ from ICT in two aspects: (1) protein A is used for labeling antibody instead of gold conjugate and (2) the sample flows vertically through the nitrocellulose membrane (NCM) as compared to lateral flow in ICT.

Flow-through tests can be used for both antigen and antibody detection. HIV TRIDOT test is a classical example (Fig. 8.13A). It detects antibodies to HIV-1 and 2 separately in patient's serum.

❖ The test system is in a cassette format, consisting of a NCM and an absorbent pad. The NCM is coated at three regions- two test regions coated with HIV-1 and 2 antigens and a third control region coated with antihuman Ig
❖ Sample and buffer reagents are added sequentially from the top following which they pass through the membrane and excess fluid is absorbed into the underlying absorbent pad
❖ As the patient's sample passes through the membrane, HIV antibodies, if present bind to the immobilized antigens (Fig. 8.13B)

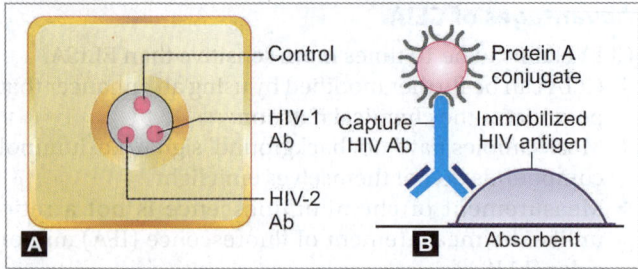

Figs. 8.13A and B: Flow-through assays: **A.** HIV TRI-DOT assay for HIV 1 and 2 antibodies detection; **B.** Principle of HIV TRI-DOT.

❖ **Test dots:** Protein-A conjugate (present in buffer) binds to the Fc portion of the HIV antibodies to give distinct pinkish purple DOT(s), separately for HIV-1 and 2 antibodies
❖ **Control dot:** Irrespective of whether the HIV antibodies are present or not, protein-A can bind to any IgG present in serum and the IgG-protein A complex can further bind to the antihuman Ig at the control line to give a pinkish purple DOT.

EXPECTED QUESTIONS

I. Write essays on:
1. Enumerate the properties and types of antigen–antibody reactions. Describe in detail about the principle, types, and applications of ELISA?
2. Describe in detail about the principle, types, and applications of agglutination reaction?

II. Write short notes on:
1. Indirect immunofluorescence assay.
2. Immunochromatographic test.

III. Multiple Choice Questions (MCQs):
1. Prozone phenomenon is due to:
   a. Excess antigen
   b. Excess antibody
   c. Hyperimmune reaction
   d. Both antigen and antibody excess

2. All are agglutination reactions, *except*:
   a. VDRL test
   b. Standard agglutination test
   c. Widal test
   d. Paul-Bunnell test

3. The following methods of diagnosis utilize labeled antibodies, *except*:
   a. ELISA
   b. CLIA
   c. Precipitation test
   d. Immunofluorescence

4. Tridot test for HIV that detects antibodies is an example for:
   a. Western blot
   b. Lateral flow assay
   c. Flow through assay
   d. Immunochromatography

Answers
1. b   2. a   3. c   4. c

Components of Immune System: Organs, Cells and Products

CHAPTER 9

CHAPTER PREVIEW

- Lymphoid Organs—Central and Peripheral Lymphoid Organs
- Lymphoid Cells—T Cells, B Cells and NK Cells
- Other Cells of Immune System
- Major Histocompatibility Complex
- Cytokines

The immune system comprises of lymphoid organs, cells of the immune system and their soluble products called cytokines **(Table 9.1)**.

LYMPHOID ORGANS

Lymphoid organs consist of central and peripheral lymphoid organs.

Central or Primary Lymphoid Organs

The central lymphoid organs are the site for the development of immune cells. Examples include bone marrow and thymus.

Bone Marrow

Almost all the cells in blood have originated from pluripotent hematopoietic stem cells of bone marrow and the process is called hematopoiesis.

- As the individual ages, hematopoietic activity in large bones decreases and after puberty, hematopoiesis is mostly confined to axial bones such as the pelvis, vertebrae, sternum, skull, and ribs
- The progenitor T and B cells originate in bone marrow. Further development of B cells occurs in the bone marrow itself, whereas the progenitor T cells migrate to the thymus for further proliferation.

Thymus

Thymus is the site of proliferation and maturation of T cells. It is highly active at birth, continues to grow for many years, reaches its peak size at puberty, and then degenerates.

Structure

It has an outer cortex and an inner medulla.

- **Cortex** is densely populated and contains thymocytes (lymphocytes of thymus), epithelial cells, and nurse cells (specialized epithelial cells with long membrane extensions that surround thymocytes).
- **Medulla** is sparsely populated and contains thymocytes, epithelial cells, interdigitating dendritic cells, and **Hassall's corpuscles** (concentric layers of degenerating epithelial cells).

Maturation of T Cells

- The cell-to-cell interaction between thymocytes, epithelial cells, dendritic cells, and macrophages and the effect of thymic hormones help in the maturation of T cells in the thymus.
- Any defect in the thymus leads to a defect in the maturation of T-lymphocytes that in turn results in severe life-threatening immunodeficiency disorders.

Central Tolerance

Only 2–5% of the developing T cells become mature and released out from the thymus; remaining T cells are destroyed as they are either not capable of recognizing

Table 9.1: Structure of the immune system.

Lymphoid organs: Consist of central and peripheral lymphoid organs
• **Central or primary lymphoid organs,** e.g. thymus and bone marrow: They host the development of immune cells (hematopoiesis)
• **Peripheral or secondary lymphoid organs,** e.g. lymph node, spleen, and mucosa-associated lymphoid tissue (MALT)
Lymphoid cells: Consist of lymphocytes such as T cells, B cells and NK cells
Other cells of immune system: Include phagocytes, such as macrophage and microphages (neutrophil, eosinophil and basophil), dendritic cells, and mast cells
Cytokines: Include interleukins, interferons, tumor necrosis factors, colony-stimulating factors, etc.

major histocompatibility complex (MHC) or are believed to be self-reacting in nature.
- Destruction of such self-reacting T cells prevents the development of autoimmunity (immune response against self-antigens)
- Such tolerance to self-antigens mediated by the thymus that occurs in embryonic life is called central tolerance.

Peripheral or Secondary Lymphoid Organs

Lymph Node

Lymph nodes are small bean-shaped organs; they occur in clusters or chains, distributed along the length of lymphatic vessels. They act as filters for the microbial antigens carried to lymph nodes by activating the T and B cells.

Structure

Lymph node is divided into three parts—(1) cortex, (2) medulla (both are B cell areas) and (3) paracortex (T cell area). Cortex is surrounded by a capsule.
- **Cortex:** It contains lymphoid follicles. The lymphoid follicles are of two types:
  1. **Primary lymphoid follicles:** They are found before the antigenic stimulus. They are smaller in size and mainly contain the resting B cells
  2. **Secondary lymphoid follicles:** Following contact with an antigen, the resting B cells start dividing and become activated to differentiate into plasma cells (which produce antibodies) and memory B cells. Follicles become larger and are called secondary lymphoid follicles. They have two areas:
     i. The central area called the **germinal center** contains dividing B cells of various stages.
     ii. The peripheral zone called **mantle area** contains activated B cells.
- **Paracortical area:** It is present in between cortex and medulla. It is the **T cell area** of the lymph node.
- **Medulla:** It is the innermost area of the lymph node, rich in B-lymphocytes; mainly plasma cells.

Spleen

Spleen is the largest secondary lymphoid organ. It acts as a physiological barrier in clearing the microbial antigens through the stimulation of T and B cells.

Structure

Spleen is situated below the diaphragm on the left side of the abdomen. It is divided into two compartments—(1) central white pulp and (2) outer red pulp, surrounded by a capsule.
- **White pulp:** It is the central densely populated area, which contains T cells-rich area and a **marginal zone** consisting of B cell lymphoid follicles (primary and secondary) and macrophages.
- **Red pulp:** It is the area that surrounds the sinusoids. It is filled with red blood cells (RBCs). The older and defective RBCs are destroyed here.

As the spleen is the site of destruction of most of the microbes, functional or structural abnormalities of the spleen or splenectomy, often lead to an increased incidence of bacterial sepsis caused primarily by capsulated bacteria such as *Streptococcus pneumoniae*, *Neisseria meningitidis*, etc.

Mucosa-associated Lymphoid Tissue (MALT)

The group of lymphoid tissues lining the mucosal sites (e.g. respiratory or intestinal) is collectively known as MALT.
- They are present either as loose clusters of lymphoid cells or as organized structures such as tonsils, appendix, and Peyer's patches
- They provide immunity at the local sites by encountering the pathogen entry.

■ LYMPHOID CELLS

Cells of the immune system comprise of lymphoid cells or lymphocytes and other cells such as phagocytes (e.g. macrophages and granulocytes), etc.
- **CD molecules:** Cluster of differentiation (CD) molecules are cell surface markers useful for the identification of cells of the immune system. They have numerous functions, and often act as surface receptors; important examples are CD4 and CD8 molecules—expressed by helper T cells and cytotoxic T cells respectively.
- **Types of lymphocytes:** Based on function and cell membrane structure, lymphocytes can be of three types—(1) T lymphocytes, (2) B lymphocytes and (3) natural killer (NK) cells.

Naïve Lymphocytes and Lymphoblasts

The T and B lymphocytes can also be classified into naïve lymphocytes and lymphoblasts.

Naïve Lymphocytes

They are resting B and T lymphocytes that have not interacted with any antigen. They are also known as small lymphocytes and they have a short-life span (1–3 months).

Lymphoblasts

When the naïve cells interact with antigen in the presence of certain cytokines (e.g. interleukin-7), they become activated and transform into lymphoblasts, which eventually differentiate into effector cells or memory cells.
- **Effector cells** function in various ways to eliminate antigen.
  - They have short-life span (few days to few weeks) and they are large lymphocytes (15 µm in size).

CHAPTER 9 ❖ Components of Immune System: Organs, Cells and Products

- Antibody-producing plasma cells is effector B cells; whereas effector T cells include helper T cells and cytotoxic T cells.
- **Memory cells:** They remain dormant like naïve cells but are capable of transforming into effector cells rapidly on the subsequent antigenic challenge.
  - They have a longer life span
  - They provide long-term immunity against many pathogens.

T Lymphocytes

T cells constitute 70–80% of blood lymphocytes. They bear specialized surface receptors called T cell receptors (TCR). Their main function is antigen recognition. It can only respond to an antigen that is processed and presented by the antigen-presenting cells, such as macrophages.

T Cell Development

T cell maturation takes place in the thymus.
- The progenitor T cells originate from the bone marrow and then migrate to the thymus through the bloodstream
- Developing T cells pass through a series of stages that are marked by characteristic changes in their cell surface markers
- Most of the development events take place in the cortex of the thymus, under the influence of thymic stromal cells which secrete thymic hormones and lymphopoietic growth factor IL-7.

Types of T Cells

There are two types of T cells—(1) $CD4^+$ helper T cells and (2) $CD8^+$ cytotoxic T cells.
- **Helper T (T_H) cells:** They possess CD4 molecules as surface receptors. They recognize the antigenic peptides that are processed by antigen-presenting cells and presented along with MHC-II molecules (major histocompatibility complex)
  - Following antigenic stimulus, the helper T cells differentiate into either of the two types of cells—(1) T_H1 and (2) T_H2 subset
  - T_H1 cells secrete specific cytokines such as IL-2, interferon-gamma which modulate the cellular immune response
  - T_H2 cells secrete specific cytokines such as IL-4, IL-5, and IL-6 which modulate the humoral immune response.
- **Cytotoxic T cells:** In contrast to T_H cells, cytotoxic T cells (T_C) possess CD8 molecules and recognize the intracellular antigens (e.g. viral antigens or tumor antigens) that are processed by any nucleated cells and presented along with MHC-I. In general, T_C cells are involved in the destruction of virus-infected cells and tumor cells.

B Lymphocytes

B lymphocytes are the mediators of humoral immunity; constitute 10–15% of blood lymphocytes. B cells proliferate through various stages, first in bone marrow, and then in peripheral lymphoid organs.
- Following antigenic stimulus, the mature B cells transform into activated B cells (lymphoblasts) which further differentiate into either effector B cells, i.e. plasma cells (majority) or memory B cells
- **Plasma cells** are antibody-secreting cells
- B cells produce five classes of antibodies, which in turn have various biological functions (discussed in **Chapter 7**).

Natural Killer Cells

Natural killer (NK) cells are large granular lymphocytes that constitute 10–15% of peripheral blood lymphocytes. They are derived from a separate lymphoid lineage. Similar to cytotoxic T cells, NK cells also are involved in the destruction of virus-infected cells and tumor cells (described in **Chapter 10**).

Other Cells of Immune System

Macrophages

Macrophages play a vital role in host defense by performing two important functions— (1) phagocytosis and (2) antigen presentation.
- **Phagocytosis:** Macrophages are the principal cells involved in phagocytosis. They also remove old dying cells from the body **(Fig. 9.1)**.
  - Phagocytosis is a process by which microbes are ingested by the formation of phagosome (vacuole) and subsequently fusion of lysosome with phagosome to form phagolysosome
  - Killing of the ingested microbes by producing various lysosomal enzymes and free radicals.

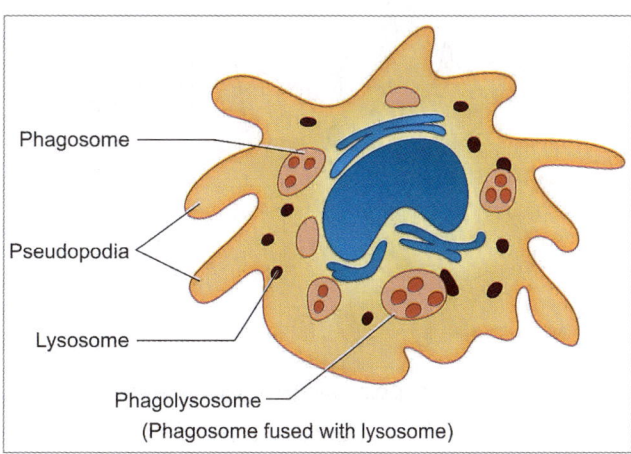

Fig. 9.1: Macrophage.

❖ **Antigen presentation:** Macrophages also promote acquired immunity, by acting as antigen-presenting cells (APCs). Macrophages capture the antigen, process it into smaller antigenic peptides, and present the antigenic peptides along with the MHC class II molecules to the helper T cells; thus, facilitating helper T cell activation. Examples of macrophages present in various body sites include—(i) Kupffer cells in the liver, (ii) microglial cells in the brain, (iii) alveolar macrophages in the lungs, etc.

Activated Macrophages

On exposure to certain cytokines such as interferon-γ, macrophages become activated.
❖ The activated macrophages have greater phagocytic ability and produce many cytokines that act against intracellular bacteria, virus-infected cells, and tumor cells
❖ They also express higher levels of MHC class II and hence can act as efficient APCs.

Dendritic Cells

Dendritic cells are specialized antigen-presenting cells of the immune system **(Fig. 9.2)**.
❖ **Naming:** They possess long membranous cytoplasmic extensions resembling dendrites of neurons; hence, they are named dendritic cells
❖ **Origin:** Dendritic cells originate from bone marrow.
❖ **Follicular dendritic cells:** They are present in lymphoid follicles. They differ from other dendritic cells, as they recognize antigen-antibody complex rather than antigen alone
❖ **Function:** Dendritic cells are nonphagocytic. They are the most efficient APCs; their main function is to capture, process and present the antigenic peptides on their cell surface to the helper T cells.

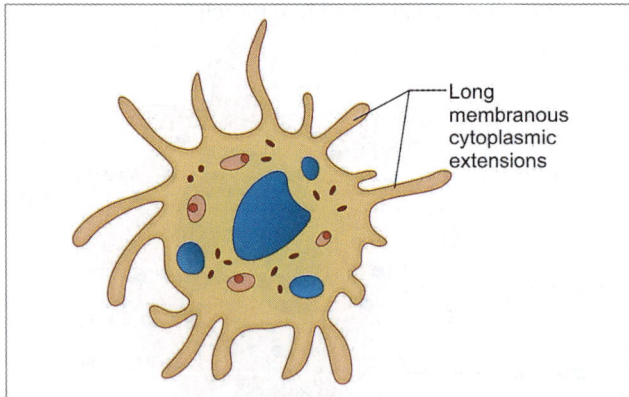

Fig. 9.2: Dendritic cell.

Granulocytic Cells

Granulocytes (e.g. neutrophils, eosinophils and basophils) are a category of white blood cells, characterized by the presence of granules in their cytoplasm.
❖ **Neutrophils:** They are often called polymorphonuclear leukocytes (PMN). Neutrophils constitute 50–70% of the circulating white blood cells (WBCs).
  ▪ They are the principal phagocytes of innate immunity
  ▪ The mechanism of microbial killing is similar to that of macrophages.
❖ **Eosinophils:** They are also phagocytic, and constitute 1–3% of total leukocytes, but the number is greatly increased in certain allergic conditions and helminthic infections
❖ **Basophils:** They are nonphagocytic granulocytes. Granules are rich in histamine and other mediators that play a major role in certain allergic responses.

Mast Cells

Mast cells are present in various body sites, such as skin, connective tissues of various organs, and mucosa (respiratory and intestinal). Like circulating basophils, mast cells also contain cytoplasmic granules rich in histamine and other active substances and play an important role in the development of certain allergic (type I hypersensitivity) reactions.

■ MAJOR HISTOCOMPATIBILITY COMPLEX

The major histocompatibility complex (MHC) is a group of genes coding for a set of host cell surface molecules that bind to peptide fragments derived from pathogens and display them on the host cell surface for recognition by the appropriate T cells.
❖ These are present in almost all human cells, but were first discovered on the surface of leukocytes; hence in humans, they are also called human leukocyte antigens (HLA)
❖ MHC molecules serve as a unique identification marker for every individual as the genetic sequence of MHC genes is different for every individual
❖ As the MHC molecules determine the compatibility between the graft and host tissues, they are named **histocompatibility antigens**.

Structure of MHC Molecule (FIG. 9.3)

MHC Class I Molecule

MHC-I proteins are located on the surface of all nucleated cells (except sperm cells) and platelets. They are absent in RBCs

CHAPTER 9 ◆ Components of Immune System: Organs, Cells and Products

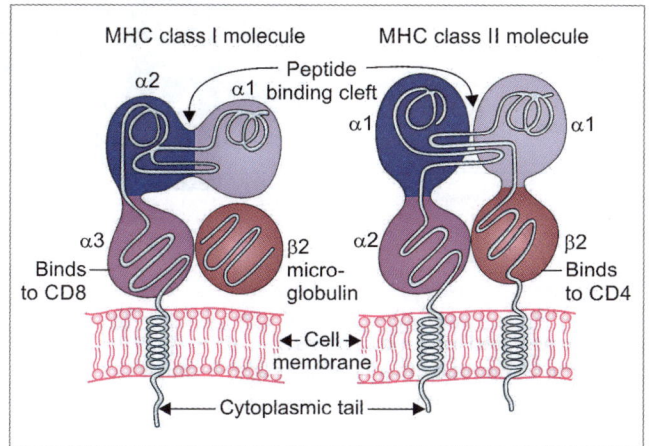

Fig. 9.3: Structure of MHC molecules.

- MHC-I molecule is composed of α chain (glycoprotein) and β2 *microglobulin*
- The α chain has three extracellular globular domains—α1, α2 and α3 and a cytoplasmic tail
- The antigen peptide binding groove of class I MHC molecule is formed by the cleft between α1 and α2 domains
- They present the peptide antigen to CD8 T cells.

MHC Class II Molecule

It comprises one α chain and one β chain. The α and β chains in turn consist of two domains each—(1) α1 and α2 and (2) β1 and β2, respectively and cytoplasmic tails.
- The antigen peptide binding groove is formed by the cleft between α1 and β1 domains
- The β2 domain interacts with the CD4 molecule of helper T cells during antigen presentation.

■ CYTOKINES

Cytokines are chemical substances that serve as messengers, mediating interaction and communication between the various cells of the immune system.

Major Classes of Cytokines

The major classes of cytokines include:
- Lymphokines—produced by lymphocytes
- Monokines—produced by monocytes and macrophages
- Interleukins—produced by WBCs and acting on the same or different WBCs
- Chemokines—involved in chemotaxis and other leukocyte behavior.

Functions of Cytokines

Though cytokines are secreted by a wide variety of cells, the major producers are T_H cells and macrophages. Cytokines produce a range of overlapping functions on the target cells/tissues, which can be broadly categorized into two groups:
1. Promote the development of cellular and humoral responses of adaptive immunity:
   - Interferon-γ
   - Cytokines such as IL-2, IL-4, IL-5.
2. Cytokines promote various responses of innate immunity:
   - Induction of inflammatory responses—by IL-1, IL-8, TNF-α
   - Regulation of hematopoiesis—by colony-stimulating factors, IL-1, IL-3, IL-7, IL-9, IL-11, etc.
   - Antiviral activity—by interferon-α and β
   - Antitumor activity—by TNF-α and β
   - Pyrogenic activity—by TNF-α, IL-1 and IL-6.

EXPECTED QUESTIONS

I. **Write essay on:**
   1. Describe in detail about the structure and function of various lymphoid organs and cells of immune system.

II. **Write short notes on:**
   1. Major histocompatibility antigen.
   2. Cytokines.

III. **Multiple Choice Questions (MCQs):**
   1. **T cell area of lymph node is:**
      a. Cortex
      b. Medulla
      c. Paracortical area
      d. All of the above
   2. **All of these are antigen-presenting cells (APCs), *except*:**
      a. T cells
      b. B cells
      c. Dendritic cells
      d. Macrophage
   3. **Cell type which lacks HLA antigen is:**
      a. Monocyte
      b. Thrombocyte
      c. Neutrophil
      d. Red blood cell
   4. **Defect in spleen predisposes to all the following infection, *except*:**
      a. *Staphylococcus aureus*
      b. *Streptococcus pneumoniae*
      c. *Neisseria meningitides*
      d. *Haemophilus influenzae*

Answers
1. c   2. a   3. d   4. a

CHAPTER 10

Immune Responses: Cell-mediated and Antibody-mediated

CHAPTER PREVIEW
- Antigen Presentation
- Helper T Cells (Activation and Differentiation)
- Cell-mediated Immune Response
- Humoral/Antibody-mediated Immune Response

INTRODUCTION

Immune response refers to the highly coordinated reaction of the cells of the immune system and their products. It has two arms: (i) humoral-mediated and (ii) cell-mediated immune response.

Humoral or Antibody-mediated Immune Response (AMI)

It protects the host by secreting *antibodies*; that can bind and neutralize microbial antigens circulating free or present on the surface of the host cells and in the extracellular spaces but have no role against intracellular antigens.

Cell-mediated Immune Response (CMI)

It plays a crucial role in protecting against intracellular microbes as well as tumor cells. Although CMI is mainly T cell-mediated (especially cytotoxic T cells); however, various other effector cells such as natural killer (NK) cells, macrophages, and granulocytes are also components of CMI.

Initial events before CMI/AMI

Certain initial events must take place before the induction of either CMI or AMI. These events are common and they occur irrespective of the type of immune response that will follow. These events include:
- Antigen presentation to helper T cells
- Activation and differentiation of helper T cells into either T_H1 or T_H2 subsets.

ANTIGEN PRESENTATION

For the induction of immune responses, recognition of antigens by T cells is essential. T cells cannot recognize the microbial antigens directly, but they do so only after the antigen is processed into smaller antigenic peptides containing specific epitopes which are subsequently combined with MHC molecules (class I or II) and presented on the host cell surface. Antigen presentation differs depending on the nature of the antigen.

❖ **Intracellular antigens:** These antigens include *M. tuberculosis*, viral antigens and tumor antigens, etc. that are present inside any infected host cells. They are processed into smaller antigenic peptides, which are complexed with the MHC-I proteins located on the host cell surfaces and are presented to CD8 T cells **(Fig. 10.1)**.

❖ **Exogenous antigens:** The extracellular microbial antigens are taken up by antigen-presenting cells (APCs), processed into smaller antigenic peptides, and are presented along with the MHC-II proteins, located on their surface. APCs present peptide antigens to CD4 T cells. Examples of APCs include macrophages, dendritic cells, and B cells **(Fig. 10.2)**.

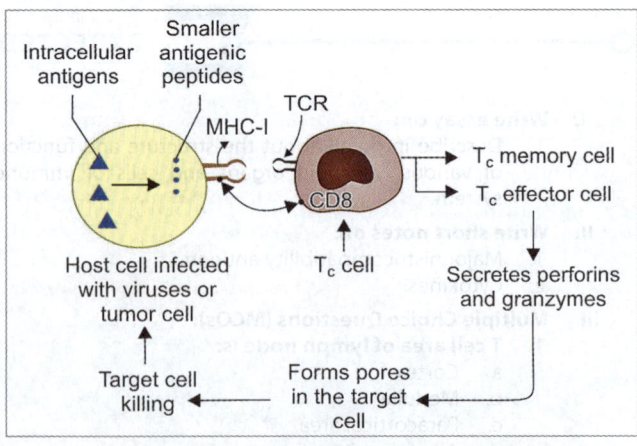

Fig. 10.1: Activation and differentiation of T_c cells.
(MHC, major histocompatibility complex; T_c cell, cytotoxic T lymphocyte; TCR, T cell receptor)

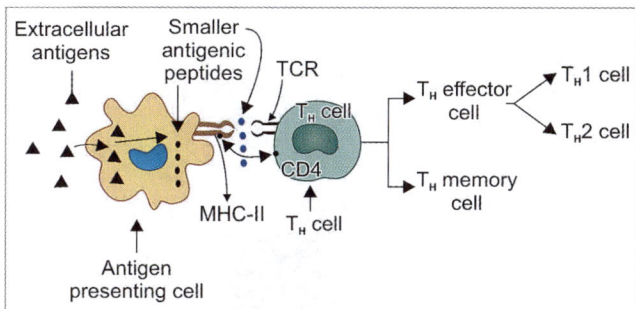

Fig. 10.2: Activation of T_H cell by interacting with APC.
(APC, antigen-presenting cell; MHC, major histocompatibility complex; T_H cell, helper T lymphocyte; TCR, T cell receptor)

■ HELPER T CELLS

Helper T (T_H) cells are the central key that regulate the type of immune response (CMI or AMI) that is going to occur.
* Activated helper T cells differentiate into either T_H1 or T_H2 subsets
* Induction of T_H1 cells secrete cytokines that stimulate cell-mediated response, whereas if T_H2 cells are differentiated, they secrete certain cytokines that in turn stimulate the B cells to produce antibodies, which lead to humoral-mediated response.

Activation and Differentiation of Helper T Cells

Activation and differentiation of helper T cells involve the following steps **(Fig. 10.2)**.
* **Activation of T_H cells:** It involves binding of antigenic peptide complexed with MHC-II on the surface of APCs to TCR (T cell receptor) present on the surface of T_H cells. CD4 molecules of T_H cells also interact with MHC-II molecule
* **Differentiation of T_H cells:** Activated T_H cells secrete an increased amount of IL-2, and subsequently differentiate into memory and effector T_H cells. The effector T_H cells further differentiate into either T_H1 or T_H2 subsets.

Effector T_H Cells

The differentiation of effector T_H cells into either T_H1 or T_H2 subsets is very crucial as they secrete distinct cytokines that further mediate specific functions.
* **T_H1 cells:** Cytokines secreted by T_H1 cell (e.g. IL-2, IFN-γ) stimulate T_C cells and induce CMI.
  ■ Interleukin 2 (IL-2): Promotes activation of T_H and T_C cells
  ■ Interferon-γ (IFN-γ): It activates the resting macrophages into activated macrophages and inhibits T_H2 cell proliferation.
* **T_H2 cells:** Cytokines secreted by T_H2 cells such as IL-4, IL-5, and IL-6 stimulate B cells producing antibodies (humoral immune responses). They also inhibit T_H1 cell differentiation. In addition, IL-5 enhances the proliferation of eosinophils.

■ CELL-MEDIATED IMMUNE RESPONSE

The term cell-mediated immune response (CMI) refers to the destruction of cells carrying intracellular microbes and other abnormal cells, such as tumor cells. CMI mediates the following immunological functions:
* Provides immunity against microbes residing in the intracellular milieu:
  ■ For obligate intracellular organisms, CMI remains the only effective immune response. Examples include all viruses, some bacteria (*Mycobacterium*, *Chlamydia*, and *Rickettsia*), some parasites (*Plasmodium*), and some fungi (*Pneumocystis*)
  ■ For facultative intracellular organisms (e.g. *Salmonella*), humoral immunity is active as long as the organism is extracellular. Once they come to intracellular milieu, CMI takes the leading role.
* Provides immunity against tumor cells and other damaged and altered cells
* Mediates delayed hypersensitivity (type IV hypersensitivity)
* Plays a key role in transplantation immunity and graft-versus-host (GVH) reaction.

Effector Cells of CMI

CMI can be mediated by both antigen-specific and nonspecific effector cells. They perform their function by directly killing the target cells (e.g. virus-infected cells or tumor cells).
* **Specific effector cell:** The most important mediator of CMI is cytotoxic T cell which is antigen-specific
* **Nonspecific effector cells:** Many nonspecific effector cells such as macrophages, NK cells, neutrophils, and eosinophils also contribute to CMI. They use antibodies as receptors to recognize the target cells for killing.

Cytotoxic T Lymphocytes

CD8 cytotoxic T lymphocytes (T_C) are the principal effector cells of CMI, involved in the destruction of target cells such as virus-infected host cells and tumor cells. The CMI mediated by T_C cells involves the following steps **(Fig. 10.1)**.
* **Activation of T_C cells:** It involves binding of antigenic peptide (of viral or tumor antigen) complexed with MHC-I on the host cell surface to TCR (T cell receptor) present on the surface of T_C cells. CD8 molecules of T_C cells also interact with MHC-I molecules
* **Target cell lysis:** The activated T_C cells produce two types of lethal enzymes; called perforins and granzymes.

Perforins produce pores in the target cell membrane; through which granzymes are released inside and induce host cell death by apoptosis.

Natural Killer Cells

Natural killer cells are large granular lymphocytes that constitute 10–15% of peripheral blood lymphocytes. They are derived from a separate lymphoid lineage.

- **Innate immunity:** NK cells are cytotoxic but are antigen nonspecific as they are part of innate immunity. They respond against virus-infected cells and tumor cells much earlier and exert CMI till the T_C cells are activated and take over the function
- **Activation of NK cells:** NK cells do not get activated against normal host cells carrying MHC-I molecules on their surface. However, in virus infected cells and tumor cells, the MHC-I expression is remarkably reduced. In such cases, NK cells get activated through its receptors such as CD16 and CD56
- **Target cell lysis:** Mechanism of target cell lysis by NK cells is similar to that of T_C cells, i.e. via secreting perforins and granzymes. Perforins form pores on target cells, through which granzymes enter and lyse the target cells.

NK cells Versus T_C Cells

NK cells although exert their function (target cell lysis) by a mechanism like that of T_C cells, they differ from T_C cells in many other aspects such as:

- **Natural killer cell markers:** NK cells lack the T cell markers such as CD8 molecules (hence are also called null cells), instead possess specific surface markers such as CD16 and CD56
- **No MHC restriction:** NK cells can recognize the ligands (antigens) without MHC presentation
- **Innate immunity:** NK cells are part of innate immunity; they do not require prior exposure to a microbial antigen
- **No memory:** NK cells unlike T_C cells do not differentiate into memory cells
- NK cells also mediate their function via ADCC (described below).

Antibody-dependent Cell-mediated Cytotoxicity (ADCC)

Several nonspecific cytotoxic cells express receptors (FcR) on their surface that can bind to the Fc region of any immunoglobulin.

- Following contact with a target cell coated with an antibody, these FcR-bearing cells can bind to Fc portion of the antibody coated on the target cells, and subsequently cause lysis of the target cell

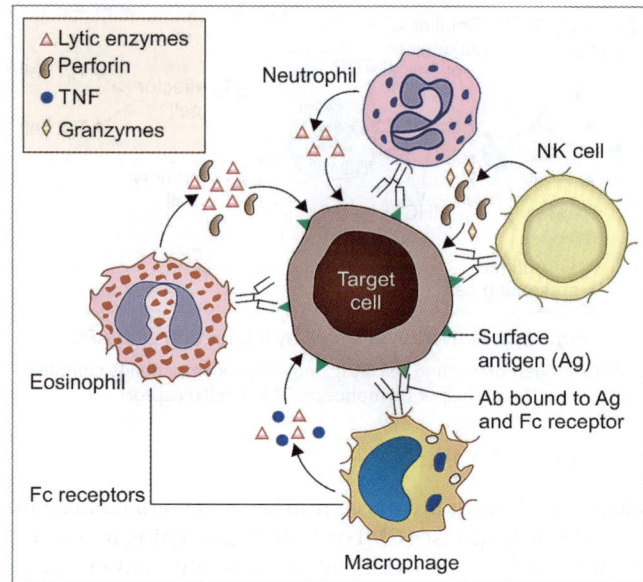

Fig. 10.3: Cytotoxic factors released by various cells in ADCC.

- Although these cytotoxic cells are nonspecific for the antigen, the specificity of the antibody directs them towards the specific target cells. This type of cytotoxicity is referred to as **antibody-dependent cell-mediated cytotoxicity (ADCC)**
- **Cells:** ADCC is exhibited by various cells such as NK cells, macrophages, monocytes, neutrophils, and eosinophils. They release various lethal factors into the target cells **(Fig. 10.3)**.
    - NK cells secrete perforins, and granzymes
    - Neutrophils release lytic enzymes
    - Eosinophils can release lytic enzymes and perforins; they play an important role in providing immunity against helminths
    - Macrophages produce lytic enzymes and tumor necrosis factor (TNF).

HUMORAL/ANTIBODY-MEDIATED IMMUNE RESPONSE

Antibody-mediated immune response (AMI) provides protection to the host by **secreting antibodies** that prevent invasion of microbes present on the surface of the host cells and in the extracellular environment but has no role against intracellular microbes. AMI occurs through the following three sequential steps:

1. Activation of B cells following contact with the microbial antigen (B cells act as APCs)
2. Proliferation and differentiation of B cells into effector cells (antibody producing plasma cells) and memory cells

CHAPTER 10 ◆ Immune Responses: Cell-mediated and Antibody-mediated

3. **Effector function:** Production of antibodies by plasma cells which in turn counteract with the microbes in many ways, such as neutralization, opsonization, complement activation, etc.

Activation of B Cells

Activation of B cells occurs through the following steps:

- **Antigen presentation:** The first and foremost step that occurs is the recognition of microbial antigen by B cell membrane immunoglobulin receptors (IgM) followed by receptor-mediated endocytosis of antigen
- Then the antigen is processed into smaller antigenic peptides that are presented in complex with MHC-II to activated T_H cells. This leads to the activation of B cells.

Proliferation and Differentiation of B Cells

The naive B cells are present in the primary lymphoid follicles of the peripheral lymphoid organs such as lymph nodes and spleen. Following antigenic exposure, the naive B cells are activated and then they proliferate. Eventually, the primary lymphoid follicles transform into secondary lymphoid follicles, where the B cell differentiation takes place **(Fig. 10.4)**.

- The activated B cells first differentiate into larger dividing cells called **centroblasts**, which further transform into smaller nondividing cells called **centrocytes** by expressing membrane Ig
- The centrocytes with high-affinity membrane Ig undergo maturation by binding to a special type of dendritic cell called **follicular dendritic cell**
- Then the mature centrocytes undergo **class switchover** so that they will be capable of producing various classes of Ig
- **Differentiation of centrocytes:** After undergoing class switchover, the selected centrocytes differentiate into effector cells (plasma cells) and memory cells
- **Plasma cells** are large antibody-secreting cells; that produce secretory Ig enormously but do not bear membrane Ig
- **Memory cells** bear high-affinity membrane Ig. They are long-lived cells that respond to the secondary antigenic stimulus.

Effector Functions of AMI

Antibodies secreted from plasma cells mediate several biological functions through their Fc portions that bind to Fc receptors (FcRs) expressed by many cell types.

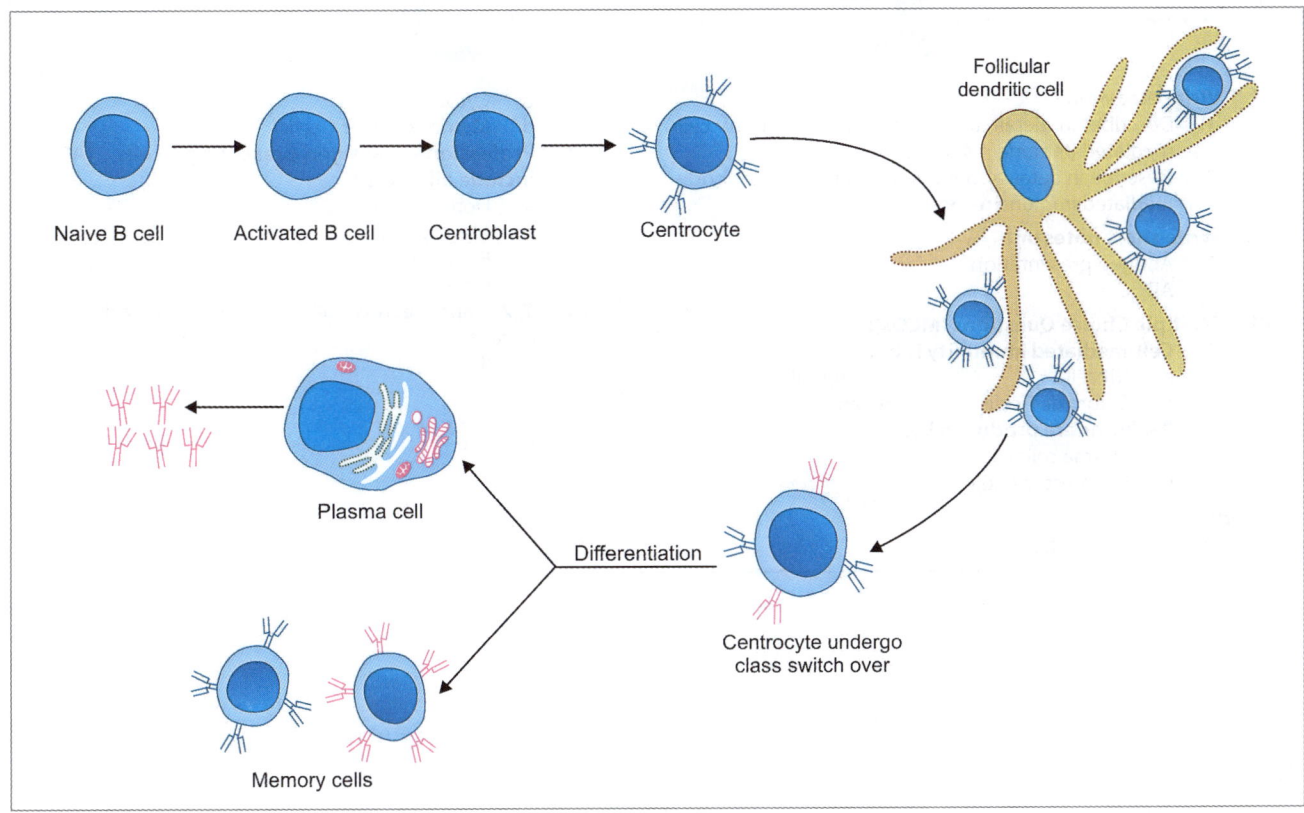

Fig. 10.4: Differentiation of B cells in secondary lymphoid follicles.

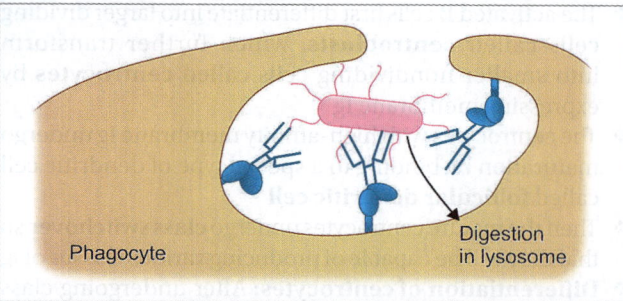

Fig. 10.5: Opsonization of bacteria and phagocytosis.

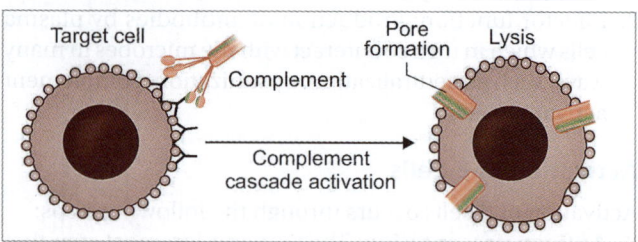

Fig. 10.6: Complement-mediated cytolysis.

- ❖ **Promotes opsonization:** FcRs present on phagocyte surface recognize antibody-coated microbes, and bind to them and which leads to enhanced phagocytosis **(Fig. 10.5)**
- ❖ **Mediates mucosal immunity:** IgA in the gut lumen provides mucosal immunity by neutralizing the microbes at local mucosal sites in the intestinal tract and respiratory tract, etc.
- ❖ **Activates complement-mediated inflammation and cytolysis:** Antigen-antibody complex activates the classical complement pathway **(Fig. 10.6)**. The final complement factors (C5-C9), also called **membrane attack complex** has lethal activity by forming pores on the target cells.
- ❖ **Promotes ADCC:** Though ADCC is principally cell-mediated (described under the CMI section); antibodies direct the cells to reach to the target cells. ADCC is important to provide immunity against:
  - Helminths (eosinophil-IgE mediated)
  - Tumor cells and virus-infected cells (NK cell-IgG mediated).

EXPECTED QUESTIONS

I. Write essay on:
1. Describe in detail about the mechanism of cell-mediated immune response.
2. Describe in detail about the mechanism of antibody-mediated immune response.

II. Write short notes on:
1. Antigen presentation.
2. ADCC.

III. Multiple Choice Questions (MCQs):
1. Cell-mediated immunity is by:
   a. NK cell   b. Eosinophil
   c. Cytotoxic T cells   d. All above
2. Perforins are produced by:
   a. Plasma cells
   b. Suppressor T cells
   c. Cytotoxic T cells
   d. Memory helper T cells
3. Professional antigen-presenting cells (APCs) include all, *except*:
   a. Dendritic cells
   b. Macrophages
   c. Fibroblasts (skin)
   d. B cells
4. T_H2 cells secrete all the following cytokines, *except*:
   a. IL-2
   b. IL-4
   c. IL-5
   d. IL-6

Answers
1. d   2. c   3. c   4. a

Hypersensitivity Reactions

CHAPTER 11

CHAPTER PREVIEW
- Definition and Classification
- Type I Hypersensitivity Reaction
- Type II Hypersensitivity Reaction
- Type III Hypersensitivity Reaction
- Type IV Hypersensitivity Reaction

The purpose of immune response is to eliminate the foreign antigens that have entered into the host. In most instances, immune response leads to only a subclinical or localized inflammatory response which just eliminates the antigen without causing significant damage to the host. However, at times, this response becomes abnormal; leading to an exaggerated inflammatory response that causes extensive tissue damage or sometimes even death.

DEFINITION AND CLASSIFICATION

The term hypersensitivity (HSN) or allergy refers to the injurious consequences in the sensitized host, following contact with specific antigens. Gell and R Coombs classified HSN reactions into four types **(Table 11.1)**.

- ❖ **Immediate HSN reactions:** These reactions occur immediately, within minutes to few hours of antigen contact, as a result of an abnormal exaggerated humoral response (antibody-mediated). This can be further classified into three types (HSN type I, II, and III), based on the type of effector mechanisms

- ❖ **Delayed HSN reaction:** It occurs after few days of antigen contact, as a result of an abnormal cell-mediated immune response. This is also called type IV HSN reaction. It is mediated by a specific subset of T_H cells called delayed hypersensitivity T cells or T_{DTH} cells.

TYPE I HYPERSENSITIVITY REACTION

Type I HSN reaction involves the production of IgE by sensitized B cells following contact with an allergen which in turn induces mast cell degranulation. Type I reaction occurs in various clinical conditions such as anaphylaxis and asthma.

Mechanism of Type I Hypersensitivity

Type I HSN reaction occurs through two phases; the sensitization and effector phases, both occurring with an interval of 2–3 weeks **(Fig. 11.1)**.

Sensitization Phase

This occurs when an individual is exposed for the first time to the sensitizing or priming dose of an allergen.

Table 11.1: Features of various types of hypersensitivity reactions.

	Type I	Type II	Type III	Type IV
Immune response altered	Humoral	Humoral	Humoral	Cell-mediated
Immediate or delayed	Immediate	Immediate	Immediate	Delayed
The duration between the appearance of symptoms and antigen contact	2–30 minutes	5–8 hours	2–8 hours	24–72 hours
Antigen	Soluble	Cell surface bound	Soluble	Soluble or bound
Mediator	IgE	IgG	Ag-Ab complex	T_{DTH} cell
Effector mechanism	Mast cell degranulation	ADCC Complement-mediated cytolysis	Complement activation and inflammatory response	Macrophage activation leads to phagocytosis or cell cytotoxicity

(ADCC, antibody-dependent cellular cytotoxicity)

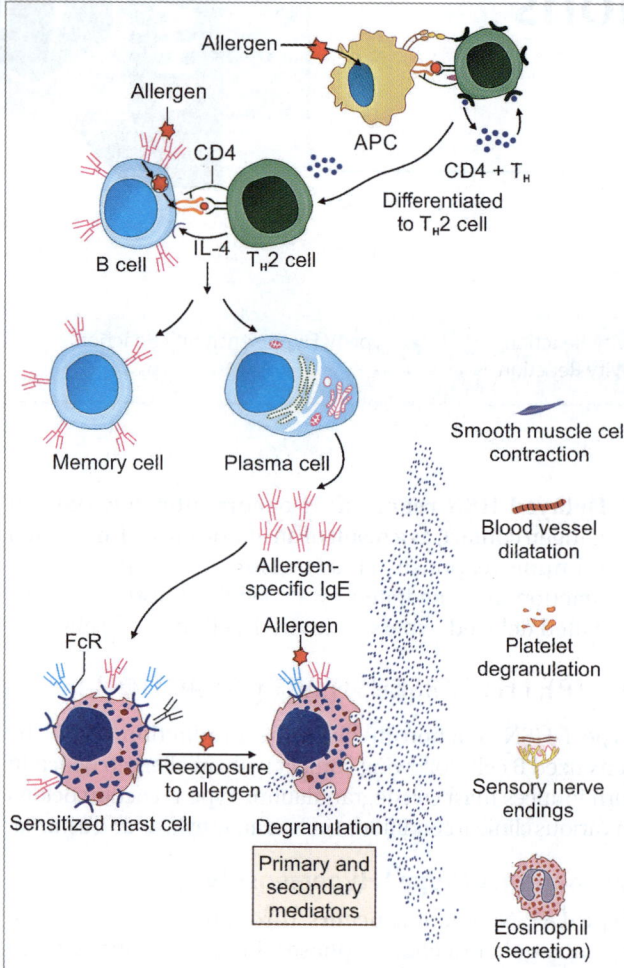

Fig. 11.1: Mechanism of type I hypersensitivity reaction.

- In susceptible individuals, very minute doses can be sufficient to sensitize the host cells
- The antigenic peptides are presented by antigen-presenting cells to the CD4 helper T cells
- Activated T_H cells are differentiated into T_H2 cells which in turn secrete interleukin 4 (IL-4)
- IL-4 induces the B cells to differentiate into IgE producing plasma cells and memory cells
- Secreted IgE migrates to the target sites, and coat on the surface of mast cells. Such sensitized mast cells (coated with IgE) will be waiting for interaction with the subsequent antigenic challenge.

Effector Phase

When the same allergen is introduced subsequently (shocking dose), it directly encounters with the IgE antibodies coated on mast cells.

- IgE cross-linkage initiates the mast cell activation and degranulation. Granules in turn release several pharmacologically active chemical mediators that lead to various manifestations of type-1 reaction
- **Degranulation occurs in two phases:** Mast cells undergo degranulation in two phases:
  1. *Primary mediators:* The preformed chemical mediators which are already synthesized by mast cells are immediately released, e.g. histamine and serotonin
  2. *Secondary mediators:* The mast cells synthesize them following stimulation by allergen and release, e.g. prostaglandins and leukotrienes.
- **Pharmacological actions:** The chemical mediators perform several pharmacological actions, such as bronchial and other smooth muscle contraction, increased vascular permeability, and vasodilation
- **Symptoms:** These actions in combinations, produce symptoms such as breathlessness, hypotension, and shock leading to death at times.

Manifestations of Type I Reaction

There are various manifestations of type I HSN reaction.
- **Systemic anaphylaxis:** It is an acute medical emergency condition, characterized by severe dyspnea, hypotension, and vascular collapse leading to death at times. A wide range of allergens trigger anaphylaxis in susceptible humans.
- **Localized anaphylaxis (atopy):** Here, the reaction is limited to a specific target tissue or organ, mostly the epithelial surfaces at the entry sites of allergen. They always run in families. Examples include: Allergic rhinitis (or hay fever), asthma, food allergy (e.g. nuts, eggs, seafood, etc.), atopic dermatitis (allergic eczema) and drug allergy (e.g. penicillin, sulfonamides, etc.)

Detection of Type I Hypersensitivity

Type I HSN reaction can be demonstrated by various tests such as:
- Skin prick test
- Detection of total serum IgE antibody by various enzyme immunoassay
- Detection of allergen-specific IgE by various immunoassay formats.

Treatment

Treatment of type I HSN reaction includes:
- Avoidance of contact with known allergens
- **Hyposensitization:** Repeated exposure to increased subcutaneous doses of allergens can reduce or eliminate the allergic response to the same allergen

- ❖ Monoclonal anti-IgE antibody
- ❖ Drugs such as antihistamines, epinephrine (adrenaline), and cortisone.

TYPE II HYPERSENSITIVITY REACTION

In type II reactions, the host injury is mediated by **antibodies** (IgG or rarely IgM), which interact with various types of antigens, such as:
- ❖ Host cell surface antigens (e.g. RBC membrane antigens like blood group and Rh antigens)
- ❖ Extracellular matrix antigens, or
- ❖ Exogenous antigens absorbed on host cells (e.g. a drug coating on the RBC membrane).

Various clinical conditions where type II HSN reactions occur are as follows:
- ❖ Complement-dependent reaction, e.g. ABO or Rh incompatibility, hemolytic anemia (autoimmune or drug-induced)
- ❖ Antibody-dependent cellular cytotoxicity (ADCC)
- ❖ Antibody-dependent cellular dysfunction, e.g. Graves' disease and myasthenia gravis.

TYPE III HYPERSENSITIVITY REACTION

Type III HSN reactions develop as a result of the excess formation of immune complexes (Ag-Ab complexes) which initiate an inflammatory response through activation of the complement system leading to tissue injury. Type III reactions occur either in localized or generalized forms.
- ❖ **Localized or arthus reaction**: It is defined as a localized area of tissue necrosis due to vasculitis resulting from acute immune complex deposition at the site of inoculation of antigen
  - In skin: Following insect bites
  - In lungs: Farmer's lungs, following inhalation of actinomycetes.
- ❖ **Systemic reaction:** Here, the small-sized soluble Ag-Ab complexes are carried in circulation and deposited in various distant sites. Examples include:
  - Connective tissue disorders such as systemic lupus erythematosus and rheumatoid arthritis
  - **Serum sickness:** This condition is not seen nowadays, it was seen in the past, following serum therapy, i.e. administration of foreign serum, e.g. horse anti-tetanus serum, to treat tetanus cases.

TYPE IV HYPERSENSITIVITY REACTION

Type IV HSN reactions differ from other types in various ways:
- ❖ **Delayed type:** It is delayed-type (occurs after 48–72 hours of antigen exposure)
- ❖ T_{DTH} **cells:** It is cell-mediated; characteristic cells called T_{DTH} cells (delayed type of hypersensitivity T cells) are the principal mediators of type IV reactions
- ❖ **Activated macrophages:** Tissue injury occurs predominantly due to activated macrophages
- ❖ **Mechanism:** The type IV HSN reaction occurs in two phases:
  1. *Sensitization phase:* This is the initial phase of 1–2 weeks, that occurs following antigenic exposure. The antigen-presenting cells process and present the antigenic peptides to the helper T cells. T_H cells are differentiated to form T_{DTH} cells
  2. *Effector phase*: The T_{DTH} cells, on subsequent contact with the antigen, secrete a variety of cytokines (e.g interferon-γ) which attract and recruit various inflammatory cells (e.g. macrophages) at the site of DTH reaction.
- ❖ **Granuloma formation:** Pathology of type IV reaction involves granuloma formation: Granuloma consists of an inner zone of epithelioid cells, typically surrounded by a collar of lymphocytes and a peripheral rim of fibroblasts and connective tissue
- ❖ **Common examples** of type IV reaction include:
  - Skin tests such as tuberculin test and lepromin test
  - Contact dermatitis, following exposure to nickel, etc.

EXPECTED QUESTIONS

I. Write short notes on:
  1. Type I hypersensitivity reaction.
  2. Type II hypersensitivity reaction.
  3. Immune complex-mediated hypersensitivity reaction.
  4. Type IV hypersensitivity reaction.

II. Multiple Choice Questions (MCQs):
  1. Type I hypersensitivity is mediated by which of the following immunoglobulins?
     a. IgA
     b. IgG
     c. IgM
     d. IgE
  2. All are early hypersensitivity reactions, *except*:
     a. Type I HSN
     b. Type II HSN
     c. Type III HSN
     d. Type IV HSN

Answers
1. d   2. d

Autoimmunity, Immunodeficiency Disorders, Transplant and Tumor Immunology

CHAPTER 12

CHAPTER PREVIEW
- Autoimmunity
  - Immunological Tolerance
  - Mechanisms of Autoimmunity
  - Autoimmune Diseases
- Immunodeficiency Diseases
  - Primary Immunodeficiency Diseases
  - Secondary Immunodeficiencies
- Transplant Immunology
- Tumor Immunology

■ AUTOIMMUNITY

Autoimmunity is a condition in which the body's own immunologically competent cells or antibodies act against its self-antigens resulting in structural or functional damage.

Normally immune system does not react to its antigens due to a protective mechanism called tolerance.

Immunological Tolerance

Immunological tolerance is a state in which an individual is incapable of developing an immune response against his own tissue antigens. It is mediated by two broad mechanisms—central tolerance and peripheral tolerance.

Central Tolerance

This refers to the deletion of self-reactive T and B lymphocytes during their maturation in central lymphoid organs thymus and bone marrow respectively. This usually occurs in the embryonic life. If some self-reactive T and B lymphocytes escape from central tolerance, they are destroyed by peripheral tolerance.

Peripheral Tolerance

Peripheral tolerance is provided by several backup mechanisms that occur in the peripheral tissues to counteract the self-reactive T cells that escape central tolerance.
- ❖ **Ignorance:** The self-reactive T cells might never encounter the self-antigen and remain in a state of ignorance
- ❖ **Cellular anergy:** It refers to the unresponsiveness of T cells to an antigenic stimulus, which occurs because of failure to produce the co-stimulatory signals
- ❖ **Phenotypic skewing:** Self-reactive T cells interacting with APCs presented with self-antigens, after activation secrete nonpathogenic cytokines, hence failing to induce autoimmune response
- ❖ **Regulatory T cells (T_{reg} cells):** T_{reg} cells can down-regulate the self-reactive T cells by secreting certain cytokines (e.g. IL-10)
- ❖ **Sequestration of self-antigen:** Certain self-antigens can escape immune recognition by sequestration in immunologically privileged sites, e.g. corneal proteins, testicular antigens, and antigens from the brain.

B cells can also exhibit peripheral tolerance. The self-reacting B cells are destroyed at the spleen by several mechanisms.

Mechanisms of Autoimmunity

Autoimmunity results due to the breakdown of one or more of the mechanisms of immunological tolerance.
- ❖ **Breakdown of T cell anergy:** This may occur in the presence of tissue necrosis and local inflammation. This mechanism is postulated for—multiple sclerosis and rheumatoid arthritis
- ❖ **Failure of AICD:** Failure of autoreactive activated T cells to undergo activation-induced cell death (AICD). It is observed in systemic lupus erythematosus (SLE) patients
- ❖ **Loss of T_{reg} cells**-mediated suppression of self-reactive lymphocytes
- ❖ **Release of sequestered antigens:** Injury to the organs leads to the release of sequestered antigens which are very well capable of mounting an immune response. Spermatozoa and ocular antigens released after trauma or surgery can cause post-vasectomy orchitis and post-traumatic uveitis

- **Molecular mimicry:** Some microorganisms share antigenic determinants (epitopes) with self-antigens, and an immune response against such microbes would produce antibodies that can cross-react with self-antigen. For example, acute rheumatic fever results due to antibodies formed against streptococcal antigens (M protein), cross-react with cardiac antigens, due to antigenic cross-reactivity
- **Polyclonal lymphocyte activation:** Several microorganisms and their products are capable of causing polyclonal activation of T cells or B cells.
  - Polyclonal T cell activation by superantigens released from microbes (e.g. *Staphylococcus aureus*)
  - Polyclonal B cell activation by products of various microbes such as Epstein-Barr virus, HIV, etc.
- **Bystander activation:** It is the nonspecific activation of bystander self-reactive T_H1 cells. Activation of microorganism-specific T_H1 cells leads to cytokine influx which causes an increased infiltration of various nonspecific T cells at the site of infection.

Autoimmune Diseases

The immunological attack of self-reacting T lymphocytes or autoantibodies on tissues leads to the development of various autoimmune diseases. There are broad ranges of autoimmune diseases that can either be localized into a single organ/cell type or may involve many organs and cause systemic manifestations **(Table 12.1)**.

Laboratory Diagnosis of Autoimmune Diseases

Autoimmune diseases are diagnosed by the detection of various autoantibodies in serum of the patients:
- **Autoimmune hemolytic anemia:** Diagnosed by the Coombs test, in which the red cells are incubated with an anti-human IgG antiserum. If IgG autoantibodies are present on the red cells, the cells are agglutinated by the antiserum
- **SLE** is diagnosed by: Detection of autoantibodies against various nuclear antigens by indirect immunofluorescence assay and ELISA. Examples include—antinuclear antibody (ANA), anti-double stranded DNA (dsDNA)

Table 12.1: Autoimmune diseases and immune response produced with their clinical manifestations.		
Single organ or cell type autoimmune diseases		
Disease	**Self-antigen present on**	**Type of immune response and important features**
Autoimmune hemolytic anemia	RBC membrane proteins	Autoantibodies to RBC antigens trigger complement mediated lysis
Graves' disease	Thyroid-stimulating hormone (TSH) receptor	Anti-TSH-autoantibody (stimulates thyroid follicles, leading to hyperthyroid state)
Myasthenia gravis	Acetylcholine receptors	Blocking type of autoantibody directed against Ach receptors present on motor nerve endings leads to progressive weakening of the skeletal muscles
Hashimoto's thyroiditis	Thyroid proteins and cells	Autoantibodies and T_{DTH} cells targeted against thyroid antigens leads to suppression of the thyroid gland
Post-streptococcal glomerulonephritis	Kidney	Streptococcal antigen-antibody complexes are deposited in the glomerular basement membrane
Systemic autoimmune diseases		
Systemic lupus erythematosus (SLE)	Autoantibodies are produced against various tissue antigens such as DNA, nuclear protein, RBC and platelet membranes	• **Immune complexes** (self Ag-autoAb) are formed; which are deposited in various organs • **Major symptoms:** Fever, butterfly rash over the cheeks, arthritis, etc.
Rheumatoid arthritis (RA)	Autoantibodies against the host IgG antibodies are produced called **RA factor** and cyclic citrullinated peptide	• Autoantibodies bind to circulating IgG, forming IgM-IgG complexes that are deposited in the joints and can activate the complement cascade • **Major symptoms:** Arthritis (chronic inflammation of the joints)
Multiple sclerosis	Brain (white matter)	Self-reactive T cells produce characteristic inflammatory lesions in the brain that destroy the myelin sheath of nerve fibers; leading to numerous neurologic dysfunctions

- **Rheumatoid arthritis is diagnosed by:** The detection of two important autoantibodies-RA factor (by latex agglutination test) and anti-cyclic citrullinated peptide (anti-CCP). *Rose-Waaler test* to detect RA factor is of historical importance, no longer used now.

IMMUNODEFICIENCY DISORDERS

Immunodeficiency is a state where the defense mechanisms of the body are impaired, leading to enhanced susceptibility to microbial infections as well as to certain forms of cancer.

Immunodeficiency diseases are broadly classified as primary or secondary.
- Primary immunodeficiency diseases result from inherited defects affecting immune system development
- Secondary immunodeficiency diseases are secondary to some other disease processes that interferes with the proper functioning of the immune system (e.g. infection, malnutrition, aging, immunosuppression, autoimmunity or chemotherapy).

Primary Immunodeficiency Diseases

Most primary immunodeficiency diseases are genetically determined and result from deficiency of either humoral/cellular immunity or both or due to defects in host defense mechanisms (mediated by complement proteins and cells such as phagocytes or NK cells) **(Table 12.2)**.
- Patients with defects in humoral immunity, complement, or phagocytosis typically suffer from recurrent infections with pyogenic bacteria
- On the other hand, those with defects in cell-mediated immunity are prone to infections caused by viruses, fungi, and intracellular bacteria.

Secondary Immunodeficiencies

Secondary immunodeficiencies, also known as acquired immunodeficiencies, are due to the secondary effects of other diseases, such as:
- Malnutrition
- Aging (suppression of the immune system with age)
- Patients with several infections that suppress the immune system causing lymphocyte depletion, e.g. HIV (human immunodeficiency virus) infection
- Underlying cancers (leukemia, lymphoma, multiple myeloma)
- Patients on immunosuppressive medications
- Patients receiving chemotherapy or radiation therapy for malignancy.

Table 12.2: Classification of primary immunodeficiency diseases.

Humoral immunodeficiency (B cell defects)
- Bruton disease (X-linked agammaglobulinemia)
- Common variable immunodeficiency
- Isolated IgA deficiency
- Hyper-IgM syndrome

Cellular immunodeficiencies (T cell defects)
- DiGeorge syndrome (thymic hypoplasia)
- Chronic mucocutaneous candidiasis
- Purine nucleoside phosphorylase (PNP) deficiency

Combined immunodeficiencies (B and T cell defects)
- Severe combined immunodeficiencies
- Wiskott–Aldrich syndrome
- Ataxia telangiectasia
- Nezelof syndrome

Disorders of phagocytosis
- Chronic granulomatous disease
- Myeloperoxidase deficiency
- Chediak–Higashi syndrome
- Leukocyte adhesion deficiency
- Lazy leukocyte syndrome
- Job's syndrome or hyper-IgE syndrome

Disorders of complement
- Complement component deficiencies
- Complement regulatory protein deficiencies

TRANSPLANT IMMUNOLOGY

Transplantation refers to the transfer of a graft or transplant (cells, tissues, or organs) from one site to another. The individual from whom the transplant is taken is referred to as the **donor**; while the individual to whom it is transplanted is called the **recipient**. Common examples of organ or tissue transplanted are kidney, heart, and skin grafts, etc.

Classification of Transplants

Based on the genetic relationship between the donor and the recipient, transplants can be classified into:
- **Autograft:** It is a self-tissue transferred from one part of the body site to another in the same individual. Examples include transferring healthy skin to a burned area in burn patients and the use of healthy blood vessels of the same person to replace blocked coronary arteries
- **Isograft or syngeneic graft:** It is a tissue transferred between genetically identical individuals (e.g. monozygotic twins)

- **Allograft:** It is a tissue transferred between genetically non-identical members of the same species (e.g. kidney or heart transplant)
- **Xenograft:** It is a tissue transferred between different species (e.g. the graft of a baboon heart into a man).

In humans, allografts are the most commonly used graft in transplant centers; hence our further discussion will be confined to allografts.
- Transplantation antigens are the antigens of allografts against which the recipient would mount an immune response
- MHC molecules (major histocompatibility antigens) are the most important transplantation antigens.

Types of Graft Rejection

Graft rejection is classified based on the time taken for the rejection **(Table 12.3)**.
- **Hyperacute rejection:** This occurs within minutes to hours of transplantation and is characterized by thrombosis of graft vessels and ischemic necrosis of the graft.
    - It is mediated by **circulating antibodies** that are specific for antigens on the graft endothelial cells and that are present before transplantation
    - It is seen in people with previous blood transfusions, pregnancy, or organ transplantation.
- **Acute graft rejection:** It occurs within days or weeks after transplantation.
    - It is due to an active immune response of the host stimulated by alloantigens in the graft
    - It is mediated by cytotoxic T cells, which directly destroy the graft cells and also antibodies that mediate injury to graft vessels by complement activation.
- **Chronic graft rejection:** It occurs over months or years, leading to progressive loss of graft function.
    - It manifests as fibrosis of the graft and by gradual narrowing of graft blood vessels called graft arteriosclerosis
    - It is mainly mediated by T cells causing delayed-type hypersensitivity reaction and also by antibodies.

Table 12.3: Comparison of various types of graft rejection.		
Graft rejection	**Time taken for rejection**	**Immune mechanisms involved**
Hyperacute	Minutes to hours	Preformed antibodies (anti-ABO and/or anti-HLA)
Acute	Weeks to months	Cytotoxic T cell-mediated Antibody-mediated
Chronic	Months to years	Chronic DTH mediated Antibody-mediated

Graft-Versus-Host Reaction

GVH reaction is a condition where graft mounts an immune response against the host (i.e. recipient) and rejects the host, in contrary to the usual situation where the recipient mounts an immune response against the graft antigens. GVH reaction occurs when:
- The graft must contain immunocompetent T-cells (e.g. stem cells or bone marrow or thymus transplants)
- The recipient should possess transplantation antigens that are absent in the graft
- The recipient may be immunologically suppressed and therefore cannot mount immune response against the graft.

Prevention of Graft Rejection

Tests to Determine Histocompatibility

Prior to transplantation, various laboratory tests should be carried out to assess the histocompatibility between the donor and recipient.
- **ABO blood group compatibility** testing by blood grouping and cross-matching
- **HLA typing:** In this test, donor's antigens expressed on the surface of leukocytes or their gene to that of the recipient are matched. The HLA compatibility is determined by:
    - Phenotypic methods, such as microcytotoxicity and mixed lymphocyte reaction
    - Genotypic methods, such as PCR detecting HLA genes or PCR-RFLP (restriction fragment length polymorphism).

Immunosuppressive Therapy

Graft rejection is treated with therapeutic regimens consisting of one or combination of various immunosuppressive therapies
- Corticosteroids
- Monoclonal antibodies against—IL-2Rα receptor antibodies (Basiliximab); CD20 antibodies (Rituximab) and TNFα (Infliximab).

TUMOR IMMUNOLOGY

Tumor immunology involves the study of antigens on tumor cells and the immune response to these antigens. Two types of tumor antigens have been identified on tumor cells:
1. Tumor-specific transplantation antigens (TSTAs)
2. Tumor-associated transplantation antigens (TATAs).

Tumor-specific Transplantation Antigen (TSTA)

Tumor-specific transplantation antigens (TSTA) are present only on tumor cells and are absent in normal cells of the body.

- TSTAs are induced on tumor cells either by chemical or physical carcinogens and also by viral carcinogens.
- In chemically/physically induced tumors, the TSTA is tumor-specific. Different tumors possess different TSTA, even though induced by the same carcinogen. Methylcholanthrene and ultraviolet light are examples of chemical and physical carcinogens that have been extensively studied
- In contrast, the TSTA of virus-induced tumors is virus-specific; all tumors produced by one virus would possess the same antigen. Examples include Epstein-Barr virus which causes nasopharyngeal carcinoma and several types of lymphoma.

Tumor-associated Transplantation Antigens

Tumor-associated transplantation antigens (TATAs) are not unique to tumor cells and may also be expressed by normal cells, but at a very low level. Their level gets exponentially high in tumor cells. Examples include (Table 12.4):
- **Oncofetal antigens:** They are the proteins that are expressed on normal cells during fetal life, but not expressed in the adult normally
    - Reactivation of the embryonic genes that encode these proteins in tumor cells results in their expression on the fully differentiated tumor cells

Table 12.4: TATAs used as tumor markers for diagnosis of cancers.

Tumor markers	Tumor types
Oncofetal proteins	
Alpha-fetoprotein (AFP)	Hepatoma Testicular cancer
Carcinoembryonic antigen (CEA)	Gastrointestinal cancers Lung, ovarian cancers
Secreted tumor antigens	
CA125	Ovarian cancers Other epithelial cancers
CA19-9	Various carcinomas
Prostate-specific antigen	Prostate cancer
β2-microglobulin	Multiple myeloma
Hormones	
β-subunit of chorionic gonadotropin	Hydatidiform mole Choriocarcinoma Testicular cancers

- Examples include alpha-fetoprotein (AFP) and carcinoembryonic antigen (CEA).
- **Non-oncofetal TATAs:** Examples include carbohydrate antigens (CA125, CA19-9), prostate-specific antigen and macroglobulin.

EXPECTED QUESTIONS

I. **Write essay on:**
   1. Define autoimmunity. Classify various autoimmune diseases and briefly explain various mechanisms involved in the development of autoimmunity with suitable examples.

II. **Write short notes on:**
   1. Graft-versus-host reaction.
   2. Tumor antigens.

III. **Multiple Choice Questions (MCQs):**
   1. **Lens antigens of the eye are a type of:**
      a. Sequestered antigens
      b. Neoantigens
      c. Cross-reacting antigens
      d. None of the above
   2. **Autoimmunity can be caused due to all of the following, *except*:**
      a. Breakdown of T cell anergy
      b. Polyclonal lymphocyte activation
      c. Negative selection of T cells in the thymus
      d. Release of sequestered antigens
   3. **Anti-citrullinated peptide antibodies (ACPA) are diagnostic for:**
      a. Systemic lupus erythematosus
      b. Rheumatoid arthritis
      c. Sjögren syndrome
      d. Scleroderma
   4. **Graft rejection due to preformed antibodies occurs in:**
      a. Hyperacute rejection
      b. Acute rejection
      c. Subacute rejection
      d. Chronic rejection

Answers
1. a   2. c   3. b   4. a

Immunoprophylaxis and Immunization Schedule

CHAPTER 13

CHAPTER PREVIEW
- Active Immunoprophylaxis
- Passive Immunoprophylaxis
- National Immunization Schedule

Immunoprophylaxis against microbial pathogens can be classified into active immunoprophylaxis (or vaccination) and passive immunoprophylaxis (or immunoglobulin administration).

VACCINATION (ACTIVE IMMUNOPROPHYLAXIS)

Vaccine is an immunobiological preparation that provides specific protection against a given disease. Following vaccine administration, the immunogen (active ingredient of the vaccine) stimulates the immune system of the body to produce active immunity in the form of protective antibody and/or immunocompetent T cell response.

Vaccines may be of various types based on their method of preparation by using live modified organisms, inactivated or killed organisms, extracted or cellular fractions, toxoids, subunit or combinations of all these. Vaccines of future prospects include DNA vaccine and viral vector vaccine.

Live Attenuated Vaccine

Live vaccines, such as BCG **(Table 13.1)** are prepared from live (usually attenuated) organisms.
- The live attenuated organisms lose their ability to induce full blown disease, but retain their immunogenicity
- **Attenuation** is achieved by passing the live organisms serially through a foreign host, such as chick embryo/tissue culture or live animals
- Live vaccines in general, are more potent immunizing agents compared to killed vaccines
- They are capable of inducing mucosal immunity by stimulating secretory IgA antibody production at the local mucosal sites.

Precautions while using Live Attenuated Vaccines
- **Contraindications:** Live vaccines should not be administered in individuals with immunodeficiency diseases

Table 13.1: Example of commonly used vaccines.

Bacterial	Viral
Live attenuated vaccines	
BCG vaccine	Measles vaccine
Typhoral vaccine	Mumps vaccine
	Rubella vaccine
	Live attenuated influenza vaccine
	Chickenpox vaccine
	Oral polio vaccine (OPV)
	Rotavirus vaccine
	Yellow fever 17D vaccine
	Hepatitis A vaccine
	Japanese B encephalitis vaccine (14-14-2 strain)
Killed/inactivated vaccine	
Typhoid vaccine	Injectable polio vaccine (IPV)
Cholera vaccine	Killed influenza vaccine
Pertussis vaccine	Rabies vaccine
Plague vaccine	Covaxin for COVID-19
Toxoid vaccine	**Subunit vaccine**
DT (Diphtheria toxoid) TT (Tetanus toxoid)	Hepatitis B vaccine HPV (Human papillomavirus) vaccine
Cellular fraction	**DNA/RNA vaccine**
Meningococcal vaccine	COVID-19 vaccines such as Moderna or Pfizer vaccines
Pneumococcal vaccine	**Viral vector vaccine**
Haemophilus influenzae type b (Hib) vaccine	Covishield vaccine (COVID-19)
Combined vaccine	
DPT vaccine (Diphtheria, pertussis and tetanus)	Mumps, measles, rubella (MMR) vaccine
Pentavalent vaccine (DPT + Hib + Hepatitis B)	

Note: Details about individual vaccine is discussed in the respective chapters.

or any conditions that suppresses the immunity, such as leukemia, lymphoma, malignancies, on corticosteroid or any other immunosuppressive drug therapy
- **Pregnancy** is another contraindication, unless the risk of infection exceeds the risk of harm to the fetus by giving the live vaccine
- When **two live vaccines** are required to be given; they should be administered with an interval of at least 4 weeks
- **Dosage:** Most live vaccines are given in single dose format as effective immunity is achieved with a single dose. Exception is oral polio vaccine (OPV) which is given as multiple doses at spaced intervals to achieve effective immunity
- **Risk of gaining the virulence:** The attenuation of the live vaccine has to be done in an effective way otherwise there is always a risk of gaining the virulence back
- **Storage:** Live vaccines must be stored cautiously to retain effectiveness, especially the OPV and measles vaccine.

Inactivated or Killed Vaccine

It consists of organisms, which are grown in culture under controlled conditions and then killed using methods, such as heat or formaldehyde.
- They are generally safer but less efficacious than live vaccines
- Compared to the live vaccines, killed vaccines require large doses, adjuvants, and multiple doses to confer immunity. In most cases, a booster dose is also needed
- Adjuvants increase the immunogenicity of the vaccine antigen (e.g., alum is used as adjuvant in DPT vaccine)
- Killed vaccines are usually administered in subcutaneous or intramuscular routes. The only absolute contraindication is a severe local or general reaction to the previous dose.

Various characteristics of killed and live vaccines are given in **Table 13.2**.

Toxoid Vaccine

The exotoxins produced by certain bacteria can be detoxicated to form toxoid by treating with acidic pH, formalin or by prolonged storage.
- Toxoid is a form of toxin that loses its virulence property but retains immunogenicity
- When a toxoid preparation is given as vaccine, it induces formation of neutralizing antibodies that are capable of neutralizing the toxin moiety produced during an infection; rather than acting upon the organism
- Examples include diphtheria toxoid (from *Corynebacterium diphtheriae*) and tetanus toxoid (from *Clostridium tetani*).

Table 13.2: Characteristics of killed and live vaccines.

Characteristics	Killed vaccine	Live vaccine
Number of doses	Multiple	Single*
Need for adjuvant	Yes	No
Duration of immunity	Shorter	Longer
Effectiveness of protection	Lower	Greater
Mimics natural infection	Less closely	More closely
Immunoglobulins produced	IgG	IgA and IgG
Mucosal immunity	Absent	Induced
Cell-mediated immunity	Poor	Induced
Reverts back to virulent form	No	Possible
Stability at room temperature	High	Low
Immunodeficiency and pregnancy	Safe	Unsafe

*Exception is oral polio vaccine (OPV), which is given as multiple doses at spaced intervals to achieve effective immunity.

Extracted or Cellular Fractions Vaccine

Vaccines, in certain instances, are prepared from extracted cellular fractions; examples include meningococcal vaccine, pneumococcal vaccine and *Haemophilus influenzae* type b vaccine—all are prepared from the capsular polysaccharide antigens of the respective organism.

Subunit Vaccines

For certain viruses, only a particular subunit of the virus is necessary to initiate the immunity, e.g. hepatitis B surface antigen (HBsAg) is the immunogenic component of hepatitis B virus. So, this viral component alone can be used as vaccine rather than the whole virus.
- Examples of subunit vaccines include hepatitis B vaccine and human papillomavirus (HPV) vaccine
- DNA recombinant technology is used for the preparation of such sub-viral components.

Combinations

If more than one immunizing agents are included in a vaccine preparation, it is called combined vaccine. The aim of the combined vaccine is to—
- Simplify administration and
- Augment the immunogenicity of the immunogen. For example, in DPT vaccine, the pertussis component acts as an adjuvant, which increases the immunogenicity of both diphtheria toxoid and tetanus toxoid.

Newer Vaccine Approaches

DNA or RNA Vaccine

DNA or RNA vaccines have recently been marketed. They have many advantages such as cost effectiveness and mounting a stronger and wider range of immune response.

The small pieces of DNA or RNA containing genes from the pathogenic microorganism are injected into the host. The gene of interest gets integrated with the host cell genome and starts transcribing the proteins against which the host mounts an immune response. The classical examples are COVID-19 vaccines such as Moderna or Pfizer vaccines.

Viral Vector Vaccines

The classical example is Covishield vaccine for COVID-19. These vaccines use a safe virus (e.g., Adenovirus) to encode the desired gene (e.g., S gene). Such vaccine when injected cannot cause disease but serves as a platform to produce proteins (e.g., spike proteins) that will stimulate the host immune system.

Cold Chain

"Cold chain" refers to a system of transport, storage, and handling of vaccines, starting at the manufacturer level and ending with the site of administration of the vaccine to the client. The optimum temperature for refrigerated vaccines is between +2°C and +8°C. For frozen vaccines the optimum temperature is –15°C or lower. In addition, protection from light is a necessary condition for some vaccines. Improper cold chain maintenance is one of the most common causes of vaccine failure; especially oral polio vaccine which is the most sensitive vaccine to heat; must be stored at –20°C.

❖ Vaccines which must be stored in the freezer compartment are polio and measles vaccines
❖ Vaccines which must be stored in the cold part but never allowed to freeze are—DPT, TT, Td, BCG, hepatitis B, *H. influenzae* type b and diluents.

Vaccine Vial Monitor

Vaccine vial monitor is a tool to monitor the stability/potency of a vaccine and to check the efficiency of cold chain.

It is heat sensitive label lining the vaccine vial. It contains an outer blue circle and an inner white square. With time and exposure to higher temperature, the inner square changes its color gradually from white towards blue, whereas the outer circle is not heat sensitive; it remains blue throughout **(Table 13.3 and Fig. 13.1)**.

NATIONAL IMMUNIZATION SCHEDULE (NIS)

Immunization is one of the most logical and cost effective strategies of any country for the prevention of childhood sicknesses and disabilities and is thus a basic need for all children. The following is the national

Table 13.3: Staging of vaccine vial monitor.

	Inner square	Outer circle	Vaccine
Stage 1	White	Blue	Can be used
Stage 2	Light blue	Blue	Can be used
Stage 3	Blue	Blue	Discard
Stage 4	Dark blue	Blue	Discard

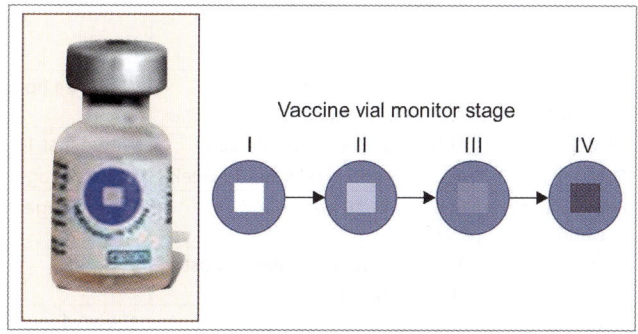

Fig. 13.1: Various stages of vaccine vial monitor (vaccine is usable up to stages I and II and should be discarded for stages III and IV).

Source: Pondicherry Institute of Medical Sciences, Puducherry (*with permission*).

immunization schedule recommended by the Ministry of Health, Government of India and it includes those vaccines that are given free of cost to all children of our country **(Table 13.4)**.

PASSIVE IMMUNOPROPHYLAXIS (IMMUNOGLOBULINS)

Passive immunoprophylaxis is given in the form of commercially available ready made **immunoglobulins** prepared against the pathogenic microorganism. Unlike vaccines, immunoglobulins act faster, without involvement of host immune apparatus.

Passive immunization is useful in the following circumstances:
❖ For immunocompromised individuals who cannot synthesize antibodies
❖ For post-exposure prophylaxis to achieve an immediate effect.

For the treatment of toxin mediated diseases to ameliorate the effect of toxin. Antibiotics cannot neutralize the toxin; hence, they cannot be used for the treatment of toxin mediated diseases.

Passive immunoprophylaxis available against various microbial diseases is given in **Table 13.5**.

Table 13.4: National Immunization Schedule (NIS) for infants, children and pregnant women.

Vaccine	When to give	Maximum age	Dose	Dilution	Route	Site
For pregnant women						
TT/Td-1	Early in pregnancy		0.5 mL	No	IM	Upper arm
TT/Td-2	4 weeks after TT/Td-1*	<36 weeks of pregnancy (if missed, can be given later)	0.5 mL	No	IM	Upper arm
TT/Td- Booster	If received 2 TT/Td doses in a pregnancy within the last 3 years*		0.5 mL	No	IM	Upper arm
For infants						
BCG	At birth or as early as possible	Till 1 year	0.05 mL (0.1 mL for >1 month)	Saline	ID	Left upper arm
Hepatitis B - Birth dose	At birth or as early as possible	Within 24 hour	0.5 mL	No	IM	Anterolateral side of mid-thigh
OPV-0	At birth or as early as possible	Within first 15 days	2 drops	No	Oral	Oral
OPV 1, 2 and 3	At 6 weeks, 10 weeks and 14 weeks	5 years of age	2 drops	No	Oral	Oral
Pentavalent# 1, 2 and 3	At 6 weeks, 10 weeks and 14 weeks	1 year of age	0.5 mL	No	IM	Anterolateral side of mid-thigh
PCV^ (3 doses)	At 6 weeks and 14 weeks, booster at 9-12 months	–	0.5 mL	–	IM	Anterolateral side of mid-thigh
Rotavirus##	At 6 weeks, 10 weeks and 14 weeks	1 year of age	5 drops	No	Oral	Oral
IPV	Two fractional doses at 6 and 14 weeks of age	1 year of age	0.1 mL	No	ID	Right upper arm
Measles /MR 1st Dose	9 completed months–12 months	5 years of age (only measles vaccine)	0.5 mL	Sterile water	SC	Right upper arm
JE - 1**	9 completed months–12 months	15 years of age	0.5 mL	Phosphate buffer	SC	Left upper arm
Vitamin A (1st dose)	At 9 completed months, given along MR vaccine	5 years of age	1 mL (1 lakh IU)	No	Oral	Oral
For children						
DPT booster-1	16–24 months	7 years of age	0.5 mL	No	IM	Anterolateral side of mid-thigh
MR 2nd dose$	16–24 months	5 years of age	0.5 mL	Sterile water	SC	Right upper arm
OPV Booster	16–24 months	5 years of age	2 drops	No	Oral	Oral
JE-2	16–24 months	–	0.5 mL	Phosphate buffer	SC	Left upper arm
Vitamin A*** (2nd to 9th dose)	16–18 months. Then one dose every 6 months up to the age of 5 years	5 years of age	2 mL (2 lakh IU)	No	Oral	Oral
DPT Booster-2	5–6 years	7 years of age	0.5 mL	No	IM	Upper arm
TT/Td	10 years and 16 years		0.5 mL	No	IM	Upper arm

*****TT/Td:** Tetanus toxoid (TT) is given alone, or in combination with adult diphtheria toxoid (Td). The second or booster dose is ideally given before 36 weeks of pregnancy, but should be given even if presented late in pregnancy or during labor.
******JE Vaccine** is introduced in selected endemic districts after the campaign: UP, Bihar, Assam, West Bengal and Karnataka.
******* The 2nd to 9th doses of Vitamin A can be administered to children 1–5 years old during biannual rounds, in collaboration with ICDS (Integrated Child Development Services).
#**Pentavalent** vaccine- contains combination of DPT, hepatitis B and *H.influenzae* type b vaccines.
Interval between two doses of pentavalent vaccine or OPV should never be less than 1 month.
##**Rotavirus vaccine:** Given in selected states such as Andhra Pradesh, Assam, Haryana, Himachal Pradesh, Jharkhand, Madhya Pradesh, Odisha, Rajasthan, Tamil Nadu, Tripura and Uttar Pradesh.
^**Pneumococcal conjugate vaccine (PCV):** Given in selected states such as Bihar, Himachal Pradesh, Madhya Pradesh, Uttar Pradesh (12 districts) & Rajasthan (9 districts).
Children who have not been received a single vaccine coming after 1 year: Will be given 3 doses of DPT at an interval of 4 weeks; Measles-1st dose, JE-1st dose (wherever applicable) up to 2 years of age.
(IM, intramuscular; SC, subcutaneous; ID, intradermal; TT/Td, Tetanus and adult diphtheria toxoid; BCG, Bacillus Calmette-Guerin; PCV, Pneumococcal conjugate vaccine)

CHAPTER 13 ◆ Immunoprophylaxis and Immunization Schedule

Table 13.5: Passive immunoprophylaxis.

Immunoglobulin preparations	Source	Indications
Diphtheria antitoxin	Equine	Treatment of respiratory diphtheria
Tetanus immune globulin (TIG)	Equine, Human	Treatment of tetanus as PEP, for people not adequately immunized with tetanus toxoid
Botulinum antitoxin	Equine, Human	Treatment of botulism
Varicella-zoster immune globulin (VZIG)	Human	PEP for immunosuppressed contacts of acute cases or newborn contacts
Rabies immunoglobulin (RIG)	Equine, Human	Treatment of rabies and PEP in people not previously immunized with rabies vaccine
Hepatitis B immunoglobulin (HBIG)	Human	PEP for percutaneous or mucosal or sexual exposure Newborn of mother with HBsAg +ve
Rubella	Human	Women exposed during early pregnancy
Measles	Human	Infants or immunosuppressed contacts of acute cases exposed <6 days previously

(PEP, post-exposure prophylaxis)

EXPECTED QUESTIONS

I. **Write short notes on:**
 1. Live vaccines vs. killed vaccines.
 2. National Immunization Schedule.
 3. Passive immunoprophylaxis.

II. **Multiple Choice Questions (MCQs):**
 1. All of the following are live attenuated vaccines, *except*:
    a. MMR
    b. Yellow fever 17D
    c. Salk polio
    d. Sabin polio
 2. All the following vaccines are given at birth, *except*:
    a. BCG
    b. Hepatitis B
    c. DPT
    d. OPV
 3. **Example for subunit vaccine is:**
    a. *H. influenza* b vaccine
    b. Hepatitis B vaccine
    c. Meningococcal vaccine
    d. Pertussis vaccine
 4. **Vaccine administered intradermally is:**
    a. MMR
    b. DPT
    c. BCG
    d. Salk polio vaccine

Answers
1. c   2. c   3. b   4. c

Immunohematology

CHAPTER 14

CHAPTER PREVIEW
- Blood Group Systems (ABO and Rh)
- Safe Blood Transfusion Practices
- Transfusion Reactions
- Transfusion-transmitted Infections

Among the 33 recognized blood group systems, the ABO system is the oldest system to be discovered (Karl Landsteiner, 1900). The other blood group systems include Rh, MN, P, Lutheran, Lewis, Kell, Duffy, etc.

ABO BLOOD GROUP SYSTEM

The ABO blood group system comprises four blood groups, each is determined by the presence or absence of two antigens A and B on the surface of the red blood cell (RBC) membrane and their corresponding antibodies in serum. The principle followed is if a blood group antigen is present on the RBC then the corresponding antibody would be absent in serum. Examples are given in **Table 14.1**.

Natural Isoantibodies

Anti-A and anti-B isoantibodies are called natural antibodies because they are seen to arise without any apparent antigenic stimulation.

They are IgM in nature (pentameric), produced by the age of 6 months, and persist thereafter.

Distribution of Blood Groups in India

In India, because of the diversity of race, religion and creed, the distribution of blood groups within the population is not uniform. A recent study done in North India showed that group B is the most common (35%), followed by groups O (30%), A (21%) and AB (14%).

RH-BLOOD GROUP SYSTEM

Rh-blood group is the most important blood group system in humans after the ABO system. It was so named because the antibody against this Rh-blood group antigen was first prepared in Rhesus monkeys by Landsteiner and Wiener.

- The commonly used terms Rh-factor, refer to the D antigen. Rh-positive and Rh-negative denote the presence or absence of Rh-antigen on the surface of RBCs. Unlike the ABO system, there are no natural Rh-antibodies in our blood
- In India, about 95% of individuals have Rh-positive blood group; the remainder (5%) are Rh-negative
- Rh-blood group system has an important role in blood transfusion.

SAFE BLOOD TRANSFUSION PRACTICES

Safe blood transfusion practices require that the following conditions are satisfied in choosing a donor:
- The recipient's plasma should not contain any antibodies that will damage the donor's RBCs
- The donor plasma should not have any antibodies that will damage the recipient's RBCs
- The donor red cells should not have any antigen that is lacking in the recipient RBCs. If the transfused cells possess a 'foreign antigen' it will stimulate an immune response in the recipient.

Selection of Blood Group for Blood Transfusion

Ideally, the donor and recipient should belong to the same ABO group. However, in emergencies, the O blood group

Table 14.1: Distribution of ABO antigens and antibodies in RBCs and serum.

Blood group	Antigen on RBC	Isoantibodies in serum
A	A	Anti-B
B	B	Anti-A
AB	AB	None
O	None	Anti-A and anti-B

can be used for transfusion for any ABO group individuals (universal donors) and AB blood group individuals can receive blood units from any blood group donors (universal recipients).

TRANSFUSION REACTIONS

Transfusion reactions are the complications arising following blood transfusion; which may be of two types—(1) immunological and (2) nonimmunological.

Immunological Complication

The immunological reactions that occur following an incompatible blood transfusion include—**acute hemolytic reactions.** They are rare and occur as a result of mismatched blood transfusion. The RBCs undergo intravascular hemolysis or they may be coated by antibodies and engulfed by phagocytes, removed from circulation, and subjected to extravascular lysis.

Nonimmunological Complications

These include—various **transfusion-transmitted infections.** These may include viruses, bacteria, and protozoa. The list of various infectious agents transmitted via blood transfusion is as follows:

- **Viruses**
  - Human immunodeficiency virus (HIV)
  - Hepatitis B, C and rarely D viruses
  - Cytomegalovirus (CMV)
  - Human T-lymphotropic virus.
- **Bacteria**
  - *Treponema pallidum*
  - *Leptospira interrogans*
  - *Borrelia burgdorferi.*
- **Protozoa**
  - *Plasmodium* species
  - *Babesia* species
  - *Leishmania donovani*
  - *Toxoplasma gondii*
  - *Trypanosoma cruzi.*

EXPECTED QUESTIONS

I. **Write short note on:**
  1. Transfusion reactions.

II. **Multiple Choice Questions (MCQs):**
  1. All of the following parasitic agents can be transmitted through blood transmission, *except*:
     a. *Plasmodium* species
     b. *Babesia* species
     c. *Cryptosporidium*
     d. *Toxoplasma gondii*

  2. All of the following viral agents can be transmitted through blood transmission, *except*:
     a. HIV
     b. Hepatitis B virus
     c. Hepatitis C virus
     d. Varicella-zoster virus

Answers
1. c   2. d

Hospital Infection Control

SECTION 3

SECTION OUTLINE

15. Healthcare-associated Infections
16. Sterilization and Disinfection
17. Biomedical Waste Management
18. Needle Stick Injury (Occupational Exposure)
19. Environmental Surveillance (Bacteriology of Water, Air, Surface, and Food)
20. Antimicrobial Stewardship

Healthcare-associated Infections

CHAPTER 15

> **CHAPTER PREVIEW**
> - Introduction
> - Major HAI Types
> - Prevention of HAIs
> - Standard Precautions
> - Transmission-based Precautions
> - Hospital Infection Control Committee

■ INTRODUCTION

Healthcare-associated infections (HAIs) can be defined as any infections acquired in the hospital by a patient admitted after 48 hours of admission. This also includes:
- Infections, that are acquired in the hospital, but symptoms appear after discharge
- Needle stick injury transmitted infections (*refer* **Chapter 18**).

As the site of healthcare facility has increasingly shifted from inpatient hospital care-based service to the ambulatory setting, the relevance of traditional terminologies such as "hospital-associated or nosocomial" infections have diminished.

Factors Affecting HAIs

At any given time 7% of patients in developed and 10% in developing countries acquire at least one HAI. Treatment of these HAIs adds a huge economic burden to the hospital. The principal factors that determine the likelihood that a given patient would acquire HAIs are:
- **Immune status:** Most admitted patients have impaired immunity and therefore are more prone to acquire infection.
- **Hospital environment:** The hospital environment harbors a greater magnitude of organisms than that of the community.
- **Hospital organisms:** Most of the organisms present in the hospital environment are multidrug-resistant.
- **Interventions** such as insertion of a central line, urinary catheters, or endotracheal tube, may introduce infection; mostly the patient's endogenous flora.
- **Transfusion:** It has a risk of transmitting infectious agents such as HIV, hepatitis B and C viruses.

Sources of Infection

Nosocomial infections are either exogenous or endogenous in origin.
- **Endogenous source:** This refers to the patient's own microbial flora which may invade the patient's body during some surgical or instrumental manipulations.
- **Exogenous sources** are infected hospital environment (surface or equipment), healthcare workers (hand flora), or other patients.

Organisms Implicated in HAIs

The ESKAPE pathogens are the major cause of nosocomial infections and represent the vast majority of multidrug resistant isolates present in a hospital.
- ***E**nterococcus faecium*
- ***S**taphylococcus aureus*
- ***K**lebsiella pneumoniae*
- ***A**cinetobacter baumannii*
- ***P**seudomonas aeruginosa*
- ***E**scherichia coli* and ***E**nterobacter* species.

Other infections that can spread in hospitals include:
- SARS-CoV-2 (COVID-19)
- Nosocomially-acquired *Mycobacterium tuberculosis*
- *Legionella pneumophila*
- *Candida albicans*
- *Clostridium difficile* diarrhea
- Blood-borne infections transmitted through needle prick injury or mucocutaneous exposure to blood include HIV, hepatitis B and C viral infections.

Modes of Transmission

Microorganisms spread in the hospital through several modes such as contact, droplet, and airborne transmissions.

They are discussed subsequently in this chapter under transmission-based precautions.

MAJOR HAI TYPES

Though several types of HAIs exist, there are four most common types (listed below) which are often monitored to estimate the burden of HAIs in a hospital. Out of these, the first three are together called device-associated infections (DAIs).
- ❖ Catheter-associated urinary tract infection (CAUTI)
- ❖ Central line-associated bloodstream infection (CLABSI)
- ❖ Ventilator-associated pneumonia (VAP)
- ❖ Surgical site infection (SSI).

Catheter-associated Urinary Tract Infection

UTI accounts for the majority of HAIs. It can be: catheter-associated (CAUTI) and noncatheter-associated; the former being the more common type:
- ❖ **Risk factors** that predispose patients to acquire a nosocomial UTI include: (i) advanced age, (ii) female gender, (iii) severe underlying disease, (iv) placement of a urinary catheter for >2 days and (v) breach in the catheter care (poor infection control practices)
- ❖ **Organisms:** Gram-negative rods cause the majority of hospital-acquired UTIs and *E. coli* is the most common organism implicated. Gram-positive bacteria such as *S. aureus* and enterococci can occasionally cause CAUTI.

Central Line Associated Bloodstream Infection

Central line-associated bloodstream infection (CLABSI) is the fourth common cause of HAIs.
- ❖ **Organisms:** Coagulase-negative staphylococci, and *S. aureus* are increasingly reported to cause CLABSI recently, followed by gram-negative rods and *Candida*
- ❖ **Risk factors** that predispose to acquire a CLABSI include:
    - *Patient-related*: Age (<1 year and >60 years), malnutrition, low immunity, severe underlying disease, loss of skin integrity (burn or bedsore), prolonged stay in ICUs.
    - *Device related:* Presence of central line
    - *HCW (healthcare worker) related:* Poor infection control practices like hand hygiene.

Ventilator-associated Pneumonia

Ventilator-associated pneumonia (VAP) is the second common cause of HAIs next to UTI.
- ❖ **Risk factors** for developing hospital-acquired pneumonia include:
    - *Device-related:* Endotracheal intubation
    - *Patient-related:* (i) Prolonged ICU stay leading to increased risk of colonization of hospital MDROs and (ii) aspiration of oropharyngeal flora due to various reasons such as semiconscious state, supine position, etc.
    - *HCW related:* Poor infection control practices such as poor hand hygiene.
- ❖ **Organisms:** Gram-negative rods such as *Acinetobacter* species and *Pseudomonas* species account for majority of VAP.

Surgical Site Infection (SSI)

Surgical site infection is defined as an infection that develops at the surgical site within 30 days of surgery (within 90 days for breast, cardiac, and joint surgeries).
- ❖ Though SSI is a major threat in hospitals, it is often underreported because 50% of SSIs develop after the discharge
- ❖ **Organisms:** Surgical site wounds are classified as clean, clean-contaminated, contaminated, or dirty
    - *For clean wound:* The skin flora of the surgical team or the environmental organisms are the major pathogens; the most common being *S. aureus*
    - *For other types:* The patient's endogenous flora (anaerobes and gram-negative rods) are the common agents.
- ❖ **Risk factors** for nosocomial wound infection include:
    - Advanced age, obesity, malnutrition, diabetes
    - Infection at a remote site that spreads through the bloodstream
    - Preoperative shaving of the site
    - Inappropriate timing of prophylactic antimicrobial agent.

Note: Antimicrobial prophylaxis is usually given to the patient to prevent the seeding of organisms on the surgical site. It is given 1 hour before the incision, usually along with the induction of anesthesia.

PREVENTION OF HAIS

The preventive measures for HAIs can be broadly categorized into: (i) standard precautions and (ii) transmission-based or specific precautions.

STANDARD PRECAUTIONS

Standard precautions are a set of infection control practices used to prevent transmission of diseases, which should be followed while handling all patients, specimens, and sharps, regardless of whether they are infected or not. Components of standard precautions include:
- ❖ Hand hygiene (*details explained later*):
    - Wash hands promptly after contact with infective material.
    - Use no touch technique wherever possible.

- ❖ **Personal protective equipment (PPE):** *See below for details*
- ❖ **Biomedical waste:** All biomedical waste including sharp should be segregated and disposed of appropriately (*refer* **Chapter 17**)
- ❖ **Spillage cleaning:** Clean up spills of infective material promptly
- ❖ **Disinfection of patient-care items:** Ensure that all patient-care items such as instruments, devices, and linens are disinfected before reuse.
- ❖ **Environmental cleaning of surface and floor** (*refer* **Chapter 19**)
- ❖ **Sharp:** Safe use and disposal of sharp (*refer* **Chapter 17**)
- ❖ Respiratory hygiene and cough etiquette.

Hand Hygiene

The hands of the HCWs are the main source of transmission of infections in a hospital. Hand hygiene is therefore the most important measure to prevent HAIs.

Types of Hand Hygiene Methods

Hand Rub

Alcohol-based (70–80% ethyl alcohol) and chlorhexidine (0.5–4%) based hand rubs are available. The duration of contact has to be at least for 20–30 seconds.

- ❖ **Advantage:** After a period of contact, it gets evaporated on its own, hence drying of hands is not required separately
- ❖ **Indications:** Hand rub is indicated during routine patient care activities or taking rounds in the wards or ICUs—whenever an opportunity for hand hygiene arises, except when the hands are visibly soiled with blood or other specimens.

Hand Wash

Antimicrobial soaps (liquid, gel, or bars) are available containing 4% chlorhexidine. If facilities are not available, then even ordinary soap and water can also be used. The duration of contact has to be at least 40–60 seconds. Hand washing is indicated in the following situations:

- ❖ When the hands are visibly soiled with blood, excreta, pus, etc.
- ❖ Before and after eating
- ❖ After going to the toilet
- ❖ Before and after shift of the duty
- ❖ When giving care to a patient with diarrhea.

Surgical Hand Scrub (3–5 min)

This is indicated before any surgical procedure and between cases; by using 4% chlorhexidine hand wash. The duration of contact has to be at least for 3–5 minutes.

Indications (Five Moments for Hand Hygiene)

The WHO has published standard guidelines describing the situations or opportunities when hand hygiene is indicated in healthcare sectors **(Fig. 15.1)**—known as 'My Five Moments for Hand Hygiene'; which include:

1. Before touching a patient
2. Before clean/aseptic procedures
3. After body fluid exposure/risk
4. After touching a patient
5. After touching the patient's surroundings.

Steps of Hand Rubbing and Hand Washing

WHO has also laid down the guidelines describing the appropriate steps involved for effective hand rubbing and hand washing **(Fig. 15.2)**.

Personal Protective Equipment (PPE)

Personal protective equipment is used to protect the HCWs from exposure to blood and/or body fluids and protect the patient from the HCWs during invasive procedures.

- ❖ The various PPE used in healthcare settings are gloves, mask/respirator, gown/plastic apron/coverall, goggles or face shield, shoe cover, and head cover **(Figs. 15.3A to N)**
- ❖ Selection of appropriate PPE is based on:
  - The level of risk associated with contamination of skin, mucous membranes, and clothing by blood and

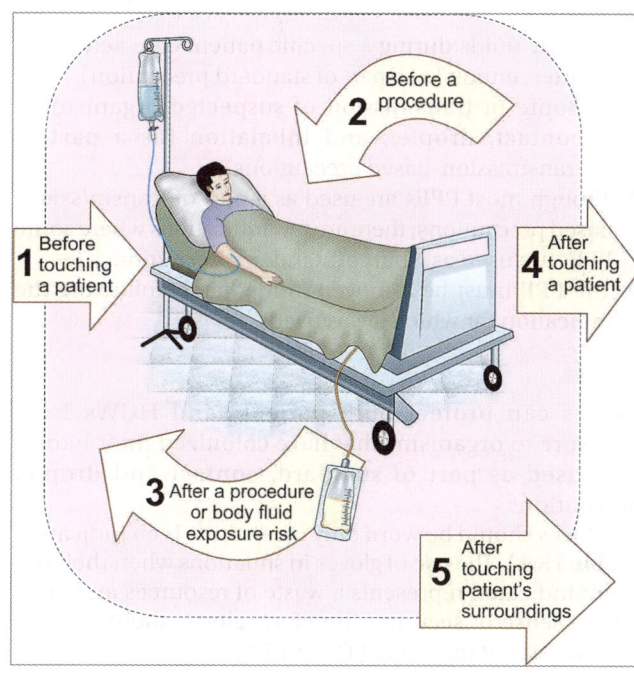

Fig. 15.1: My five moments for hand hygiene.
Source: World Health Organization (WHO) (*with permission*).

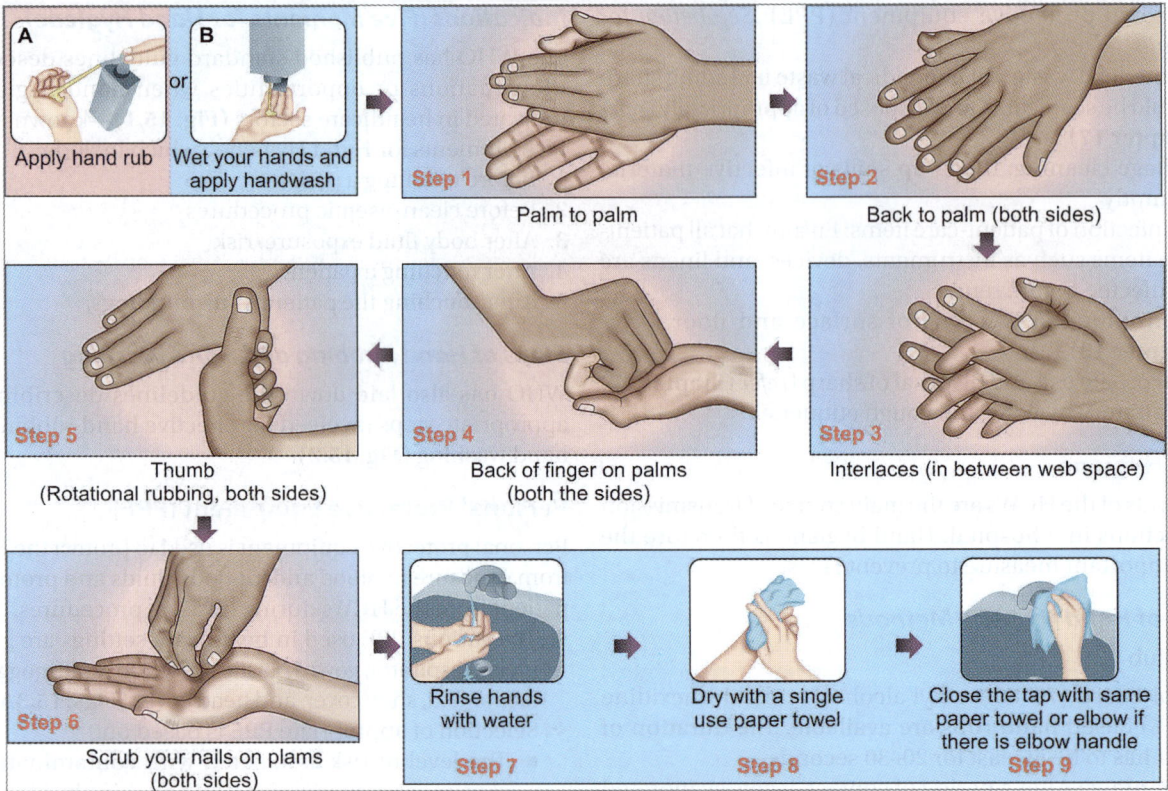

Fig. 15.2: Steps of hand rubbing and hand washing (WHO): Hand rub steps 1 to 6 (20–30 seconds); Hand wash steps 1 to 9 (40–60 seconds).

body fluids during a specific patient care activity or intervention (as a part of standard precaution)
- Route of transmission of suspected organisms—contact, droplet, and inhalation (as a part of transmission-based precautions).
❖ Though most PPEs are used as a part of transmission-based precautions; there are few indications where some PPEs are used as a part of standard precaution
❖ The PPE must be removed immediately following the indication for which it was used.

Gloves

Gloves can protect both patients and HCWs from exposure to organisms that have colonized their hands. It is used as part of standard, contact and droplet precautions.

Gloves should be worn only when there is an indication **(Table 15.1)**. The use of gloves in situations when their use is not indicated represents a waste of resources and gives a false sense of security. Therefore, gloves should not be used when not indicated **(Table 15.1)**.

Hand Hygiene and Use of Gloves

Glove is not a substitute for hand hygiene. In no way does the glove use modify hand hygiene indications or replace hand hygiene. The following measures should be adapted during glove use:
❖ **Hand hygiene before gloves use:** This is to prevent possible cross-contamination of gloves with HCW's flora
❖ **Hand wash after glove use:** To prevent cross-contamination, hands must be washed immediately after the removal of gloves as it creates a moist, warm, and occlusive environment between the skin and the glove which is a 'safe-haven' for microorganisms. Furthermore, microtears can occur in gloves which may lead to the transmission of organisms if the HCW has had contact with blood or body fluid
❖ **Change:** Gloves should be worn for a single patient care activity and not beyond. Gloves must be changed between patient contacts and between separate procedures on the same patient
❖ **No hand hygiene over the gloved hand:** Gloved hands should neither be wiped with any form of hand rub nor washed with soap and water.

The technique for donning and doffing gloves has been depicted in **Figures 15.4 and 15.5**.

Surgical (3-ply) Mask and Respirators

Respiratory protection is essential when there is a risk of transmission of droplets and aerosols. There are two types

CHAPTER 15 ♦ Healthcare-associated Infections

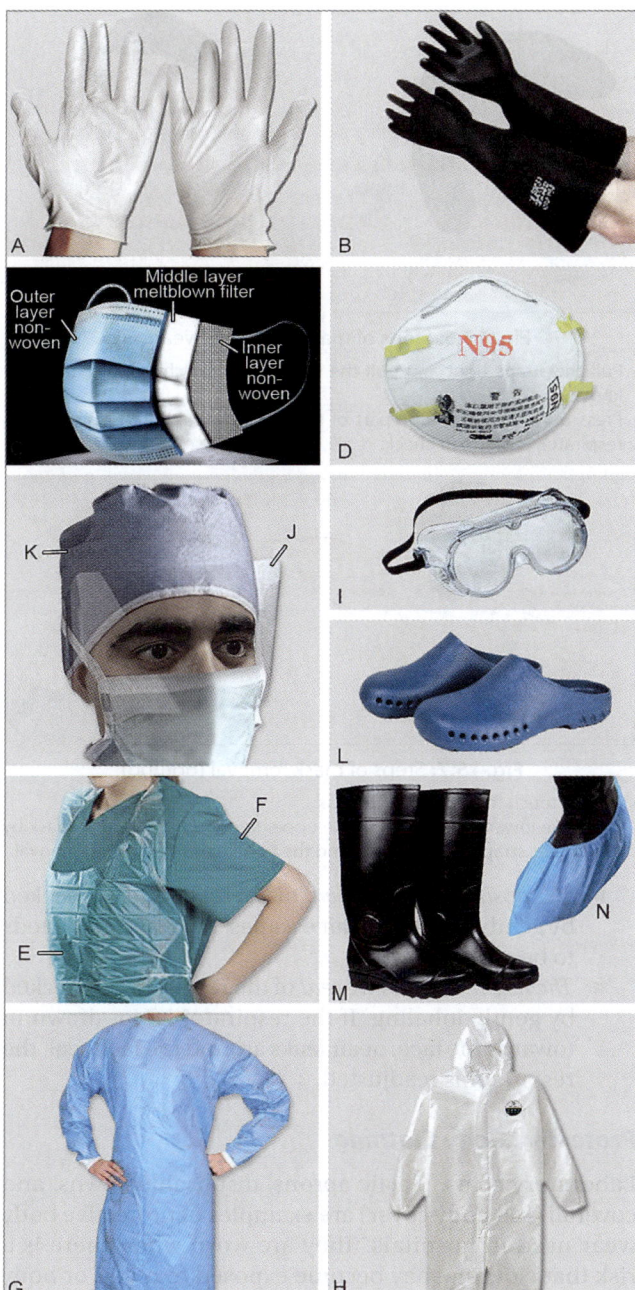

Figs. 15.3A to N: Personal protective equipment (PPE): A. Gloves; B. Heavy duty gloves; C. Surgical mask; D. N95 respirator; E. Plastic apron; F. Linen gown; G. Disposable gown; H. Coverall; I. Goggles; J. Face shield; K. Cap; L. Shoes; M. Gum boot; N. Shoe cover.

of PPE available for respiratory protection: surgical masks and respirators.

Surgical Mask (3-ply Mask)

Surgical masks (also called medical masks or 3-ply masks) are loose-fitting, single-use items that cover the nose and mouth.

Table 15.1: Indications for appropriate use of glove.

Indications for glove use
- As a part of standard precautions
  - Before a sterile procedure
  - Anticipation of contact with blood or body fluid
- As a part of contact precautions: Contact with a patient (and his/her immediate surroundings)
- Heavy duty gloves: To protect from sharp injuries, mainly used by biomedical waste handlers

Indications for glove removal
- As soon as gloves are damaged
- Gloves are meant for single-use and must be changed in between patients or patient care activities
- When there is an indication for hand hygiene

Clinical situations where the use of gloves is not recommended
- For routine patient care activities if there is no anticipated risk to blood/body fluid or no indication for contact precautions
- Examples: Measuring blood pressure, temperature, and pulse, while administering medications (oral or injections), during maintenance of IV cannula, during dressing and transporting patient, writing in the patient's case sheet, etc.

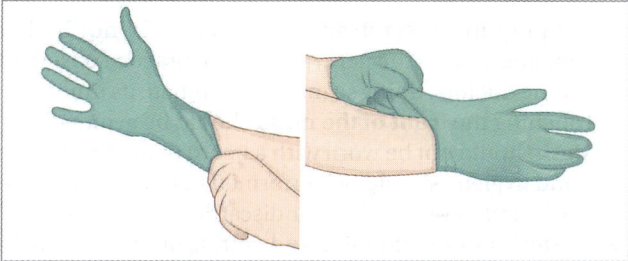

Fig. 15.4: Steps of gloves donning (wearing).

1. Donning of the first glove: Wear by touching and pulling only the edge of the cuff.
2. Donning of the second glove: Avoid touching the forearm skin by pulling the external surface of the second glove with the finger of the gloved hand.

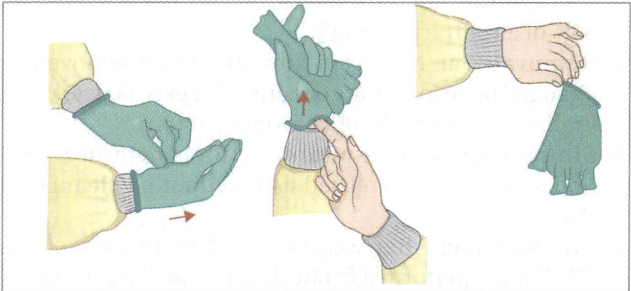

Fig. 15.5: Steps of gloves removal (doffing).

Do not touch the outside of the gloves (contaminated):
- Using a gloved hand, grasp the palm area of the other gloved hand and peel off the first glove.
- Hold removed glove in gloved hand slide fingers of ungloved hand under the other glove at wrist and peel off the second glove over the first glove.
- The first glove will remain inside the pouch of the second glove.
- Perform hand hygiene after removal.

- They are used as part of standard precautions to prevent splashes or sprays from reaching the mouth and nose of the person wearing them
- They also provide some protection from respiratory secretions and are worn when caring for patients on droplet precautions.
- **Composition:** It has three layers **(Fig. 15.3C)**:
  1. Outer hydrophobic layer that can repel droplets and blood
  2. Middle filter layer, made up of melt-blown material
  3. Inner hydrophilic layer, to absorb secretions.

Instructions

When using a surgical mask, the following measures should be considered:
- **Shelf-life:** Single-use only; should be discarded or changed after 4-6 hours of use or earlier if it becomes soiled or wet.
- **Donning:** Place the mask carefully, ensuring it covers the mouth and nose, adjust to the nose bridge, and tie it securely to minimize any gaps between the face and the mask
- **Hanging mask syndrome:** Masks should not be left dangling around the neck, a common practice observed among doctors, doing so may contaminate its inner side
- Touching the **front of the mask** should be avoided.
- Mask should not be worn with a beard or unshaven face
- Hand hygiene should be performed before donning the mask, and upon touching or discarding a used mask.
- The technique of donning and doffing of surgical masks has been depicted in **Figures 15.6 and 15.7**.

Respirator (N95 Respirator)

N95 respirator is a device designed to protect the wearer from airborne microorganisms (e.g. *M. tuberculosis*). There are many types of respirators:
- N95 refers to 'not resistance to oil and ability to filter off 95% of airborne particles'
- **Removal:** The N95 respirator should be removed or changed once in 8 hours or earlier if it gets clogged, wet, or dirty on the inside, or deformed, or torn
- **Single-use:** N95 respirator is for single-use only and should not be reused as it cannot be cleaned or disinfected
- **Fit checking:** After wearing the N95 respirator, the HCW must perform a fit check to ensure if it is properly fitted. No clinical activity should be undertaken until a satisfactory fit check has been achieved. It includes the following steps:
  - *Sealing:* The respirator is compressed to ensure a seal across the face, cheeks, and the nasal bridge

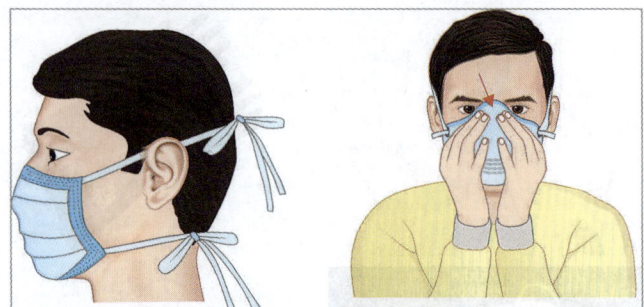

Fig. 15.6: Steps of mask donning (wearing).

- Pull the straps tight and pull the mask to below chin and then apply knots.
- Press on the nasal bridge part of the mask to seal tightly and for N95 respirator, perform fit check.

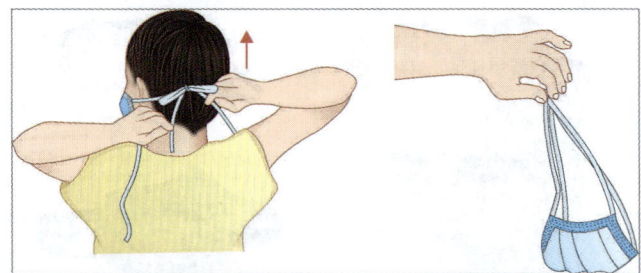

Fig. 15.7: Steps of mask removal (doffing).

- Do not touch front part of the mask.
- Untie the lower knot first, then the upper knot and remove the mask by holding its straps, without touching the front; hand wash after removal.

  - *The positive pressure seal* of the respirator is checked by gently exhaling. If air escapes, the respirator needs to be adjusted
  - *The negative pressure seal* of the respirator is checked by gently inhaling. If the respirator is not drawn in towards the face, or air leaks around the face seal, the respirator is readjusted.

Protective Body Clothing

Laboratory coats, plastic aprons, disposable gowns, and coverall (full body cover) are examples of protective body wear used in hospitals. They are worn when there is a risk that clothing may become exposed to blood or body fluids.
- **Laboratory coats:** They are used as a part of a standard precaution by all laboratory staff which protect their clothing and skin from the splash of blood or body fluid; however, they are not fluid-resistant
- **Plastic aprons:** Worn when there is a low risk of contamination of blood/body fluid. They are fluid-resistant and for single-use only, i.e. used for one procedure or one patient care activity **(Fig. 15.3E)**

- ❖ **Disposable gowns:** They are long-sleeved, fluid resistant; indicated when there is a moderate risk of contamination with blood/body fluid **(Fig. 15.3G)**
- ❖ **Coverall:** It comprises a gown with pants and a hood, which covers the whole body including the head. Coverall should be used in the following situations:
  - Anticipated risk of splashing with a large volume of blood/ body fluid (e.g. cardiac surgeries)
  - Anticipated risk of extensive skin-to-skin contact with a patient known to harbor organisms of contact transmission (e.g. lifting a patient with uncontrolled diarrhea)
  - Handling patients infected with pathogens of high mortality (e.g. Nipah or Ebola) or in the laboratory while handling their specimens **(Fig. 15.3H)**.
- ❖ **Donning:** The gown should be fully covered, with torso from neck to knees, arms to end of the wrist, and then wrapped around the neck. It should be fastened in the back of the neck and waist **(Fig. 15.8)**
- ❖ **Doffing:** Once the task is performed, the gown must be removed immediately after use by unfastening the gown ties taking care that sleeves should not contact the body while reaching for the ties **(Fig. 15.9)**.

Protective Eye/Face Wear

Protective eyewears (goggles, or face shields) are used to protect the mucous membranes of the eyes, nose, and mouth
- ❖ Prevents exposure to blood and/or body fluids that may be splashed, sprayed, or splattered into the face during clinical procedures
- ❖ Eyewear must be worn during procedures that are likely to generate droplets or aerosols of blood and/or high-risk body fluids **(Figs. 15.3I and J)**.

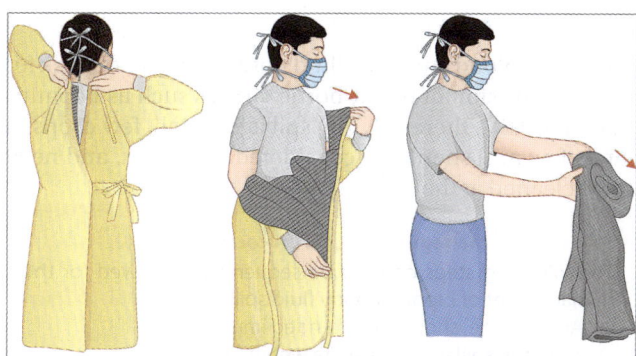

Fig. 15.9: Steps of gown removal (doffing). Do not touch the front part of the gown.

- Unfasten gown ties, taking care that sleeves don't touch the body when reaching for ties.
- Pull the gown away from neck and shoulders, touching inside of gown only.
- Turn gown inside out and roll into a bundle and discard.
- Perform hand hygiene after removal.

Head Cover and Shoe Cover

- ❖ **Headcover or cap (Fig. 15.3K)** is used when spillage of blood is suspected, e.g. during major cardiac surgeries, etc.
- ❖ **Shoe covers include:** (1) Surgical shoes (slippers) and shoe covers **(Figs. 15.3L and N)**: Used mainly in ICUs and operation theaters to protect HCWs from organisms present on the floor and (2) Gumboots: Used for anticipated risk of sharp injuries (e.g. for biomedical waste handlers, laundry staff, and housekeeping staff) **(Fig. 15.3M)**.

Donning and Doffing

To minimize the risk of transmission of infection, donning (wearing) and doffing (removing) of PPE must be performed in a particular sequence.

> Donning (wearing): Gown first → Mask or respirator → Goggles or face shield → Gloves
> Doffing (removing): Gloves first → Gown → Face shield or goggles → Mask or respirator.

Doffing is extremely important as even a minor breach in the doffing procedure would subject the HCW to a huge risk of acquiring the infection. This could be a potential reason why many HCWs got infected during the COVID-19 pandemic.
- ❖ All PPE should be removed just before exiting the patient room **except a respirator**, which should be removed after leaving the patient room and closing the door
- ❖ Discard into appropriate BMW bins:
  - Yellow bag: Gown/coverall, mask/respirator, shoe cover, and cap
  - Red bag: Plastic apron, goggles/face shield, gloves.

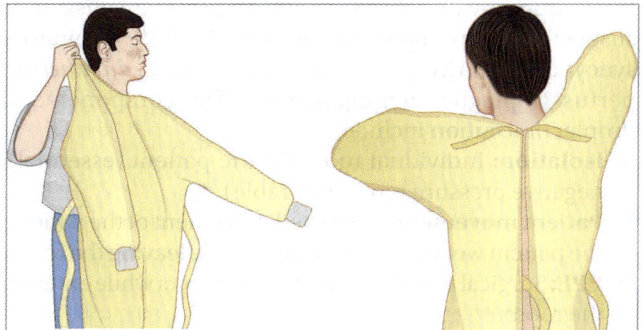

Fig. 15.8: Steps of gown donning (wearing).
- Fully cover torso from neck to knees, arms to the end of wrists, and wrap around the back.
- Fasten it on the back of the neck and waist.

Blood Spill Management

Spillage of blood and body fluid poses a substantial risk for the transmission of blood-borne viruses such as hepatitis B, C, and HIV. Therefore, any spillage (small, few drops to large, few mL) should be considered infectious, and need to be cleaned at the earliest.

> **Steps of spill management (CDC protocol, Fig. 15.10)**
> The following steps need to be sequentially followed for the management of blood or body fluid spillage.
> ❑ Any spillage, should be attended immediately
> ❑ Mark the spill area, place the wet floor signage
> ❑ Wear appropriate PPE (gloves and gown) as mentioned in the spill kit
> ❑ Confine the spill and wipe immediately with an absorbent towel or cloth, which is spread over the spill to solidify the blood or body fluid. Then it is disposed of as infectious waste
> ❑ Clean with hypochlorite (freshly prepared)
>   ➤ For large spills (>10 cm size): Use 1:10 dilution of 5% hypochlorite (5000 ppm), i.e. 0.5%
>   ➤ For small spills (<10 cm size): Use 1:100 dilution of 5% hypochlorite (500 ppm), i.e. 0.05%
> ❑ Allow the disinfectant to remain wet on the surface for at least a contact time of 10 min
> ❑ Rinse the area with clean water to remove the disinfectant residue.

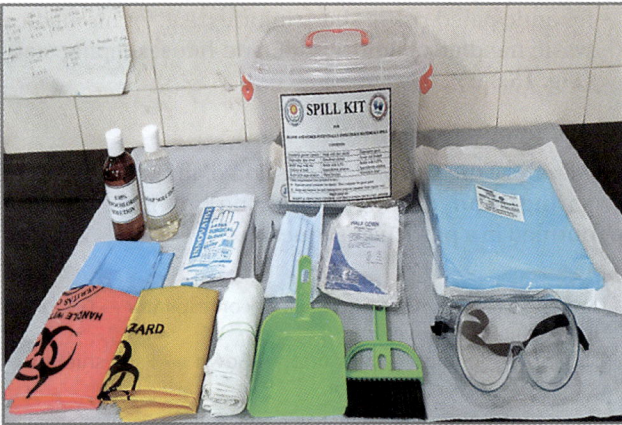

Fig. 15.10: Blood spill kit.
Source: Hospital Infection Control and Prevention Unit, Department of Microbiology, JIPMER, Puducherry (*with permission*).

■ TRANSMISSION-BASED PRECAUTIONS

These are the additional precautions taken over and above the standard precautions when a disease of a specific transmission is suspected and where standard precautions may not be sufficient to prevent the transmission of infection. Based on the specific modes of transmission; there are three types of transmission-based precautions.

Contact Precautions

It is required when disease with contact transmission is suspected; for example,
❖ Patients with enteric infections and diarrhea which cannot be controlled
❖ Highly contagious skin lesions
❖ *Clostridium difficile* infection
❖ Hepatitis A and E virus
❖ Multidrug-resistant organisms (MDROs) isolated in a hospital setting, for example,
  ■ MRSA (Methicillin-resistant *S. aureus*)
  ■ VRE (Vancomycin resistant enterococci)
  ■ CRE (Carbapenem resistant *Enterobacterales*).

The components of contact precaution include:
❖ **Isolation:** Individual room for the patient (optional); otherwise cohorting of patients (desirable). Cohorting involves placing the patients infected with the same pathogen together in the same room or the same cubicle in a ward
❖ **Patient movement:** The patient should be confined to the room. If the transfer is required, then hand hygiene and appropriate PPE must be used and the patient's colonized area must be covered
❖ **PPE:** Staff must wear gloves and gowns on entering the room
❖ **Patient dedicated equipment:** Equipment such as blood pressure cuffs, nebulizers, and stethoscopes must be used for single patient and must be disinfected before re-use
❖ **Hand washing** should be done before and after contact with the patient, and on leaving the room
❖ **Environmental cleaning** (floor, clothes, toilet) and equipment cleaning, with appropriate disinfectant is essential.

Droplet Precautions

It is required when disease with droplet transmission is suspected; for example, influenza, COVID-19, respiratory syncytial virus, *Mycoplasma*, parainfluenza, *C. diphtheriae*, pertussis, plague, meningococcus. The components of droplet precaution include:
❖ **Isolation:** Individual room for the patient (essential), negative pressure room (desirable).
❖ **Patient movement:** Restricted movement of the patient; the patient wears a surgical mask while leaving the room.
❖ **PPE:** Surgical mask for healthcare workers while entering the room.

Airborne Precautions

It is required when disease with airborne transmission is suspected; for example, pulmonary TB, chickenpox, and measles. The components of airborne precaution include:

CHAPTER 15 ♦ Healthcare-associated Infections

- ❖ **Isolation:** Individual rooms should be provided with adequate ventilation with a negative pressure facility (essential).
- ❖ **Patient movement:** The patient should be confined to the room all the time.
- ❖ **PPE:** Staff should wear high-efficiency masks (N95 masks) while entering the room. Patients may wear surgical masks all the time.

■ HOSPITAL INFECTION CONTROL COMMITTEE

The hospital infection control program is organized and run by the Medical Superintendent (MS), for which he/she constitutes the Hospital Infection Control Committee (HICC). The HICC provides a forum for multidisciplinary input, cooperation, and information sharing, required for hospital infection control and prevention. The HICC is advisory to the MS and makes its recommendations to the MS.

> **HICC Constitution**
> The hospital infection control committee (HICC) should include wide representations from relevant departments, as follows:
> ❑ Chairperson, usually the Medical Superintendent
> ❑ Secretary, mostly the head of the Department of Microbiology
> ❑ Hospital Infection Control Officer (HICO)
> ❑ Hospital Infection Control Nurses (HICNs)
> ❑ Head of all the clinical (all medical and surgical) departments
>
> *Contd...*

> *Contd...*
> ❑ Nursing Superintendent
> ❑ In-charge of Central Sterile Supplies Department (CSSD)
> ❑ In-charge of biomedical waste management
> ❑ In-charge of pharmacy, linen and laundry, and kitchen

Functions of HICC

The HICC supervises the implementation of the hospital infection control program. The various functions of the committee include:

- ❖ **HAI surveillance:** Maintains surveillance of hospital-acquired infections such as CA-UTI, CLABSI, VAP, and SSI
- ❖ **Antimicrobial stewardship program (AMSP):** Develops antibiotic policies, monitors the antibiotic usage
- ❖ **Policies:** Reviews and updates on the hospital infection control policies and guidelines from time to time
- ❖ **Education:** Conducts teaching sessions for healthcare workers regarding matters related to HAIs
- ❖ **Staff health:** Monitors employee health activities regarding matters related to HAIs such as needle stick injury prevention, hepatitis B vaccination, etc.
- ❖ **Outbreak management:** Develops strategies to identify infectious outbreaks, and their source and implements preventive and corrective measures
- ❖ **HICC meetings:** HICC shall meet regularly not less than once a month or as often as required.

EXPECTED QUESTIONS

I. Write short notes on:
1. Modes of transmission of healthcare-associated pathogens.
2. Prevention of healthcare-associated infections.
3. Hand hygiene.
4. Standard precautions.

II. Multiple choice questions (MCQs):
1. Hand rub should not be used in which condition?
   a. Before touching patient
   b. After touching patient
   c. After touching patient's surrounding
   d. Hands are visibly soiled
2. The ESKAPE pathogens include all, *except*:
   a. *Enterococcus faecium*
   b. *Streptococcus pyogenes*
   c. *Klebsiella pneumoniae*
   d. *Acinetobacter baumannii*
3. 'My Five Moments for Hand Hygiene' include all, *except*:
   a. Before touching a patient
   b. After touching a patient
   c. After body fluid exposure/risk
   d. Before touching the patient's surroundings
4. Which of the following protective equipment (PPE) is indicated while giving care to a patient on contact precautions?
   a. Gloves and mask
   b. Gloves and gown
   c. Mask and gown
   d. Only gloves

Answers
1. d   2. b   3. d   4. b

Sterilization and Disinfection

CHAPTER 16

CHAPTER PREVIEW
- Definitions
- Sterilants
- High-level Disinfectants
- Intermediate-level Disinfectants
- Low-level Disinfectants
- Cleaning Agents
- Environmental Cleaning
- Methods to Test Efficacy of Sterilant/Disinfectant

INTRODUCTION

The sterilization and disinfection practices in a hospital is of paramount importance in preventing transmission of healthcare-associated infections.

Definitions

Sterilization, disinfection and cleaning are three separate but interrelated terminologies, all aiming at removing or destroying the microorganisms from materials or from body surfaces. However they vary in their efficacy of destroying the microorganisms **(Table 16.1)**.

Sterilization

Sterilization is a process by which all living microorganisms including viable spores, are either destroyed or removed from an article, surface or medium. The agents which achieve sterilization are called as sterilants **(Table 16.2)**.

Disinfection

It refers to a process that destroys or removes most if not all pathogenic organisms but may or may not destroy bacterial spores. They are normally used only on inanimate objects, not on body surfaces. The agents which achieve disinfection are called disinfectants **(Table 16.2)**.

Type of Disinfectants

Depending upon their efficacy, the disinfectants are further classified into three categories.

- ❖ **High-level disinfectants (HLD)** are capable of killing bacterial spores when used in sufficient concentration under suitable conditions. They can kill all other microorganisms
- ❖ **Intermediate-level disinfectants (ILD)** destroy all microorganisms, but not bacterial spores
- ❖ **Low-level disinfectants (LLD)** destroy vegetative bacteria and enveloped viruses; variable action on nonenveloped viruses, and fungi, but no action on tubercle bacilli and spores.

Note: **Antiseptics** are a type of disinfectants which are safe to apply on body surfaces (skin and mucosa) resulting in the destruction of organisms present on the body surfaces. This type of disinfection is termed as **asepsis**.

Cleaning (Decontamination)

Cleaning refers to the reduction in the pathogenic microbial population to a level at which items are considered safe without protective attire. It can be achieved by manual cleaning with soap and detergents to eliminate debris or organic matter from the medical devices or surfaces **(Table 16.2)**.

In a healthcare facility, most of the sterilization practices for surgical instrument and other critical care items are carried out in **Central Sterile Supply Department (CSSD)**. CSSD is an integrated place in hospitals that performs sterilization of medical devices, equipment and consumables; that are used for aseptic procedures. The processing area of CSSD consists of four unidirectional

Table 16.1: Level of sterilant/disinfectants according to their microbicidal action.

Level of disinfectant/ sterilant	Bacterial spores	Tubercle bacilli	Non-enveloped viruses	Fungi	Vegetative bacteria	Enveloped viruses
Sterilant	Yes	Yes	Yes	Yes	Yes	Yes
Disinfectant						
High level	+/−	Yes	Yes	Yes	Yes	Yes
Intermediate level	No	Yes	Yes	Yes	Yes	Yes
Low level	No	No	+/−	+/−	Yes	Yes

CHAPTER 16 ❖ Sterilization and Disinfection

Table 16.2: Classification of agents used in the hospital for achieving sterilization, disinfection and cleaning.

Agents	Physical methods	Chemical methods
Sterilants		

Agents of sterilization	• Heat-based methods (>100°C):
	  1. Steam sterilizer (autoclave),
	  2. Dry heat sterilizer (hot air oven)
	• Filtration
	• Radiation: Ionizing and non-ionizing (infrared)
	• Others: Incineration, microwave
		• Ethylene oxide (ETO) sterilizer
		• Plasma sterilizer

Disinfectants		
High-level disinfectants	No physical methods in this category	• Aldehydes–glutaraldehyde, orthophthaldehyde, formaldehyde • Peracetic acid • Hydrogen peroxide
Intermediate-level disinfectants	• Heat-based methods: <100°C (pasteurization, inspissation) and at 100°C (boiling, steaming and tyndallization) • Radiation: Non-ionizing (ultraviolet)	• Alcohols–ethyl alcohol and isopropyl alcohol • Phenolics–phenol, cresol, lysol • Halogens–iodine and chlorine
Low-level disinfectants	No physical methods in this category	• Quaternary ammonium compound (QAC) • Chlorhexidine
Cleaning		
Agents of cleaning	Automated washers such as ultrasonic washers, washer-disinfector and automated cart washers	• Enzymatic solution • Detergent • Soap (antimicrobial or plain soap)

zones starting from an unsterile area to a sterile area separated by a physical barrier:

1. **Decontamination area,** where items are collected and then decontaminated/cleaned
2. **Packaging area:** Here, the items (medical devices) are enclosed in materials to allow the penetration of the sterilant during sterilization
3. **Sterilization area:** The packed medical devices are subjected to sterilization process by steam sterilizer, or ethylene oxide sterilizer (ETO)
4. **Sterile storage area:** After sterilization, the sterilized items are stored in this area.

Factors Influencing Efficacy of Sterilant/Disinfectant

The efficiency of a sterilant/disinfectant is affected by various factors.

- ❖ **Organism load**: As the bioburden increases, the contact time of the disinfectant also needs to be increased
- ❖ **Nature of organisms**: Organisms vary greatly in their resistance to disinfectants and sterilants

> The decreasing order of resistance of microorganisms to various agents used for sterilization or disinfection is as follows.
> Prions > bacterial spores > coccidian oocyst > mycobacteria > non-enveloped viruses > fungi > vegetative bacteria > enveloped viruses

- ❖ **Concentration:** The agents should be used at their optimal concentration to produce the desired antimicrobial action
- ❖ **Contact time:** It is the most crucial factor for a disinfectant to be effective. It refers to the time period, which a disinfectant is in direct contact with the surface or item to be disinfected. Lower exposure time doesn't achieve effective killing
- ❖ **Temperature:** The activity of most agents increases as the temperature increases. However, inappropriate higher temperatures may degrade the agent
- ❖ **Stability:** Some agents are unstable at in-use concentration, e.g. hypochlorite, and should be freshly prepared each day
- ❖ **Local pH:** The pH influences the antimicrobial activity
- ❖ **Relative humidity** is an important factor influencing the activity of gaseous disinfectant such as ethylene oxide (ETO)
- ❖ **Organic matter** such as pus, serum, blood, and stool can interfere with the antimicrobial activity of some disinfectants, (e.g. hypochlorites and QAC). This can be overcome by mechanically cleaning the instrument or surface/floor before it is subjected for sterilization/disinfection
- ❖ **Biofilm:** Formation of biofilm is another mechanism which prevents the entry of disinfectant/sterilant to act on the microorganisms which are embedded inside the biofilm.

Property of an Ideal Sterilant/Disinfectant

An ideal disinfectant/sterilant should have various properties—(i) broader microbicidal activity, (ii) fast acting, (iii) not affected by environmental factors such as organic matter, (iv) nontoxic, (v) compatible with surfaces/materials to which it is used, (vi) odorless or pleasant odor, (vii) economical and (viii) environmental friendly.

Spaulding's Classification of Medical Devices

Spaulding's classifies the medical devices into three categories according to the degree of risk for infection involved in use of the items **(Table 16.3)**.

The various agents used in the hospital for achieving sterilization, disinfection and cleaning are enlisted in **Table 16.2** and are discussed below.

STERILANTS

Steam Sterilizer (Autoclave)

Principle

Steam sterilizer functions similar to a pressure cooker and follows the general laws of gas.
- Water boils when its vapor pressure equals that of the surrounding atmosphere
- When the atmospheric pressure is raised, the boiling temperature is also raised
- At normal pressure, water boils at 100°C but when the pressure inside a closed vessel increases, the temperature at which water boils also increases.

Mechanism of action: Moist heat destroys microorganisms by irreversible coagulation, denaturation of enzymes and structural proteins.

Components of Steam Sterilizer (Autoclave)

Steam sterilizer is a pressure chamber; consists of a cylinder, a lid and an electrical heater.
- **Pressure chamber:** It consists of:
  - A large **cylinder** (vertical or horizontal) made up of gunmetal or stainless steel, in which the materials to be sterilized are placed
  - A **steam jacket** (water compartment).
- **Lid:** It bears the following:
  - A discharge tap for the passage of air and steam
  - A pressure gauge (sets the pressure at a particular level)
  - A safety valve (to remove the excess steam).
- **Electrical heater**: It is attached to the jacket; that heats the water to produce steam.

Procedure

The materials to be sterilized are placed inside the cylinder. The steam jacket is filled with sufficient water, lid is closed and the electrical heater is put on. The sterilization process can be divided into three phases.
- **Conditioning phase:** After the water boils, the air in the chamber is completely displaced by the steam produced. The steam pressure rises inside and when it reaches the desired set level (15 pounds per square inch), the safety valve opens and excess steam escapes out
- **Exposure phase:** The holding period is counted from this point of time, which is about 15 minutes in most cases
- **Exhaust phase:** After the holding period, the electrical heater is switched off and the steam sterilizer is allowed to cool till it reaches atmospheric pressure.

> **Sterilization Conditions**
> The steam sterilizer can be set to provide higher temperatures by adjusting the pressure provided to the vessel.
> ❑ Cycle duration varies (3 to 18 min) depending on the sterilization temperature (121°C–135°C)
> ❑ The most commonly used sterilization condition is 121°C for 15 min at a pressure of 15 pounds (lbs) per square inch (psi).

Uses of Steam Sterilizer (Autoclave)

Steam sterilizer is the most commonly used sterilization method in the hospital. It is used for:
- All critical and semi-critical items that are heat and moisture resistant: surgical instruments, anesthetic equipment, dental instruments, implanted medical devices and surgical drapes and linens

Table 16.3: Spaulding's classification of medical devices.

Risk category	Definition	Recommended method	Medical equipment or surfaces
Critical device (high risk)	Items that enter a normally sterile site	Sterilization	Surgical instruments, implants/prosthesis, rigid endoscopes, syringes, needles
Semi-critical device (intermediate risk)	Items in contact with mucous membranes or body fluids	Disinfection (HLD)	Respiratory equipment, non-invasive flexible endoscopes, bedpans, urine bottles
Non-critical (low-risk)	Items in contact with intact skin	Disinfection (ILD or LLD)	Non-critical patient items[1] Non-critical environmental surfaces[2]

[1]**Non-critical patient items**—examples include blood pressure cuffs, ECG electrodes, thermometer and stethoscopes
[2]**Non-critical environmental surfaces**—e.g. medical equipment, computers, bedrails, food utensils, bedside tables, patient furniture and floor
(HLD, high-level disinfectant; ILD, intermediate-level disinfectant; LLD, low-level disinfectant)

CHAPTER 16 ◆ Sterilization and Disinfection

- Culture media preparation
- Biomedical waste treatment (e.g. plastic waste and sharps).

Precautions

- It should not be used for sterilizing waterproof materials such as oil and grease or dry materials such as glove powder
- The chamber should not be overfilled and the material should not touch the sides or top of the chamber
- Separate steam sterilizers should be used for treatment of biomedical waste.

Types of Steam Sterilizer

Steam sterilizers are available in various sizes and dimensions.
- **Horizontal type** (large volume capacity) **(Figs 16.1A and B)**: It is used in CSSD, large-size laboratories and for biomedical waste treatment
- **Vertical type** (small volume capacity) **(Fig. 16.1C)**: It is used for small-size laboratories.

Advantages

Steam sterilizer has the following advantages:
- It is low cost than ETO and plasma sterilizers
- Sterilization cycles are fast compared to ETO sterilizers
- It is nontoxic and leaves no by-product behind (unlike ETO).

Disadvantages

Disadvantages of steam sterilizer include:
- Heat can damage acrylics and styrene, PVC material and corrode some metals
- Higher temperature for a prolonged time can harm or shorten the life of instruments.

Sterilization Control

The effectiveness of the sterilization achieved by steam sterilizer can be monitored by:
- **Biological indicator:** Spores of *Geobacillus stearothermophilus* are the best indicator. Their spores are killed in 12 minutes at 121°C
- **Chemical indicators**
  - External pack control, e.g. autoclave tape
  - Bowie-Dick test
  - Internal pack control.
- **Physical indicators:** For example, digital displays on the equipment displaying temperature, time and pressure.

Ethylene Oxide (ETO) Sterilizer

Ethylene oxide (ETO) is one of the widely used gaseous chemical sterilants in CSSD.

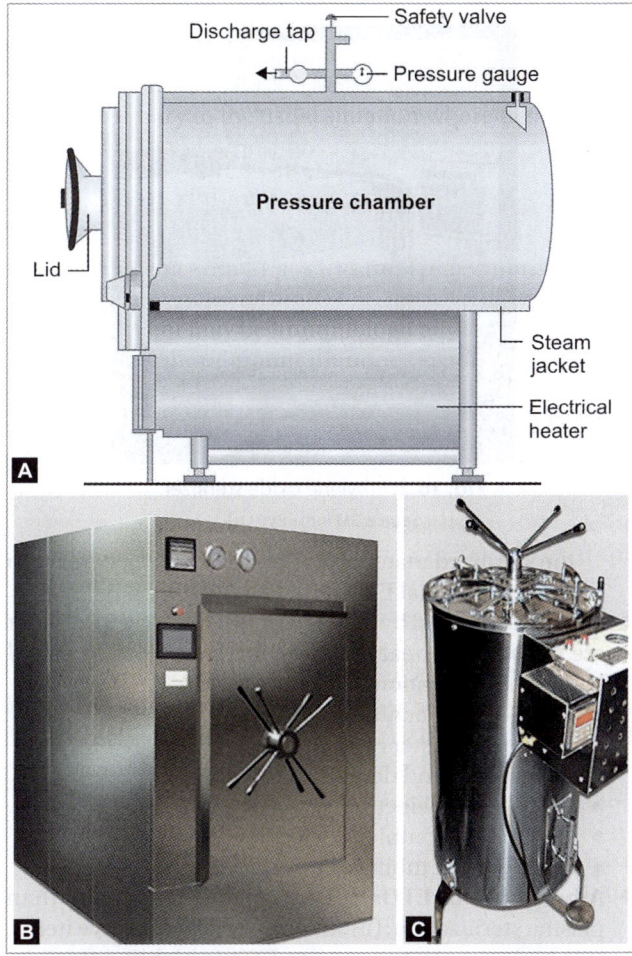

Figs. 16.1A to C: Steam sterilizer (autoclave): **A.** Schematic diagram; **B.** Horizontal autoclave; **C.** Vertical autoclave.

- **Mechanism of action:** ETO has broad microbicidal action including spores; causes alkylation of cell components such as cell proteins, DNA and RNA
- **Sterilization cycle:** It is carried out in a special equipment called ethylene oxide sterilizer **(Fig. 16.2)**. The process comprises of three stages:
  - *Preconditioning:* At first, air is removed from the chamber and vacuum is created. Then the physical conditions (temperature, pressure and humidity) for sterilization are set in the chamber
  - *Sterilization:* ETO is allowed to enter the chamber. At ETO concentration of 700 mg/liter and 40–80% relative humidity, sterilization is achieved in 4–5 hours at 38°C or 1 hour at 55°C
  - *Aeration (Degassing):* The ETO residues left on surgical instruments and tubing may be toxic to the patients and staff. Therefore, extensive aeration of

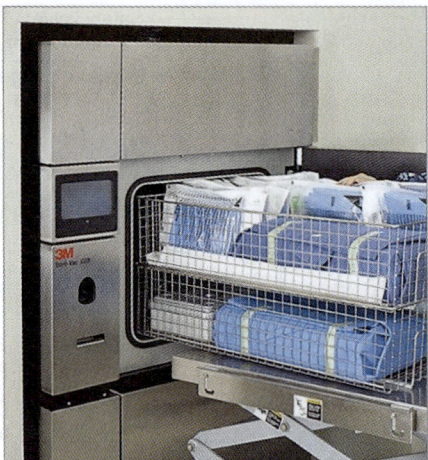

Fig. 16.2: Ethylene oxide sterilizer.
Source: 3M India Pvt. Ltd.

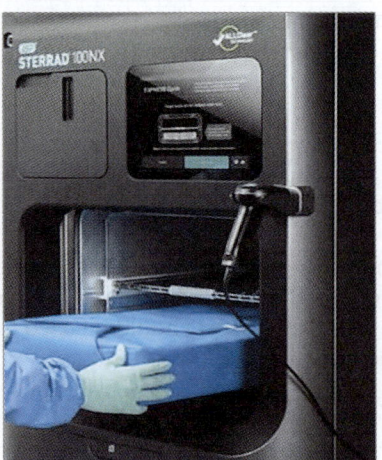

Fig. 16.3: Plasma sterilizer (Sterrad).
Source: Johnson & Johnson Pvt. Ltd.

the sterilized materials for 8–12 hours is necessary to remove residual ETO.
- ❖ **Uses:** ETO is used by CSSD to sterilize critical items that are moisture or heat sensitive and cannot be sterilized by steam sterilization. Examples include:
  - Heart-lung machine components
  - Sutures, catheters and stents
  - Respirators and dental equipment
  - Devices with electronic components
  - Assembled complex devices
  - Multi-lumen tubings, etc.
- ❖ **Advantages of ETO:** (i) Large chamber capacity than plasma sterilization, (ii) suitable for heat sensitive items, (iii) high penetration power-ETO is highly diffusible, penetrates areas that cannot be reached by steam and (iv) non-corrosive to plastic, metal and rubber materials
- ❖ **Disadvantages:** (i) ETO is highly inflammable, irritant, explosive and carcinogenic, (ii) ETO is usually supplied in a 10–20% concentration; mixed with inert gases like either CO_2, (iii) long duration of cycle (12–14 hours) and (iv) high cost of instrument and consumables
- ❖ **Sterilization control:** Spores of *Bacillus atrophaeus* is used as biological indicator to check the effectiveness of sterilization. Physical and chemical indicators are same as discussed for autoclave.

Plasma Sterilization

Plasma refers to a gaseous state consisting of ions, photons, free electrons and free radicals (such as O and OH). Plasma sterilizer is a special device used to create the plasma state (commercial brands, such as *Sterrad*). It has the following steps **(Fig. 16.3)**.
- ❖ **Vacuum:** First, the chamber is evacuated to create a vacuum
- ❖ **Chemical sterilant:** Next step is injection of chemical sterilant hydrogen peroxide (H_2O_2) solution from a cassette, which gets vaporized in the sterilization chamber to a concentration of 6 mg/L
  - The H_2O_2 vapor diffuses through the chamber (50 minutes), exposes all surfaces of the load to the sterilant
  - Low temperature is maintained 37-44°C throughout the cycle.
- ❖ **Gas plasma:** In the next step, an **electrical field** is applied to the chamber to create a gas plasma. H_2O_2 breaks into free radicals such as hydroxyl (OH^-) and hydroperoxyl (HO_2) which initiate microbicidal action, which subsequently interact with essential cell components (e.g. enzymes, nucleic acids)
- ❖ **Finally,** the excess gas is removed
- ❖ **Cycle duration:** It has a cycle time of 75 min. The newer versions have shorter cycles of 52 min and 24 min
- ❖ **Sterilization control:** Spores of *Geobacillus stearothermophilus* is used as a biological indicator to check the effectiveness of sterilization. Physical and chemical indicators are the same as discussed for the autoclave.

Uses of Plasma Sterilizer

It is used by CSSD for sterilization of materials and devices that cannot tolerate high temperature and humidity of steam sterilizer, such as some plastics, electrical devices, and corrosion-susceptible metals such as arthroscope, micro and vascular instruments, spine sets and laparoscope.

Precautions/Disadvantages

The following precautions should be followed while using plasma sterilizer.
- ❖ Items should be dried before loading
- ❖ Linen or paper or cellulose or liquid cannot be processed
- ❖ It may not penetrate well, especially in channels or devices designed with long lumens

- It has a small chamber, therefore cannot be used for bulk items
- High cost of equipment and packing materials.

Dry Heat Sterilizer (Hot Air Oven)

This method is used for materials that might be damaged by moist heat or that are impenetrable to the moist heat (e.g. glass wares, powders, petroleum products, sharp instruments).
- **Procedure:** It has a sterilization chamber, which is electrically heated and has a fan or a motor to ensure adequate and even distribution of hot air in the chamber **(Fig. 16.4)**
  - Dry heat acts by oxidation of cell constituents
  - The most common cycles used are 170°C for 60 minutes, 160°C for 120 minutes, and 150°C for 150 minutes.
- **Advantages:** (i) It is non-toxic and does not harm environment, (ii) low operating costs, (iii) penetrates well into materials, (iv) noncorrosive for metals
- **Disadvantages:** The high temperatures are not suitable for most materials
- **Sterilization control:** Spores of *Bacillus atrophaeus* is used as biological indicator as they are more resistant to dry heat than are *Geobacillus stearothermophilus* spores.

Filtration

Filtration acts by removing microorganisms, not by killing, rather only filters them out.

There are two types of filters.
- **Depth filters:** They retain particles throughout the depth of the filter, rather than just on the surface **(Fig. 16.5A)**. They are used as drinking water purifiers.
- **Membrane filters:** They are the most widely used filters in hospitals. They retain all the particles on the surface that are larger than their pore size **(Figs. 16.5B and 16.6)**
- Membrane filtration has two wider applications in hospital settings—filtration of air and water.

Filtration of Air

- **Surgical (3-ply) mask and respirators:** They are simplest examples of filters being used for purification of air.
- **HEPA filters** (High-efficiency particulate air filters):
  - HEPA filter removes 99.97% of particles that have a size of 0.3 µm or more
  - HEPA filters in hospitals are used in biological safety cabinets, airflow system, operation theatre, and isolation rooms.
- **ULPA filters** (ultra-low particulate/penetration air): An ULPA filter can remove from the air at least 99.999% of dust, pollen, mold, bacteria and any airborne particles with a size of 0.12 µm or larger.

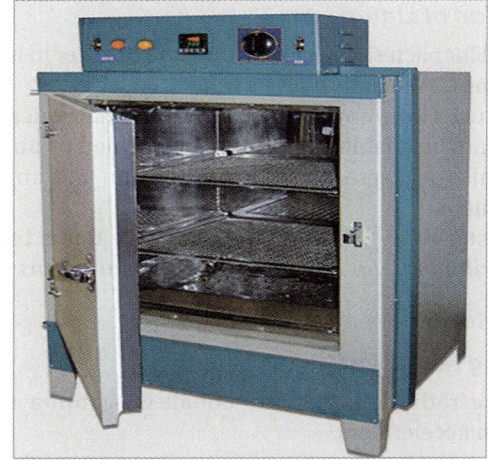

Fig. 16.4: Dry heat sterilizer (hot air oven).

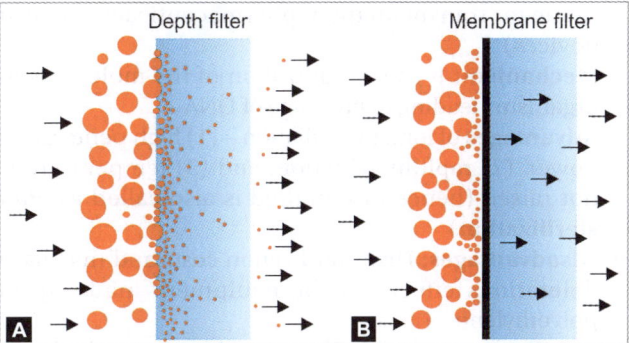

Figs. 16.5A and B: Filtration methods: **A.** Depth filters; **B.** Membrane filters.

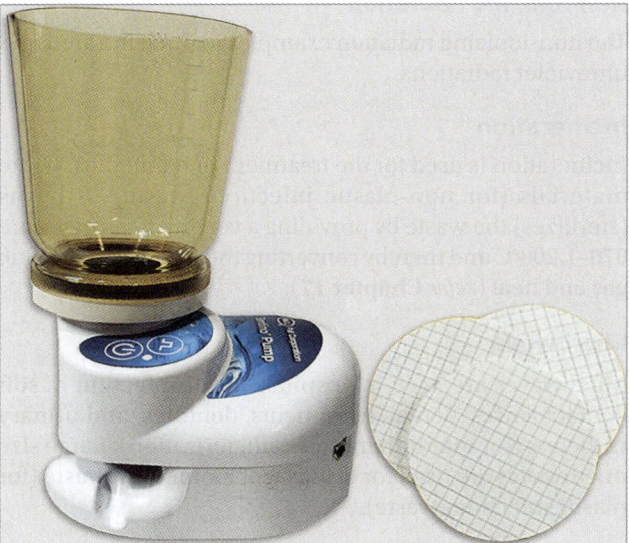

Fig. 16.6: Filter apparatus with membrane filter.
Source: Department of Microbiology, JIPMER, Puducherry.

Filtration of Liquid

- Used for bacteriological examination of water in hospital settings, especially dialysis water
- Also used to remove bacteria from pharmaceutical fluids that are heat labile and cannot be purified by any other means—e.g. sera, sugar, toxin, vaccine and antibiotic solutions.

The sterilization control of membrane filters includes *Brevundimonas diminuta* and *Serratia marcescens*.

Radiation

Ionizing Radiation

Ionizing radiations include cobalt 60 gamma rays or electron accelerators.

- **Use:** It is a low-temperature sterilization method that has been used for a number of medical products (e.g. tissue for transplantation, pharmaceuticals, medical devices)
- **Mechanism:** It causes ionization of the molecules in organisms leading to breakage of DNA
- **Advantages** of ionizing radiation—(1) high penetrating power, (2) rapidity of action, and (3) temperature is not raised (hence this method is also called as **cold sterilization**)
- **Disadvantages:** High sterilization costs and may have deleterious effects on the equipment made up of polyethylene
- **Sterilization control:** Efficacy of ionizing radiation is tested by using *Bacillus pumilus*.

Non-ionizing Radiation

The non-ionizing radiation examples include infrared and ultraviolet radiations.

Incineration

Incineration is used for the treatment of biomedical waste materials (for non-plastic infectious waste). It burns (sterilizes) the waste by providing a very high temperature 870–1,200°C and thereby converting the waste into ash, flue gas and heat (*refer* **Chapter 17**).

Microwave

Microwaves are used in hospitals for disinfection of soft contact lenses, dental instruments, dentures, and urinary catheters (for intermittent self-catheterization). Large size microwaves are used for disposal of biomedical waste (for plastic infectious waste).

■ HIGH-LEVEL DISINFECTANTS (HLD)

HLD agents are capable of killing bacterial spores when used in sufficient concentration under suitable conditions. They can kill all the other microorganisms.

Aldehyde

Formaldehyde, glutaraldehyde and ortho-phthalaldehyde are the commonly used disinfectants. They combine with nucleic acids, proteins and inactivate them, probably by cross-linking and alkylating the molecules.

Glutaraldehyde

- **Semicritical items:** It remains active in the presence of organic matter and is non-corrosive to equipment. Therefore, glutaraldehyde is the most common HLD used for semicritical equipment, such as endoscopes and cystoscopes
    - It is used at 2% or 2.4% concentration (e.g. Cidex). It disinfects objects within 20 minutes but may require longer time to kill spores (10–14 hours)
    - It is available in inactive form; has to be activated by alkalinization before use. Once activated, it remains active only for 14 days.
- **Aerial disinfection and cleaning:** It is also used for fogging and cleaning of floor and surfaces of critical areas such as operation theatre (e.g. Bacillocid Extra)
- **Advantages:** It remains active in the presence of organic matter, has excellent material compatibility
- **Disadvantages:** It has a pungent odor, can produce eye irritation, occupational asthma and contact dermatitis.

Ortho-phthalaldehyde (0.55%)

This can also be used for disinfection of semicritical items, has many advantages over glutaraldehyde—(1) it does not require activation, (2) better odor, (3) less eye irritation, (4) acts faster (5–10 min). However, it does not kill spores effectively and stains skin gray.

Formaldehyde

Although it is an excellent HLD, the health-care uses of formaldehyde are limited because it produces irritating fumes and pungent odor and also a potential carcinogen. It was used for fumigation of closed areas, such as operation theatre, but now this is an obsolete practice.

Peracetic Acid

Peracetic acid is used in automated machines. It is also available for manual immersion; 0.1–0.2%, used for 5–15 min.

- **Use:** It can be used to sterilize medical (e.g. endoscopes, arthroscopes), surgical, and dental instruments. Peracetic acid in combination with hydrogen peroxide has been used for disinfecting hemodialyzers
- **Disadvantages:** Expensive, has material compatibility issues, causes chemical irritation and eye damage.

Hydrogen Peroxide (H_2O_2)

H_2O_2 works by producing destructive hydroxyl free radicals that can attack various cell components.

- **Uses:** H_2O_2 has several usages at various concentrations. It is sporicidal only at >4–5%
  - 3% H_2O_2 is used for environmental surface disinfection, fogging and for wound cleaning
  - 3–6% H_2O_2 is used to disinfect soft contact lens, tonometer biprisms, ventilators, fabrics, and endoscopes, etc.
  - 6–7.5% H_2O_2 is used as chemical sterilant in plasma sterilization
  - Vaporized H_2O_2 is used for industrial sterilization of medical devices and for decontamination of large and small area.
- **Advantages:** It is rapid in action, nontoxic, has detergent properties with good cleaning ability, and is active in the presence of organic material
- **Disadvantages** include—expensive, has material compatibility issue (contraindicated for use on copper, brass, zinc, aluminium), can produce chemical irritation and corneal damage. It should be properly stored in dark containers.

INTERMEDIATE-LEVEL DISINFECTANTS

Alcohol

Ethyl alcohol and isopropyl alcohol are the most popular alcohols used in hospitals.
- **Action:** They are rapidly bactericidal to most organisms except spores. The cidal activity drops sharply when diluted below 50% concentration. They act by denaturation of proteins
- **Uses:** Alcohol (60–80%) is used for various purposes
  - **Alcohol based handrub** (ABHR), e.g. Sterillium, a popular commercial product
  - Disinfecting **smaller non-critical instruments** such as thermometers, which are immersed in alcohol for 10–15 minutes
  - Disinfection of **small medical items/surfaces** such as rubber stoppers of multiple-dose medication vials or vaccine bottles and hubs of the central line
  - Disinfection of **external surfaces of equipment** such as stethoscopes, ventilators, manual ventilation bags, ultrasound machines, etc.
  - Disinfection of **non-critical surfaces** such as laboratory bench, medication preparation areas.
  - **Spirit** (70% alcohol): Used a skin antiseptic
- **Disadvantages:** (i) Flammable and must be stored in a cool, well-ventilated area, (ii) Evaporate rapidly, making exposure time difficult to achieve and (iii) Inactivated by organic matter.

Phenolics

The phenol and its derivatives (called phenolics) are produced by distillation of coal tar.

- **Mechanisms:** Phenolics act as protoplasmic poison, disrupt the cell wall and precipitate the cell proteins
- **Used as disinfectants:** Cresol, and lysol are the common phenolics used for disinfecting environmental surfaces (e.g. bedside tables, bedrails, and laboratory surfaces) and noncritical medical devices. They are toxic to skin, hence not used as antiseptics. **5% phenol** is mycobactericidal, used for disinfection of sputum specimen
- **Used as antiseptics:** Certain phenolics are compatible with skin and are widely used as antiseptics. The classical example is chloroxylenol (the active ingredient of the commercial brand, Dettol)
- **Advantages:** Phenolics are the only ILD that retain activity in the presence of organic materials
- **Disadvantages:** They can cause hyperbilirubinemia in infants and therefore should not be used in nurseries.

Halogens

Among the halogens, iodine and chlorine have antimicrobial activity. They exist in free state, and form salt with sodium and other metals.

Iodine

Iodine acts by disruption of protein and nucleic acid.
- **Preparations:** Two iodine preparations are available.
  - **Tincture of iodine:** It is a preparation of iodine (2%) in potassium iodide. It used as antiseptic for wound cleaning, but can cause staining and skin allergy
  - **Iodophor (e.g. povidone iodine):** It is prepared by complexing iodine with carrier (povidone) which helps in sustained-release of iodine. It is nonstaining and free of skin toxicity. Some popular brands available are Wescodyne and Betadine.
- **Uses:** Iodophors are used both as antiseptics and disinfectant at different concentrations. Therefore, antiseptic iodophors are not suitable for use as disinfectants and vice-versa
  - **Used as antiseptics**
    - 5% topical solution and ointment is used for wound cleaning
    - 7.5% is used for hand scrub
    - 10% is used for surgical skin preparation
    - 1% is used as an oral antiseptic, for mouth wash.
  - **Used as disinfectant** for medical equipment, such as hydrotherapy tanks and thermometers.

Chlorine and Hypochlorite

Chlorine is one of the most commonly available disinfectant in hospital.
- **Preparations:** Chlorine occurs as—(1) free chlorine and (2) hypochlorite.

- **Mechanisms:** All preparations yield hypochlorous acid (HClO), which causes oxidation of cellular materials and destruction of vegetative bacteria and fungi
- **Uses (free chlorine):** Chlorine is used for disinfection of municipal water supplies and swimming pool water. It is also employed in the dairy and food industries
- **Uses (sodium hypochlorite):** It is available at 5.25–6.15%, which is equivalent to 50,000 ppm of available chlorine. It should be used in appropriate dilutions (by adding with water) for disinfection of various hospital supplies. The contact time is about 10–20 minutes
    - Large blood spill: 0.5% (1:10 dilution or 5,000 ppm) is used
    - Small blood spill: 0.05% (1:100 dilution, or 500 ppm) is used
    - Pre-treatment of liquid waste before disposal: 1% (1:5 dilution, 10,000 ppm) is used
    - Surface disinfectant: 0.5% (1:10 dilution or 5,000 ppm) is used
    - *C. difficile* (diarrheal stool): Hypochlorite is sporicidal only >0.5% (5000 ppm).
- **Advantages:** Hypochlorites are broad spectrum, rapid in its action, non-flammable, low cost and are widely available
- **Disadvantages:** (1) Inactivated by organic matter, which can be overcome by adding excess chlorine, (2) Toxic to skin and mucosa, and carcinogenic, (3) Daily preparation—hypochlorite is unstable, evaporates on exposure to sunlight or air. Hence, it has to be prepared daily and stored in opaque container, (4) Leaves residue, requires rinsing or neutralization and (5) Offensive odors.

Heat-based Methods

The following heat-based methods can act as ILD, kill all organisms except the spores.
- **Pasteurization:** Developed by Louis Pasteur and is used for destroying the food-spoiling organisms in milk and fruit juice and thereby extending their shelf-life. In hospitals, pasteurization is used to disinfect respiratory and anesthesia equipment, by immersing in hot water (70°C for 30 min)
- **Inspissation:** The egg-based culture media such as Lowenstein–Jensen medium are sterilized by heating at 80–85°C for 30 minutes on three successive days so that the spores can be killed
- **Boiling at 100°C:** Boiling of the items in water for 15 minutes may kill most of the vegetative forms but not the spores, hence not suitable for sterilization of surgical instruments
- **Steaming at 100°C:** When the autoclave is used without closing the pressure valve, the temperature does not rise beyond 100°C. It may be useful for disinfecting those items which cannot withstand the high temperature of autoclave
- **Tyndallization** or intermittent sterilization: The gelatin, egg, serum containing media are sterilized by heating at 100°C for 20 minutes on 3 successive days (similar to inspissation).

Ultraviolet (UV) Radiation

Ultraviolet (UV) radiation is a form of non-ionizing radiation that is emitted by the sun and artificial sources such as mercury vapor bulbs.
- **Mechanism of action:** Causes destruction of nucleic acid through induction of thymine dimers. Bacteria and viruses are more easily killed by UV light but not spores
- **Uses:** UV radiation has been employed for:
    - Disinfection of drinking water, titanium implants and contact lenses
    - Disinfection of air and/or surfaces as in operating rooms, isolation rooms, and biologic safety cabinets
    - Sun-rays also contain UV rays, which may disinfect organisms present on environmental surfaces.
- **Disadvantages:** The effectiveness is influenced by organic matter. In isolation rooms, it may cause skin erythema and keratoconjunctivitis in patients and visitors.

LOW-LEVEL DISINFECTANTS

Low-level disinfectants (LLD) destroy vegetative bacteria and enveloped viruses, variable action on nonenveloped viruses, and fungi, but no action on tubercle bacilli and spores.

Quaternary Ammonium Compound (QAC)

QAC are commonly used in ordinary environmental sanitation of noncritical surfaces, such as floors, furniture, and walls. Some products are also used for disinfecting non-critical medical equipment that contacts intact skin (e.g. blood pressure cuffs). QAC are also good cleaning agents as they have surfactant like action.
- **Mechanism:** They act by inactivation of energy-producing enzymes, denaturation of essential cell proteins, and disruption of the cell membrane
- **QAC formulations:** Benzyl ammonium chloride is the most popular QAC used in the healthcare. It does not act in the presence of hard water. The newer generation of QACs (e.g. didecyl dimethyl ammonium bromide) remain active in hard water and are better compatible.

Chlorhexidine Gluconate (CHG)

CHG is a biguanide disinfectant, acts by disruption of cytoplasmic membrane.

- **Uses:** CHG is widely used in antiseptic products, at various concentrations
  - **Hand hygiene product:** Hand rub (0.5%), hand wash (4%) (e.g. Microshield, a commercial product)
  - **Mouthwash** (0.1–0.2%)
  - **Body wash** solutions (used before surgery)
  - **Skin disinfectant** before surgery (2 %)
  - **Antiseptic** for wound cleaning: Commercially available as **Savlon** which is a combination of CHG 0.3%, cetrimide and isopropyl alcohol.
- **Advantages:** The wide use of CHG is due to its residual activity (prolonged action than alcohol hand rub) and is less irritant
- **Disadvantages:** It is slower in action, activity is pH dependent and is greatly reduced in the presence of organic matter. It produces dermatitis on prolonged use as handrub.

CLEANING AGENTS

Most disinfectants act well only when the instrument or the surface is free from organic matter such as dirt, blood, or other specimens.
- Therefore, cleaning is a very important step which needs to be performed before the disinfectants are applied
- An ideal cleaning agent should have the following properties: easily emulsifiable, saponifiable, water softening, non-toxic and have surfactant like action.

Cleaning Products

Broadly two types of cleaning agents are available.
1. **Enzymatic (proteolytic) cleaners:** They remove protein from surfaces
2. **Cleaning chemicals (detergents):** These agents act by reducing surface tension and dissolving fat and organic matter. Detergents used for surface and floor cleaning are different than that used for instrument cleaning.

ENVIRONMENTAL CLEANING

Environmental cleaning of the floor and surface of hospitals play a vital role in controlling the spread of infections. The general principles of environmental cleaning are as follows.
- **Cleaning followed by disinfections:**
  - **Cleaning:** Always cleaning with a detergent is performed first, before applying disinfectant
  - **Disinfection:** CDC recommends to use low- to intermediate-level disinfectants for environmental cleaning such as QAC, hypochlorite and improved hydrogen peroxide.
- **Cleaning sequence:** Cleaning should be performed in correct sequence to prevent recontamination
  - **Cleaner to dirtier:** The cleaner areas are cleaned first, followed by the dirtier areas; for e.g. low-touch surfaces should be cleaned first followed by high-touch surfaces
  - **High to low:** Top area should be cleaned first, then proceed towards bottom (e.g. bedrails → bed legs and table surfaces → floors)
  - **Inward to outwards:** Clean the farthest point from the door first and then proceed towards the door.
- **Frequency of cleaning for common situations:**
  - Non-critical surfaces and floors can be cleaned 2-3 times a day
  - Mattress used for patients should be cleaned weekly and after discharge
  - Doors, windows, walls and ceiling should be cleaned once a month and spot-cleaning when soiled
  - **High touch areas** such as doorknobs, elevator buttons, telephones, bedrails, light switches, computer keyboards, monitoring equipment should be cleaned more frequently, every 3–4 hours.

Disinfection of Operation Theatre

Environmental cleaning in operation theatre (OT) minimizes patients' and HCWs' exposure to potentially infectious microorganisms.
- **Surface disinfection:** Cleaning should be performed first with a cleansing agent, followed by disinfection by using an aldehyde-based disinfectant. Disinfection of OT is carried out in the following situations
  - First cleaning of the day (before cases begin)
  - In between cases (cleaning 3 to 4 feet perimeter around the OT table)
  - Terminal cleaning of OT after the last case
  - Detailed wash-down of the OT complex once a week
  - During renovation or construction of OT or nearby places.
- **Fogging:** Also called aerial disinfection, involves spraying of a disinfectant (e.g. glutaraldehyde, H_2O_2 or QAC based product) with the help of a fogger machine
  - The procedure takes around 1-2 hours, during which OT should be closed down and personnel need to be vacated
  - Indication: Routine periodic fogging is not recommended, but is indicated only when any outbreak of infection is suspected or any change in infection control practice implemented or during renovation or construction of OT or nearby places.

METHODS TO TEST EFFICACY OF STERILANT/DISINFECTANT

Tests for Chemical Disinfectants

Chemical disinfectants used in hospitals and laboratories must be tested periodically to ascertain its potency and efficacy. Various methods are available.

- **Rideal and Walker test or Phenol coefficient test**: It tests the efficacy of a phenolic disinfectant to kill *Salmonella* Typhi, when compared with that of phenol
- **Chick Martin test**: It is a modification of Rideal and Walker test, in which the disinfectant acts in the presence of organic matter (e.g. dried yeast, feces, etc.) to simulate the natural conditions
- **Capacity (Kelsey-Sykes) test**: It tests the capacity of a disinfectant to retain its activity when the microbiological load keeps increasing. It is used to test new disinfectants procured in hospitals to know which dilutions are suitable for use
- **In-use (Kelsey-Maurer) test**: It simulates real-time situation. It is used to determine whether an in-use solution of disinfectant in hospital is microbiologically contaminated.

Tests for Sterilizers (Indicators)

The efficacy of sterilizers can be assessed by using physical, chemical and biological indicators.

- **Physical Indicator:** These are the digital displays of the sterilizer equipment showing parameters such as temperature, time and pressure, etc.
- **Chemical indicator:** They use heat or chemical sensitive materials which undergo a color change if the sterilization parameter (e.g. time, steam quality and temperature) for which it is issued is achieved. Example include—Bowie-Dick test (for steam sterilizer)
- **Biological indicator (BI):** It is the most reliable indicator as it uses bacterial spores to check the effectiveness of sterilization. The spores are highly resistant and will be destroyed only when the effective condition is achieved. Example include—spores of *Geobacillus stearothermophilus* for steam sterilizer and gas plasma sterilizer.

Common sterilization agents/disinfectants used in the hospital and their applications have been enlisted in **Table 16.4**.

Table 16.4: Common sterilization agents/disinfectants used in the hospital and their applications.		
Agents		**Applications/Uses**
Sterilants	Steam sterilizer (autoclave)	• Used by CSSD for the sterilization of all critical and semi-critical items that are heat and moisture-resistant: e.g., surgical, anesthetic, dental instruments, implanted medical devices, and surgical drapes and linens • Used by microbiology laboratory for culture media preparation • Biomedical waste treatment (e.g. plastic waste and sharps)
	Ethylene oxide (ETO) sterilizer	It is used by CSSD to sterilize **heat-sensitive critical items** such as: • Heart-lung machine components, respirators, dental equipment • Sutures, catheters, stents, multi-lumen tubings, etc.
	Plasma sterilization	Used by CSSD for the sterilization of some plastics, electrical devices, and corrosion-susceptible metals such as arthroscopes, micro, and vascular instruments, spine sets, and laparoscope
High-level disinfectants	Glutaraldehyde (2%)	• Used for semi-critical items such as **endoscopes and cystoscopes** as it is non-corrosive to metals • Air and surface disinfection: It is also used for fogging, cleaning floors and surfaces of critical areas such as operation theatres (e.g. Bacillocid extra)
	Ortho-phthalaldehyde (0.55%)	It can also be used for sterilization of endoscopes and cystoscopes and has the advantage over glutaraldehyde as it does not require prior activation
	Peracetic acid (0.1–0.2%)	It can be used to sterilize medical (e.g. endoscopes, arthroscopes), surgical, and dental instruments
	Hydrogen peroxide	• 3% H_2O_2 is used for environmental surface disinfection and fogging • 3–6% H_2O_2 is used to disinfect soft contact lenses, tonometer biprisms, ventilators, fabrics, and endoscopes, etc. • 6–7.5% H_2O_2 is used as a chemical sterilant in plasma sterilization
Intermediate-level disinfectants	Alcohols	• It is used as surgical spirit (70%) in **hand rubs or, as antiseptics.** • Used for disinfection of small non-critical items like thermometers, stethoscopes, etc. • Used for disinfection of external surfaces of equipment such as ventilators, manual ventilation bags, ultrasound machines, etc. • Spray and wipes are used for surface disinfection (e.g. laboratory bench, etc.)
	Phenolic compounds	• Used as **surface disinfectants** in hospitals: e.g. **Cresol and Lysol** • 5% phenol is used for the disinfection of sputum • Used as antiseptics: Chloroxylenol, commercially available as **Dettol** • Active in presence of organic matter

Contd...

CHAPTER 16 ◆ Sterilization and Disinfection

Contd...

Agents		Applications/Uses
	Povidone iodine	Used as a skin antiseptic for wounds, pre-operatively and also before venepuncture
	Chlorine	• It is used for the disinfection of potable water supplies • It is used also as a bleaching agent to remove the stain from clothes
	Sodium hypochlorite	• Used as laboratory **disinfectant in discarding jars (1%),** for blood spillages (0.5%), and as a surface disinfectant: 0.5% • Disinfection of laundry items (0.1%) • Pre-treatment of liquid waste before disposal: 1%
Low-level disinfectants	Quaternary ammonium compounds	• Used as a surface disinfectant for noncritical surfaces, such as floors, and walls • In combination with glutaraldehyde: Used as a surface disinfectant for critical surfaces • Disinfecting non-critical medical equipment (e.g. blood pressure cuffs) • QAC are also good cleaning agents as they have surfactant-like action
	Chlorhexidine Gluconate (CHG)	• It is used as a **hand rub (0.5%), hand wash (4%),** body wash solutions, skin disinfectant before surgery (2%), and for wound cleaning • It is commercially available as **Savlon** which is a combination of CHG 0.3%, cetrimide, and isopropyl alcohol

EXPECTED QUESTIONS

I. Write essays on:
1. Define sterilization and disinfection. Describe principle and uses of steam sterilizers.
2. What are chemical sterilants? Discuss their application in healthcare settings.

II. Write short notes on:
1. Membrane filters.
2. Application of glutaraldehyde in healthcare setting.

III. Multiple Choice Questions (MCQs):
1. Which of the following disinfectant is used in plasma sterilization?
    a. Formaldehyde
    b. Glutaraldehyde
    c. Hydrogen peroxide
    d. Ethylene oxide
2. *Geobacillus stearothermophilus* is used as indicator for efficacy of:
    a. Hot air oven
    b. Autoclave
    c. Filtration
    d. Ultraviolet rays
3. Endoscope is sterilized by:
    a. Glutaraldehyde
    b. Formaldehyde
    c. Autoclaving
    d. Hot air oven
4. Which of the following disinfectant is used for hand wash?
    a. Ethylene oxide
    b. Formaldehyde
    c. Chlorhexidine
    d. Povidone iodine
5. Which of the following is used for disinfection of blood spillage area?
    a. Phenol
    b. Hypochlorite
    c. Lysol
    d. Formaldehyde

Answers
1. c 2. b 3. a 4. c 5. b

Biomedical Waste Management

CHAPTER 17

CHAPTER PREVIEW
- Biomedical Waste Rule
- Waste Segregation in Hospitals
- Treatment and Disposal Methods
- Blood Spill Management

INTRODUCTION

The waste generated from the hospital carries a higher potential for infections and injuries. Therefore, it is essential to have safe and reliable methods of segregation and disposal of hospital waste.

Definition

Biomedical wastes (BMW) are defined as wastes that are generated during the laboratory diagnosis, treatment or immunization of human beings or animals, or in research activities pertaining thereto, or in the production of biologicals.

Waste Generated in Hospitals

In developing countries, the waste generated in hospitals falls into two categories:
1. **General (non-hazardous solid waste, 80%):** A large amount of waste falls in the general waste category, which may be disposed of with the usual domestic and urban waste management system. They do not cause any harm to humans. They are not considered as BMW. They should not be mixed with BMW
2. **Biomedical waste:** This includes infectious waste (10%) and chemical/radioactive waste (5%).

Hazards Associated with BMW

Inappropriate and inefficient disposal of BMW can lead to infectious hazards, malignancies, malformations, and environmental (air, land and water) pollution not only to the current generation but also for future generations. The various hazards are:
- ❖ **Hazards from infectious wastes:** This is the component of hospital waste that produces maximum hazards
  - Pathogens in the infectious waste may infect HCWs by entering through ingestion, inhalation or direct skin-to-skin contact and can cause various type of infections such as gastrointestinal, respiratory, skin infections, etc.
  - **Hazards from infectious sharps**—leads to transmission of blood borne viruses (hepatitis B, C and HIV).
- ❖ **Hazards from chemical wastes:** They include laboratory reagents, disinfectants, and waste with high content of heavy metals, e.g. mercury from broken thermometers. Most chemicals are toxic, corrosive, explosive and flammable; can cause various physical injuries including chemical burns
- ❖ **Pharmaceutical waste:** It includes expired, unused and contaminated drugs, vaccines, sera, etc. Exposure to these agents may cause several adverse effects depending upon the nature of the pharmaceutical waste
- ❖ **Hazards from cytotoxic waste:** Cytotoxic drugs used in the treatment of cancers and autoimmune disorders are extremely hazardous to the environment and human health owing to their mutagenic, teratogenic, or carcinogenic properties
- ❖ **Hazards from radioactive waste:** They include materials contaminated with radionuclides
  - They are produced as a result of procedures performed by radiology and nuclear medicine departments
  - They are genotoxic, in higher doses can cause severe injuries, including tissue destruction, necessitating the amputation of body parts.

Situation in India

According to the Ministry of Environment and Forests (MoEF), the gross generation of BMW in India is about 484 TPD (tons per day). Unfortunately, only 447 TPD is treated, and 37 TPD (8%) is left untreated. Karnataka tops the chart among all the states in generation of BMW followed by Maharashtra.

CHAPTER 17 ❖ Biomedical Waste Management

Waste Management Hierarchy

The waste management hierarchy is largely based on the concept of the "3Rs", namely reduce, recycle and recover. If none of these methods is available, then the last method opted is disposal.

- **Prevent or reduce** the production of waste as far as possible
- **Reuse and recycle** the waste
- **Recover the waste** items for secondary use, for example waste is converted to fuel for generating electricity
- **Treatment:** Wastes that cannot be recycled or recovered, can be subjected to incineration. Treatment is also necessary for the biomedical waste before sending for recycling or recovery as these wastes are potentially infectious. This is usually carried out by the autoclave or microwave (explained later)
- **Disposal** of the waste in landfill or dump yard. This is the least preferable option among all waste management strategies.

■ BIOMEDICAL WASTE RULE, INDIA

The Ministry of Environment and Forests (MoEF) has formulated biomedical waste rule in 1998; had classified the waste into 10 categories, which used to be segregated into five color-coded containers. There was considerable overlapping between categories which created ambiguity and confusion.

The new BMW guideline was published in 2016 with an amendment added in 2018 and 2019. According to this new rule, there are four categories of BMWs, each is segregated by a single color-coded container **(Table 17.1)**.

Table 17.1: Biomedical Waste Management Rule, India, 2016 (including the amendment added in 2018 and 2019).

Category	Type of waste	Type of Bag/container	Treatment/disposal options
Yellow	a. Human anatomical waste	Yellow colored non-chlorinated plastic bags	Incineration/plasma pyrolysis/deep burial
	b. Animal anatomical waste		
	c. Soiled waste		Incineration/plasma pyrolysis/deep burial/autoclaving or hydroclaving + shredding/mutilation
	d. Expired/discarded medicines—pharmaceutical waste, cytotoxic drugs	Yellow colored containers/non-chlorinated plastic bags with cytotoxic label	Sent back to manufacturer/CBMWTF for incineration (cytotoxic drugs at temperature >1,200°C)
	e. Chemical solid waste	Yellow colored containers/nonchlorinated plastic bags	Incineration or plasma pyrolysis or encapsulation
	f. Chemical liquid waste such as discarded disinfectants, infected body fluids and secretions, liquid from house-keeping related activities	To be discharged into separate collection system, which leads to effluent treatment system Not to be discarded into yellow bag	Pre-treated[1] before mixing with other waste water
	g. Discarded linen waste contaminated with blood/body fluids, mask, cap, gown and shoe cover	Non-chlorinated yellow plastic bags/suitable packing material	Non-chlorinated chemical disinfection[2] followed by incineration/plasma pyrolysis
	h. Microbiology, other clinical laboratory waste, blood bags, live attenuated vaccines	Autoclave safe plastic bag/container	Pre-treat to sterilize with non-chlorinated chemicals[2] on-site as per NACO/WHO guidelines (Blue book 2014) + incineration
Red	**Infectious plastic waste** Disposable items such as tubing, bottles, intravenous tubes and sets, catheters, urine bags, syringes (without needles and fixed needle syringes) and vacutainer with their needles cut, gloves, plastic apron and goggles	Red colored non-chlorinated plastic bags or containers	• Autoclaving/microwaving/hydroclaving + shredding • Mutilation/sterilization + shredding Treated waste sent to authorized recyclers or for energy recovery

Contd...

Contd...

Category	Type of waste	Type of Bag/container	Treatment/disposal options
White (Translucent)	**Waste sharps including metal sharps** Needles, syringes with fixed needles, needles from needle tip cutter or burner, scalpels, blades, or any other contaminated sharp (used or discarded)	Puncture-proof, leak-proof, tamper-proof containers	Autoclaving/dry heat sterilization followed by: • Shredding or mutilation or encapsulation in metal container or cement concrete or • Sanitary landfill or • Designated concrete waste sharp pit
Blue	a. **Glasswares:** Broken or discarded and contaminated glass including medicine vials and ampoules except those contaminated with cytotoxic wastes, microscope slides b. **Metallic body implants** Dental implants, other body implants and plates	Puncture proof and leak-proof container	Disinfection can be carried out by: • Soaking the washed glass waste after cleaning with detergent and sodium hypochlorite treatment (1–2%) or • Autoclaving/microwaving/hydroclaving and then it is sent for recycling

Note:
- Biomedical waste rule does not specify any specific color coded bag for general waste segregation in hospital. Depending upon the local policy, hospitals choose any color coded bag for general waste (e.g. JIPMER uses black bag for general waste).
- [1]**Chemical treatment:** Hypochlorite should be used at 1–2% concentration having 30% residual chlorine with contact time of 20 minutes.
- [2]**Non-chlorinated chemicals** include 5% phenol, 5% cresol or 5% lysol.
- The chlorinated plastic bags (except blood bags) and gloves should be phased out and replaced by non-chlorinated bags and gloves.
- Every health care facility should have their own STP (sewage treatment plant).
- Barcoding system should be introduced to monitor the segregation compliance.

(NACO, National AIDS Control Organization; WHO, World Health Organization; CBMWTF, Common bio-medical waste treatment facility)

Steps of BMW Management

The management of BMW can overall be summarized into five simple steps.
1. Waste segregation (at the point of generation) into color-coded containers
2. Pre-treatment for laboratory liquid waste
3. Transport of waste from generation site to central storage area of the hospital
4. Transport of waste from central storage area to common bio-medical waste treatment facility (CBMWTF)
5. Treatment and/or disposal (within 48 hours of generation).

Waste Segregation in Hospitals

Waste segregation refers to the basic separation of different categories of waste generated at source in the hospital and thereby reducing the risks as well as the cost of handling and disposal.

According to BMW Rule (2016), segregation of waste should be done by using containers of four different colors—each is designated for segregation of a particular waste category (*see* **Table 17.1**).
- Yellow bag—for infectious non-plastic waste
- Red bag—for infectious plastic waste
- White or translucent sharp container (puncture-proof box)—for metal sharps
- Blue container (puncture-proof box)—for broken glass items and metal implants.

The following general principles need to be followed during segregation, transport and storage of BMW.
- **Waste receptacles:** The waste receptacles should have the following properties
  - **Plastic bags** must be labeled with biohazard logos (**Fig. 17.1**) and should be non-inflammable, autoclave stable and non-chlorinated with a thickness of ≥50 μm
  - **Containers** should have well-fitting lids, either removable by hand or preferably operated by a foot pedal
  - **Sharp box** should be puncture-proof, leak-proof and tamper-proof impermeable container.

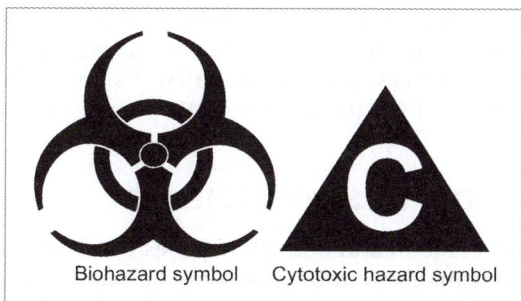

Fig. 17.1: Logos used for segregation of biomedical waste.

- **Importance of segregation**: Segregation is the most crucial step in BMW management. Wrong segregation may lead to serious consequences such as:
  - Needle stick injury transmitting hepatitis B or HIV (if sharp items are segregated in to yellow or red bags)
  - Production of carcinogens (if plastic items are wrongly segregated into yellow bag and subjected to incineration, leads to production of carcinogenic furans).
- **Securement:** All the bags used for waste collection need to be sealed once they are filled to 3/4th of their capacity
- **Labeling:** Bags and containers should be labeled properly with the date and place
- **Pre-treatment:** The laboratory liquid waste should always be pre-treated either with chemical (1–2% hypochlorite) or autoclave before segregating into appropriate containers
- **Transport:** The waste should be transported within 24 hours by **dedicated trolley** to the central BMW storage facility of the hospital. Separate routes should be used for transport to prevent exposure to staff and patients and to minimize the passage of loaded carts through patient care and other clean areas. Interim storage of the waste at ward is strongly discouraged
- **Central storage area:** This is a temporary storage facility present within a hospital where different types of waste should be brought for safe retention until it is treated or collected for transport to CBMWTF
- **Personal protective equipment (PPE):** HCWs handling BMW during transport or in the storage area should wear appropriate PPE such as heavy duty gloves, 3-ply mask, gowns and gumboots.

Treatment and Disposal Methods

As per the mandate of the BMWM rules, 2016, the final disposal and recycling must be performed at common biomedical waste treatment facility (CBMWTF). Only when there is no CBMWTF within 75 km, the hospital can create its own the disposal facility. The following are the methods used for treatment/disposal of BMW.

- **Incineration:** It has been the method of choice for the disposal of BMW. It is a high temperature (800–1,200°C) dry oxidation process that reduces organic and combustible waste into nonorganic incombustible matter, resulting in a very significant reduction of waste volume and weight. It is used for those wastes that cannot be reused or recycled (e.g. microbiological waste, human and animal anatomical waste, etc.)
- **Autoclave:** It is mainly used for the treatment of infectious plastic and sharp waste.
- **Chemical disinfection** using hypochlorite 1–2%. It is more suitable for liquid waste such as discarded blood and body fluids and also for hospital sewage.
- **Effluent Treatment Plant (ETP):** The liquid waste (effluent) generated in the hospital, is first subjected to chemical treatment and then is drained into effluent treatment plant (ETP).
- **Microwaving:** Large size microwaves are used for disposal of BMW—mainly infectious plastics and sharp wastes.
- **Hydroclaving:** It is a low-temperature steam sterilizer, involving steam treatment with fragmentation and drying of waste.
- **Shredder:** It is a process by which wastes are de-shaped or cut into smaller pieces so as to make the wastes unrecognizable.
- **Deep burial** is a pit dug about two meters deep. It needs to be half-filled with waste, and then covered with lime within 50 cm of the surface, before filling the rest of the pit with soil.
- **Sharp pit:** It is an alternative method for disposal of the sharp wastes generated from the facility.
- **Encapsulation:** It involves filling the containers with waste, adding immobilizing material and sealing the containers, to prevent the access to unscrupulous activities.
- **Inertization:** It involves mixing waste with cement and other substances before disposal to minimize the risk of toxic substances contained in the waste migrating to surface or groundwater.
- **Plasma pyrolysis** uses ionized gas in the plasma state to convert electrical energy to temperatures of several thousand degrees using plasma arc torches or electrodes. This methods destroys pathogens completely.

Disposal of Cytotoxic Drug Waste

Expired cytotoxic drugs to be returned back to the manufacturer or supplier or CBMWTF for incineration at >1,200°C or encapsulation or plasma pyrolysis at >1,200°C.

Disposal of General Waste (Solid Waste)

They constitute the large component of hospital waste (80%). They are not biomedical waste; their disposal can be carried out by several strategies.
- **Composting:** It is the decomposition of organic matter by microorganism in warm moist environment
- **Waste-to-energy:** By various methods such as incineration, pelletization, biomethanation, etc.
- Recycling of the waste
- Landfilling in dump yard (least preferred method).

MONITORING OF BMW MANAGEMENT

Monitoring is an essential component of managing biomedical waste in the hospital. BMW management committee should be formed in a healthcare facility, which serves several functions—(1) to oversee the implementation of BMW practices, (2) to educate HCWs about BMWM practices, and (3) to monitor BMW management in a hospital.

BLOOD SPILL MANAGEMENT

Spillage of blood and body fluid poses a substantial risk for the transmission of blood-borne viruses such as hepatitis B, C, and HIV. Therefore, any spillage (small, few drops to large, few mL) should be considered infectious, and need to be cleaned at the earliest. *Refer* **Chapter 15** for details (**Fig. 15.10** and highlight box for steps of spill management, CDC protocol).

EXPECTED QUESTIONS

I. Write short notes on:
   1. Categories of biomedical waste.
   2. Disposal methods available for biomedical waste.
   3. Type of containers used for disposal of biomedical waste.

II. Multiple Choice Questions (MCQs):
   1. **Anatomical waste should be segregated in which color bags?**
      a. Yellow   b. Red
      c. Blue   d. Black
   2. **Microbiological waste should be segregated in which color bags?**
      a. Yellow   b. Red
      c. Blue   d. Black
   3. **Sharps should be segregated in which color box?**
      a. Yellow   b. Red
      c. Blue   d. White
   4. **Plastic infectious items should be segregated in which color bag?**
      a. Yellow   b. Red
      c. Blue   d. White
   5. **Before segregation of microbiological wastes, pre-treatment with what concentration of hypochlorite is recommended?**
      a. 1–2%   b. 5%
      c. 10%   d. 15%
   6. **Blood bag should be segregated in which color bags?**
      a. Yellow   b. Red
      c. Blue   d. Black
   7. **Gloves should be segregated in which color bags?**
      a. Yellow   b. Red
      c. Blue   d. Black

Answers
1. a   2. a   3. d   4. b   5. a   6. a   7. b

Needle Stick Injury (Occupational Exposure)

CHAPTER 18

CHAPTER PREVIEW
- Prevention of Needle Stick Injury
- Post-exposure Management

INTRODUCTION

An occupational exposure is defined as:
- Percutaneous injury, e.g. needle stick injury (NSI) or other sharp injury
- Splash injury:
  - Contact with the mucous membrane (e.g. eye or mouth)
  - Contact with non-intact skin (abraded skin or afflicted with dermatitis)
  - Contact with the intact skin when the duration is prolonged (e.g. several minutes or more).

An occupational injury is often loosely termed as needle stick injury though it includes injury through needle or other sharps and splashes.

Agents transmitted:
Hepatitis B virus (HBV), hepatitis C virus (HCV) and HIV are three major blood-borne viruses (BBVs) that are transmitted through NSI. The risk of transmission is highest for HBV (30%) followed by HCV (3%) and HIV (0.3%).

Infectious specimens for NSI:
- *Potentially infectious body fluids* include blood, genital secretions (semen, vaginal secretions) and all body fluids (CSF, synovial fluid, pleural fluid, peritoneal fluid, pericardial fluid, amniotic fluid)
- *The following are not considered potentially infectious*, unless visibly contaminated with blood: Feces, nasal secretions, saliva, sputum, sweat, tears, urine and vomitus.

Factors that influence the risk of contracting infection following NSI:
The risk of infection following exposure depends on the following factors:
- Type of needle (hollow bore needle has a higher risk than solid needle)
- Device visibly contaminated with blood
- Depth of injury (higher is the depth, more is the risk)
- Volume of blood involved in the exposure
- Viral load present in the blood at the time of exposure
- Timely performing first aid
- Timely start of appropriate post-exposure prophylaxis (PEP) for HBV and HIV.

PREVENTION OF NEEDLE STICK INJURY

Precautions During Handling Needles

The following measures should be taken during handling needles to prevent occupational exposures:
- **Standard precautions** must be followed such as hand hygiene and appropriate use of personal protective equipment (PPE) (e.g. gloves, gowns, masks, and goggles) while handling blood or body fluids
- **Work surfaces** must be disinfected with 0.5% sodium hypochlorite solution
- **HBV vaccination:** Health care workers (HCWs) must be immunized against HBV and protective titer must be documented
- **Spill management:** Spillage of blood and other body fluids must be promptly cleaned and surface disinfected with 0.5% sodium hypochlorite solution
- **Disposable needles** should be used. Needles should never be reused
- **Never recap needles:** If unavoidable, single hand-scoop technique may be followed **(Figs. 18.1A and B)**
- **Disposal after use:** Needles must be disposed into the sharp box immediately after use. Needles/sharps should not be left on trolleys and bedside tables
- **Engineering control measures:** Various devices are specially designed with safety features to prevent NSI such as retractable lancets, safety lock syringe with a protective sheath and needleless IV systems.

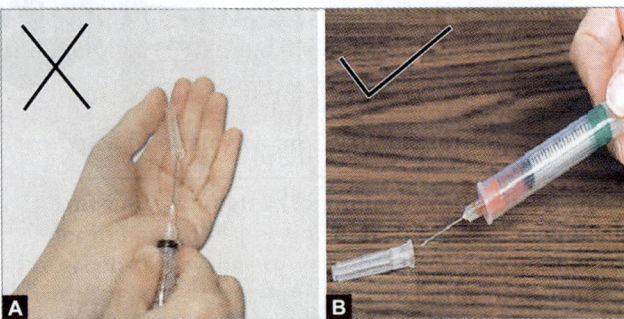

Figs. 18.1A and B: Recapping of needle: **A.** Wrong method; **B.** Correct method (single hand 'scoop' technique).

POST-EXPOSURE MANAGEMENT

Steps of Post-exposure Management

The following are the sequential steps to be followed following an occupational exposure (**Table 18.1**):
1. **First aid:** First aid has to be started as early as possible (**Table 18.2**)
2. **Report to the designated nodal center:** Every hospital must have a nodal center for the management of NSI. In most hospitals, HICC office acts as a nodal center, other hospitals may designate staff clinic or casualty for the purpose. Nodal centers perform the following functions as mentioned below (steps 3–9)
3. **Take first dose of PEP for HIV:**
    - The first dose of PEP for HIV should be taken as early as possible. Effect is maximum if taken <2 hours and effect is nil if taken after 72 hours of exposure
    - **NACO recommendation:** Fixed dose combination of TLD regimen (Tenofovir + Lamivudine + Dolutegravir) is the preferred regimen (**Table 18.3**)
    - If the HIV negative status of the source is documented in patient's case record or in the hospital information system, then the first dose of PEP is not required
    - If test report is not available, then administer the first dose regimen immediately without waiting for the laboratory result.
4. **Testing for BBVs:** The following tests are done for both source and HCW. The test format should be a rapid method (immunochromatographic test or flow through assay) and result should be available within 1–2 hours
    - Anti-HIV antibody detection
    - HBsAg detection
    - Anti-HCV antibody detection
    - Anti-HBs antibody (done for HCW if previously vaccinated for HBV and titer not tested).
5. **Decision on post-exposure prophylaxis** (PEP) for HIV and HBV is taken based on standard guidelines (NACO for HIV and CDC for HBV) as described in **Tables 18.3** and **18.4** respectively.
6. **Informed consent and counseling:** Almost every person feels anxious after exposure. They should be counseled and provided with psychological support
    - They should be informed about the risks and benefits of PEP medications
    - PEP is not mandatory. If the exposed person refuses to take the PEP, it should be documented. However, he should be made to understand about the risk of acquiring infection if PEP is not taken.
7. **Documentation and recording of exposure:**
    - A *structured proforma* should be used to collect the detail information related to exposure such as date, time, and place of exposure, type of procedure done, type of exposure, duration of exposure, source status, volume and type of specimen involved
    - *Consent form:* For prophylactic treatment, the exposed person must sign a consent form. If the individual refuses to initiate PEP, it should be documented. The designated officer for PEP should keep this document.
8. **Follow-up testing** of HCWs for BBVs should be done if the source status is positive/unknown
    - *HIV testing follow-up is done:* At 6 weeks, 3 months and 6 months after exposure

Table 18.1: Steps of post-exposure management.

1. First aid
2. Report to designated nodal center
3. Take first dose of PEP for HIV
4. Testing for BBVs
5. Decision on PEP for HIV and HBV
6. Documentation and recording of exposure
7. Informed consent and counseling
8. Follow-up testing of HCWs
9. Precautions during the follow-up period

(PEP, post-exposure prophylaxis; HCW, health-care worker; BBV, blood-borne virus)

Table 18.2: First Aid: Management of exposed site.

Do's	Don'ts
Earlier the first aid, lesser is the chance of transmission of BBVs • For splash injury: Irrigate thoroughly the site (e.g. eyes or mouth or other exposed area) vigorously with water at least for 5 minutes • Spit fluid out immediately if gone into mouth and rinse the mouth several times • If wearing contact lenses, leave them in place while irrigating. Once the eye is cleaned, remove the contact lens and clean them in a normal manner	• Do not panic • Do not place the pricked finger into the mouth reflexively • Do not squeeze blood from wound • Do not use antiseptics and detergents

CHAPTER 18 ◆ Needle Stick Injury (Occupational Exposure)

Table 18.3: Revised NACO Guidelines for post-exposure prophylaxis (PEP), 2021.

Exposure code (EC)	Source HIV status code (SC)	PEP Recommendation
1, 2 or 3	Negative	Not warranted
1	1	Not warranted
1	2	PEP is recommended Duration of PEP: 28 days **TLD Regimen:** Fixed dose combination (FDC) of Tenofovir (300 mg) + Lamivudine (300 mg) + Dolutegravir (50 mg)—as a single tablet, once daily for 4 weeks
2	1	
2	2	
3	1 or 2	
2 or 3	Unknown (in area with high prevalence)	

Source material: Blood, body fluids or other potentially infectious material (CSF, synovial, pleural, pericardial and amniotic fluid, and pus) or an instrument contaminated with any of these substances

Exposure code:
1. **EC-1 (Mild exposure):** Mucous membrane/non-intact skin exposure with small volumes, or less duration
2. **EC-2 (Moderate exposure):**
   - Mucous membrane/non-intact skin with large volumes/splashes for several minutes or more duration OR
   - Percutaneous superficial exposure with solid needle or superficial scratch
3. **EC-3 (Severe exposure):** Percutaneous exposure with:
   - Large volume transfer
   - By hollow needle, wide bore needle or deep puncture
   - Visible blood on device
   - Needle used in patient's artery or vein

Source HIV Status Code (SC):
1. **SC-1:** HIV positive, asymptomatic or low viral load (<400 copies/mL)
2. **SC-2:** HIV positive, symptomatic (advanced AIDS or primary HIV infection), high viral load
3. **SC Unknown:** Status of the patient is unknown and neither the patient nor his/her blood is available for testing
4. **HIV negative:** Tested negative according to NACO strategy

The first dose of PEP
Should be started within 2 hours (for greater impact) and definitely within 72 hours. No need to provide PEP if exposure occurred >72 hours

PEP is not required in the following situations:
1. If exposed person is HIV positive: Exposed individuals who are known or discovered to be HIV positive should not receive PEP. They should be referred to ART clinic for counseling and initiation of ART
2. If the exposure is on an intact skin
3. If source is HIV negative
4. Exposure with low-risk specimens like tear, saliva, urine, stool, vomitus, nasal secretion, sweat, etc.
5. For exposures with EC-1 and SC-1
6. Source unknown if HIV prevalence is low
7. In case of delay in reporting the exposure by >72 hours, PEP initiation becomes optional

Side effects and compliance to PEP:
- Common side effects are:
  - At the initial phase of the course: Nausea, diarrhea, muscular pain, headache or fatigue
  - Later during the course: Anemia, leukopenia or thrombocytopenia
- For most side effects except jaundice or liver tenderness, **PEP should never be discontinued**.
- Compliance of >95% to the PEP schedule is required to maximize the efficacy of PEP. Hence, the person should be counseled to continue the PEP and to take medication to minimize the side effects of PEP.

Note: Regimen for exposure in pregnant women is essentially same as that of non-pregnant persons.
(NACO, National AIDS Control Organization; ART, antiretroviral therapy)

- HBV and HCV follow-up testing is done at 6 months after exposure.
9. **Precautions during the follow-up period:** If the source status is positive/unknown, then the following precautions should be adopted by the HCW during the follow-up period, especially the first 6–12 weeks
   - Refraining from blood, semen, organ donation
   - Abstinence from sexual intercourse or use of latex condom till both baseline and 3 months HIV tests are found negative
   - Women should not breastfeed their infants
   - The exposed person is advised to seek medical evaluation for any febrile illness that occurs within 12 weeks of exposure.

Table 18.4: Post-exposure prophylaxis (PEP) for hepatitis B.		
HCW status	If source is positive or unknown for HBsAg	If source is negative for HBsAg
If the exposed person is completely vaccinated and the antibody titer is protective (≥10 mIU/mL)	No further treatment is required: • Regardless of the HBV status of the source* • Regardless if the titer falls down later*	
If the exposed person is completely vaccinated and the titer is not protective (<10 mIU/mL)	HBIG-1 dose should be started immediately; maximum within 7 days Vaccine: Start the second series (3 doses)	Vaccine: Start the second series (3 doses)
If the exposed person is not vaccinated or partially vaccinated	HBIG-1 dose should be started immediately; maximum within 7 days Vaccine: Complete the vaccine series from the last dose given (do not restart)	Vaccine: Complete the vaccine series from the last dose given (do not restart)
Nonresponders (If the exposed person is vaccinated for 2 series, i.e. 6 doses and the titer is not protective)	HBIG-2 doses at 1 month apart (0.06 mL/kg or 10–12 IU/kg)	Nothing is required

Note:
- HCW is said to be protected when titer rises (anti-HBs ≥10 mIU/mL), after three or more doses of vaccination. Rise of titer after one or two doses of vaccine should not be considered as protective.
- HCWs who are not protected must be checked for their HBsAg status at baseline and follow-up testing 6 months later, regardless of their vaccination status.
- Anti-HBs antibody titer should be checked only after 2 months of last dose of vaccine and 6 months after HBIG administration; otherwise, it will give erratic results.
- HBIG and HBV vaccine can be administered simultaneously but at different sites.
- HBIG provides a temporary protection for 3–6 months.
- Previous report of Anti-HBs titer is acceptable only if it is documented. Verbal reports should not be considered.

* In a previously protected person, the memory B cells will start producing antibodies soon after the antigenic challenge, hence revaccination by booster doses is not recommended even if the titer falls down later.
Adapted from CDC guideline, 2013.
(HBIG, hepatitis B immunoglobulin; HCW, health-care worker; HBsAg, hepatitis B surface antigen)

EXPECTED QUESTIONS

I. **Write short notes on:**
   1. Sequential steps to be followed after a needle stick injury.
   2. Post-exposure prophylaxis for HIV.
   3. Post-exposure prophylaxis for hepatitis B.

II. **Multiple Choice Questions (MCQs):**
   1. **The decreasing order of risk of transmission following occupational exposure:**
      a. HIV>HBV>HCV
      b. HBV>HIV>HCV
      c. HBV>HCV>HIV
      d. HCV>HBV>HIV
   2. **All are potentially highly infectious specimen for occupational injury; *except*:**
      a. Blood
      b. Semen
      c. CSF
      d. Saliva
   3. **The sequence of steps to be followed after accidental exposure to blood/fluid:**
      a. First aid → Reach to nodal center and try to get report of source status → Take first dose of PEP for HIV → Testing of source and HCW status for BBVs → Prophylactic treatment for HIV and HBV
      b. Reach to nodal center and try to get report of source status → First aid → Take first dose of PEP for HIV → Testing of source and HCW status for BBVs → Prophylactic treatment for HIV and HBV
      c. Take first dose of PEP for HIV → Testing of source and HCW status for BBVs → First aid → Reach to nodal center and try to get report of source status → Prophylactic treatment for HIV and HBV
      d. Prophylactic treatment for HIV and HBV → Take first dose of PEP for HIV → Testing of source and HCW status for BBVs → First aid → Reach to nodal center and try to get report of source status
   4. **The best protection will be achieved if first dose of PEP for HIV is taken within:**
      a. 2 hours of exposure
      b. 6 hours of exposure
      c. 12 hours of exposure
      d. 72 hours of exposure
   5. **Following needle stick injury, the tests for HIV, HBV and HCV are done for:**
      a. For source only
      b. For healthcare workers only
      c. Both for source and healthcare workers
      d. None of the above

Answers
1. c 2. d 3. a 4. a 5. c

Environmental Surveillance (Bacteriology of Water, Air, Surface, and Food)

CHAPTER 19

CHAPTER PREVIEW
- Water Surveillance
- Air Surveillance
- Surface Surveillance
- Food Surveillance

The environment in the hospital plays an important role in the occurrence of healthcare-associated infections. The various environmental sources from which microorganisms can be transmitted to patients and healthcare workers include water, air, food and environmental surfaces. Therefore, monitoring of microbiological quality of water, food, air and surfaces are of paramount importance for safe hospital environment.

■ INDICATIONS

Microbiological sampling of air, water, and environment is an expensive and time-consuming process. CDC recommends to perform targeted microbiological sampling of air, water and surfaces for defined indications, as given below.
1. **Outbreak investigation:** To determine whether environmental microorganisms are the source of the outbreak
2. **To evaluate the change in infection control practice:** For example, to assess a new method introduced for equipment sterilization
3. **Construction:** During construction or renovation work in the hospital premises, or commissioning newly constructed space in special care areas (OTs), it is necessary to assure that the environment is clean
4. **Research purpose:** To study the environmental microbial contamination and to compare with HAI rates in health care facility.

■ WATER SURVEILLANCE

Waterborne Pathogens

Hospital water and water-containing devices may serve as a reservoir of healthcare associated waterborne pathogens. Microbial contamination of water in healthcare settings is broadly of two types.

Category 1 (Enteric Pathogens)

This results from fecal contamination of drinking water supplies. This group of waterborne pathogens are common in community settings than in hospitals. These agents are transmitted by ingestion of contaminated water. Most of them cause diarrheal outbreaks, while few agents cause extraintestinal illness. Examples include:
- **Bacteria:** Gram-negative bacilli such as *Salmonella, Shigella, Vibrio cholerae*
- **Viruses:** Rotavirus, norovirus, hepatitis A and E viruses
- **Parasites:** *Entamoeba histolytica, Giardia lamblia, Cryptosporidium, Cyclospora,* etc.

Category 2 (Common Hospital Pathogens)

These include multidrug resistant gram-negative bacilli (MDR-GNB), legionellae, etc.
- This group of waterborne pathogens are more important in hospital-setting and can contaminate various hospital water reservoirs such as potable water, dialysis water, etc.
- They are transmitted by various routes such as ingestion, contact, aspiration, etc.
- Waterborne outbreaks in healthcare setting caused by these pathogens have been a serious threat to critically ill or immunocompromised patients.

Test of Drinking Water Contaminated with Enteric Pathogens

Hospital drinking water should be free of enteric pathogens and safe for drinking. Therefore, water supplies should be regularly tested.
- However, it is impractical to detect the presence of all types of enteric pathogen in water because they are usually present in minute quantity; such as *Shigella, Salmonella,* etc.
- Instead, it is wise to test the water supplies for those microorganisms which indicate that fecal contamination

has taken place. These organisms are called as indicator organisms.

Indicator Organisms

Indicator organisms are usually the commensal bacteria of intestine. Their presence in water supplies indicates that there may be a contamination of sewage with enteric pathogens and the water supplies needs to be disinfected. These organisms should be present in excess number and also they should be more resistant to the stresses of aquatic environment and disinfection processes.

There are a number of intestinal commensals, used as indicator organisms, of which important ones are as follows.
- ❖ Fecal (thermotolerant) *Escherichia coli*: It does not survive in water for long time, and therefore is the *best indicator of recent fecal contamination of water*
- ❖ Coliform (other than *Escherichia coli*): Indicates remote contamination—either by fecal (presumptive) or soil and vegetation
- ❖ Other indicator organisms are less reliable of fecal pollution of water, which include fecal streptococci, *Clostridium perfringens*, *Pseudomonas aeruginosa*, and bacteriophages.

Collection and Transport of Water Sample

Water specimen should be collected in a screw-capped wide sterile container.
- ❖ **Volume:** At least 150–200 mL of water should be collected
- ❖ **Neutralizer:** Sodium thiosulfate is added to neutralize the bactericidal effect of residual chlorine present in water if any
- ❖ **Sampling points** in hospitals must represent different sources from which water is obtained such as potable water from pipelines, endoscopy rinse water, dialysis water, dental chair unit waterline, etc.
- ❖ **Sampling method from the tap:** Care should be taken while collecting water to minimize extraneous contamination. Hand washing should be performed and gloves should be worn before collection **(Fig. 19.1)**
- ❖ **Tap swabs:** Sterile swab is inserted into the nozzle of the tap carefully, without touching the outer tap surface. The swab is then rubbed around–that is, moved backwards and forwards and up and down, as much as possible, on the inside surface of the tap outlet or flow straightener **(Fig. 19.1)**.

There are two methods employed for detection of microbial contamination of water—(1) Multiple-tube method and (2) membrane filtration method.

Multiple-tube Method

It is the most common method used for water surveillance. It is so named as it involves mixing of specific volume

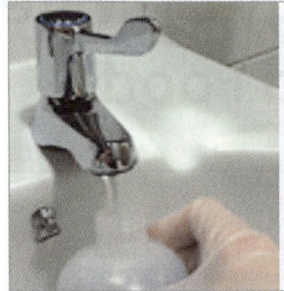
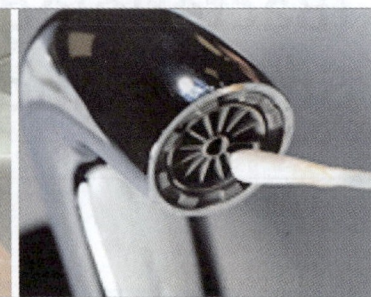

Fig. 19.1: Water sampling methods.

(100 mL) of water samples, divided into multiple tubes containing a special culture medium—MacConkey purple broth.
- ❖ **Procedure:** As per WHO guideline, for testing of unpolluted water samples the following method should be followed **(Fig. 19.2)**
  - 50 mL of water is added to one bottle having 50 mL of culture medium
  - 10 mL of water is added to each of five tubes containing 10 mL of culture medium.
- ❖ **Positive result:** After incubated for 24–48 hours, the medium turns to yellow from purple (due to lactose fermentation), along with turbidity of the medium and gas collected in the Durham's tube. This indicates the the presence of coliform bacteria. However, it cannot differentiate between fecal *E. coli* and other coliform bacteria
- ❖ **Differential coliform count (Eijkman test):** Subsequently fecal *E. coli* can be differentiated from other coliform bacteria by
  - Detection of lactose fermentation with the production of acid and gas at 44°C, and
  - Demonstrating a positive indole test at 44°C.

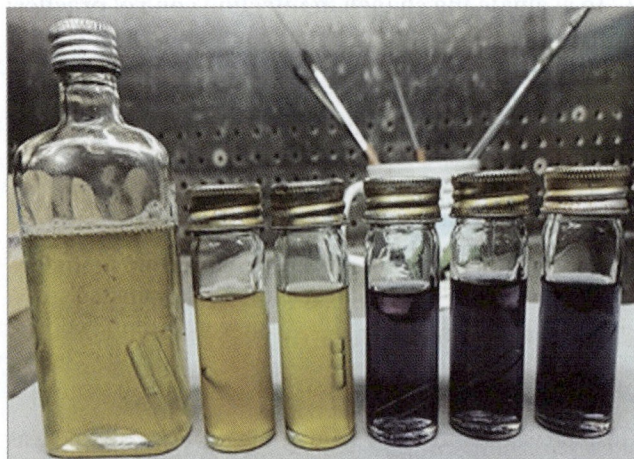

Fig. 19.2: MacConkey purple broth for multiple tube method (one 50 mL and five 10 mL tubes are needed for testing unpolluted water); if negative, media appears purple; if positive, media turn yellow.

Source: Department of Microbiology, JIPMER, Puducherry (*with permission*).

CHAPTER 19 ◈ Environmental Surveillance (Bacteriology of Water, Air, Surface, and Food)

Table 19.1: Classification of quality of drinking water supply.

Quality of drinking water supply	Most probable number (MPN)/100 mL of water	
	Coliform count/100 mL	Thermotolerant *E. coli* count/100 mL
Excellent	0	0
Satisfactory	1–3	0
Intermediate	4–9	0
Unsatisfactory	≥10	≥1

- **Determination of MPN:** The number of tubes giving positive reaction is compared with specialized statistical table (called McCrady table) to determine the most probable number (MPN) of coliform count present per 100 mL of water. This is called as presumptive coliform count
- **Quality of water supply:** Depending upon the MPN/100 mL, the quality of the water specimen can be interpreted as excellent, satisfactory, intermediate or unsatisfactory **(Table 19.1)**.

Membrane Filtration Method

This method is based on the filtration of a known volume (e.g. 100 mL) of water through a cellulose membrane of pore size 0.2 or 0.45 μm.
- **Advantages:** Membrane filtration is the recommended method for—(1) testing dialysis water, (2) for testing clean water, where the bacterial count in water is expected to be low and (3) for testing a large volume of water
- **Disadvantages:** It is not suitable for turbid water. Expensive than multiple tube method.

Test of Water Contaminated with Healthcare Associated Pathogens

Most of the healthcare associated pathogens are recovered by membrane filtration method, followed by plating on to a suitable culture medium.

Endotoxin Detection

Endotoxins are the component of the cell wall of gram-negative bacteria. Dialysis water, devices, etc. contaminated with endotoxin can elicit a variety of inflammatory responses in our body and thereby cause serious toxic effects. Therefore, apart from bacteriological testing, the dialysis water used for hemodialysis is also tested for the presence of endotoxin.
- **Methods:** Three methods are available— (i) gel clot assay (Limulus amebocyte lysate assay), (ii) turbidimetric method, and (iii) chromogenic technique
- **Permissive level:** Water used to prepare dialysate and to reprocess hemodialyzers should contain endotoxin unit <0.25 EU/mL.

■ AIR SURVEILLANCE

Air is an important vehicle of transmission of many pathogenic organisms. Therefore, the examination of air to detect the number of bacteria carrying particles is important particularly in critical areas such as operation theatres (OTs), bone marrow transplant units, etc.

Indication (CDC Recommendations)

Routine air sampling (i.e. random or periodic sampling) is not recommended. CDC recommends targeted air surveillance, which should be carried out for the following indications:
- Investigation of an outbreak
- For research purpose
- After reconstruction or newly constructed buildings
- After fogging (to monitor the quality)
- For short-term evaluation of a change in infection control practice.

Evaluation of the Quality of Air in OT

Evaluation of the quality of air includes both microbiological and non-microbiological (physical) parameters.

Microbiological Parameters

There are two principle means of monitoring the microbiological parameters present in the air, passive monitoring and active sampling.

Passive Monitoring (Settle Plate) Method

Standard Petri dishes containing culture media (e.g. blood agar) are exposed to the air for a given time and then the plates are incubated at 37°C for 24 hours aerobically.
- **1, 1, 1 method:** The ideal recommendation is the 1, 1, 1 method where the plates are placed at different locations in the OT one meter away from the side walls, one meter above the floor and for a duration of 1 hour
- **Disadvantages:** (1) It cannot detect smaller particles or droplets suspended in the air, (2) This method cannot quantify the volume of air sampled.

Active Monitoring (Slit Sampler Method)

In active monitoring, a microbiological air sampler (e.g. sieve impactor) is used. It has a vacuum pump, and a perforated lid **(Fig. 19.3B)**, in which an agar plate can be placed.
- The vacuum pump physically draws a known volume of air through the perforated lid and allows it to impact on the agar plate (e.g. blood agar)
- Following incubation, the quantity of microorganisms present in the culture plate is measured in terms of CFU/m^3 of air **(Fig. 19.3A)**
- Active monitoring is applicable when the concentration of microorganisms is not very high, such as in an operating theatre, bone marrow transplant unit, etc.

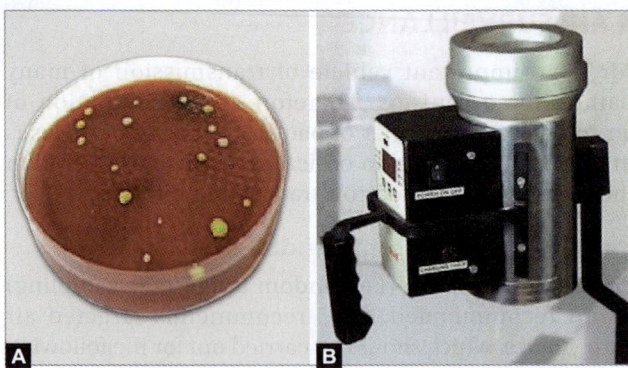

Figs. 19.3A and B: A. Air sampler method showing blood agar with bacterial colonies; **B.** Air sampler (HiMedia).
Source: Department of Microbiology, JIPMER, Puducherry (*with permission*).

Air Particle Counters

Air particle counters have been developed recently, that are capable of detecting airborne particles containing microorganisms in real time. Most of the HEPA filtered OT should satisfy ISO 6 level of clean room standard, which refers that the room should maintain <35,200 particles of 0.5 µm in size per cubic meter.

Non-microbiological Parameters

The number of bacteria in air at any given point of time depends upon various non-microbiological parameters such as air changes per hour, air velocity, positive pressure environment, temperature and relative humidity inside OT, etc. Therefore, there should be periodic monitoring of non-microbiological parameters.

■ SURFACE SURVEILLANCE

Environmental surface sampling has been used to determine (a) reservoirs of potential environmental pathogens and (b) the sources of the environmental contamination.

* **Locations:** It is required for high-risk locations such as operation theatres and ICU settings
* **Sites for sampling (high touch areas):** Surface sampling is taken from sites where there is high-risk of contaminations
* **Indications (CDC recommendation):** Surface sampling is indicated during an outbreak investigation
* **Method:** Moistened sterile swabs (soaked in sterile saline) are used to collect the samples from high-risk areas and then inoculated on to blood agar for the recovery of aerobic bacteria
* **Reporting:** Only pathogenic organisms isolated are reported. A semi-quantitative report (as heavy, moderate or light growth) should be provided. Contaminants such as aerobic spore bearers are not reported
* **Newer techniques** such as luminometer and glow gel techniques are available which are easy to perform though expensive.

■ FOOD SURVEILLANCE

There are a number of food-borne pathogens, transmitted by various sources of food. They pose a significant public health problem causing morbidity and mortality. Therefore, food surveillance is essential to control the standards of hygiene practices followed and also to investigate outbreaks of food poisoning.

Viable Plate Count

Viable plate count (or standard plate count) is the standard method followed for bacteriological examination of food.
* **Food sampling:** (1) 10 g of food material is taken in a sterile container and is homogenized in 90 mL of sterile diluent, e.g. Ringer's solution. (2) For the food contaminated only on its surface, such as intact vegetable or fruit, 100 g of food is taken in a sterile container containing 100 mL of sterile water and then shaken well so that all bacteria present on its surface will come out and are dissolved in water
* **Food processing:** Serial dilutions of homogenate or diluent is made, and then plated onto appropriate medium. The coliform count on MacConkey broth and differential count detecting thermotolerant *E. coli* can be made by the methods as described for water analysis.

EXPECTED QUESTIONS

I. Write short notes on:
1. Water surveillance.
2. Air surveillance.

II. Multiple Choice Questions (MCQs):
1. Which is the best indicator organism of fecal contamination of water?
   a. Fecal *E. coli*   b. Staphylococcus
   c. Pseudomonas   d. Vibrio cholerae
2. Evaluation of the quality of air in OTs can be performed by all the following methods, *except*:
   a. Settle plate   b. Slit sampler
   c. Particle count   d. Multiple tube method

Answers
1. a   2. d

Antimicrobial Stewardship

CHAPTER 20

CHAPTER PREVIEW
- Implementation of Antimicrobial Stewardship Program
- Rational use of Antimicrobial Agents
- Hospital Antibiogram

INTRODUCTION

Antimicrobial stewardship program (AMSP) provides strategies for rationalizing the use of antimicrobials in the hospital.

Definition

Centers for disease control and prevention (CDC) has defined antimicrobial stewardship as use of the right antimicrobial agent, for the right patient, at the right time, with the right dose, route and frequency, causing the least harm to the patient and future patients.

Why AMSP is Needed?

Antimicrobial stewardship program in a hospital is required for the following reasons.
- ❖ **The rising threat of antimicrobial resistance (AMR):** Extensive use of antimicrobials is the single most important factor for the bacteria to undergo mutation, which leads bacteria to become resistant to antimicrobials and then the resistant strain flourish exponentially in the presence of selective pressure of antimicrobials.
- ❖ **Misuse and over-use of antimicrobials** such as use without a prescription, overuse for self-limiting infections, non-bacterial infections, or treatment of colonizer/contaminant
- ❖ **Widespread use of antimicrobials in other sectors** such as animal, agriculture, etc.
- ❖ **Limited availability of newer drugs** because of poor antimicrobial research, as there is a high-risk of developing resistance to the newer drugs.

IMPLEMENTATION OF ANTIMICROBIAL STEWARDSHIP PROGRAM

The key steps of implementation of AMSP in a hospital is as follows.

Administrative Support (Leadership)

The most important prerequisite for implementing AMSP is a strong administrative support.

Formulating AMS Team

Antimicrobial stewardship team (AMS team) is a multi-disciplinary committee which is responsible for framing, implementing and monitoring the compliance to antimicrobial policy of the hospital. Members of AMS team include infectious disease physician, microbiologist, clinical pharmacists, infection control officer and officer in-charge of pharmacy.

Infrastructure Support

Infrastructure support is essential to initiate appropriate pathogen-directed antimicrobial agent at the earliest.
- ❖ **Support from the microbiology laboratory**
  - *Automations:* Facility for automated culture (e.g. BacT/ALERT), identification (MALDI-TOF) and sensitivity (e.g. VITEK) should be available
  - *Biomarkers* such as procalcitonin and C-reactive protein (CRP) must be available (discussed subsequently)
  - *Molecular tests:* Facility to perform rapid molecular tests must be available
  - *Emergency laboratory:* Emergency lab functioning round the clock is a marker of a quality microbiology laboratory.
- ❖ **Hospital information system (HIS):** Fully functional HIS including laboratory information system will augment the stewardship program by many folds
- ❖ Supporting manpower availability.

Framing Antimicrobial Policy

Every hospital should frame their own hospital antimicrobial policy which is usually a pocket handbook, comprising of system/syndrome wise indications for antimicrobial choice and their dosage.

Implementing AMS Strategies

Two types of strategies are available for implementing AMSP.
1. **Front-end strategies (formulary restriction):** These refer to limited dispensing of restricted antimicrobials (e.g. colistin) by the hospital pharmacy, procurement of which requires prior authorization by the AMS team
2. **Back-end strategies (prospective audit and feedback):** It involves daily rounds conducted by the AMS team, which discusses the cases with the clinical team and provides advice on the rational use of antimicrobial therapy.

Education and Training

Similar to any other health care program, AMSP also needs continuous education, training, motivation and assessment of the health care providers. Developing antimicrobial stewardship is a behavioral change within the person. Hence, adequate motivational education is a must to bring in such change.

RATIONAL USE OF ANTIMICROBIAL AGENTS

When prescribing antimicrobial agents, the clinicians should consider the following advice.

Prescribe Only when Indicated

Prescribe antibiotics only when it is indicated. There are various conditions where antibiotics are not required such as diarrhea, upper respiratory tract infections or when alternative diagnosis is suspected/confirmed.

Culture of Cultures

Antibiotics should always be started only after site-specific specimens are collected for culture. If specimens are collected after antibiotic start, then cultures become false-negative and thus it will not help in targeted therapy.

Empirical vs Targeted Therapy

Empirical therapy: Empirical antibiotics should not be given randomly, but based on three important elements.
- The infective syndrome likely to be present
- The common etiological bacterial agents for that infective syndrome
- The local antibiogram for those organisms, indicating the antimicrobial resistance pattern.

Targeted or pathogen-directed therapy: The empirical therapy should be modified subsequently, based on antimicrobial susceptibility test (AST) report. The modifications may be of two types—escalation or de-escalation.

Escalation vs De-escalation Approach

There are two approaches by which antimicrobial agents are prescribed—escalation and de-escalation.
- **Escalation approach** is chosen if the local antimicrobial resistance pattern is unlikely and/or the patient is clinically stable. The empirical therapy is started with a narrow-spectrum antibiotic (e.g. ceftriaxone for *E. coli*). If AST report shows resistance, then can be escalated to a higher rank antibiotic subsequently (e.g. meropenem for *E. coli*).
- **De-escalation approach** is chosen if the local antimicrobial resistance pattern is expected to be high and/or patient is critically ill. Empirical therapy is started with broad-spectrum antibiotics (e.g. meropenem for *E. coli*). If AST report shows susceptible, it can be de-escalated to a narrow-spectrum antibiotic subsequently (e.g. ceftriaxone for *E. coli*).

Site-specific Antimicrobials

Only those antimicrobials should be prescribed which are active at the infection site. Antibiotics such as chloramphenicol, macrolide and clindamycin should be avoided in UTI; as they do not achieve adequate urinary concentrations.

Avoid Administration Errors

Antimicrobials must be administrated at the correct dose (as per the age/body weight), and frequency and duration of therapy. Renal adjusted dose to be given according to creatinine clearance.

MIC-guided Therapy

The AST can be performed by disk diffusion or by MIC (minimum inhibitory concentration)–based method; the latter being more accurate and reliable. There are certain situations, where the antibiotic treatment is MIC-guided. In cinical conditions such as endocarditis, pneumococcal meningitis/pneumonia, etc. MIC guided therapy has a great role.

Timely Stoppage of Antimicrobial

Antimicrobial agent must be stopped at appropriate time, which may be determined by clinical improvement or after obtaining negative culture or by use of biomarkers.

Biomarkers-guided Therapy

Biomarkers such as procalcitonin (PCT) or C-reactive protein (CRP) may be used for predicting bacterial infection. PCT is more reliable marker than CRP.

CHAPTER 20 ◆ Antimicrobial Stewardship

Procalcitonin (PCT)
It is a peptide precursor of the hormone calcitonin, secreted at very low level (<0.05 ng/mL) normally by the body, but the level goes up by manifolds in bacterial infection. The various diagnostic application of PCT include:
- To differentiate bacterial vs viral infection
- For predicting bacterial infections such as local or systemic infection (e.g. in bacterial sepsis, procalcitonin levels will be >10 ng/mL)
- Helps to decide whether to continue antibiotics in culture-negative cases
- Helps to decide whether to stop antibiotics
- Severity: PCT levels parallel with the severity of the bacterial infections.

Table 20.1: Hospital antibiogram of gram-negative bacteria for the year 2020, expressed in terms of susceptibility rate.

	Ciprofloxacin	Amikacin	Ceftazidime	Piperacillin-tazobactam	Meropenem	Colistin
E. coli	25	85	55	75	82	99
Klebsiella	15	75	35	65	70	85
Pseudomonas	32	80	60	80	80	99
Acinetobacter	29	70	10	18	20	99

Misuse of Antimicrobials
The misuse of antimicrobials should be avoided. Example include—avoid use of two or more antibiotics having overlapping antibacterial spectra or ineffective antibiotic.

■ HOSPITAL ANTIBIOGRAM

An **antibiogram** is an overall profile of antimicrobial susceptibility testing results of a specific microorganism to a battery of antimicrobial agents **(Table 20.1)**. It is the responsibility of the department of Microbiology to construct a hospital antibiogram and share it with clinicians. It has the following uses.

❖ Antibiogram guides the clinicians in selecting the best empirical antimicrobial treatment in the event of pending culture and susceptibility results
❖ It is also an useful tool for detecting and monitoring trends in antimicrobial resistance within the hospital
❖ Antibiograms can also be used to compare susceptibility rates across institutions and track resistance trends and thereby contributing to the national AMR surveillance database.

EXPECTED QUESTIONS

I. Write short notes on:
1. Strategies of antimicrobial stewardship program.
2. Hospital antibiogram.

II. Multiple Choice Questions (MCQs):
1. Maximum consumption of antibiotics occurs for:
   a. Human therapeutic use
   b. Human non-therapeutic use
   c. Animal therapeutic use
   d. Animal non-therapeutic use

2. In which of the following infectious disease, antibiotics are required?
   a. Diarrhea
   b. Influenza
   c. Dengue
   d. None of the above

Answers
1. d   2. d

Systematic Bacteriology

SECTION 4

SECTION OUTLINE

Gram-positive Cocci
21. *Staphylococcus*
22. *Streptococcus*, Pneumococcus and *Enterococcus*

Gram-negative Cocci
23. *Neisseria*: Meningococcus and Gonococcus

Gram-positive Bacilli
24. *Corynebacterium*
25. *Bacillus*
26. Anaerobes: *Clostridium* and Non-sporing Anaerobes
27. Mycobacteria: *M. tuberculosis*, Nontuberculous Mycobacteria and *M. leprae*
28. Miscellaneous Gram-positive Bacilli (Actinomycetes and *Listeria*)

Gram-negative Bacilli
29. Enterobacterales (*Escherichia coli, Klebsiella, Shigella, Salmonella* and Others)
30. *Vibrio*
31. *Pseudomonas, Acinetobacter* and Other Nonfermenters
32. Fastidious Gram-negative Bacilli: *Haemophilus, Brucella* and *Bordetella*
33. Miscellaneous Gram-negative Bacilli: *Campylobacter, Helicobacter, Legionella, Pasteurella*, Agents of Bacterial Vaginosis, Rat-bite Fever
34. Spirochetes: *Treponema, Borrelia* and *Leptospira*
35. Rickettsiae, Chlamydiae and *Mycoplasma*

Staphylococcus

CHAPTER 21

CHAPTER PREVIEW

- *Staphylococcus aureus*
- Coagulase-negative Staphylococci (CoNS)

■ INTRODUCTION

Gram-positive cocci are classified into two families—Micrococcaceae and Streptococcaceae, differentiated by the catalase test. Micrococcaceae are catalase positive, gram-positive cocci arranged in tetrads or clusters; whereas Streptococcaceae are catalase negative gram-positive cocci, arranged in pairs or chains.

Family Micrococcaceae comprises of genera—*Micrococcus* and *Staphylococcus*.

- ❖ *Micrococcus* species are skin commensals, usually not associated with human infections. They are 1–1.8 μm size, arranged in tetrads
- ❖ *Staphylococcus* species are arranged in clusters. This is due to cell division occurs in multiple planes with the daughter cells remain attached together.

■ STAPHYLOCOCCUS

Staphylococcus was named after the Greek word, *Staphyle* means 'a bunch of grapes' and *kokkos* means 'berry shaped'. Staphylococci can be classified into *S. aureus*, the most pathogenic species to man and other species called coagulase-negative staphylococci (CoNS) that are less pathogenic to man.

Staphylococcus aureus

Staphylococcus aureus is the most common gram-positive cocci infecting humans. *S. aureus* is named based on the characteristic golden yellow pigmentation of its colonies. It can cause both community and nosocomial acquired infections that may range from relatively milder skin and soft tissue infections to life-threatening systemic infections.

Virulence Factors

The pathogenic potential of *S. aureus* is due to the expression of several virulence factors which include:

- ❖ **Toxins** such as hemolysins (e.g., α, β, γ, δ), exfoliative toxin, enterotoxin, and toxic shock syndrome toxin
- ❖ **Extracellular enzymes** such as coagulase (principle virulence factor), heat-stable thermonuclease, staphylokinase, hyaluronidase, etc.
- ❖ **Cell wall-associated factors** such as :
  - ■ **Thick peptidoglycan layer:** It confers rigidity and maintains the shape
  - ■ **Teichoic acid:** Helps in adhesion of cocci to mucosal surfaces and inhibits opsonization
  - ■ **Cell surface adhesins** such as clumping factor, fibronectin binding adhesins
  - ■ **Protein A:** It is anti-complementary and chemotactic.

Pathogenesis

Pathogenesis of *S. aureus* involves the following steps:

- ❖ **Colonization:** *S. aureus* colonizes on various body surfaces, such as anterior nares, oropharynx, axilla and perineal skin
- ❖ **Introduction into the tissue:** Organisms are introduced into the tissues as a result of minor abrasions. Then they adhere to the tissue surfaces by various adhesins, e.g. clumping factor
- ❖ **Invasion:** *S. aureus* can invade into the tissues by elaborating enzymes, such as serine proteases, hyaluronidases, and lipases
- ❖ **By evasion of host defense mechanisms** such as: Antiphagocytic activity mediated by protein A, inhibition of leukocyte migration, etc.
- ❖ **Metastatic spread:** Finally, *S. aureus* spreads to various distant sites by hematogenous spread.

Clinical Manifestations

The clinical spectrum of *S. aureus* includes (**Figs. 21.1A and B**):

- ❖ Skin and soft tissue infections such as folliculitis, furuncle, cellulitis, abscess, impetigo, etc.

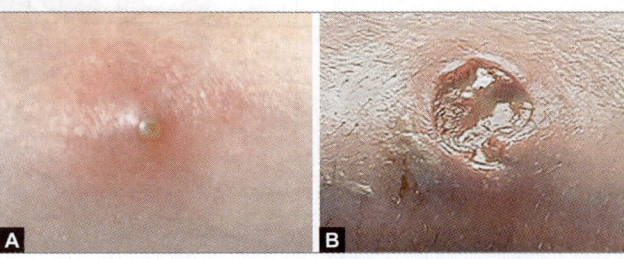

Figs. 21.1A and B: A. Staphylococcal folliculitis; **B.** Staphylococcal abscess (ruptured).
Source: Centers for Disease Control and Prevention (CDC), Atlanta (*with permission*).

- Musculoskeletal infections such as osteomyelitis, septic arthritis, and pyomyositis
- Respiratory tract infections such as pneumonia
- Bacteremia, sepsis, and infective endocarditis
- Urinary tract infections (UTI).

Toxin-mediated infections: *S. aureus* can also cause several toxin-mediated diseases such as:

- **Scalded skin syndrome:** Mediated by exfoliative toxin (or epidermolytic toxin), characterized by localized tender blisters and bullae formation and exfoliation of the skin
- **Food poisoning:** Mediated by enterotoxin. It is a *preformed toxin* (i.e. secreted in food before consumption) so that it can act rapidly. As a result, the *incubation period is short* (1–6 hours)
- **Toxic shock syndrome:** Mediated by toxic shock syndrome toxin (TSS)
  - It is common among women using vaginal tampons during menstruation
  - The toxin is absorbed into circulation to cause a potentially fatal multisystem disease with erythematous rashes.

HAI: Overall, *S. aureus* is a leading cause of healthcare-associated infections (HAI). The hospital staff are the potential carriers of *S. aureus*. Hospital strains are often multidrug-resistant, spread to patients either from hospital staff/other patients/environment or also from patients' skin flora.

Laboratory Diagnosis (Table 21.1)

The various specimens collected depend on the nature of the lesion such as pus, wound swab, sputum, midstream urine, and blood.

- **Direct smear microscopy:** Reveals gram-positive cocci (1 μm) in clusters and pus cells **(Fig. 21.2A)**
- **Culture:** Incubation at 37°C for 24h reveals the following growth:

Table 21.1: Laboratory findings of *S. aureus* and coagulase negative staphylococci.

Organism	Catalase	Gram-positive cocci	Culture finding on blood agar	Other tests
S. aureus	Positive	Arranged in clusters	Pinhead-shaped colonies with a narrow zone of complete (β) hemolysis and golden yellow pigmentation	Coagulase test: positive
CoNS	Positive	Arranged in clusters	Pinhead-shaped colonies without hemolysis and no pigmentation	Coagulase test: negative

(CoNS, coagulase-negative staphylococci)

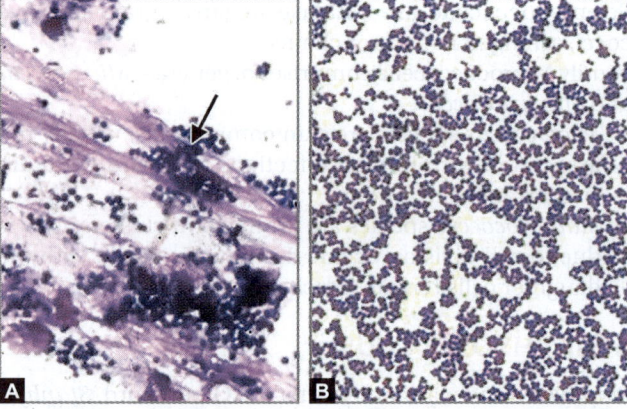

Figs. 21.2A and B: A. Direct smear: arrow showing gram-positive cocci in clusters with pus cells; **B.** Culture smear showing gram-positive cocci in clusters.
Source: Department of Microbiology, JIPMER, Puducherry (*with permission*).

- Nutrient agar—colonies are 1–3 mm in size, circular, smooth, convex, opaque and easily emulsifiable. Most strains produce golden-yellow non-diffusible **pigments** (made up of β-carotene) **(Fig. 21.3A)**
- Blood agar—shows pin-head colonies with a narrow zone of complete (β) hemolysis **(Fig. 21.3B)**
- **MacConkey agar:** Small pink colonies are produced due to lactose fermentation
- Selective media such as mannitol salt agar (nutrient agar with 7.5% NaCl)—produces yellow colonies.
- **Culture smear microscopy** from the colonies reveals gram-positive cocci in clusters **(Fig. 21.2B)**

CHAPTER 21 ◆ Staphylococcus

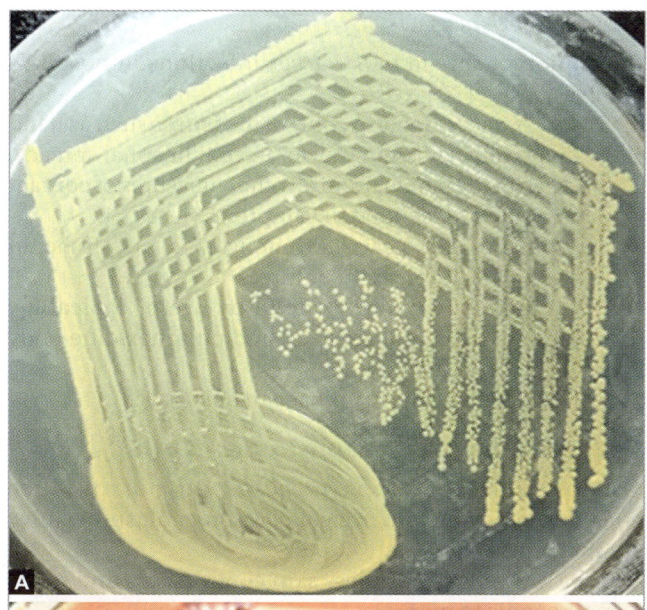
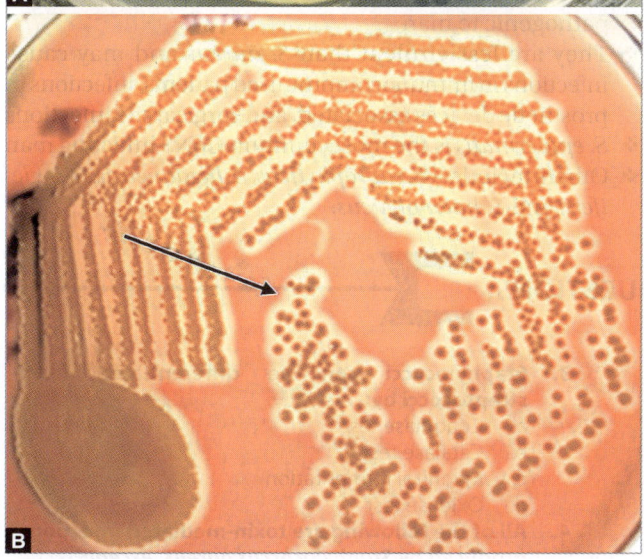

Figs. 21.3A and B: Colonies of *S. aureus*: **A.** Nutrient agar—shows golden-yellow pigmented colonies; **B.** Blood agar—arrow shows a narrow zone of beta-hemolysis surrounding the colonies.

Source: Department of Microbiology, Pondicherry Institute of Medical Sciences, Puducherry (*with permission*).

- **Biochemical identification:** Various tests which help in the identification of *S. aureus* are:
  - Catalase test—positive (differentiates staphylococci from streptococci)
  - Coagulase test—positive (differentiates *S. aureus* from CoNS). Two test formats are available: slide coagulase and tube coagulase tests (described below in highlight box)
  - Protein A detection (differentiates *S. aureus* from CoNS).

Coagulase Test
It is the most commonly performed biochemical reaction for identification of *S. aureus*.

Tube Coagulase Test
It detects free coagulase secreted by *S. aureus*.
- **Procedure:** Colony of *S. aureus* is emulsified in plasma in a test tube and incubated at 37°C for 4 hours
  - **Positive test** is indicated by formation of a clot that does not flow when the test tube is tilted **(Fig. 21.4A)**
  - The **negative tubes** (no clot formation) should be incubated overnight and re-examined as some strains may produce a delayed clot **(Fig. 21.4B)**
- This test is different from slide coagulase test, which is mediated by clumping factor.

Slide Coagulase Test
It detects clumping factor (i.e., bound coagulase).
- **Procedure:** A colony of *S. aureus* is emulsified with a drop of normal saline on a slide to form a milky white suspension. Then a loopful of plasma is added and mixed properly
- **Positive result:** It is indicated by formation of coarse clumps **(Fig. 21.4C)**; whereas it remains as milky-white suspension if test is negative.

- ❖ **Automated identification systems** such as VITEK and MALDI-TOF can be performed for rapid and accurate identification of *S. aureus*
- ❖ **Typing of *S. aureus*:** It is especially useful in outbreaks such as food poisoning affecting a larger community. Typing methods include—bacteriophage typing (based on their susceptibility to bacteriophages), antibiogram typing, sequence based typing, etc.
- ❖ **Antimicrobial susceptibility testing** can be performed by disk diffusion method (on Mueller–Hinton agar) or MIC-based method (VITEK).

TREATMENT — S. aureus

S. aureus is primarily treated by anti-staphylococcal penicillins such as cloxacillin.

However, for MRSA infections (see below), vancomycin is the drug of choice. Others include clindamycin, doxycycline, co-trimoxazole, or linezolid, etc.

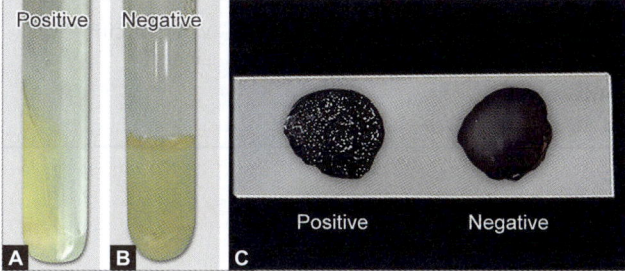

Figs. 21.4A to C: Coagulase test: **A.** Tube coagulase test (positive); **B.** Tube coagulase test (negative); **C.** Slide showing coagulase test.

Source: Department of Microbiology, Pondicherry Institute of Medical Sciences, Puducherry (*with permission*).

MRSA

Methicillin-resistant *S. aureus* (MRSA) is a resistant phenotype, that has been increasingly reported over the last few decades. It shows resistance to all β-lactam antimicrobials and thus possesses a great therapeutic challenge. It is widespread in hospital settings, causing several outbreaks.

- **Mechanism:** Mediated by a gene called **mecA gene**, which alters penicillin-binding protein (PBP) present on *S. aureus* cell wall to PBP2a.
  - PBP is an essential protein needed for the cell wall synthesis of bacteria. β-lactam drugs bind and inhibit this protein, thereby inhibiting the cell wall synthesis
  - The altered PBP2a of MRSA strains have less affinity for β-lactam antibiotics; hence, MRSA strains are resistant to all β-lactam antibiotics
- **Epidemiology:** MRSA rate is very high, accounting for 30-40% of *S. aureus* infections in India
- **Detection of MRSA** is done by following methods:
  - By susceptibility test using cefoxitin disk (30 μg) or oxacillin (MIC based method). These antibiotics are used as a surrogate marker for the detection of MRSA
  - PCR detecting *mecA* gene
  - Latex agglutination test detecting PBP2a.
- **Treatment:** Vancomycin or linezolid are recommended for serious infections, whereas doxycycline or cotrimoxazole can be given for non-life-threatening infections.

Control Measures

Prevention of spread of *S. aureus* infections in hospitals involves:
- Ensure proper **infection control measures** such as hand hygiene (most efficient way to prevent hospital spread), isolation of the patients and all other measures of **contact precautions** (described in **Chapter 15**)
- **Screening of MRSA carriers** among hospital staff should be done when there is an outbreak
- **Treatment of carriers** is done by use of topical 2% mupirocin (for nasal carriers) and chlorhexidine body bath (for skin carriers)
- **Stoppage of antibiotic misuse** in hospitals.

Coagulase-negative Staphylococci (CoNS)

Other species of *Staphylococcus* do not produce coagulase enzyme and are called as coagulase-negative staphylococci (CoNS).
- They are usually harmless skin commensals and rarely pathogenic to man
- They are less virulent than *S. aureus* and may cause infections in immunocompromised patients, infections in prosthetic devices associated, and surgical site infections
- *S. epidermidis* is the most common CoNS infecting man
- Others include—*S. saprophyticus, S. lugdunensis, S. schleiferi,* and *S. haemolyticus.*

EXPECTED QUESTIONS

I. Write an essay on:
1. Discuss the manifestations, laboratory diagnosis, and treatment of staphylococcal infections.

II. Write short note on:
1. Methicillin-resistant *Staphylococcus aureus* (MRSA).

III. Multiple Choice Questions (MCQs):
1. Scalded skin syndrome is mediated by:
   a. Hemolysin b. Coagulase
   c. Enterotoxin d. Exfoliative toxin
2. All of the above can be given for the treatment of MRSA, *except*:
   a. Meropenem b. Vancomycin
   c. Cotrimoxazole d. Linezolid
3. Staphylococci can be differentiated from streptococci by:
   a. Coagulase test
   b. Catalase test
   c. Mannitol fermentation
   d. Oxidase test
4. All of the following are toxin-mediated infections produced by *Staphylococcus aureus*, *except*:
   a. Scalded skin syndrome
   b. Cellulitis
   c. Food poisoning
   d. Toxic shock syndrome

Answers
1. d 2. a 3. b 4. b

Streptococcus, Pneumococcus and Enterococcus

CHAPTER 22

CHAPTER PREVIEW
- Streptococcus
- Pneumococcus
- Enterococcus

■ INTRODUCTION

Family Streptococcaceae are catalase negative gram-positive cocci, arranged in pairs or chains (due to single plane of division). *Streptococcus*, *Enterococcus* and pneumococcus are the important members of this family.

Streptococci are part of normal flora. However, some are important human pathogens, such as *Streptococcus pyogenes* causing pyogenic infections, *S. agalactiae* causing meningitis in newborn and *S. pneumoniae* causing pneumonia and meningitis in all age groups.

■ STREPTOCOCCUS

Streptococci can be classified based on the pattern of hemolysis they produce on blood agar.
- ❖ **α or partial hemolysis**: Greenish discoloration surrounding the colonies; e.g. Viridans streptococci and *S. pneumoniae*
- ❖ **β or complete hemolysis**: Yellowish discoloration surrounding the colonies; e.g. β-hemolytic streptococci such as *S. pyogenes* and *S. agalactiae*
- ❖ **γ hemolysis**: No hemolysis surrounding the colonies; e.g. *Enterococcus* (now reclassified under separate family Enterococcaceae).

Lancefield grouping (Fig. 22.1): The β-hemolytic streptococci are further classified based on the C-carbohydrate antigen in the cell wall into 20 serological groups. The majority of streptococci causing human infection include—group A streptococci (*S. pyogenes*) and group B streptococci (*S. agalactiae*).

Streptococcus pyogenes

Streptococcus pyogenes (group A *Streptococcus*) is one of the leading cause of pyogenic infections in humans.

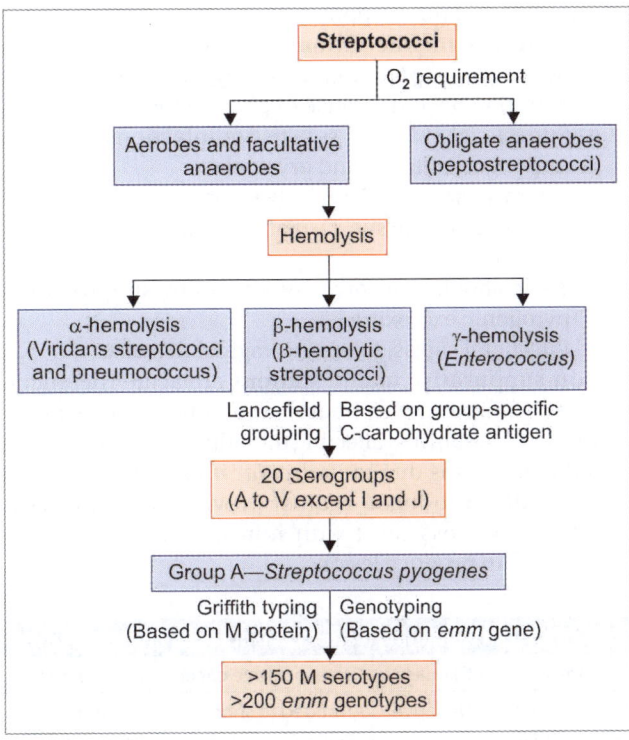

Fig. 22.1: Classification of family Streptococcaceae.

Virulence Factors

The virulence factors of *S. pyogenes* include:
- ❖ Cell wall antigens such as C-carbohydrate antigens, lipoteichoic acid, M protein (see highlight box for details), capsule (composed of hyaluronic acid), etc.
- ❖ Toxins such as streptococcal pyrogenic exotoxin and hemolysins
- ❖ Various enzymes such as streptokinase, streptodornase, hyaluronidase (spreading factor), etc.

> **M protein**
> It is the principal virulence factor of group A *Streptococcus*.
> ❏ It inhibits complement mediated opsonization by phagocytes
> ❏ It complexes with fibrinogen and bind to neutrophils, leading to release of inflammatory mediators which induce vascular leakage; causing streptococcal toxic shock syndrome
> ❏ Some M protein types are cross-reactive to human myocardial antigens and play an important role in the pathogenesis of acute rheumatic fever.

Clinical Manifestations

Streptococcus pyogenes is associated with a variety of suppurative and non-suppurative manifestations.
- ❖ **Suppurative manifestations** include:
  - Sore throat (pharyngitis): *S. pyogenes* is the most common bacterial cause of pharyngitis in children
  - Superficial skin and soft-tissue infections: Such as impetigo, cellulitis, and erysipelas
  - Necrotizing fasciitis: Involves extensive necrosis of subcutaneous tissue, fascia, and muscles
  - Bacteremia
  - Toxic shock syndrome (mediated by streptococcal pyrogenic exotoxin)
  - Puerperal sepsis, following vaginal delivery.
- ❖ **Non-suppurative manifestations** are acute rheumatic fever (affecting the heart) and post-streptococcal glomerulonephritis (affecting the kidney). The underlying pathogenesis is due to *molecular mimicry*; where, the antibodies produced against previous streptococcal infections cross-react with human tissues (heart or kidneys) to produce lesions.

Laboratory Diagnosis (Table 22.1)

The specimen to be collected depends on the site of the infection. Common specimens are pus, throat swab, blood, etc.
- ❖ **Direct smear microscopy:** Reveals pus cells with gram-positive cocci (0.5–1 μm) in chains **(Fig. 22.2A)**.
- ❖ The specimens are inoculated onto various media and incubated overnight at 37°C aerobically in presence of 5–10% CO_2. *S. pyogenes* is fastidious, does not grow on MacConkey agar and nutrient agar. It grows only in media enriched with blood or serum.
  - **Blood agar:** Colonies are small 0.5–1 mm, pinpoint, with a wide zone of β-hemolysis **(Fig. 22.3A)**
  - **Selective media** such as crystal violet blood agar can be used.

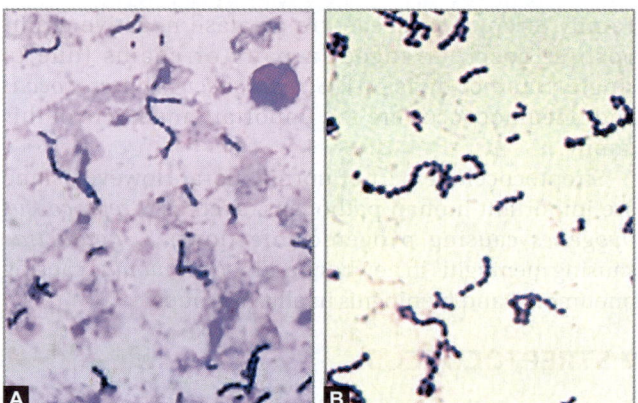

Figs. 22.2A and B: Streptococci: **A.** In Gram-stained smear of pus; **B.** In culture smear showing gram-positive cocci in short chains.
Source: Department of Microbiology, Pondicherry Institute of Medical Sciences, Puducherry (*with permission*).

Table 22.1: Differentiating features of laboratory findings of streptococci, pneumococcus, *Enterococcus*.

Organism	Catalase	Gram-positive cocci	Culture finding on blood agar	Other tests
β-hemolytic streptococci	Negative	Arranged in short chains	Pinpoint colonies with a wide zone of complete (β) hemolysis	**S. pyogenes:** Bacitracin (S), CAMP test negative **S. agalactiae:** Bacitracin (R), CAMP test positive
Viridans streptococci	Negative	Arranged in long chains	Minute α-hemolytic (green-colored) colonies	Bile solubility test: negative Inulin: not fermented Optochin: resistant
S. pneumoniae	Negative	Arranged in pairs, lanceolate-shaped	Draughtsman-shaped or carrom coin-shaped colonies with partial (α) hemolysis	Bile solubility test: positive Inulin: fermented Optochin: sensitive
Enterococcus	Negative	Arranged in pairs, spectacle eye-shaped	Small, translucent, non-hemolytic colonies	Bile esculin test: positive *E. faecalis:* Arabinose not fermented *E. faecium:* Arabinose fermented

(S, sensitive; R, resistant; CAMP test, Christie-Atkins-Munch-Peterson test)

CHAPTER 22 — Streptococcus, Pneumococcus and Enterococcus

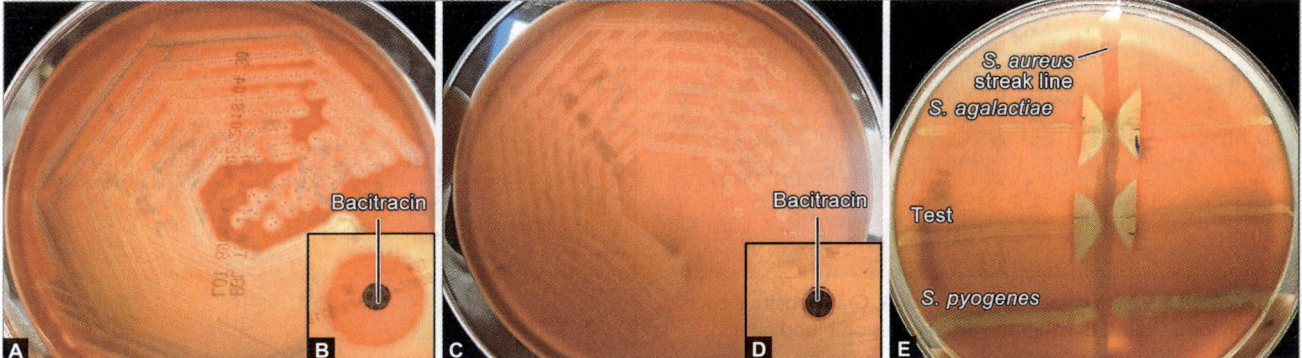

Figs. 22.3A to E: *Streptococcus pyogenes*: **A.** Growth on blood agar with wide zone of beta-hemolysis around the pinpoint colonies; **B.** Bacitracin sensitive. **C to E:** *Streptococcus agalactiae*: **C.** Growth on blood agar with wide zone of beta-hemolysis around the colonies; **D.** Bacitracin resistant; **E.** CAMP test positive.
Source: Department of Microbiology, JIPMER, Puducherry (*with permission*).
(CAMP, Christie, Atkins, and Munch-Peterson test)

- **Culture smear** microscopy from the colonies reveals gram-positive cocci in short chains **(Fig. 22.2B)**
- **Biochemical identification:** Various tests which help in the identification of *S. pyogenes* are:
    - Catalase negative
    - Susceptible to bacitracin **(Fig. 22.3B):** Group A *Streptococcus* is sensitive to bacitracin 0.04 U disk (any zone of inhibition around the disk is considered as positive test).
    - CAMP (Christie, Atkins, and Munch-Peterson) test: Negative **(Fig. 22.3E)**.
- **Lancefield grouping** shows group A *Streptococcus*
- **Automated ID systems** such as VITEK and MALDI-TOF can be performed for rapid and accurate identification of *S. pyogenes*
- **Serology:** ASO (anti-streptolysin O) antibodies and anti-DNase B antibodies are elevated
- **Antimicrobial susceptibility testing** can be performed by disk diffusion method (on Mueller–Hinton blood agar) or MIC-based method (VITEK).

TREATMENT — S. pyogenes

The infections caused by *S. pyogenes* are primarily treated by penicillin. Erythromycin can be given in case of penicillin allergy.

Streptococcus agalactiae

Streptococcus agalactiae colonizes the female genital tract and therefore the infection is common in neonates and in pregnancy.
- It has been recognized as a major cause of neonatal sepsis and meningitis
- Infections in pregnancy can lead to peripartum fever, endometritis, and puerperal sepsis
- Similar to *S. pyogenes*, it also produces β-hemolytic pinpoint colonies (mucoid and slightly larger, **Fig. 22.3C**), gram-positive cocci in chains, and catalase negative
- But it differs from *S. pyogenes*, being bacitracin resistant **(Fig. 22.3D)**, CAMP test positive (see below) and Lancefield grouping showing group B *Streptococcus* **(see Fig. 22.1 and Table 22.1)**
- Penicillin/ampicillin plus gentamicin are the drug of choice for all *S. agalactiae* infections.

CAMP Test
- CAMP factor (named after the discoverers—Christie, Atkins-Munch-Petersen) is a phospholipase produced by group B streptococci that enhances the hemolysis of *S. aureus*
- When group B streptococci is streaked on blood agar plate perpendicular to *S. aureus*, an enhanced arrowhead shaped hemolysis is produced at their junction, pointing towards *S. aureus* streak line **(Fig. 22.3E)**.

Viridans streptococci

Viridans streptococci are commensals of the mouth and upper respiratory tract.
- However, occasionally they can cause infections such as dental caries, subacute bacterial endocarditis, prolonged bacteremia among neutropenic patients undergoing cancer chemotherapy and suppurative infections
- They appear as long chains of gram-positive cocci and produce minute α-hemolytic colonies on blood agar **(Figs. 22.4A and B)**

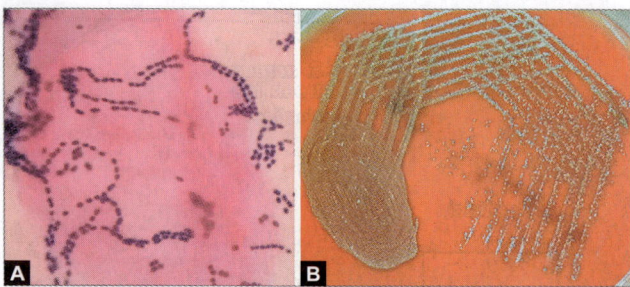

Figs. 22.4A and B: Viridans streptococci: **A.** Gram-positive cocci in long chains; **B.** α-hemolytic colonies on blood agar.

Source: Department of Microbiology, PIMS, Puducherry (*with permission*).

❖ They can be differentiated by pneumococci, being resistant to optochin and insoluble in bile
❖ They are usually susceptible to penicillin and vancomycin.

Streptococcus pneumoniae (Pneumococcus)

Streptococcus pneumoniae, commonly referred to as pneumococcus is the leading cause of lobar pneumonia, otitis media in children, and meningitis in all ages.

❖ **Clinical manifestations:** *S. pneumoniae* can cause both invasive infections such as lobar pneumonia, bloodstream infection, pyogenic meningitis, septic arthritis and non-invasive infections such as otitis media and sinusitis
❖ **Risk factors** for pneumococcal infection include—children less than two years, splenectomy, underlying comorbid conditions (e.g. chronic lung, kidney, and liver disease), etc.
❖ **Laboratory diagnosis:** Clinical specimens include CSF, blood, sputum, etc. depending on the system involved. Specimens should be processed immediately. In case of delay, CSF specimen should be kept at 37°C (*see* **Table 22.1**).
  - *Gram stain:* Direct microscopy of smears made from specimens show numerous pus cells and **lanceolate or flame**-shaped grampositive cocci (1 µm) in pairs, surrounded by a clear halo (due to capsule) (**Fig. 22.5**).
  - *India ink preparation* for capsule demonstration: Capsule is seen as a clear halo.
  - *Antigen detection:* Detection of capsular antigens in CSF by latex agglutination test
  - *Culture:* On blood agar, pneumococci produce characteristic draughtsman or carom coin-shaped α-hemolytic colonies (**Fig. 22.6A**) and on chocolate agar, it produces greenish discoloration (bleaching effect)
  - *Identification:* Pneumococcus shows—(i) a positive bile solubility test, (ii) susceptibility to optochin (produce 14 mm or more wider zone of inhibition (**Fig. 22.6B**) and (iii) positive for inulin fermentation. Automated ID systems (e.g. MALDI-TOF or VITEK) can also be used for identification

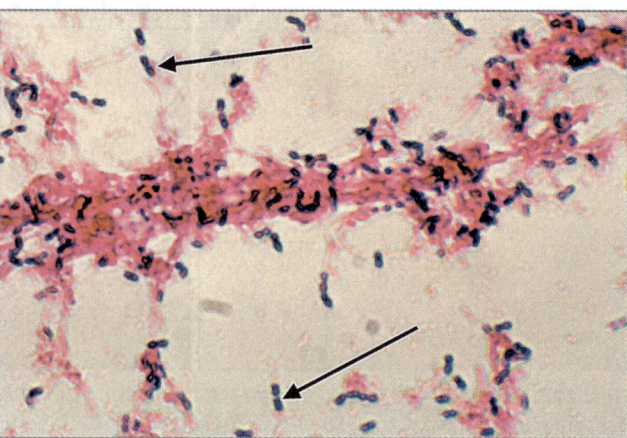

Fig. 22.5: Pneumococci in Gram stained smear of sputum [lanceolate shaped gram-positive cocci in pair surrounded by clear halo (capsule)].

Source: Public Health Image Library, ID#/2896/Dr Mike Miller/Centers for Disease Control and Prevention (CDC), Atlanta (*with permission*).

- **Typing of *S. pneumoniae*** is done by **(i) Quellung reaction** (sputum specimen is treated with type-specific antiserum, along with methylene blue dye; capsule becomes swollen, sharply delineated and refractile) and (ii) serotyping by latex agglutination test
- **Antimicrobial susceptibility testing:** It can be performed by disk diffusion method (on Mueller–Hinton blood agar) or MIC-based method (VITEK).
❖ **Treatment:** Meningitis and bacteremia cases respond well to penicillin-G. Ceftriaxone or vancomycin can be given in case of penicillin resistance

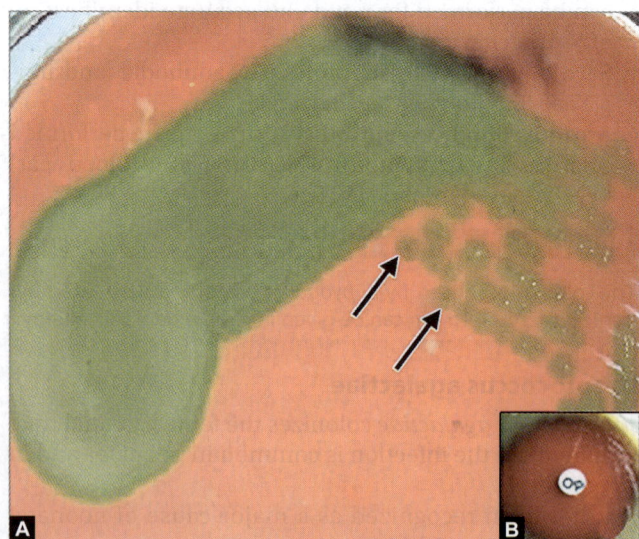

Figs. 22.6A and B: Properties of pneumococci: **A.** α-hemolytic draughtsman-shaped colonies on blood agar; **B.** Sensitive to optochin.

Source: Department of Microbiology, Pondicherry Institute of Medical Sciences, Puducherry (*with permission*).

- Meningitis cases require early treatment as are associated with high fatality
- Pneumonia cases can be treated with oral amoxicillin or levofloxacin or IV ceftriaxone.
❖ **Infection control measures** such as droplet precautions should be followed in hospitals (*refer* **Chapter 15**)
❖ **Vaccine**: There are two vaccines available for pneumococcus:
  - 23-valent pneumococcal polysaccharide vaccine (PPSV23)—given to high-risk adults such to old age, immunodeficiency, splenic dysfunction, etc., but not to children. It is less immunogenic and provides short-term immunity
  - Pneumococcal conjugate vaccine (PCV13)—given both to children and high-risk adults. It is more immunogenic and provides longer immunity.

■ ENTEROCOCCUS

Enterococcus was initially grouped under group D *Streptococcus*, but later, have been reclassified as a separate genus *Enterococcus*. Enterococci are part of the normal flora of the human intestine. *E. faecalis* and *E. faecium* are the common species infecting man.

❖ **Virulence factors include:**
  - Aggregation substances or pheromones help in clumping of adjacent cells to facilitate plasmid exchange (transfers drug resistance)
  - Extracellular surface protein (ESP) helps in adhesion to bladder mucosa (causes UTI)
❖ **Clinical manifestations:** Enterococci can cause various infections ranging from UTI, chronic prostatitis, bacteremia, endocarditis, intra-abdominal, pelvic and soft tissue infections, surgical site infections, late onset neonatal sepsis, meningitis, and pneumonia.
❖ **Laboratory diagnosis:** Enterococci have the following laboratory features **(Table 22.1)**.
  - *Gram stain:* They appear oval-shaped gram-positive cocci in pairs; at an angle to each other
  - *Culture:* Produce non-hemolytic translucent colonies on blood agar. On MacConkey agar it produces minute magenta pink colonies
  - They can grow in presence of extreme conditions such as—6.5% NaCl, 40% bile, pH 9.6, 45°C and 10°C
  - *Identification:* Enterococci show a positive bile esculin hydrolysis test. *E. faecalis* is negative and *E. faecium* is positive for arabinose fermentation test. Automated ID systems can also be used for identification
  - **Antimicrobial susceptibility testing:** It can be performed by disk diffusion method (on Mueller–Hinton agar) or MIC-based method (VITEK).
❖ **Treatment**: Enterococci can be treated with ampicillin ± gentamicin, vancomycin, and fosfomycin (for *E. faecalis* only).

Vancomycin resistant enterococci (VRE) have also been isolated; where linezolid is the treatment of choice. *E. faecium* is found to be more resistant to vancomycin than *E. faecalis*.

EXPECTED QUESTIONS

I. **Write an essay on:**
  1. Discuss the manifestations, laboratory diagnosis, and treatment of *Streptococcus pyogenes* infection.

II. **Write short notes on:**
  1. Laboratory diagnosis and treatment of pneumococcal infections.
  2. Write briefly on clinical spectrum and laboratory diagnosis of enterococci infections.

III. **Multiple Choice Questions (MCQs):**
  1. **CAMP test is useful in identification of:**
     a. *S. pyogenes* b. *S. agalactiae*
     c. *S. pneumoniae* d. Viridans streptococci
  2. ***Streptococcus pyogenes* can be differentiated from *S. agalactiae* by testing susceptibility to:**
     a. Optochin b. Bacitracin
     c. Polymyxin d. Novobiocin
  3. **Pneumococcus can be identified by testing susceptibility to:**
     a. Polymyxin b. Novobiocin
     c. Optochin d. Bacitracin
  4. **Carrom coin appearance of colonies is seen for:**
     a. *S. pyogenes*
     b. Viridans streptococci
     c. *S. agalactiae*
     d. *S. pneumoniae*
  5. **Which of the following is the property of enterococci?**
     a. Bacitracin sensitive
     b. CAMP positive
     c. Bile esculin hydrolysis
     d. Optochin sensitive

Answers
1. b 2. b 3. c 4. d 5. c

Neisseria: Meningococcus and Gonococcus

CHAPTER 23

CHAPTER PREVIEW
- Meningococcus
- Gonococcus

Members of genus *Neisseria* are catalase and oxidase positive, non-motile, aerobic gram-negative diplococci. Two species are pathogenic to humans—(1) *N. meningitidis* (causes pyogenic meningitis) and (2) *N. gonorrhoeae* (causes gonorrhea), both differ from each other in various aspects **(Table 23.1)**.

NEISSERIA MENINGITIDIS

N. meningitidis (or meningococci) are capsulated gram-negative diplococci—one of the important causes of pyogenic meningitis.

Virulence Factors

Pathogenesis of meningococcal infection is due to the expression of several virulence factors.
- Important virulence factors are—polysaccharide capsule, endotoxin, and outer membrane proteins

Table 23.1: Differences between *Neisseria meningitidis* and *Neisseria gonorrhoeae*.

N. meningitidis	N. gonorrhoeae
Capsulated	Noncapsulated
Lens-shaped/half moon-shaped (diplococci with adjacent sides flattened)	Kidney-shaped (diplococci with adjacent sides concave)
Ferments glucose and maltose	Ferments only glucose
Rarely have plasmids	Usually possess plasmids, coding for drug-resistant genes
Exist in both intra- and extracellular forms	Predominantly exist in intracellular form
Colony—circular	Colony—varies in size with irregular margin
Habitat—nasopharynx	Habitat—genital tract (urethra, cervix), rarely pharynx

- Based on the capsular polysaccharide, meningococci can be typed into several serotypes
- Serotypes A, B, C, X, Y and W135 cause invasive disease.

Clinical Manifestations
- Meningococcus is transmitted by droplet inhalation
- The majority of infections result in a nasopharyngeal carriage
- In susceptible children, it spreads through the hematogenous route to CNS to cause pyogenic meningitis
- Systemic spread can cause fatal septicemia and complication such as Waterhouse–Friderichsen syndrome—characterized by adrenal hemorrhage, disseminated intravascular coagulation, purpuric rashes, and shock.

Epidemiology

Meningococcus causes several patterns of invasive disease ranging from sporadic infection, to endemic, and explosive epidemics
- The serogroups distribution varies among various regions of the world
- The sub-Saharan belt of Africa is the most prevalent area.

Laboratory Diagnosis
- **Specimen collection:** Useful specimens are CSF and blood for cases and nasopharyngeal swab for carriers. All specimens should be transported and processed immediately. If there is a delay should be kept in incubator at 37°C, never refrigerated
- **CSF examination:** CSF is divided into three portions:
  - **First portion** of CSF is centrifuged and the supernatant is used for capsular antigen detection by latex agglutination test and also used for biochemical analysis. The sediment is used for direct Gram staining.

CHAPTER 23 ❖ Neisseria: Meningococcus and Gonococcus

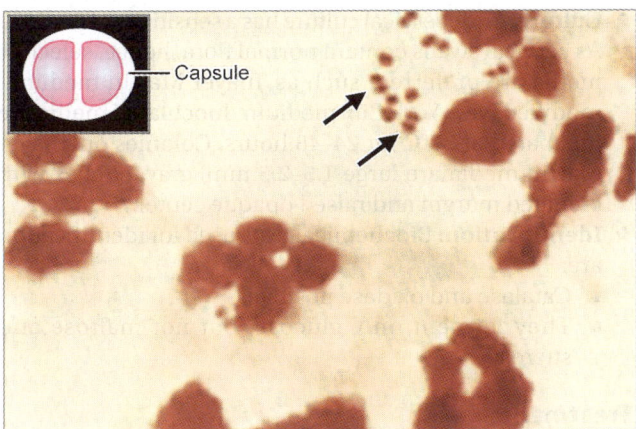

Fig. 23.1: Meningococci in CSF smear (gram-negative diplococci, lens-shaped) (arrows showing).
Source: Centers for Disease Control and Prevention (CDC), Atlanta (*with permission*).

- **Second portion of CSF:** It is inoculated onto blood agar and chocolate agar.
- **Third portion of CSF:** It is inoculated into BHI broth, incubated overnight and then subcultured onto blood agar and chocolate agar.
❖ **Gram stain** reveals gram-negative diplococci (0.8 μm in size), capsulated, lens-shaped **(Fig. 23.1)**
❖ **Culture:** Meningococci are very delicate and fastidious; do not grow in basal media.
  - Useful culture media are—blood agar and chocolate agar (for CSF specimen), blood culture bottles (for blood specimen), and Thayer Martin media or New York City medium (to suppress the growth of normal flora, for nasopharyngeal swab).
  - Culture plates are incubated for 24–48 hours at 37°C under 5–10% CO_2.
  - Meningococcus colonies are small (1 mm), round, convex, gray, non-hemolytic, translucent at 24hr of incubation.
  - Meningococci are very delicate and fastidious; do not grow in basal media.
❖ **Identification:** It is catalase and oxidase positive, ferments glucose and maltose.
❖ **Molecular diagnosis:** By PCR to detect meningococcal DNA in CSF or blood.

Treatment
Third-generation cephalosporins such as ceftriaxone are the drug of choice. Meningitis cases are associated with high fatality and therefore warrant early treatment.

Prevention
❖ **Vaccines:** Capsular polysaccharide vaccine and conjugated capsular vaccine are available for meningococcus
❖ **Infection control measures** such as droplet precautions should be followed in hospitals (*refer* **Chapter 15**).

■ NEISSERIA GONORRHOEAE

Neisseria gonorrhoeae causes a sexually transmitted infection (STI), known as 'gonorrhea' and commonly manifests as cervicitis, and urethritis.

Virulence Factors
Virulence factors produced by *N. gonorrhoeae* are:
❖ **Pili:** It helps in adhesion to host cells and prevent bacteria from phagocytosis
❖ **Outer membrane protein:** They form transmembrane channels (pores) which help in exchange of molecules across gonococcal surface
❖ **IgA1 protease:** It protects the organism from the action of mucosal IgA antibody
❖ **Lipo-oligosaccharide (LOS):** It has marked endotoxic activity.

Clinical Manifestations
Gonorrhea commonly manifests as:
❖ **In males:** Acute urethritis, characterized by purulent urethral discharge
❖ **In females:** Mucopurulent cervicitis is the most common presentation
❖ **In both sexes:** Anorectal and pharyngeal gonorrhea
❖ **Among neonates:** Transmission during delivery from the maternal genital tract to the baby can cause conjunctivitis *(ophthalmia neonatorum)* in the newborn
❖ **Disseminated gonococcal infection:** Presents as polyarthritis, and endocarditis.

Laboratory Diagnosis
❖ **Specimen collection:** Urethral swabs (for males) and endocervical swabs (for females) are the ideal specimens.
  - Specimens should be transported immediately.
  - If not possible, then it should be collected in charcoal-coated swabs kept in **Stuart's** transport medium or charcoal containing medium (**Amies** medium).
❖ **Direct microscopy:** Gram staining of urethral exudates reveals gram-negative intracellular kidney-shaped diplococci **(Fig. 23.2)**.

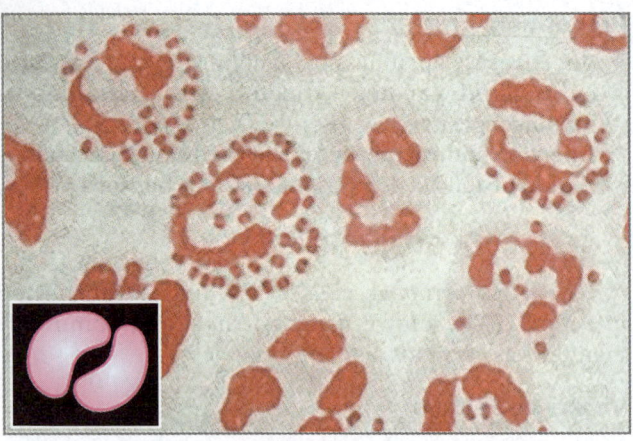

Fig. 23.2: Gonococcus (gram-negative diplococci, kidney-shaped).
Source: Public Health Image Library, ID# /2108, Centers for Disease Control and Prevention (CDC), Atlanta *(with permission).*

- **Culture:** Endocervical culture has a sensitivity of 80–90%. As cervical swabs contain normal flora, hence, selective media are preferred, such as Thayer Martin medium, modified New York City medium. Inoculated media are incubated at 37°C for 24–48 hours. Colonies on Thayer Martin media are large 1.5–2.5 mm, gray, convex with crenated margin and raised opaque center.
- **Identification:** Biochemical tests used for identification are:
  - Catalase and oxidase positive
  - They ferment only glucose, but not maltose and sucrose.

Treatment

Third-generation cephalosporin such as ceftriaxone is the drug of choice. Both sexual partners should be treated.

 EXPECTED QUESTIONS

I. **Write short notes on:**
   1. Clinical manifestations and laboratory diagnosis of meningococcal meningitis.
   2. Clinical manifestations and laboratory diagnosis of gonorrhea.

II. **Multiple Choice Questions (MCQs):**
   1. **Serotyping of meningococci are based on:**
      a. Outer membrane proteins
      b. Endotoxin
      c. Capsular polysaccharide
      d. Transferrin binding proteins
   2. **Gonococci can be differentiated by meningococci by following sugar fermentation test:**
      a. Glucose
      b. Sucrose
      c. Mannitol
      d. Maltose
   3. **The most common mode of transmission of gonorrhea is:**
      a. Sexual transmission
      b. Injection
      c. Blood transfusion
      d. Inhalation
   4. **Transport media used for gonococci is:**
      a. VR medium
      b. Pike's medium
      c. Stuart's medium
      d. Cary-Blair medium

Answers
1. c   2. d   3. a   4. c

Corynebacterium

CHAPTER 24

CHAPTER PREVIEW
- Corynebacterium diphtheriae
- Other Coryneform Bacteria

■ INTRODUCTION

Corynebacteria are club-shaped irregularly stained gram-positive bacilli **(Fig. 24.1A)** (Greek word *koryne*, meaning club). *C. diphtheriae* is the most important species pathogenic to man; other species called *diphtheroids* are mainly skin commensals, and occasionally can be pathogenic to man.

■ CORYNEBACTERIUM DIPHTHERIAE

Corynebacterium diphtheriae is the causative agent of **diphtheria**—a contagious disease, characterized by pseudomembrane formation over the tonsil. It commonly affects unvaccinated children. It typically shows two characteristic features such as:

1. **Chinese letter or cuneiform arrangement:** They appear as V- or L-shaped in smear, because the bacterial cells divide and daughter cells tend to lie at acute angles to each other. This type of cell division is called **snapping type of division (Fig. 24.1B)**
2. **Metachromatic granules:** They are present at ends or poles of the bacilli (*refer* highlight box given below).

Metachromatic Granules
Also called polar bodies or Babes–Ernst bodies or volutin granules.
- They are storage granules of the organism, composed of polymetaphosphates
- Granules are stained strongly gram-positive compared to remaining part of the bacilli. The granules take up bluish purple metachromatic color when stained with Loeffler's methylene blue
- However, they are better stained with special stains, such as Albert's, Neisser's and Ponder's stain **(Fig. 24.1C)**
- Granules are well developed on enriched media, such as blood agar or Loeffler's serum slope.

Virulence Factors (Diphtheria Toxin)

The pathogenesis of diphtheria is mediated by diphtheria toxin; which acts by inhibiting protein synthesis. **Diphtheria toxin** is a bacteriophage coded toxin, comprises of two fragments—A and B.
- *Fragment B* binds to the host cell receptors and helps in the entry of fragment A

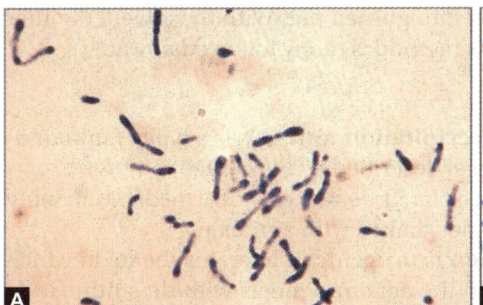 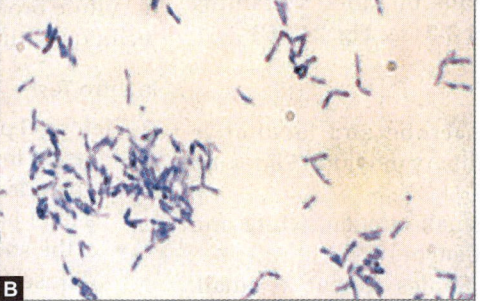 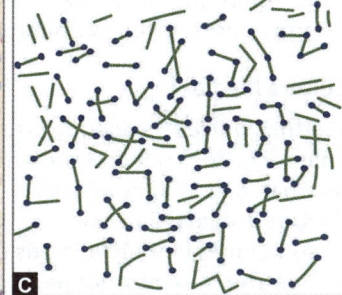

Figs. 24.1A to C: *Corynebacterium diphtheriae*: **A.** Club-shaped bacilli in methylene blue-stained smear; **B.** Gram-stained smear shows V- or L-shaped bacilli with cuneiform arrangement; **C.** Albert's stain shows dark blue metachromatic granules at the ends of the green bacilli (schematic).
Source: Public Health Image Library, A. ID# /7323/P.B. Smith; B. ID# /1943, Centers for Disease Control and Prevention (CDC), Atlanta (*with permission*).

❖ *Fragment A* is the active fragment, that gets internalized into the host cell and causes inhibition of protein synthesis by inhibiting elongation factor 2 (EF-2).

Pathogenesis and Clinical Manifestations
- **Mode of transmission:** Occurs through inhalation of respiratory droplets (by coughing or sneezing)
- **Spread:** Organism does not invade, multiplies only at the local site, and secrets toxin. It is the toxin that enters the circulation and goes to various sites to produce various clinical manifestations.
- **Clinical manifestations** are:
  - **Respiratory (faucial) diphtheria** is the most common form; characterized by—the presence of a tough leathery grayish white pseudomembrane, formed over the tonsils
  - The **other manifestations** are cutaneous diphtheria and less commonly, toxic systemic complications such as myocarditis and neurologic manifestations.

Laboratory Diagnosis
Laboratory diagnosis consists of isolation of the bacilli and toxin demonstration.

Isolation and Identification of Diphtheria Bacilli
Specimen
Useful specimens include: (1) throat swab (one or two) containing fibrinous exudates, (2) a portion of pseudomembrane, (3) nose or skin specimens (if infected).

Direct Smear Microscopy
- **Gram stain:** *C. diphtheriae* appear as irregularly stained club-shaped gram-positive bacilli of 3–6 μm length, typically arranged in **Chinese letter** or **cuneiform** arrangement (V- or L-shaped) (*see* **Fig. 24.1B**)
- **Albert's stain:** It is more specific for *C. diphtheriae;* they appear as green bacilli with bluish black metachromatic granules at the poles. Details of Albert's staining procedure is given in **Chapter 3.2** (*see* **Fig. 24.1C**).

Culture Media
C. diphtheriae is fastidious, aerobe and facultative anaerobe; does not grow on ordinary medium. Plates are incubated at 37°C aerobically.
- **Blood agar:** Colonies are small circular, white and sometimes hemolytic (mitis biotype)
- **Loeffler's serum slope:** Colonies appear as small, circular, glistening, and white with a yellow tinge in 6–8 hours. Growth can be detected as early as 6–8 hours. It is the best medium for the production of metachromatic granules **(Fig. 24.2A)**

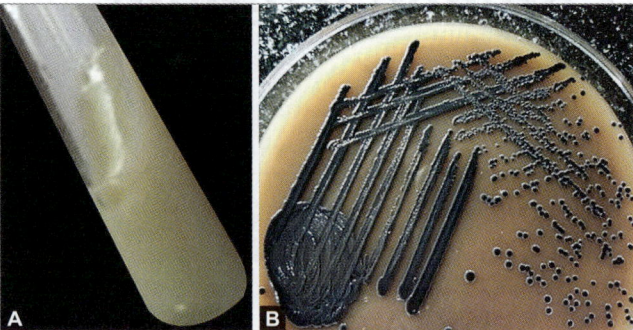

Figs. 24.2A and B: A. Loeffler's serum slope; **B.** Potassium tellurite agar shows black-colored colonies.
Source: A. Department of Microbiology, JIPMER, Puducherry; B. Department of Microbiology, Pondicherry Institute of Medical Sciences, Puducherry (*with permission*).

- **Potassium tellurite agar (PTA):** *C. diphtheriae* reduces tellurite to metallic tellurium which gets incorporated into the colonies giving them black color **(Fig. 24.2B)**. It is a selective media and it inhibits the throat commensals. Colonies appear only after 48 hours of incubation.

Identification
Species identification of *C. diphtheriae* is made by:
- **Biochemical tests:**
  - *Corynebacterium* is catalase positive but oxidase negative and nonmotile
  - Sugar fermentation test using Hiss's serum sugar media: Diphtheria bacilli ferment glucose and maltose (by all biotypes) and starch (by only gravis biotype), with the production of acid but no gas.
  - Urease test negative.
- **Automated identification systems** such as MALDI-TOF or VITEK.

Toxin Demonstration
In Vivo Test (Animal Inoculation)
In vivo toxin demonstration can be done by inoculation of culture broth into **guinea pig**. With the advent of other techniques, this method is rarely followed nowadays.

In Vitro Test
- **Elek's gel precipitation test:** This is a type of immunodiffusion in gel described by Elek (1949)
  - The strain isolated is streaked onto a media containing a filter paper soaked with antitoxin
  - If the strain is toxigenic, it liberates the toxin which diffuses in the agar and meets with the antitoxin to produce an arrow-shaped precipitation band
  - This test can also be used to know the relatedness between the strains isolated during an outbreak. The precipitate bands of outbreak isolates (streaked

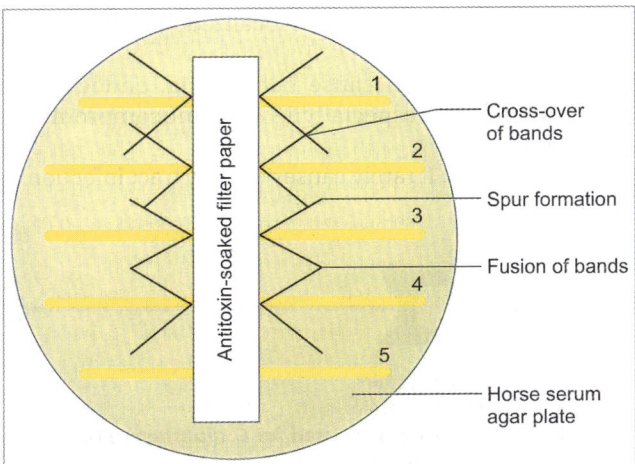

Fig. 24.3: Elek's gel precipitation test.

adjacent) when meet with each other, three patterns may be observed **(Fig. 24.3)**:
1. Cross-over with each other—indicates unrelated strain
2. Spur formation—indicates partially related strain
3. Fused with each other—indicates identical strain.
- **Other in vitro tests** include:
  - Detection of *Tox* gene by PCR
  - Detection of diphtheria toxin by ELISA or immunochromatographic test (ICT).

Epidemiology
The incidence of diphtheria is greatly reduced after the introduction of widespread immunization. However, there are reports of a resurgence of cases in older children with incomplete booster doses. India still accounts for the maximum number of cases globally. The main source of infection is the carriers (nasal and throat), which is common in children.

> **TREATMENT**   Diphtheria
>
> Diphtheria is a medical emergency, and should be treated at the earliest. The treatment regimen comprises:
> - **Anti-diphtheritic serum:** Passive immunization with anti-diphtheritic horse serum is the treatment of choice as it neutralizes the toxin
> - **Antibiotics such as penicillin or erythromycin:** It has a role if given early in treatment before toxin release. Antibiotics are also useful for the treatment of carriers.

Prophylaxis

Infection Control Measures
Patient should be placed in isolation room and all the steps of droplet precaution should be followed for the prevention of transmission of *C. diphtheriae* in hospitals (*refer* **Chapter 15**).

Post-exposure Prophylaxis
For close contacts (e.g. household), booster dose of diphtheria vaccine and penicillin G (single dose) or erythromycin (7–10 days) is recommended.

Vaccination
The diphtheria vaccine (toxoid) is given under the national immunization schedule as a combined vaccine along with pertussis and tetanus (DPT vaccine).
- **Children:** A total of seven doses are given.
  - Three doses of pentavalent vaccine (DPT + hepatitis B+ *Haemophilus influenzae* b) at 6, 10, and 14 weeks of birth, followed by two booster doses of DPT at 16–24 months and 5 years, and
  - Another two booster doses of Td (tetanus toxoid, adult dose of diphtheria toxoid) at 10 years and 16 years.
- **A pregnant woman** also should receive two doses of Td at one month interval
- **Site:** DPT is given deep intramuscularly (IM) at the anterolateral aspect of the thigh
- **Thiomersal** (0.01%) is used as a preservative
- **Storage:** DPT should be kept at 2–8°C; if accidentally frozen then it has to be discarded
- **Protective titer:** Following vaccination, an antitoxin titer of ≥0.01 IU/mL is said to be protective.

Diphtheroids
Diphtheroids or coryneforms usually exist as normal commensals in the throat, skin, conjunctiva and other areas. They can be differentiated from *C. diphtheriae*

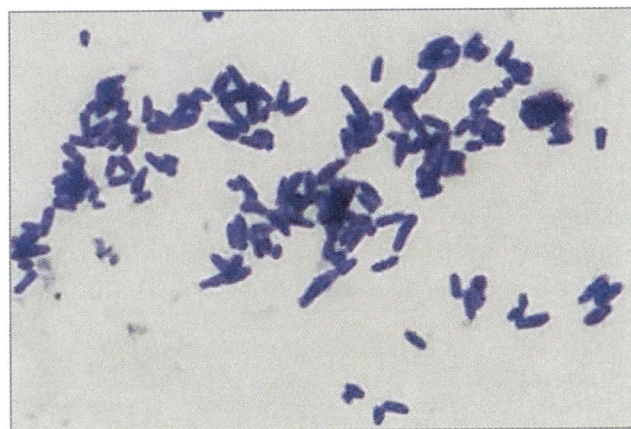

Fig. 24.4: Diphtheroids—palisade arrangement of gram-positive bacilli.
Source: Department of Microbiology, JIPMER, Puducherry (*with permission*).

by many features such as: (i) Stains more uniformly, (ii) palisade arrangement (arranged in parallel rows) **(Fig. 24.4)**, and (iii) absence of metachromatic granules.

Common coryneforms that are rarely pathogenic to man are:

❖ *C. ulcerans* and *C. pseudotuberculosis* produce ulcerations in throat

❖ *C. minutissimum:* It causes a localized infection of skin (axilla and groin)

❖ *C. jeikeium:* It can cause bacteremia, endocarditis and meningitis, especially in immunocompromised patients.

❖ *C. urealyticum:* It rarely causes urinary tract infection.

EXPECTED QUESTIONS

I. **Write short notes on:**
   1. Laboratory diagnosis of diphtheria.
   2. DPT vaccines.

III. **Multiple Choice Questions (MCQs):**
   1. Production of early metachromatic granules can be seen best in which of the following media:
      a. Nutrient agar
      b. Chocolate agar
      c. Loeffler's serum slope
      d. Potassium tellurite agar
   2. Metachromatic granules of *Corynebacterium diphtheriae* can be stained by all of the following special stains, *except*:
      a. Neisser's stain
      b. Ziehl–Neelsen stain
      c. Albert's stain
      d. Ponder's stain
   3. Selective medium used for *C. diphtheriae* is:
      a. Blood agar
      b. Chocolate agar
      c. LJ medium
      d. Potassium tellurite agar
   4. Which of the following site is most commonly affected by *C. diphtheriae*?
      a. Skin
      b. Conjunctiva
      c. Faucial
      d. Kidney

Answers
1. c   2. b   3. d   4. c

Bacillus

CHAPTER 25

CHAPTER PREVIEW
- *Bacillus anthracis*
- Other *Bacillus* Species of Human Importance

Gram-positive spore forming bacilli belong to two genera:
1. *Bacillus:* They are obligate aerobes; having non-bulging spores.
2. *Clostridium:* They are obligate anaerobes with bulging spores.

Bacillus species are gram-positive spore-bearing bacilli. The important pathogens are *B. anthracis* (causes anthrax) and *B. cereus* (causes food poisoning). Other *Bacillus* species (called as anthracoid bacilli) are common laboratory contaminants.

BACILLUS ANTHRACIS

Bacillus anthracis is the causative agent of an important zoonotic disease called **anthrax**. They are gram-positive, large rectangular rods (3–10 μm × 1–1.6 μm) arranged in chains, non-motile and capsulated bearing non-bulging oval spores.

Virulence Factors and Pathogenesis

The pathogenesis of anthrax is mediated by two important virulence factors—
1. **Capsule:** It is polypeptide in nature, and acts by inhibiting phagocytosis
2. **Anthrax toxin:** It has three fragments; edema factor, protective factor and lethal factor.

Clinical Manifestations

B. anthracis is transmitted in three modes—contact, inhalation and ingestion. Accordingly anthrax in humans manifests in three forms:
1. **Cutaneous anthrax** (Hide porter's disease): It is the most common form (95%), characterized by black eschar surrounded by non-pitting edema called **malignant pustule (Fig. 25.1)**.
2. **Pulmonary anthrax:** Wool sorter's disease (as commonly seen in workers of wool factory), characterized by hemorrhagic mediastinitis
3. **Intestinal anthrax** is very rare.

Laboratory Diagnosis

There is a high-risk of laboratory acquired infection of anthrax, hence utmost precautions should be taken and specimens should be processed in appropriate biological safety cabinets.

Specimen Collection

The specimens should be collected before starting antibiotic treatment. The useful specimens are:
- Pus, swab or tissue from the malignant pustule
- Sputum in pulmonary anthrax
- Blood (in septicemia)
- CSF (in hemorrhagic meningitis)
- Gastric aspirate, feces or food (in intestinal anthrax).

Direct Demonstration

- **Gram staining:** Reveals gram-positive, large rectangular rods (3–10 μm × 1–1.6 μm). Spores are usually not seen in clinical samples **(Fig. 25.2A)**

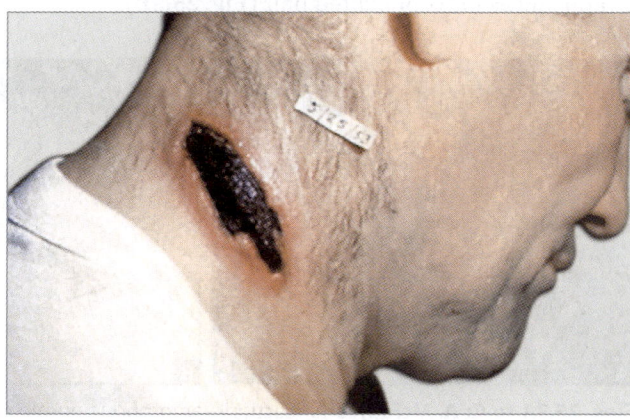

Fig. 25.1: Malignant pustule.
Source: Public Health Image Library, ID# 1934/Centers for Disease Control and Prevention (CDC), Atlanta (*with permission*).

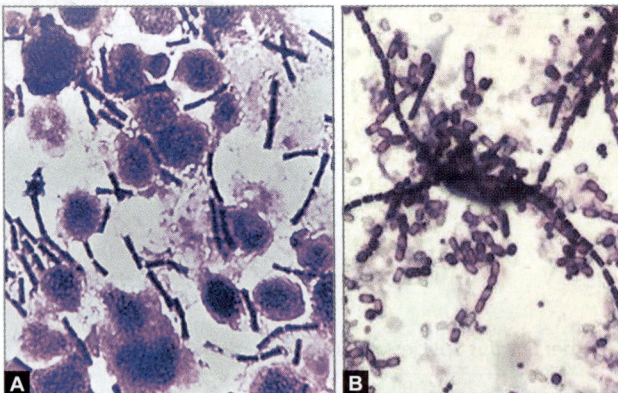

Figs. 25.2A and B: Gram stain of *B. anthracis*: **A.** Direct smear-shows gram-positive, large rectangular bacilli and pus cells; **B.** Culture smear-shows gram-positive bacilli with non-bulging spores (bamboo stick appearance).
Source: A. Public Health Image Library/ID#: 1811, Centers for Disease Control and Prevention (CDC), Atlanta (*with permission*); B. Department of Microbiology, JIPMER, Puducherry (*with permission*).

- ❖ **McFadyean's reaction:** It shows amorphous purple capsule surrounding blue bacilli (polychrome methylene blue stain) **(Fig. 25.3A)**
- ❖ **Ascoli's thermoprecipitation test:** It is a ring precipitation test, performed when specimens are received in the putrid form.

Culture

Bacillus anthracis is aerobic, non-fastidious, grows in ordinary media.
- ❖ **Nutrient agar:** Colonies are 2–3 mm in size, irregular, round, opaque, with a frosted glass appearance
- ❖ **Medusa head appearance:** When colonies are viewed under low power microscope, the edge of the colony which is composed of long interlacing chains of bacilli, appears as locks of matted hair **(Fig. 25.3B)**
- ❖ **Blood agar:** It produces dry wrinkled, non-hemolytic colonies **(Fig. 25.3C)**
- ❖ **Gelatin stab agar:** Growth occurs as inverted fir tree appearance (due to liquefaction of gelatin)
- ❖ **Selective media (PLET medium):** It consists of polymyxin, lysozyme, EDTA and thallous acetate.

Culture Smear

- ❖ **Gram staining:** Reveals **bamboo stick appearance**, i.e. long chain of gram-positive bacilli with non-bulging spores (appear as empty space) **(Fig. 25.2B)**.
- ❖ **Spores:** They can be demonstrated by using special stains, such as hot malachite green (Ashby's method) or modified acid-fast staining using 0.25% sulfuric acid (spores are acid-fast).

> **TREATMENT** — Anthrax
>
> Ciprofloxacin or doxycycline are the drugs of choice, given for:
> ☐ 7–10 days for treatment of anthrax
> ☐ 60 days for post-exposure prophylaxis (along with anthrax vaccine)

Prevention

The general control measures include:
- ❖ Disposal of animal carcasses by deep burial in lime pits
- ❖ Decontamination (usually by autoclaving) of animal products
- ❖ Protective clothing and gloves for handling potentially infectious materials.

Vaccine

Two important vaccines are available for anthrax:
1. Live attenuated, non-capsulated spore vaccine
2. Adsorbed (alum precipitated) toxoid vaccine containing the protective factor.

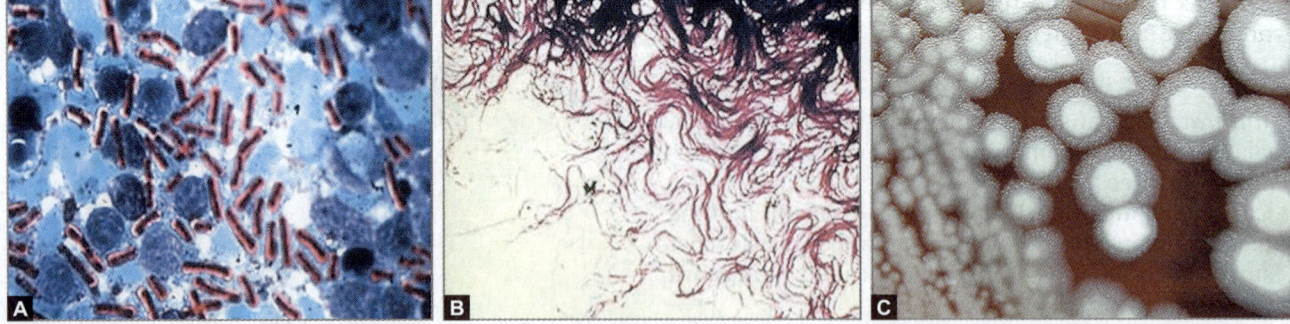

Figs. 25.3A to C: A. McFadyean's reaction—amorphous purple capsule surrounding blue bacilli (polychrome methylene blue stain); **B.** Medusa head colonies of *Bacillus anthracis* on nutrient agar (10x magnification); **C.** Non-hemolytic dry wrinkled colonies of *Bacillus anthracis* on blood agar.
Source: A. Department of Pathobiology, University of Guelph, Canada; B. Dr J Glenn Songer, Iowa State University, USA; C. Public Health Image Library/ID#: 1897/Dr Larry Stauffer, Centers for Disease Control and Prevention (CDC), Atlanta (*with permission*).

OTHER BACILLUS SPECIES OF HUMAN IMPORTANCE

Bacillus species other than the anthrax bacillus, are collectively called **anthracoid bacilli**.
- Except *B. cereus*, most of them are non-pathogenic and are common contaminants in laboratory cultures
- They have a general resemblance to anthrax bacilli such as producing dry wrinkled colonies and in smear they appear as chains of spore-bearing gram-positive bacilli.

Bacillus cereus

Bacillus cereus is a normal habitant of soil, also widely isolated from food items. It is an important agent of food poisoning in man; mediated by producing two types of toxins—
1. **Emetic toxin:** causes emetic type of food poisoning.
   - It is a preformed toxin (like *S. aureus* enterotoxin), that acts immediately after food intake, and therefore the incubation period is short (1–6 hours)
   - Associated with the consumption of contaminated fried rice with emetic toxin.
2. **Diarrheal toxin:** causes a diarrheal type of food poisoning. Organism secretes this toxin only after entering the intestine, hence the incubation period is longer (8–16 hours).

Laboratory Diagnosis

Bacillus cereus is motile, non-capsulated gram-positive bacilli. It can be isolated from feces by using selective media such as: MYPA (mannitol, egg yolk, polymyxin B, phenol red and agar).

Bacillus (Spores) used as Sterilization Control

Bacillus species are used as biological indicators to check the efficacy of sterilization process. For example;
- *Geobacillus stearothermophilus* (formerly *Bacillus stearothermophilus*) is used for autoclave, hydrogen peroxide gas plasma sterilizer and liquid acetic acid sterilizer
- *Bacillus atrophaeus* is used for ethylene oxide sterilizer and dry heat sterilizer.

EXPECTED QUESTIONS

I. **Write short notes on:**
   1. Clinical forms of anthrax.
   2. Laboratory diagnosis of anthrax.
   3. *Bacillus cereus*.

II. **Multiple Choice Questions (MCQs):**
   1. **Gram-stain morphology of *Bacillus anthracis* is:**
      a. Tennis racket appearance
      b. Drum stick appearance
      c. Bamboo stick appearance
      d. Spectacle glass appearance
   2. **"Malignant pustule" is a term used for:**
      a. An infected malignant melanoma
      b. A carbuncle
      c. A rapidly spreading rodent ulcer
      d. Anthrax of the skin
   3. **Selective medium for *B. cereus*:**
      a. PLET medium
      b. Loeffler's serum slope
      c. Potassium tellurite agar
      d. MYPA medium
   4. **Incubation period for *B. cereus* food poisoning following consumption of contaminated fried rice:**
      a. 1–6 hours
      b. 8–16 hours
      c. 24 hours
      d. >24 hours

Answers
1. c   2. d   3. d   4. a

Anaerobes: Clostridium and Non-sporing Anaerobes

CHAPTER 26

> **CHAPTER PREVIEW**
> - *Clostridium* Species
> - Non-sporing Anaerobes

■ INTRODUCTION

Anaerobic bacteria that cannot grow in presence of oxygen are called as **obligate anaerobes** and anaerobes that do not utilize oxygen but tolerate its presence are called as **aerotolerant anaerobes**. Anaerobes need special requirements to grow in culture such as:

- **Anaerobic condition:** This can be achieved by various methods such as:
  - McIntosh and Filde's anaerobic jar
  - GasPak system
  - Anoxomat system
  - Anaerobic glove box
  - Pre-reduced anaerobically sterilized (PRAS) media.
- **Medium with low redox potential:** This can be achieved by adding to the media with reducing substances such as unsaturated fatty acid, ascorbic acid, glutathione, cysteine, glucose, sulfites and metallic iron.

The obligate anaerobic bacteria infecting man can be grouped into spore-bearing (e.g. *Clostridium*) and non-sporing anaerobes (described later in the chapter).

■ CLOSTRIDIUM SPECIES

Clostridia are gram-positive bacilli with bulging spores, commonly found as saprophytes in soil and commensals in the intestine of man and animals. However, few members can cause a variety of infections in humans.

- *Clostridium perfringens*: causes gas gangrene
- *Clostridium tetani*: causes tetanus
- *Clostridium botulinum*: causes botulism
- *Clostridioides difficile*: causes pseudomembranous colitis.

Clostridium perfringens

C. perfringens is commensal in the large intestine of human beings and also a soil saprophyte.

- It is capsulated, non-motile, gram-positive bacillus
- It bears subterminal bulging spores; but does not produce spores in tissues or in culture media
- It is invasive as well as toxigenic. It is the causative agent of **gas gangrene**, a rapidly spreading edematous myonecrosis.

Pathogenesis

The pathogenesis is due to its invasiveness and liberation of a variety of toxins including α-toxin (lecithinase), which is the principal virulence factor. Other toxins produced include—beta (β), epsilon (ε), and iota (ι), etc.

Clinical Manifestations

Clostridium perfringens infections are mostly polymicrobial involving other clostridia species. Various manifestations include:

- **Clostridial wound infections:** It occurs in three stages—(i) simple wound contamination, (ii) anaerobic cellulitis, (iii) anaerobic myositis or gas gangrene

> **Gas gangrene**
> It is rapidly spreading, edematous myonecrosis, occurring in association with severely crushed wounds contaminated with pathogenic clostridia:
> - **Agents:** *C. perfringens* is the most common causative agent (60%), followed by *C. novyi* and *C. septicum* (20–40%)
> - **Predisposing factors:** Crushing injuries of muscles (e.g. road traffic accidents or bullet injuries) lead to interruption in the blood supply and anoxic muscle necrosis
> - **Clinical manifestations include:** The incubation period is about 10–48 hours. Characterized by sudden onset of excruciating pain at the affected site, rapid development of a foul-smelling thin serosanguineous discharge and gas bubbles **(crepitus)** in the muscle planes.

- **Clostridial enteric infections** such as food poisoning, necrotizing enterocolitis, and gangrenous appendicitis

- ❖ Skin and soft-tissue infections
- ❖ Bacteremia.

Laboratory Diagnosis

- ❖ **Specimen:** Ideal specimens are necrotic tissues, muscle fragments and exudates from deeper part of the wound. Specimens should be put into Robertson's cooked meat broth and transported immediately to the laboratory.
- ❖ **Direct microscopy:** Thick, stubby, boxcar-shaped gram-positive bacilli without spore are suggestive of *C. perfringens* **(Fig. 26.1)**
- ❖ **Culture:** Culture media such Robertson cooked meat (RCM) broth, egg yolk agar, etc. are used, which are incubated anaerobically by GasPak or Anoxomat, etc.
- ❖ **Identification:** *C. perfringens* is identified by:
  - Target hemolysis: On blood agar, *C. perfringens* produces an inner narrow zone of complete hemolysis, surrounded by a much wider zone of incomplete hemolysis (double zone of hemolysis)
  - Nagler's reaction: Opalescence surrounding the streak line on egg yolk agar
  - Reverse CAMP test: *C. perfringens* is streaked over the center of blood agar plate and *Streptococcus agalactiae* is streaked perpendicular to it. Presence of enhanced zone of hemolysis (arrow-shaped) pointing towards *C. perfringens* indicates the test is positive
  - In litmus milk, it produces **"stormy clot reaction"** due to fermentation of lactose producing acid and vigorous gas.
  - Automated ID method such as MALDI-TOF is the current method of choice for rapid and accurate identification.

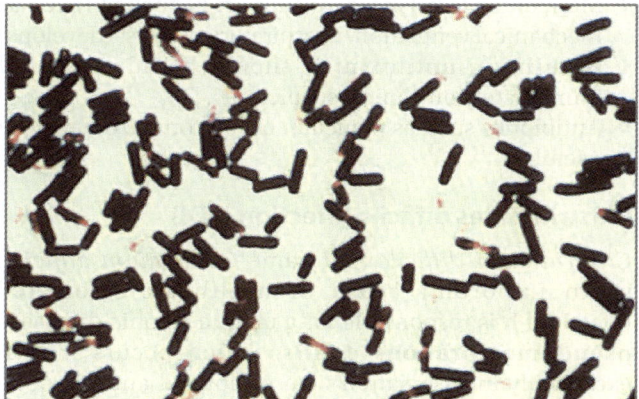

Fig. 26.1: Gram-stained smear of *Clostridium perfringens*.
Source: Public Health Image Library/ID# 11196, Don Stalons/Centers for Disease Control and Prevention (CDC), Atlanta (*with permission*).

> **TREATMENT** — Gas gangrene
>
> Surgical debridement is the mainstay of treatment. All devitalized tissues should be widely resected to remove conditions that produce an anaerobic environment. Other treatment modalities include:
> - Hyperbaric oxygen
> - Antibiotics such as penicillin plus clindamycin
> - Passive immunization with anti-α-toxin antiserum.

Clostridium tetani

Clostridium tetani is an obligate anaerobic, gram-positive bacillus with terminal round spore (drum stick appearance). It is ubiquitous in nature, widely distributed in soil, and hospital environment. It is the causative agent of 'tetanus'—an acute disease, manifested by skeletal muscle spasm and autonomic nervous system disturbance.

- ❖ **Transmission:** Tetanus bacilli enter through wounds (accidents or surgical incision) or neonates through umbilical stumps
- ❖ **Pathogenesis:** It produces a powerful neurotoxin *tetanospasmin*, which blocks the release of neurotransmitters glycine and GABA (gamma-aminobutyric acid) from the inhibitory neuron terminals, thereby causing spastic contraction of muscles **(Fig. 26.2A)**
- ❖ **Clinical manifestation:** The incubation period is about 6–10 days. Muscles of the face and jaw are often affected first (called trismus or lockjaw) followed by painful muscle spasms → leading to descending spastic paralysis
  - *Abnormal posture:* The patient may develop an opisthotonos position due to generalized spastic contraction of the extensor muscles **(Fig. 26.2B)**
  - *Autonomic disturbance* may occur leading to alerted blood pressure, tachycardia, intestinal stasis, sweating, etc.
- ❖ **Epidemiology:** Tetanus is more common in developing countries including India, which is attributed various risk factors such as—(i) warm climate, (ii) rural area with fertile soil, and (iii) unhygienic surgeries or deliveries.
- ❖ **Laboratory diagnosis:** Excised tissue bits from the necrotic depths of wounds are more reliable than wound swabs
  - *Gram staining* reveals gram-positive bacilli with terminal and round spores (drum stick appearance) **(Fig. 26.2C)**
  - *Culture:* (i) On Robertson cooked meat broth, *C. tetani*, being proteolytic turns the meat particles

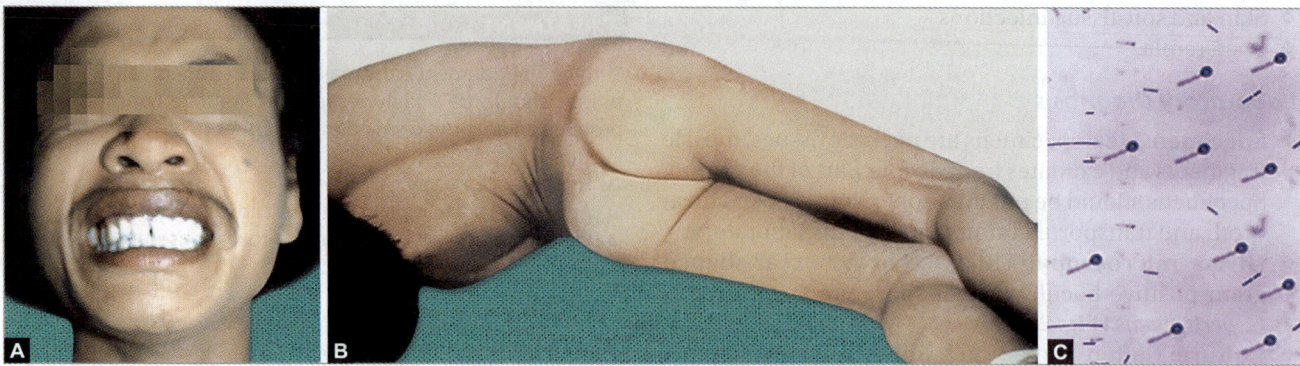

Figs. 26.2A to C: A. Lockjaw and facial spasms; **B.** Patient with opisthotonos seen in tetanus; **C.** Gram-stained smear of *Clostridium tetani* showing round terminal spore-bearing gram-positive bacilli.
Source: **A.** Wikia/Hoidkempuhtust; **B.** Public Health Image Library, ID# 6373; **C.** ID# 12056/Dr Holdeman/Centers for Disease Control and Prevention (CDC), Atlanta (*with permission*).

black and produces foul odor, and (ii) on blood agar with polymyxin, it produces characteristic **swarming growth**.
- *Toxigenicity test* can be performed by in vivo mouse inoculation test on specimens such as serum and urine.
❖ **Treatment:** The treatment modalities of tetanus include:
  - Passive immunization by tetanus immunoglobulin
  - The first dose of TT (if unvaccinated)
  - Antibiotics: Metronidazole or penicillin.
❖ **Vaccine:** The tetanus toxoid (TT) vaccine is the most effective way of prevention of tetanus. TT is given along with DPT vaccine under the childhood immunization program (*refer* **Chapter 13 for details**).

Clostridium botulinum

It produces a powerful neurotoxin *botulinum toxin*, which acts by blocking the release of acetylcholine from nerve terminals and thereby causing flaccid paralysis of voluntary muscles.

Clinical Manifestations

Botulism occurs in three clinical types.
1. **Food-borne botulism:** It results from the consumption of foods (e.g. canned food) contaminated with preformed botulinum toxin
2. **Wound botulism:** It results from contamination of wounds with *C. botulinum* spores
3. **Infant botulism:** It is the most common type; (75%); usually affects infants following ingestion of contaminated food (usually **honey**). Manifestations include floppy neck, and extreme weakness (hence called **floppy child syndrome**). It is usually self-limiting.

Laboratory Diagnosis

Diagnosis of botulism includes isolation of the bacilli and demonstration of the toxin.
❖ **Isolation of the bacilli:** Food or feces can be subjected to:
  - Gram staining: Reveals gram-positive, non-capsulated bacilli with subterminal, oval, bulging spores
  - Culture using Robertson's cooked meat (RCM) broth
  - Growth may be confirmed by Gram staining and biochemical tests or by automated identification methods
❖ **Toxin demonstration** is done by mouse bioassay.

Treatment

Treatment of botulism includes:
❖ Meticulous intensive care support is needed (such as mechanical ventilation, if respiratory paralysis develops)
❖ **Botulinum antitoxin:** It should be administered immediately on clinical suspicion.
❖ Antibiotics such as penicillin or metronidazole may be useful.

Clostridioides difficile Infection (CDI)

Clostridioides difficile (old name *Clostridium difficile*) is an important cause of healthcare-associated infection. It is responsible for a unique colonic disease—**pseudomembranous colitis**, which occurs almost exclusively in association with prolonged antimicrobial use in hospitals; therefore, called as antibiotic-associated diarrhea.
❖ **Risk factors:** *Clostridioides difficile* is associated with the following risk factors:

- **Prolonged antibiotics use:** Cephalosporins, clindamycin, ampicillin and fluoroquinolones are frequently responsible for this condition
- Advanced age (>65 years)
- Immunosuppression and cancer chemotherapy
- Malignancies and gastrointestinal surgeries.
❖ **Laboratory diagnosis:** Various methods to detect CDI include:
  - Culture on special media such as CCFA (cycloserine cefoxitin fructose agar)
  - Cell culture cytotoxin neutralization assay
  - Detection of antigen (GDH, toxin A/B) in stool (by rapid test)
  - PCR detecting toxin gene (toxin A/B).
❖ **Treatment:** Oral vancomycin or metronidazole are given for treatment
❖ **Prevention:**
  - Broad spectrum antimicrobials should be stopped at the earliest
  - Infection control measures of contact precaution (*see* **Chapter 15**) should be followed such as: strict hand hygiene and patient isolation
  - Ensure proper disinfection of floor, surfaces, toilets and other soiled areas using 1% freshly prepared sodium hypochlorite solution.

■ NON-SPORING ANAEROBES

Non-sporing anaerobes are often a part of the normal flora of the mouth, GIT, and genital tract of man and animals. Medially important non-sporing anaerobes include:
❖ Gram-positive cocci: *Peptostreptococcus*
❖ Gram-negative cocci: *Veillonella*
❖ Gram-positive bacilli: *Bifidobacterium, Propionibacterium* and *Mobiluncus*
❖ Gram-negative bacilli: *Bacteroides, Prevotella, Porphyromonas, Fusobacterium.*

Bacteroides fragilis

Bacteroides fragilis is recognized as the most common commensal in the human intestine; it is also the most frequent anaerobe isolated from clinical specimens. It causes peritonitis and intra-abdominal abscess following bowel injury (most common manifestation), pelvic inflammatory disease (PID), brain abscesses, bacteremia, and empyema.

EXPECTED QUESTIONS

I. Write short notes on:
  1. Gas gangrene.
  2. Tetanus.
  3. Botulism.
  4. Antibiotic-associated diarrhea.

II. Multiple Choice Questions (MCQs):
  1. Naegler's reaction is positive for:
     a. *Clostridium perfringens*
     b. *Clostridium tetani*
     c. *Clostridium botulinum*
     d. *Clostridioides difficile*
  2. Pseudomembranous colitis is caused by:
     a. *Clostridium perfringens*
     b. *Clostridium tetani*
     c. *Clostridium botulinum*
     d. *Clostridioides difficile*
  3. The most common type of botulism:
     a. Food botulism
     b. Infant botulism
     c. Wound botulism
     d. Iatrogenic botulism
  4. Which of the following produces a toxin that inhibits release of GABA and glycine neurotransmitters?
     a. *Clostridium perfringens*
     b. *Clostridium tetani*
     c. *Clostridium botulinum*
     d. *Clostridioides difficile*
  5. The most effective way of preventing tetanus:
     a. Hyperbaric oxygen
     b. Antibiotics
     c. Tetanus toxoid
     d. Surgical debridement and toilet

Answers
1. a 2. d 3. b 4. b 5. c

Mycobacteria

CHAPTER 27

CHAPTER PREVIEW

- Mycobacterium tuberculosis
- Mycobacterium leprae
- Nontuberculous Mycobacteria

Mycobacteria are acid-fast obligate aerobes. They can be classified into:
- *Mycobacterium tuberculosis* complex: It is responsible for tuberculosis in man
- *Mycobacterium leprae* (Hansen's bacillus): causes leprosy
- Nontuberculous mycobacteria (NTM): causes cutaneous, and pulmonary infections.

MYCOBACTERIUM TUBERCULOSIS

Mycobacterium tuberculosis complex causes tuberculosis, which is one of the oldest disease of mankind and is a major cause of death worldwide. It usually affects the lungs, although other organs are also involved. India accounts for the highest burden of tuberculosis (20% of total TB cases) worldwide.

Pathogenesis

- **Transmission:** *M. tuberculosis* is mainly transmitted by inhalation of aerosols (<5 µm), generated while coughing or sneezing by infected patients
- **Bacillary load:** At least 10^4 bacilli/mL in sputum is required for an effective transmission
- A fraction of small droplet nuclei containing bacilli reaches the lungs, where the bacilli are phagocytosed by the alveolar macrophages
- *M. tuberculosis* is an obligate intracellular pathogen, that survives inside the macrophage by inhibition of phagolysosome fusion
- **CMI:** Host's cell-mediated immune response to *M. tuberculosis* is critical to contain the infection
- **Macrophage-activating response:** If the host mounts a good immune response, the activated macrophages kill the tubercle bacilli and form characteristic granuloma called tubercles
- **Tissue-damaging response:** In case bacilli are more virulent and the host mounts a delayed hypersensitivity reaction (DTH) to contain the infection, which leads to lung tissue destruction.

Clinical Forms

Tuberculosis occurs both in pulmonary and extrapulmonary forms.

Pulmonary Tuberculosis (PTB)

It is the most common type, presents either as primary PTB in children or as post-primary PTB in adults.
- **Primary PTB:** It is characterized by fibrotic nodular lesions (Ghon focus) in the lungs and associated hilar lymphadenopathy—together referred to as primary complex. The middle and lower lobes of the lungs are commonly affected
- **Post-primary PTB:** It usually occurs in adults, where the apical lobe of the lungs gets involved. Common features observed are hematogenous spread, cavitation, and caseating granuloma formation
- **Clinical features:** Patients usually present with fever, productive cough (±hemoptysis) and occasionally pleuritic chest pain, night sweating, weight loss, etc.

Extrapulmonary Tuberculosis (EPTB)

EPTB results from hematogenous dissemination of tubercle bacilli to various organs. In HIV patients, the occurrence of EPTB is much higher. The common types of EPTB include—tuberculous lymphadenitis (35%), pleural tuberculosis (20%), genitourinary tuberculosis, skeletal tuberculosis, tuberculous meningitis, gastrointestinal tuberculosis, and tuberculous skin lesions.

Epidemiology

About a quarter of the current world population is infected asymptomatically with *M. tuberculosis*, of which 5–10% develop the clinical disease during their lifetime.

- **World:** The WHO has estimated 10.6 million new cases of TB occurred in 2021 with a global incidence of 130 new cases per one lakh population per year
- Countries with high TB burden are **India,** China, Indonesia, Philippines, Pakistan, Nigeria, Bangladesh and South Africa
- **India:** In 2021, about 26 lakh cases occurred India; with highest burden from Uttar Pradesh (20% of total TB cases) followed by Maharashtra
- TB is one of the top 10 causes of death worldwide and the leading cause among infectious diseases.

Laboratory Diagnosis

The specimens collected for the diagnosis of tuberculosis depend upon the clinical forms.
- In PTB, a minimum of *two sputum specimens* are examined—**spot sample** (collected on the same day under supervision) and **early morning sample** (collected on the next day). **Sputum collection** should be done outside in an open well-ventilated space
- Whereas in EPTB, the specimens vary depending on the site involved such as pleural fluid, CSF, urine, etc.

Microscopy

Acid-fast staining is the microscopic method performed for the detection of *M. tuberculosis*.
- **Digestion and decontamination:** The sputum specimens are prior subjected to digestion (to liquefy the thick pus) and decontamination by treatment with sodium hydroxide (Petroff's method) or N-acetyl L-cysteine (NALC)
- **Thickness of the smear** prepared can be assessed by placing the smear on printed matter. The print should be just readable through the smear
- **Methods:** The various acid-fast staining methods available are:
  - *Ziehl-Neelsen (ZN) staining* (hot method) using 25% sulfuric acid as the decolorizer—*M. tuberculosis* appears as long slender, beaded, red colored acid-fast bacilli **(Fig 27.1A)**. At least 100 oil immersion fields should be examined for 10–15 minutes before giving a negative report. Details of ZN staining procedure is given in **Chapter 3.2**
  - *Kinyoun's cold acid-fast staining*—It differs from ZN stain in that—(i) heating is not required, (ii) phenol concentration in carbol fuchsin is increased, and (iii) duration of carbol fuchsin staining is more
  - *Fluorescent staining*—It uses auraminephenol solution (for 7–10 min) as primary stain, 0.5% acid alcohol (for 2 min, twice) as decolorizer and 0.1% potassium permanganate (for 30 sec) as counter stain. Then the slide is examined under fluorescent

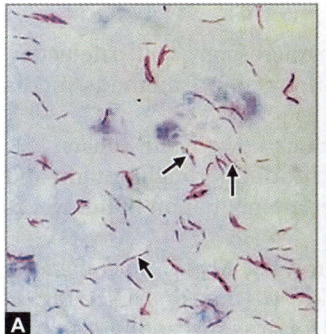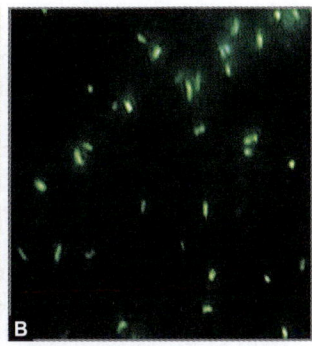

Figs. 27.1A and B: A. ZN staining of sputum smear showing long, slender and beaded red colored acid–fast bacilli; **B.** Auramine phenol staining of sputum smear—tubercle bacilli appear bright brilliant green against the dark background.

Source: Department of Microbiology, JIPMER, Puducherry (*with permission*).

LED (light-emitting diode) microscope. It is more sensitive and smears can be screened more rapidly than ZN staining. Tubercle bacilli appear bright brilliant green against the dark background **(Fig. 27.1B)**.
- **Grading** of the sputum smear is done (0 to 3+) which helps to determine the severity of disease, and infectiousness and also to monitor the response to treatment
- **Detection limit:** At least 10^4 bacilli/mL in sputum is required for the bacilli to be detected in acid-fast stained smear.

NTEP Guidelines for Grading of Sputum Smear

National Tuberculosis Elimination Programme (NTEP) of India has given guidelines for grading of **ZN stained sputum smears (Table 27.1)**. Grading of the sputum smear depends upon the quality of sputum collected. *NTEP grading is useful for:*
- Monitoring the treatment response: The grading falls following successful treatment and clinical recovery. However, the grade remains constant among the treatment defaulters or drug resistant cases
- Assessing the severity of disease: Higher is the grade, more severe is the disease.

Table 27.1: NTEP guidelines for grading of ZN stained sputum smears.

No. of AFB seen	OIF to be screened	Grading	Result
No AFB in 100 OIF	100	0	Negative
1–9/100 OIF	100	Scanty*	Positive
10–99/100 OIF	100	1+	Positive
1–10/OIF	50	2+	Positive
>10/OIF	20	3+	Positive

(AFB, acid-fast bacilli; OIF, oil immersion fields; ZN, Ziehl-Neelsen)
*Record the actual no. of bacilli seen in 100 fields, e.g. "Scanty 8".

Culture

Culture is more sensitive than microscopy, with a detection limit of 10-100 bacilli/mL. Various culture methods/media available are:

- **Conventional media** such as Lowenstein-Jensen (LJ) medium: *M. tuberculosis* produces rough, tough, and buff-colored colonies after an incubation of 6-8 weeks (Fig. 27.2A)
- **Automated culture systems,** e.g. MGIT (Mycobacteria growth indicator tube): Takes less time than LJ culture (3 weeks). It can also be used for drug susceptibility testing (Fig. 27.2B)
- **Identification** of *M. tuberculosis* in culture is made by:
  - Automated identification—by MALDI-TOF
  - Antigen detection by ICT—detecting MPT 64 antigen.

Molecular Methods

As culture is time-consuming, and microcopy is less sensitive, the diagnosis of TB greatly relies on molecular methods. Various molecular methods available are:

- **Cartridge-based nucleic acid amplification test (CBNAAT):** It is an automated real-time PCR system that has completely revolutionized the diagnosis of TB. Example includes—**GeneXpert**.
  - *Uses:* It serves two purposes—(i) detection of *M. tuberculosis* complex in the specimen, and (ii) detection of rifampicin resistance
  - *Advantages:* It is rapid, takes <2h of time, and is highly sensitive (detection limit 131 bacilli/mL of the specimen).
- **Chip-based NAAT: Truenat** is a chip-based real-time PCR system, developed in India, that works in a similar principle as GeneXpert
- **Line probe assay (LPA):** It involves probe-based detection of amplified DNA in the specimen
  - *Uses:* (i) Identification of MTB complex, (ii) detection of resistance to first-line and second-line antitubercular drugs
  - *Disadvantages:* It takes 2–3 days. It is less sensitive, and can be performed only on smear-positive specimens.

Drug Susceptibility Test (DST)

Universal-DST refers to performing DST for all TB patients—first performing CBNAAT to determine rifampicin susceptibility; followed by line probe assay (LPA) or MGIT to detect susceptibility to other antitubercular drugs.

Diagnosis of Latent Tuberculosis Infection (LTBI)

Latent tuberculosis infection (LTBI) is diagnosed by demonstration of delayed or type IV hypersensitivity reaction against the tubercle bacilli antigens.

- **Three methods** are available: (1) tuberculin skin test (or Monteux test), (2) IFN-γ release assay, and (3) Cy-TB test.
- **A positive test** indicates prior exposure to *M. tuberculosis*, but cannot differentiate between past exposure and active infection. However, in infants, it can suggest an active infection.

> **TREATMENT** — Tuberculosis
>
> Treatment of tuberculosis involves a multidrug regimen of first-line agents, given for a longer duration (6 months) and under the direct supervision:
> - Intensive phase (2 months) with four drugs (HRZE): Isoniazid, rifampicin, pyrazinamide, and ethambutol
> - Continuation phase (4 months) with three drugs (HRE): Isoniazid, rifampicin, and ethambutol
> - FDC: All drugs must be given in fixed-dose combination (FDC) tablets as per body weight
> - Daily-oral regimen: The FDC tablets should be taken orally, once a day.

Drug Resistance

Failure to adhere to the multidrug regimen is a common practice in patients, which often leads to the emergence of drug resistance in *M. tuberculosis*. The common pattern of drug resistance are:

- **MDR-TB:** Defined as resistance to both isoniazid and rifampicin with or without resistance to other first-line drugs

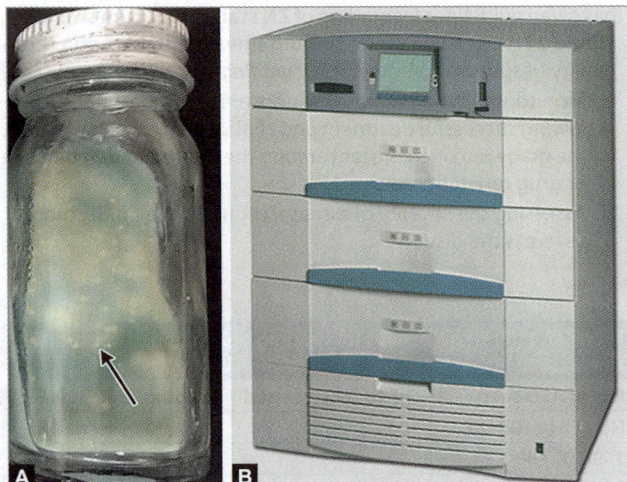

Figs. 27.2: Culture media/culture systems for *M. tuberculosis*: **A.** Lowenstein-Jensen medium (arrow showing rough, tough and buff-colored colonies); **B.** BACTEC MGIT.
Source: Department of Microbiology, JIPMER, Puducherry (*with permission*).

CHAPTER 27 ◆ Mycobacteria

❖ **XDR-TB:** Defined as MDR-TB plus resistance to second-line agents such as at least one injectable aminoglycoside and one fluoroquinolone.

National TB Elimination Programme

The National Tuberculosis Elimination Programme (NTEP) is the national program implemented in India for the control of tuberculosis. It was earlier called as Revised National Tuberculosis Control Programme (RNTCP).

Nikshay: It is a web portal for surveillance of TB, where all health care facilities need to notify all new TB cases through this web.

Infection Control Measures

Airborne precautions (e.g. negative pressure isolation room, N95 respirator, etc.) must be followed **(Chapter 15)**.

Vaccine

Bacillus Calmette-Guérin (BCG) is a live attenuated vaccine for tuberculosis.
❖ **Strain:** In India, WHO recommended Danish 1331 strain of BCG is used. It is prepared in Central BCG laboratory, Guindy, Chennai
❖ **Indication:** It is given to newborn, at birth
❖ **Administered** by intradermal route above the insertion of left deltoid. If properly given, a permanent tiny round scar is developed in 6–12 weeks of time
❖ **Protection:** BCG has a variable efficacy of 0–80% and only up to 15–20 years. However, it surely gives protection against the development of complications such as tuberculous meningitis and disseminated tuberculosis
❖ **Contraindications to BCG include:**
  ▪ HIV-positive child
  ▪ Child born to AFB positive mother
  ▪ Child with low immunity
  ▪ Pregnancy.

■ MYCOBACTERIUM LEPRAE

Mycobacterium leprae (Hansen's bacillus) causes leprosy; characterized by anesthetic skin lesions, bony deformities, and disfigurement.
❖ Due to fear, ignorance, superstitious beliefs, and characteristic disfigurement produced in the patients, leprosy remained as a social stigma over many years and patients have been socially outcasted
❖ However today, with early diagnosis and effective treatment, patients can lead a productive life in the community and the deformities can largely be prevented.

Clinical Manifestations

Based on the number of skin lesions, presence of nerve involvement and identification of bacilli in the slit-skin smear, leprosy can be classified into two categories. This classification is used by the National Leprosy Eradication Programme (NLEP), for the treatment of leprosy patients (described later).
❖ **Paucibacillary (PB) leprosy:** A case of leprosy which fulfills all the criteria—(i) 1 to 5 skin lesions, (ii) no nerve or one nerve involvement, and (iii) slit-skin smear negative for lepra bacilli at all sites
❖ **Multibacillary (MB) leprosy:** A case of leprosy that fulfills any one of the criteria—(i) >5 skin lesions or (ii) more than one nerve involvement or (iii) slit-skin smear-positive for lepra bacilli.

Leprosy is a bipolar disease. Depending upon the host cell-mediated immune response (CMI), the patient can develop various clinical forms ranging from lepromatous, borderline, or tuberculoid forms
❖ There are various **classification schemes** described in the literature such as Ridley-Jopling, Madrid, and Indian classification
❖ The **differences** between lepromatous leprosy (LL) and tuberculoid leprosy (TT) are depicted in **Table 27.2**.

Epidemiology

Unlike its superstitious beliefs, leprosy is not a highly communicable disease. Intimate and prolonged contact is

Table 27.2: Differences between lepromatous leprosy (LL) and tuberculoid leprosy (TT).

Characters	Lepromatous leprosy	Tuberculoid leprosy
Bacillary load	Multibacillary	Paucibacillary
Skin lesions	• Many, symmetrical • Margin is irregular	• One or few, asymmetrical • Margin is sharp
Nerve lesion	Appear late	• Early anesthetic skin lesion • Enlarged thickened nerves
CMI	Low	Normal
Lepromin test	Negative	Positive
Humoral immunity	Exaggerated	Normal
Macrophages	Foamy type (lipid laden)	Epithelioid type
Langhans giant cells	Not seen	Found

(CMI, cell-mediated immunity)

necessary for transmission. Only about 5% of spouses living with leprosy patients develop the disease.
- ❖ **Transmission:** *M. leprae* is transmitted mainly through:
  - Nasal droplet inhalation (common mode)
  - Contact transmission (skin).
- ❖ **Leprosy elimination:** As per WHO, leprosy is said to be eliminated if the caseload is <1 case per 10,000 population. Many countries have achieved this target including India
- ❖ **The situation in World**: Once leprosy was worldwide in distribution, but now, it is almost exclusively confined to the developing nations of Asia, and Africa
- ❖ **The situation in India**: Although India has achieved leprosy elimination in 2005, cases still occur in various pockets of India such as Bihar, Chhattisgarh, etc. India still accounts for the highest-burden of leprosy in the world.

Laboratory Diagnosis

Smear Microscopy

Smear microscopy is done to demonstrate the acid-fast bacilli in the lesions.
- ❖ **Specimens:** Total six samples are collected; four from skin (forehead, cheek, chin and buttock), one from ear lobe and nasal mucosa by nasal blow/scraping.
  - **Slit skin smear** is the technique followed to collect the skin and ear lobe specimens. The **edge of the lesion** is the preferred site. Using scalpel blade tissue pulp is obtained from below the epidermis and smeared on a slide.
  - **Nasal specimens** obtained by nasal blow or by nasal scraping
  - **Biopsy** from the thickened nerves and nodular lesions
- ❖ **Acid-fast stain** using 5% sulfuric acid: *M. leprae* appears red acid-fast bacilli arranged in cigar-like bundles to form globi, found inside the foamy macrophages **(Fig. 27.3)**.
  - **Live bacilli** will be uniformly stained with parallel sides and round ends and length is five times the width
  - **Dead bacilli** are less uniformly stained and have fragmented and granular appearance.

Other Methods

The other methods for diagnosis of leprosy include:
- ❖ **Mouse footpad cultivation:** *M. leprae* is not cultivable in culture media or in tissue culture, but can grow in mouse foot pads
- ❖ **Antibody detection** by FLA-ABS (fluorescent leprosy antibody absorption test)
- ❖ **Lepromin test:** It is a skin test similar to tuberculin test. Positive test indicates that the patient's CMI is intact and

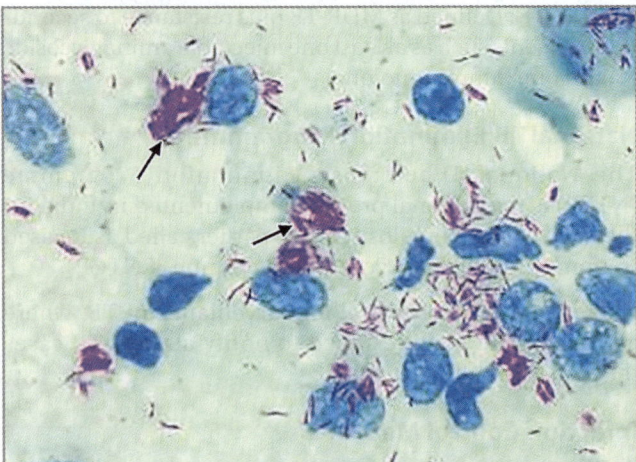

Fig. 27.3: Acid-fast stained slit skin smear showing numerous *Mycobacterium leprae* singly or in globi (arrows).
Source: Dr Isabella Princess, Apollo Hospital, Chennai (*with permission*).

good prognosis, while negative test indicates absence of CMI and poor prognosis.
- **Procedure:** Lepromin antigen is injected intradermally to forearm and reading is taken at two occasions
- **At 48hr (early or Fernandez reaction):** Induration (>10 mm) is produced at the site of inoculation which corresponds to DTH reaction to lepra antigen and indicates past exposure to lepra bacilli
- **At 21 days (late or Mitsuda reaction):** A nodule of >5 mm size is formed at the site of inoculation which subsequently ulcerates.

TREATMENT — Leprosy

Multidrug therapy (MDT) is recommended for the treatment of leprosy, because of the risk of development of drug resistance to a single drug.
- ❑ **3-drug regimen:** WHO recommends a 3-drug regimen of rifampicin, dapsone and clofazimine for all leprosy patients
- ❑ **Duration of treatment**—6 months for paucibacillary leprosy and 12 months for multibacillary leprosy
- ❑ **Follow**-up is conducted annually for 2 years for paucibacillary leprosy and 5 years for multibacillary leprosy cases.

■ NONTUBERCULOUS MYCOBACTERIA (NTM)

They are a diverse group of mycobacteria, exist either as saprophytes or commensals, but can occasionally cause opportunistic infection in man.

Classification of NTM

NTM have been classified into four groups by Runyon, based on pigment production and rate of growth.

- ❖ **Photochromogens:** Produce pigments only in light, e.g.
  - ■ *M. marinum:* It causes skin ulcers known as **swimming pool granuloma** or fish tank granuloma
  - ■ *M. kansasii:* It causes chronic pulmonary disease resembling tuberculosis.
- ❖ **Scotochromogens:** Produce pigments both in light and dark, e.g.
  - ■ *M. scrofulaceum:* It causes scrofula (cervical lymphadenitis) in children
  - ■ *M. gordonae:* It is often found as commensal in tap water.
- ❖ **Non-chromogens:** Do not produce pigments, e.g. *M. avium-intracellulare* complex (MAC). It causes opportunistic infections (especially in HIV-infected people) such as lymphadenitis, respiratory infection, and disseminated disease
- ❖ **Rapid growers:** Grow within one week, e.g. *M. chelonae, M. fortuitum,* they cause post-trauma injection abscess and catheter-related infections.

The clinical manifestations of NTM are tabulated in **Table 27.3**.

Laboratory Diagnosis

- ❖ **Specimens:** Sputum, lymph node aspirate, pus or exudate, biopsy from skin lesions are the usual specimens
- ❖ **Microscopy by ZN staining:** Shows red acid-fast bacilli which needs to be differentiated from *M. tuberculosis*
- ❖ **Culture on LJ media:** Several species of NTM grow well on LJ medium, however a few grow sparsely
- ❖ **Pigment production:** LJ media are incubated in dark and light separately for distinguishing between photochromogens and scotochromogens

Table 27.3: Clinical manifestations of nontuberculous mycobacteria (NTM).

Disease	Organisms
Pulmonary infection	*M. avium-intracellulare* (MAC) *M. kansasii, M. xenopi, M. malmoense, M. szulgai, M. abscessus*
Lymph node infection	*M. avium-intracellulare* (MAC) *M. scrofulaceum*—causes scrofula *M. malmoense*
Cutaneous infection	*M. marinum*—causes swimming pool or fish tank granuloma *M. ulcerans*—causes Buruli ulcer *M. abscessus* *M. fortuitum* and *M. chelonae*—cause injection abscess *M. avium-intracellulare* (MAC)
Disseminated infection	*M. avium-intracellulare* (MAC) *M. kansasii*

- ❖ **Identification:** Species of NTM can be differentiated from *M. tuberculosis* complex by:
  - ■ Negative for MPT64 antigen by ICT
  - ■ Biochemical tests; which are less commonly used now
  - ■ Newer methods such as MALDI-TOF and PCR assays are useful.

Treatment

NTM infections are treated with multidrug therapy. *M. avium-intracellulare* complex (MAC), *M. kansasii* and *M. marinum* infections often require multidrug therapy with clarithromycin or azithromycin, ethambutol, and a rifamycin.

EXPECTED QUESTIONS

I. **Write an essay on:**
  1. Discuss the pathogenesis, clinical manifestations and laboratory diagnosis of pulmonary tuberculosis.

II. **Write short notes on:**
  1. Clinical manifestations of leprosy.
  2. Nontuberculous mycobacteria (NTM) infections.

III. **Multiple Choice Questions (MCQs):**
  1. How much bacillary load in sputum is required for effective transmission of *M. tuberculosis*?
     a. 10 bacilli/mL
     b. 100 bacilli/mL
     c. 1,000 bacilli/mL
     d. 10,000 bacilli/mL
  2. Survival of *M. tuberculosis* inside the macrophages is due to:
     a. Inhibition of entry into the host cell
     b. Inhibition of entry into the phagosome
     c. Inhibition of phagosome-lysosome fusion
     d. Inhibits degradation by lysosomal enzymes
  3. GeneXpert can detect resistance to:
     a. Isoniazid   b. Rifampicin
     c. Pyrazinamide   d. Ethambutol
  4. Which of the following is a rapid grower mycobacteria?
     a. *M. marinum*
     b. *M. kansasii*
     c. *M. scrofulaceum*
     d. *M. chelonae*

Answers
1. d   2. c   3. b   4. d

Miscellaneous Gram-positive Bacilli

CHAPTER 28

CHAPTER PREVIEW
- Actinomycetes
- *Listeria monocytogenes*

This chapter covers gram-positive bacilli such as *Actinomycetes* and *Listeria*.

ACTINOMYCETES

Actinomycetes are gram-positive, non-motile, non-sporing, non-capsulated bacilli arranged in chains or branching filaments. Most of them are soil saprophytes or normal human commensals. Important genera include- *Actinomyces, Nocardia, Actinomadura,* and *Streptomyces*.

Actinomyces

Actinomyces are anaerobic, gram-positive branching filamentous bacilli, soil saprophytes, and commensals of the oral cavity. In humans, they cause actinomycosis. *A. israelii* is the most common species infecting man.

Clinical Manifestations (Actinomycosis)

- **Oral-cervicofacial actinomycosis:** This is the most common form, and usually presents as a painless, slow-growing, hard mass with cutaneous fistulas, a condition commonly known as **lumpy jaw (Fig. 28.1A)**.
- **Other forms:** Thoracic actinomycosis, abdominal and pelvic forms, brain abscesses, bone destruction and soft tissue infections, dental caries, and periodontal diseases (caused by *A. naeslundii* and *A. odontolyticus*).

Laboratory Diagnosis

Specimen
Specimens collected include discharge from the sinuses or fistula, rarely sputum, bronchial washings, and cervicovaginal secretions.

Direct Microscopy
Pus discharge is thoroughly washed in saline in a test tube and the sediment is collected that contains gritty, white or yellowish **sulfur granules**, of <5 mm in size. Granules are crushed between two slides and smears are made.

- **Gram-staining (Brown–Brenn modification):** It shows a central mass of gram-positive branching, filamentous

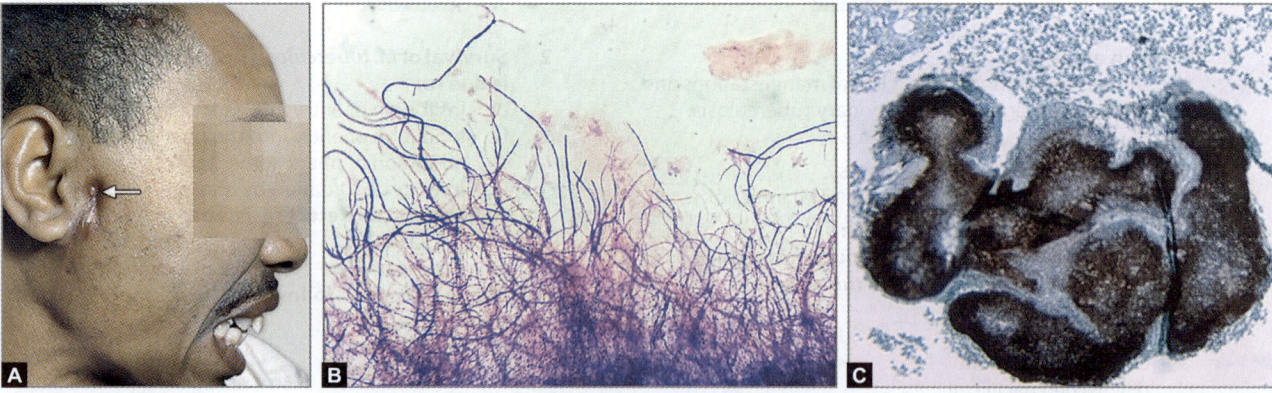

Figs. 28.1A to C: A. Actinomycosis (painless, slow-growing, hard mass with cutaneous fistula) (arrow showing); **B.** Gram-positive filamentous bacilli; **C.** Gomori's stained smear showing sun-ray appearance.
Source: A. Public Health Image Library, ID# 2856, CDC, Atlanta; B. Dr Isabella Princess, Apollo Hospitals, Chennai; C. ID# 10601/Centers for Disease Control and Prevention (CDC), Atlanta (with permission).

bacilli, radiating peripherally with hyaline, club-shaped ends **(Fig. 28.1B)**
- Histopathological staining such as hematoxylin-eosin (H and E) or Gomori's stained tissue sections reveal granules composed of eosinophilic clubs surrounding basophilic filaments and inflammatory cells (sun-rays appearance) **(Fig. 28.1C)**.

Culture
Pus containing sulfur granules are washed and cultured anaerobically at 37°C on media such as thioglycollate broth and brain heart infusion (BHI) agar. Species identification is done by:
- Biochemical reactions or automated methods
- Molecular methods, such as PCR.

Treatment
- IV penicillin G or IV ampicillin
- Surgical removal of the affected tissues may be required for extensive lesions.

Nocardiosis

Nocardia species are gram-positive branching filamentous bacilli similar to *Actinomyces*; however, they differ from the latter by being aerobic and acid-fast. *N. asteroides* and *N. brasiliensis* are the most common human pathogens.

Clinical Manifestations
Clinical manifestations of nocardiosis include–
- Pulmonary nocardiosis (lobar pneumonia)
- Extrapulmonary nocardiosis (brain abscess, abscesses of skin, kidneys, bone and muscle).
- **Actionomycetoma:** It is a chronic granulomatous condition of bacterial etiology, characterized by subcutaneous nodular swelling, multiple sinuses and discharge containing granules (described in **Chapter 58**).

Laboratory Diagnosis
Specimen
Depending on the site affected, various specimens collected such as sputum, pus from abscesses, and granules. Granules present in discharge are collected in sterile gauze or loop by pressing the sinuses from the periphery to express them out (as in the case of actinomycetoma).

Direct Microscopy
- **Gram staining:** Reveals gram-positive branching and filamentous bacilli of width 0.5–1 μm
- **Modified acid-fast staining** using 1% sulfuric acid as decolorizer (Kinyoun method): They are partially

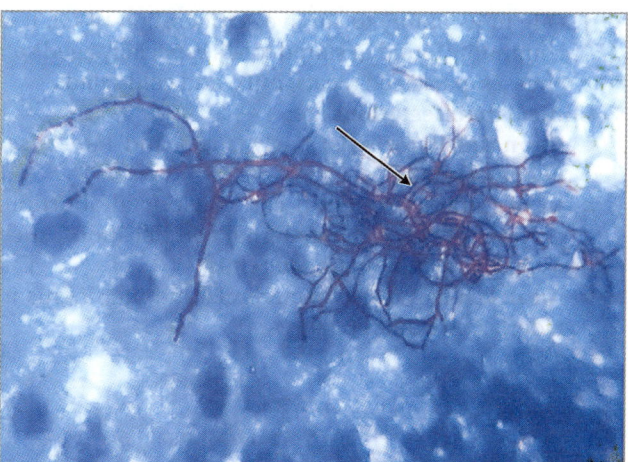

Fig. 28.2: Acid-fast filamentous branching bacilli of *Nocardia* (modified acid-fast stain).
Source: Dr Suchitra Mishra, Department of Microbiology, HiTech Medical College, Rourkela, Odisha (*with permission*).

acid-fast and appear as branching and filamentous red-colored acid-fast bacilli **(Fig. 28.2)**
- **Histopathology (H and E stain) of the granules:** Shows multilobulated with sun-ray appearance.

Culture
- Nocardiae are obligate aerobes that grow on brain heart infusion agar and Sabouraud dextrose agar (SDA). Colonies are creamy, wrinkled, pigmented (orange or pink colored), and adhere firmly to the medium.
- Lowenstein–Jensen medium: Produces moist glabrous colonies
- Species identification is made by appropriate biochemical tests or automated methods.

Treatment
- Cotrimoxazole is the drug of choice
- Aspiration or drainage of the abscesses should be carried out to limit the spread of infection.

Listeria monocytogenes

Listeria monocytogenes is a food-borne pathogen that can cause serious infections, particularly in neonates, pregnant women, and elderly people.
- **Human infection** (listeriosis): It is transmitted most commonly through contaminated food followed by vertical transmission (mother to fetus, during birth)
    - **Common food sources** include contaminated milk, soft cheeses, and several types of "ready-to-eat" foods
    - **Age:** Listeriosis is common among neonates and old aged people

- Due to its ability to survive refrigeration (4°C), it is commonly found in stored foods especially aged soft cheeses, packaged meats, milk, and cold salads.

❖ **Clinical manifestations** are:
  - **Neonatal listeriosis:** Early onset and late-onset neonatal sepsis
  - **In pregnant women:** It can cause fetal abortion, preterm delivery and maternal complications, such as flu-like symptoms, bacteremia
  - **Adults:** It can cause bacteremia and meningitis in elderly individuals (>60 years).

❖ **Laboratory diagnosis:** It includes CSF, blood and amniotic fluid culture.
  - **Gram stain** shows gram-positive short coccobacilli
  - **Differential motility:** It shows a tumbling type of motility at 25°C but non-motile at 37°C
  - **Culture:** It grows on blood agar (β-hemolytic colonies), chocolate agar and selective media, such as **PALCAM agar** (polymyxin, acriflavine, lithium chloride, ceftazidime, aesculin and mannitol).

❖ **Treatment:** Ampicillin is the drug of choice, given for 2–3 weeks in combination with gentamicin.

EXPECTED QUESTIONS

I. **Write short notes on:**
   1. Nocardiosis.
   2. Listeriosis.

II. **Multiple Choice Questions (MCQs):**
   1. Which of the following actinomycete is acid-fast?
      a. *Streptomyces*
      b. *Actinomadura*
      c. *Nocardia*
      d. *Actinomyces*

2. Drug of choice to treat nocardiosis is:
   a. Penicillin
   b. Cotrimoxazole
   c. Metronidazole
   d. Voriconazole

3. Selective culture media for *Listeria monocytogenes* is:
   a. Potassium tellurite agar
   b. TCBS agar
   c. Lowenstein–Jensen medium
   d. PALCAM agar

Answers
1. c   2. b   3. d

Enterobacterales

CHAPTER 29

CHAPTER PREVIEW
- *Escherichia coli*
- *Klebsiella*
- *Shigella*
- *Salmonella*
- Other Enterobacterales

ENTEROBACTERALES

Enterobacterales include the commensal bacteria in the human intestine called coliform bacilli. They have the following general properties:
- They are gram-negative bacilli
- Aerobes and facultative anaerobes
- Nonfastidious, can grow in basal media like nutrient agar
- Ferment glucose to produce acid with or without gas
- Reduce nitrate to nitrite
- All are catalase-positive, but oxidase test negative.

Based on the fermentation of lactose, Enterobacterales can be classified into:
- **Lactose fermenters (LF)**: Ferment lactose and produce pink colored colonies on MacConkey agar; e.g. *Escherichia, Klebsiella, Enterobacter,* and *Citrobacter*
- **Non-lactose fermenters (NLF)**: Do not ferment lactose, produce pale colonies on MacConkey agar; e.g. *Salmonella, Shigella,* Proteeae (*Proteus, Morganella, Providencia*), and *Yersinia*.

Escherichia coli

Escherichia coli is the most common pathogen encountered clinically. It is also the most common aerobe to be harbored in the gut of humans.

Virulence Factors

Virulence factors of *E. coli* may be grouped into surface antigen and toxins.
- **Surface antigens**: *E. coli* possesses four surface antigens—(1) somatic (O), (2) flagellar (H), (3) capsular antigens (K), and (4) fimbrial antigen.
  - **Somatic or O antigen**: It is a side chain present on lipopolysaccharide (LPS) antigen
  - **Flagellar or H antigen**: It is responsible for bacterial motility
  - **Capsular or K antigen**: It is the polysaccharide capsular antigen
  - **Fimbrial antigen** (pilus) is the organ of adhesion, helps in attachment and colonization.
- **Toxins**: The exotoxins secreted by *E. coli* are of several types:
  - **Enterotoxins**: They are produced by diarrheagenic strains of *E. coli*.
  - **Cytotoxic necrotizing factor 1 (CNF1)**: They are cytotoxic to bladder and kidney cells; act as virulence factor for pathogenesis of UTI.

Clinical Manifestations

Various strains of *E. coli* have been associated with various manifestations.

UTI by UPEC

Urinary tract infection (UTI) is caused by a strain of *E. coli* known as uropathogenic *E. coli* (UPEC), which is the most common cause (70–75%) of UTI. Infection to the bladder is usually spread by ascending route through the urethra, from the perineal flora.

Diarrhea (Diarrheagenic *E. coli*)

Diarrhea is caused by a strain of *E. coli* known as diarrheagenic *E. coli,* which further comprises six pathotypes.
1. **Enteropathogenic *E. coli* (EPEC)**: It causes infantile diarrhea. It is nontoxigenic and noninvasive
2. **Enterotoxigenic *E. coli* (ETEC)**: It causes traveler's diarrhea. Pathogenesis is mediated by producing toxins such as:
   - Heat labile toxin (LT): Acts by increasing cyclic AMP (similar to cholera toxin)
   - Heat stable toxin (ST): Acts by increasing cyclic GMP.
3. **Enteroinvasive *E. coli* (EIEC)**: It is not toxigenic, but invasive and causes bloody diarrhea (i.e. dysentery)

4. **Enterohemorrhagic *E. coli* (EHEC):** The most common serotype associated with EHEC is O157:H7
   - Its pathogenesis is mediated by a toxin called verocytotoxin (or Shiga-like toxin)
   - It also causes dysentery, similar to EIEC
   - Verocytotoxin damages the endothelial cells causing capillary microangiopathy which may lead to complications such as hemolytic uremic syndrome (HUS) and hemorrhagic colitis.
5. **Enteroaggregative *E. coli* (EAEC):** It causes persistent and acute diarrhea
6. **Diffusely adherent *E. coli* (DAEC):** It causes diarrhea in children aged 2–6 years.

Other Infections

Apart from UTI and diarrhea, *E. coli* can cause several pyogenic infections such as:
- **Abdominal infections:** Bacterial peritonitis (primary or secondary), visceral abscesses, such as hepatic abscess
- Pneumonia (especially in hospitalized patients—ventilator-associated pneumonia)
- Bloodstream infection (especially in hospitalized patients)
- Meningitis (especially neonatal meningitis)
- Wound and soft tissue infections such as cellulitis, infection of ulcers and wounds, especially in patient with diabetic foot.

Laboratory Diagnosis

Sample collection depends on the site of infection—urine, stool, pus, wound swab, blood, CSF, etc.
- **Direct smear microscopy:** Shows gram-negative bacilli, and pus cells
- **Culture:** Incubation at 37°C for 24h reveals the following growth:
  - Blood agar: Gray, moist colonies
  - MacConkey agar: Flat, pink LF colonies **(Fig. 29.1A)**
  - **Culture smear and motility:** Motile gram-negative bacilli **(Fig. 29.1B)**.
- **Biochemical identification:** Various biochemical tests which help in the identification of *E. coli* are:
  - Catalase positive and oxidase negative
  - ICUT tests: Indole test (positive), citrate test (negative), urease test (negative) and TSI (triple sugar iron agar) test shows acid/acid, gas present, H_2S absent **(Fig. 29.2)**.
- **Automated ID systems** such as VITEK and MALDI-TOF can be performed for rapid and accurate identification of *E. coli*
- **Antimicrobial susceptibility testing** can be performed by disk diffusion method (on Mueller-Hinton agar) or MIC-based method (VITEK). *E. coli* can rapidly develop resistance to multiple drugs. Many strains of *E. coli* are producers of β-lactamases such as ESBL (extended spectrum β-lactamases).

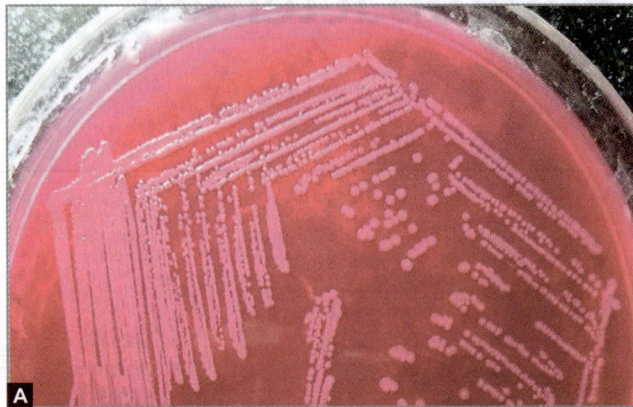
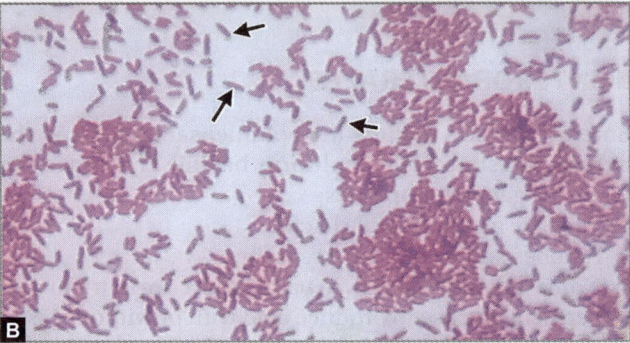

Figs. 29.1A and B: A. Flat pink lactose fermenting colonies of *E. coli* on MacConkey agar; **B.** Slender gram-negative bacilli (arrows showing).
Source: Department of Microbiology, Pondicherry Institute of Medical Sciences, Puducherry (*with permission*).

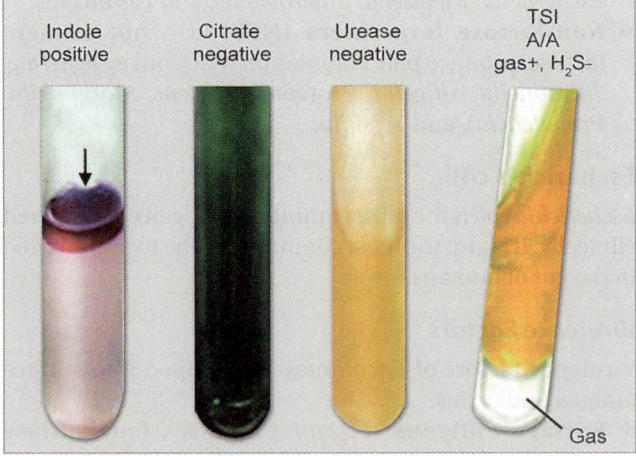

Fig. 29.2: Biochemical reactions of *Escherichia coli*.
Source: Department of Microbiology, JIPMER, Puducherry (*with permission*).

TREATMENT

E. coli and Klebsiella

Treatment is essentially based upon an antimicrobial susceptibility test report. The majority of isolates in hospitals are multi-drug resistant (MDR) and require treatment with any of the following higher antimicrobials if found susceptible:
- Carbapenems such as meropenem
- β-lactam/β-lactamase inhibitor combinations (BL/BLIs) such as piperacillin-tazobactam or cefoperazone-sulbactam
- Aminoglycosides such as amikacin
- Polymyxins such as colistin
- Others: Fosfomycin or tigecycline, etc.

Preventive Measures

Infection control measures (contact precaution) such as hand hygiene are crucial to limit the spread of infection by multi-drug resistant Enterobacterales (*refer* **Chapter 15**).

Klebsiella pneumoniae

Similar to *E. coli*, *Klebsiella pneumoniae* can cause UTI, lobar pneumonia, meningitis (in neonates), septicemia, pyogenic infections such as abscesses, and wound infections.

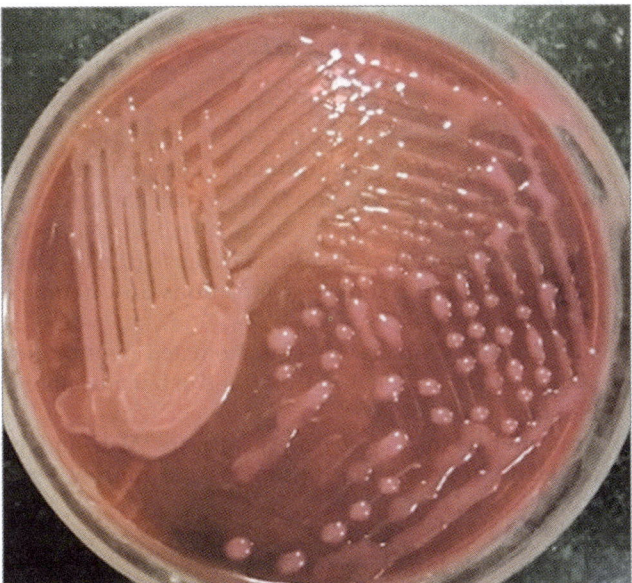

Fig. 29.3: *Klebsiella pneumoniae*; on MacConkey agar showing mucoid pink-colored lactose-fermenting colonies.
Source: Department of Microbiology, Pondicherry Institute of Medical Sciences, Puducherry (with permission).

Laboratory Diagnosis

- **Sample collection:** It depends on the site of infection—urine, pus, wound swab, blood, CSF, etc.
- **Gram staining:** It is short, plump, straight capsulated gram-negative rods.
- **Culture:** On MacConkey agar, it produces large mucoid (due to capsule), pink color, lactose fermenting colonies (**Fig. 29.3**)
- **Biochemical identification** is made as described below (**Fig. 29.4**):
  - It is catalase positive and oxidase negative
  - **ICUT tests:** Indole test (negative), citrate test (positive), urease test (positive) and TSI (triple sugar iron agar) test shows acid/acid, gas present, H_2S absent
- **Automated ID systems** such as VITEK and MALDI-TOF can be performed for rapid and accurate identification of *Klebsiella pneumoniae*.

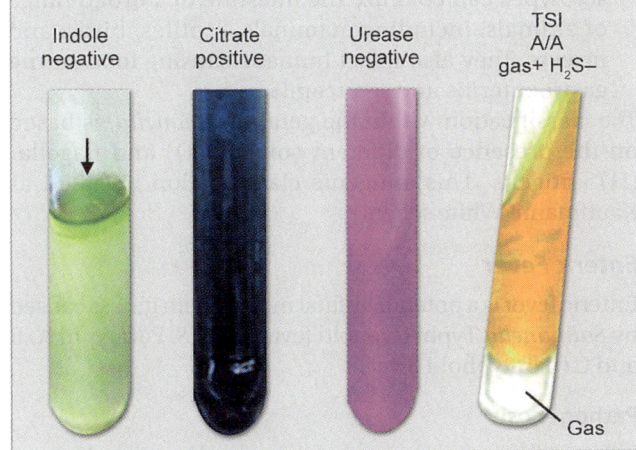

Fig. 29.4: Biochemical reactions of *Klebsiella* species.
Source: Department of Microbiology, JIPMER, Puducherry (with permission).

Treatment

Treatment is based upon an antimicrobial susceptibility test report. The majority of isolates in hospitals are multi-drug resistant (MDR). Treatment options for *K. pneumoniae* are the same as discussed for *E. coli*.

Other *Klebsiella* species include:
- ***Klebsiella granulomatis:*** It causes granuloma inguinale, a type of genitoulcerative disease
- ***K. rhinoscleromatis*** and ***K. ozaenae:*** Produce infections of the nasal cavity, called rhinoscleroma and atrophic rhinitis respectively.

Enterobacter Species

Enterobacter species are similar to *Klebsiella* in clinical manifestations and also in most of the biochemical reactions except for being motile. *E. aerogenes* and

E. cloacae are the most commonly isolated species from the clinical specimens. Treatment of *Enterobacter* infections is same as discussed for *E. coli*.

Citrobacter Species

Citrobacter species are environmental contaminants, but species such as *C. freundii* and *C. koseri* can cause human infections.
- **Manifestations:** They occasionally cause urinary tract, gallbladder and middle ear infections and neonatal meningitis
- **Identification** is made either by automated identification systems such as MALDI-TOF or VITEK or by conventional biochemical tests
- **Treatment:** Most *Citrobacter* isolates are MDR, and the guideline for treatment is the same as that used for *E. coli*.

Salmonella

Salmonellae are broadly classified into two groups, based on the clinical disease produced:
1. **Typhoidal *Salmonella*:** It includes serotypes *S*. Typhi and *S*. Paratyphi. They are restricted to human hosts, in whom they cause enteric fever.
2. **Non-typhoidal salmonellae or NTS:** The remaining serotypes can colonize the intestine of a broad range of animals, including mammals, reptiles, birds, and insects. They also infect humans causing food-borne gastroenteritis and septicemia.

The classification within the genus *Salmonella*, is based on the presence of different somatic (O) and flagellar (H) antigens. This antigenic classification is called as Kauffmann–White scheme.

Enteric Fever

Enteric fever is a potentially fatal multisystem illness caused by *Salmonella* Typhi (typhoid fever) and, *S*. Paratyphi A, B and C (paratyphoid fever).

Pathogenesis

Salmonellae are transmitted by oral route, through ingestion of contaminated food or water.
- **The infective dose of *Salmonella*** is higher than that of *Shigella*. Minimum 10^3–10^6 bacilli are needed to initiate the infection
- **Risk factors** that promote transmission include the conditions that decrease gastric acidity and intestinal integrity
- **Primary bacteremia:** The bacilli enter through a specialized epithelial cell lining the intestinal mucosa— called M cells. Following this, they are internalized by macrophages and are carried to the bloodstream
- **Spread:** Then, the bacilli disseminate throughout the body such liver, spleen, lymph nodes and bone marrow, etc. where further multiplication takes place and then seeded back into the bloodstream (**secondary bacteremia**), which leads to the onset of clinical disease.

Clinical Manifestations of Enteric Fever

The incubation period is about 10–14 days. Enteric fever is named after the mode of transmission (enteric route) of its causative agent. However, the manifestations seen are largely extraintestinal.
- **Fever (step ladder pattern of remittent fever):** Fever rises gradually to a higher level with every spike; then falls, but does not touch normal
- **Other symptoms:** Headache, chills, cough, sweating, myalgia, and arthralgia
- **Rashes (called rose spots):** Faint, salmon-colored, blanching, maculopapular rash on the trunk and chest seen in 30% of patients at the end of the first week
- **Early intestinal manifestations** such as abdominal pain, nausea, vomiting, constipation or diarrhea, and anorexia
- **Important signs** include hepatosplenomegaly, epistaxis, and relative bradycardia
- **Complications:** Gastrointestinal bleeding and intestinal perforation can occur mostly in the third and fourth weeks of illness
- **Neurologic manifestations** occur rarely which include meningitis, and neuropsychiatric symptoms such as delirium, etc.

Epidemiology

- **Host:** Humans are the only natural hosts
- **Transmission:** It is transmitted by ingestion of contaminated water and food
- **Typhi vs Paratyphi:** *S*. Typhi infection is more common than *S*. Paratyphi A (ratio is 4:1)
- **Carriage:** Untreated patients become carriers and excrete *S*. Typhi in feces or urine. Carriers are of two types:
  1. **Fecal carriers:** Typhoid bacilli multiply in the gallbladder and are excreted in the feces. Fecal carriers are more common
  2. **Urinary carriers:** Multiplication takes place in kidneys and bacilli are excreted in urine. Urinary carries are rare.

Laboratory Diagnosis

(A) Blood Culture (First week of illness)

In the first week of illness, a blood culture is recommended.
- **Conventional blood culture** is done using media such as brain heart infusion (BHI) broth (monophasic media) or BHI broth/agar (biphasic media) (*refer* **Figs. 3.2.7C and D**)

CHAPTER 29 ◆ Enterobacterales

- **Automated blood culture systems**—such as BACTEC or BacT/ALERT (*refer* **Fig. 3.2.8, Chapter 3.2**). Subcultures are made from positively flagged blood culture broth, on to blood agar and MacConkey agar.
- **Blood culture positivity** is >90% in the first week. Thereafter the positivity declines to 75% in the second week and 60% in the third week.
- **Colony appearance:**
  - **Blood agar:** Nonhemolytic moist colonies
  - **MacConkey agar:** Colonies are round, translucent, pale and non-lactose fermenting.
- If blood culture is found negative, bone marrow culture or culture from duodenal aspirate may be performed in the first week of illness.

(B) Stool/Urine Culture (in 3–4 weeks of illness)

Stool or urine culture is indicated in 3-4 weeks of illness, and also for detection of carriers:
- For **stool culture** the following media are used:
  - Enrichment broth such as Selenite F broth, tetrathionate broth, and gram-negative broth
  - Low selective medium such as MacConkey agar: Produces translucent NLF colonies **(Fig. 29.5)**
  - Highly selective media: DCA (deoxycholate citrate agar), XLD agar (xylose lysine deoxycholate), and Wilson Blair's Bismuth sulphite medium are used.
- A **urine culture** can be performed on media such as MacConkey agar.

(C) Identification

Salmonellae are motile, gram-negative bacilli.
- Identification from the colonies grown in culture is made either by automated ID system such as VITEK or by conventional biochemical tests such as—catalase, oxidase, indole, citrate, urease and TSI
- **A slide agglutination test** is performed to confirm the serotype.

(D) Widal test (Serum antibody detection)

Widal test is indicated in 2–3 weeks of illness. It is a tube agglutination test, that detects antibodies in the patient's serum against antigens of *Salmonella* Typhi and *S.* Paratyphi.
- **Antigens:** In the Widal test, four different antigens are used such as:
  - O antigen of *S.* Typhi (TO): It is cross-reactive to O antigens of *S.* Paratyphi A and B. Therefore, TO antigen can detect O antibody of *S.* Typhi, as well as *S.* Paratyphi A and B
  - H antigen of *S.* Typhi (TH)
  - H antigen of *S.* Paratyphi A (AH)
  - H antigen of *S.* Paratyphi B (BH)
- **Procedure:** Serial dilutions of patient serum are mixed with four different *Salmonella* antigens (TO, TH, AH, and BH) and the tubes are incubated in the water bath at 37°C for 24 hours
- **Result:** The result is read using a concave mirror. If corresponding antibodies are present, then an agglutination reaction will occur leading to matt formation. The absence of antibodies would lead to button formation **(Fig. 29.6)**
  - *O antibodies:* Produce granular chalky clumps when react with O Ag
  - *H antibodies:* Produce cottony woolly clumps when react with H Ag.
- **Significant titer:** H antibody titer of >1:200 is considered significant, whereas significant titer for O antibody is taken as >1:100. Low titers may be produced in cross-reacting infections and therefore should be ignored **(Fig. 29.7)**

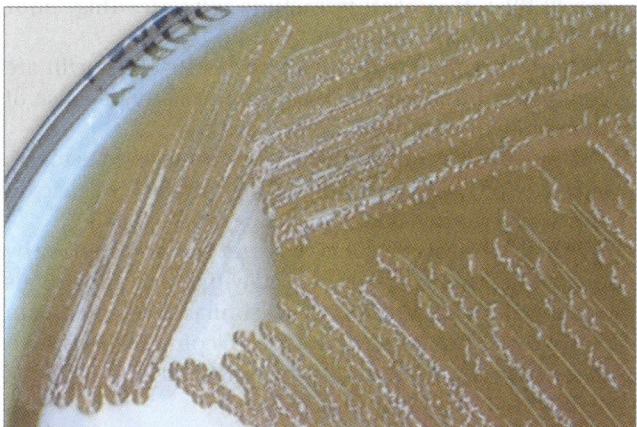

Fig. 29.5: MacConkey agar showing nonlactose fermenter colonies of *Salmonella*.
Source: Department of Microbiology, Pondicherry Institute of Medical Sciences, Puducherry (*with permission*).

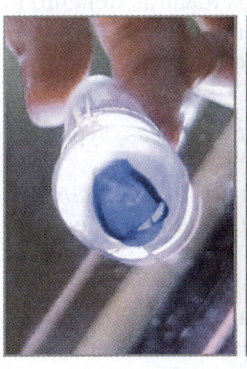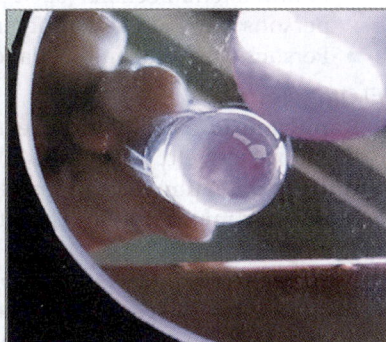

Fig. 29.6: O and H agglutination in Widal test (reading taken in a mirror).
Source: Department of Microbiology, Pondicherry Institute of Medical Sciences, Puducherry (*with permission*).

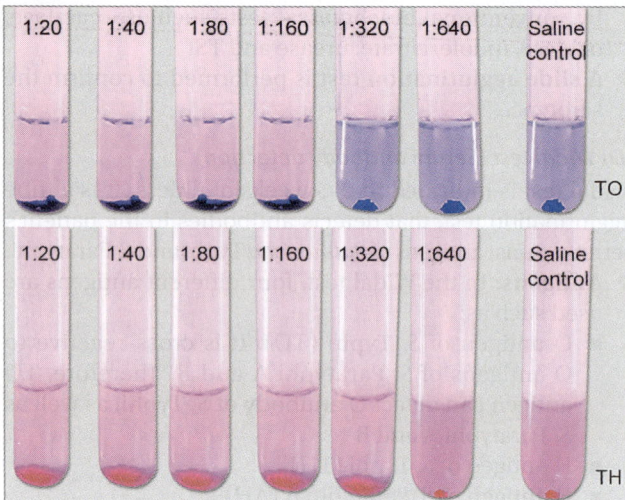

Fig. 29.7: Widal test showing titre of TO 1:160 and TH 1:320.
(TO and TH, antibody titer to *S.* Typhi O and H antigens in patient's serum)
Source: Department of Microbiology, Pondicherry Institute of Medical Sciences, Puducherry (*with permission*).

- **Interpretation:** The results are interpreted as below:
  - In *S.* Typhi infection: Antibodies to TO and TH antigens are raised
  - In *S.* Paratyphi A infection: Antibodies to TO and AH antibodies are raised
  - In *S.* Paratyphi B infection: Antibodies to TO and BH antibodies are raised.
- **False-negative:** The Widal test may produce a false-negative result in a very early stage (1st week) or due to prior antimicrobial therapy or due to prozone phenomena (antibody excess)
- **False-positive:** Widal test may produce a false-positive result in:
  - **Anamnestic response:** A transient rise of titers due to unrelated infections (such as malaria, dengue) in persons who have had prior enteric fever).
  - Persons with prior immunization (with TAB vaccine).

(E) Other Tests
- **Rapid antibody detection tests** such as Typhidot, IDLTubex test, etc.
- **Antigen detection** (in serum and urine): By ELISA
- **Molecular methods:** PCR detecting *flagellin* gene, *iro B* and *fli C* gene
- **Nonspecific findings:** For example, neutropenia
- **Antimicrobial susceptibility testing** can be performed by disk diffusion test or by MIC-based automated system (e.g. VITEK).

(F) Detection of Carriers
- **Culture:** By stool and bile culture (detects fecal carriers) and urine culture (detects urinary carriers)

- **Detection of Vi antibodies** by tube agglutination test.
- **Isolation of salmonellae from sewage:** It is carried out to trace the carriers in the communities. It can be done by sewer-swab technique and filtration method. Highly selective media, such as Wilson and Blair media are used for isolation of the bacilli.

> **TREATMENT** — Enteric fever
>
> Third-generation cephalosporins such as ceftriaxone is the drug of choice for empirical treatment.
> Alternative drugs are azithromycin, ciprofloxacin, chloramphenicol, ampicillin, and cotrimoxazole.

Vaccines for Typhoid Fever

There are two types of typhoid vaccines available currently.
1. **Vi antigen vaccine:** It is composed of purified Vi capsular polysaccharide antigen derived from *S.* Typhi strain Ty2
   - It is given as a single dose, by IM or subcutaneous route
   - The vaccine confers protection for 2 years; a booster is given every 2 years.
2. **Typhoral:** It contains live attenuated *S.* Typhi Ty21a strain
   - It is given orally as enteric-coated capsules
   - Four doses, given on alternate days
   - Revaccination is recommended every 5 years.

Shigella

Shigella is the causative agent of bacillary dysentery. It comprises four species—*S. dysenteriae, S. flexneri, S. boydii* and *S. sonnei*.
- **Transmission** of infection occurs by ingestion through contaminated fingers (most common), food, water, or rarely flies. Risk factors include overcrowding, poor hygiene, and children, etc.
- **Minimum infective dose:** As low as 10–100 bacilli are capable of initiating the disease, probably because of their ability to survive in gastric acidity
- **Pathogenesis** is due to the expression of various toxins such as—*Shigella* enterotoxin (by *S. flexneri*), Shiga toxin (by *S. dysenteriae*) and endotoxin (by all species)
- **Clinical features:** Bacillary dysentery is characterized by the passage of loose stool mixed with blood and mucus
  - Shiga toxin (*S. dysenteriae*) is similar to verocytotoxin (of EHEC) and is associated with complications such as hemolytic uremic syndrome and hemorrhagic colitis
  - Rarely, may be associated with intestinal complications such as toxic megacolon, perforations, and rectal prolapse.
- **Laboratory diagnosis:** Fresh stool is the ideal specimen. Specimens should be transported immediately.

- **Wet mount preparation** of feces shows large number of pus cells, erythrocytes and macrophages
- **Culture:** Fecal specimen is inoculated simultaneously into enrichment broth (e.g. Selenite F broth) and selective media such as DCA (deoxycholate citrate agar) or XLD (xylose lysine deoxycholate) agar
- **Culture smear and motility testing:** Gram stained smear of colonies reveals short, gram-negative bacilli and nonmotile
- **Identification** of *Shigella* from colonies is made either by automated identification systems (e.g., VITEK); or by conventional biochemical tests such as catalase positive and oxidase negative, indole test (negative), citrate test (negative), urease test (negative) and TSI (triple sugar iron agar) test shows alkaline/acid, gas absent, H_2S absent
- **Serotyping:** The species identification is done by group specific antisera and serotyping is done by using type specific antisera
- **Colicin typing** is done for *S. sonnei*.
❖ **Antimicrobial susceptibility testing** can be performed by disk diffusion test or VITEK.
❖ **Treatment** of shigellosis includes fluid replacement and antimicrobials such as ciprofloxacin or ceftriaxone.

Tribe Proteeae

Tribe Proteeae comprises three genera: *Proteus, Morganella,* and *Providencia.*
❖ Although they are saprophytes and commensals; they can also cause opportunistic infections such as urinary tract infections, wound and soft tissue infections, septicemia and nosocomial outbreaks. *Proteus* is also involved in the pathogenesis of renal stones (struvite/phosphate stones)
❖ **Laboratory diagnosis include:**
- *Proteus* produces characteristic swarming growth on blood agar **(Fig. 29.8)**
- Identification of various members are made either by automated identification systems (VITEK or MALDI-TOF); or by conventional biochemical tests such as catalase positive and oxidase negative, indole test (negative for *P. mirabilis*, positive for *P. vulgaris*), citrate test (positive), urease test (positive) and TSI (triple sugar iron agar) test shows alkaline slant/acid butt, gas present and H_2S present and phenylpyruvic acid (PPA) test (positive).
- Antimicrobial susceptibility testing can be performed by disk diffusion test or VITEK.
❖ **Treatment** is the same as discussed for *E. coli*, except that Tribe Proteeae are intrinsically resistant to certain antimicrobial agents (e.g. colistin, tigecycline, etc.) which should be avoided in the treatment

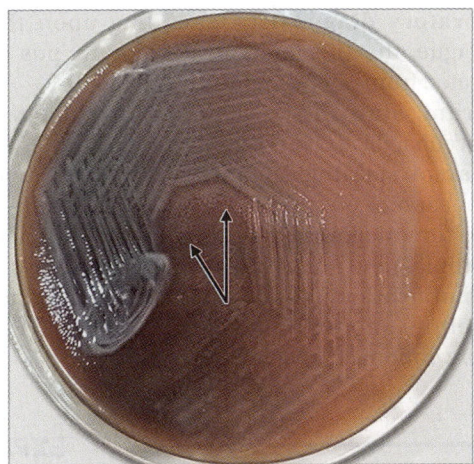

Fig. 29.8: *Proteus* on blood agar, showing swarming growth (arrows showing).
Source: Department of Microbiology, JIPMER, Puducherry (*with permission*).

❖ The somatic antigen of certain non-motile *Proteus* strains (called X strains) can be used to detect cross-reacting heterophile antibodies in sera of patients suffering from rickettsial infections (Weil-Felix reaction).

Serratia

Serratia marcescens is usually a saprophyte in the environment, and typically produces a red non-diffusible pigment called prodigiosin. However, the hospital strains of *S. marcescens* are often non-pigmented and multiple drug-resistant and are associated with various nosocomial infections.

Yersinia species

Yersinia pestis (Plague)

It is the causative agent of plague, a fulminant systemic zoonosis; transmitted from rodents by the arthropod vector, the rat flea.
❖ **Epidemiology:** Plague was one of the greatest killer known to mankind; caused several pandemics in the ancient days producing millions of deaths. In India, the Surat epidemic (in 1994) has witnessed more than 6,000 suspected plague cases with 60 deaths
❖ **Clinical forms:** Human plague occurs in three clinical forms—(1) bubonic plague (most common form, characterized by enlarged and tender regional lymph nodes), (2) pneumonic plague, and (3) septicemic plague
❖ **Agent of bioterrorism:** Because of the highly infectious nature, *Y. pestis* is currently classified as category A agent of bioterrorism.

- **Laboratory diagnosis:** Depending upon the type of plague, the specimens collected are: pus or fluid aspirated from buboes, sputum and blood
    - **Gram staining** reveals gram-negative oval coccobacilli and pus cells
    - **Wayson staining** demonstrates *bipolar* or *safety pin* appearance of the bacilli
    - **Culture media** used are: Blood agar (non-hemolytic colonies) and MacConkey agar (NLF colonies)
    - **Identification** from colonies is either by automated identification systems (e.g. MALDI-TOF) or by conventional biochemical tests.
- **Treatment:** Streptomycin or gentamicin is recommended for treatment.

Yersiniosis

Infections due to other *Yersinia* species such as *Y. enterocolitica* or *Y. pseudotuberculosis* are called yersiniosis. They are enteropathogenic and cause gastroenteritis, terminal ileitis, and mesenteric lymphadenitis.

EXPECTED QUESTIONS

I. **Write essay on:**
   1. Discuss the pathogenesis, clinical manifestations, laboratory diagnosis, and treatment of enteric fever.

II. **Write short notes on:**
   1. Diarrheagenic *E. coli*.
   2. Laboratory diagnosis of *Escherichia coli* infections.
   3. *Klebsiella pneumoniae* infections.
   4. Shigellosis.
   5. Plague.

III. **Multiple Choice Questions (MCQs):**
   1. Which of the following member of Enterobacterales is non-motile?
      a. *Salmonella*   b. *Shigella*
      c. *Serratia*   d. *E. coli*
   2. In first week of illness, enteric fever is diagnosed by:
      a. Widal test
      b. Blood culture
      c. Stool culture
      d. Urine culture
   3. Most common cause of infantile diarrhea in developing country is:
      a. EHEC   b. ETEC
      c. EPEC   d. EIEC
   4. In Widal test, large loose fluffy cotton woolly clumps, with clear supernatant fluid was noted. It indicates agglutination with:
      a. O antibodies
      b. H antibodies
      c. Vi antibodies
      d. Any of the above
   5. Plague is transmitted by:
      a. Rat flea
      b. Soft tick
      c. Hard tick
      d. Louse

Answers
1. b   2. b   3. c   4. b   5. a

Vibrio

CHAPTER 30

CHAPTER PREVIEW
- Vibrio cholerae
- Halophilic Vibrios

Vibrios are curved gram-negative bacilli that are actively motile by means of single polar flagellum. The name '*Vibrio*' is derived from its characteristic vibratory motility.

VIBRIO CHOLERAE

Vibrio cholerae is the causative agent of an acute diarrheal disease called '**cholera**' and has been responsible for seven global pandemics and several epidemics over the past two centuries. It differs from Enterobacterales being oxidase positive.

Classification of Vibrios

A unique property exhibited by all vibrios, is their growth is being stimulated in presence of salt. However, the optimum salt concentration required, varies among different vibrios. Accordingly, they are classified into:

- ❖ **Nonhalophilic vibrios:** They grow well at 1% salt concentration; not at higher salt concentrations. Example includes *V. cholerae*.
- ❖ **Halophilic vibrios:** They can tolerate and grow at higher salt concentration of up to 7–10%. Examples include *V. parahaemolyticus*, *V. alginolyticus* and *V. vulnificus*.

Gardner and Venkatraman Classification

This classification of *V. cholerae* was based on serogrouping, biotyping, serotyping and phage typing. Such typing schemes are of great epidemiological importance in tracking the outbreaks by finding out the relatedness between the isolates in different clinical specimens.

Typing

Typing of *Vibrio cholerae* can be done as follows:

- ❖ **Serogroups:** Based on the somatic O antigen, *V. cholerae* can be typed into several serogroups (>200). Out of which, serogroups O1 is the most common group to cause cholera, followed by serogroups O139
- ❖ **Biotypes:** Serogroup O1 can be typed based on biochemical reactions into two biotypes—classical and El Tor
    - Classical biotype is more virulent whereas El Tor biotype is more resistant to environmental stresses
    - Therefore classical biotype produces more severe illness, whereas El Tor biotype produces milder cases but more number of carriers.
- ❖ **Serotypes:** Serogroup O1 can be typed based on minor differences in O antigen into three serotypes—Ogawa, Inaba, Hikojima.

Epidemiology

The world has witnessed several cholera pandemics in the past; resulting in several thousands of deaths.

- ❖ **Seven pandemics** have been reported till date—first six were due to classical biotype and the seventh one was due to El Tor biotype
- ❖ **Currently**, cholera occurs as sporadic and limited outbreaks. Majority of cases are due to El Tor, but cases due to classical biotype still occur in small proportion.

Pathogenesis

Pathogenesis of *V. cholerae* is due to a potent enterotoxin, called cholera toxin and a pilus (TCP).

- ❖ **Toxin-coregulated pilus (TCP):** It helps in the adhesion of the bacilli to the intestinal epithelium
- ❖ **Cholera toxin**: It is similar to the heat-labile toxin of *E. coli*, and has two fragments A and B
    - Fragment B binds to GM1 ganglioside receptors on the intestinal epithelium
    - Fragment A is the active unit, acts by increasing cyclic AMP
    - Cyclic AMP inhibits the absorption sodium and activates the secretion chloride, which lead to the accumulation of sodium chloride and water in the intestinal lumen and finally results in watery diarrhea.

Clinical Manifestations

Cholera manifests as painless watery diarrhea, described as a **rice-water stool**.
- **Mild fluid loss** may lead to features such as weakness, postural hypotension, tachycardia, and decreased skin turgor
- **Severe dehydration** can result in renal failure and fluid loss leading to—oliguria, weak or absent pulses, sunken eyes, wrinkled ("washerwoman") skin and even coma.

Laboratory Diagnosis

Useful specimens are watery stool (for cases) or rectal swabs (for carriers).
- **Transport media:** Specimens should be sent in appropriate transport media such as VR medium (Venkatraman–Ramakrishnan), and Cary-Blair medium
- **Direct microscopy** of the stool specimen reveals:
  - Gram stain: Gram-negative rods, short curved comma-shaped (fish in stream appearance) **(Fig. 30.1)**
  - Hanging drop method: Demonstrates **darting motility**—extremely active motility with rapid changing direction.
- **Culture:** Various culture media used for *V. cholerae* are:
  - **Enrichment broth:** Alkaline peptone water, Monsur's taurocholate tellurite peptone water
  - **Selective media**: (i) Bile salt agar, (ii) Monsur's gelatin taurocholate tellurite (GTT) agar, and (iii) thiosulfate citrate bile salts sucrose (TCBS) agar
  - **TCBS agar:** It is the most common selective media used for *V. cholerae*. It can ferment sucrose and produce large yellow colonies **(Fig. 30.2B)**
  - **MacConkey agar:** *V. cholerae* produces translucent NLF colonies.
- **Culture smear and motility testing**—reveal short curved gram-negative bacilli and darting motility
- **Identification:** *V. cholerae* produces hemodigestion on blood agar. It causes nonspecific lysis of blood cells, seen as greenish clearing around the main inoculum **(Fig. 30.2A)**. Identification of *V. cholerae* from the colonies can be performed by following tests:
  - **String test:** When a colony of *Vibrio* is mixed with a drop of 0.5% sodium deoxycholate on a slide, the suspension loses its turbidity, and becomes mucoid. When tried lifting the suspension with a loop, it forms a string **(Fig. 30.2C)**.
  - **Conventional biochemical tests** such as catalase (positive), oxidase (positive), Indole test (positive), citrate test (variable), urease test (negative), and TSI (being sucrose fermenter, it shows acid/acid, gas absent, H_2S absent).
  - **Cholera red reaction:** Indole and nitrate reduction properties can be tested together by adding few drops of sulfuric acid to a peptone water culture of *Vibrio cholerae*. A reddish-pink color ring is formed.
  - **Automated methods** such as MALDI-TOF and VITEK.
- **Typing:** After being identified as *V. cholerae,* it is further subjected to various typing methods
  - *Biotyping:* To differentiate classical and El Tor
  - *Serogrouping:* To differentiate O1 and O139
  - *Serotyping:* To differentiate Ogawa, Inaba, and Hikojima serotypes of serogroup O1.
- **Antigen detection** can be done by tests such as cholera dipstick assay
- **Molecular method:** Multiplex PCR can be used to detect common diarrheal pathogens
- **Antimicrobial susceptibility testing** can be performed by disk diffusion test or by automated methods (e.g. VITEK).

> **TREATMENT** — Cholera
>
> Fluid replacement is the mainstay of treatment of cholera. Antibiotics such as macrolides (azithromycin) or doxycycline can be given to severely dehydrated patients.

Cholera Vaccine

Oral cholera vaccines (OCV) are currently in use for the prevention of cholera. They usually give short-term protection (6 months or so). Two types of OCVs are available.
1. **Killed whole-cell vaccine,** e.g. include whole-cell (WC) vaccine (e.g. Shanchol) and whole-cell recombinant B subunit vaccine (e.g. Dukoral)

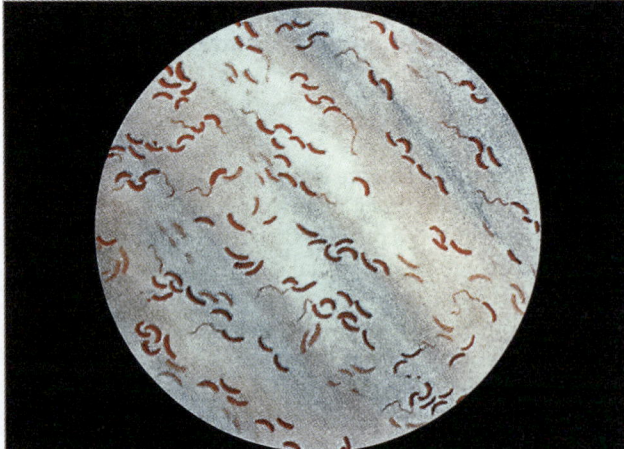

Fig. 30.1: *Vibrio cholerae* (Gram stain): Curved comma-shaped gram-negative rods (fish in stream appearance).
Source: Public Health Image Library, ID#:5324/Centers for Disease Control and Prevention (CDC) (*with permission*).

CHAPTER 30 ◆ Vibrio

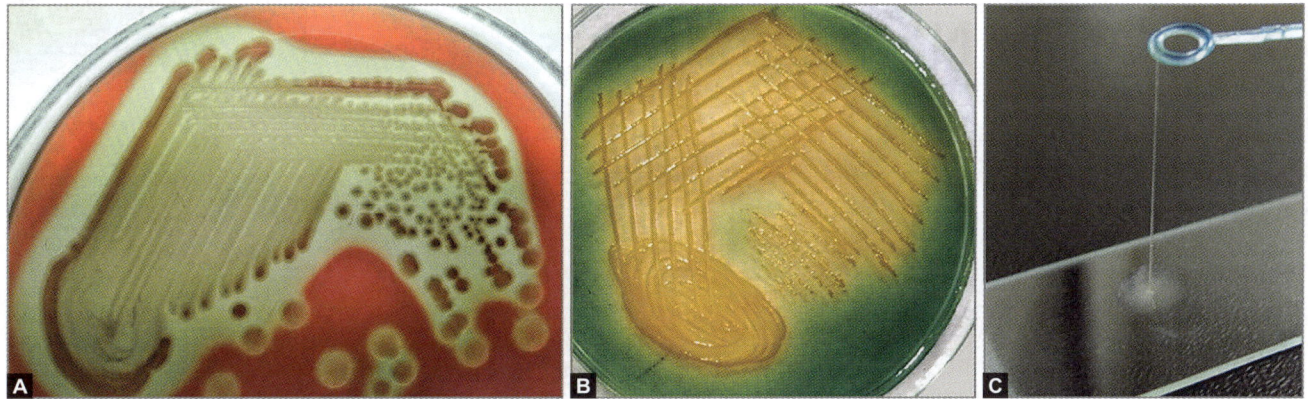

Figs. 30.2A to C: A. *Vibrio cholerae* on blood agar (hemodigestion); **B.** TCBS agar with yellow colored colonies of *Vibrio cholerae*; **C.** String test.
Source: Department of Microbiology, Pondicherry Institute of Medical Sciences, Puducherry (*with permission*).

2. **Oral live attenuated vaccines,** e.g. CVD 103-HgR vaccine.

Injectable killed vaccines which were used before are no longer used.

Halophilic Vibrio

The *Vibrio* species other than *V. cholerae* that grow in higher salt concentrations are called **halophilic *Vibrios***; examples include *V. parahaemolyticus, V. alginolyticus* and *V. vulnificus.* They cause intestinal and extraintestinal manifestations.

❖ ***Vibrio parahaemolyticus:*** It causes food-borne gastroenteritis by ingestion of raw or uncooked sea food.
  ■ It is capsulated, shows bipolar staining
  ■ On TCBS agar it produces green colonies (sucrose nonfermenter)
  ■ It swarms on blood agar and it can resist maximum of 8% NaCl
  ■ Doxycycline or macrolide are the drug of choice.
❖ ***Vibrio vulnificus:*** It produces sepsis and wound infections.
  ■ It can be cultured from blood or cutaneous lesions
  ■ It ferments lactose, which differentiates it from all other vibrios
  ■ Tetracycline, fluoroquinolones, or third-generation cephalosporins can be used for treatment.
❖ ***Vibrio alginolyticus:*** It can occasionally cause eye, ear and wound infections.
  ■ It rarely causes bacteremia in immunocompromised hosts
  ■ It can grow at salt concentrations of more than 10%
  ■ Disease is usually self-limiting.

EXPECTED QUESTIONS

I. **Write essay on:**
  1. Discuss the epidemiology, clinical manifestations, laboratory diagnosis and treatment of cholera.

II. **Write short notes on:**
  1. Laboratory diagnosis of cholera.
  2. Halophilic vibrios.

III. **Multiple Choice Questions (MCQs):**
  1. TCBS agar is used for:
     a. *Vibrio cholerae*   b. *Salmonella*
     c. *Shigella*   d. Mycobacteria
  2. Which of the following exhibits darting motility?
     a. *Salmonella*   b. *Shigella*
     c. *Vibrio cholerae*   d. *E. coli*

  3. All of the following are selective media for *Vibrio cholerae*, except:
     a. Wilson Blair bismuth sulphite medium
     b. Monsur's gelatin taurocholate tellurite agar
     c. Thiosulfate citrate bile salts sucrose agar
     d. Bile salt agar
  4. All of the following *Vibrio* species are halophilic, except:
     a. *V. cholerae*
     b. *V. parahaemolyticus*
     c. *V. alginolyticus*
     d. *V. vulnificus*

Answers
1. a   2. c   3. a   4. a

Pseudomonas, Acinetobacter and Other Nonfermenters

CHAPTER 31

CHAPTER PREVIEW
- *Pseudomonas* species
- *Acinetobacter* species
- *Burkholderia* species
- *Stenotrophomonas maltophilia*

Non-fermenting gram-negative bacilli (NF-GNB) do not ferment any sugars, but they utilize the sugars oxidatively.
❖ Most of the NF-GNB exist as environmental commensals in hospitals. They are resistant to multiple antibiotics. Examples include:
  - *Pseudomonas aeruginosa*
  - *Burkholderia cepacia*
  - *Acinetobacter baumannii*
  - *Stenotrophomonas maltophilia*
❖ Some non-fermenters are principally community associated pathogens, e.g. *Burkholderia pseudomallei*.

PSEUDOMONAS AERUGINOSA

Pseudomonas is an oxidase positive, pigment producing, non-fermenting gram-negative bacilli. It is a major pathogen responsible for most of the hospital acquired infections and also of importance in patients with cystic fibrosis.

Pathogenesis

The pathogenesis is greatly attributed to its ability to develop widespread resistance to multiple antibiotics and disinfectants and produce several virulence factors.
❖ **Toxins,** e.g. exotoxin A. It acts by inhibiting protein synthesis
❖ **Enzymes,** e.g. phospholipases, elastases, etc.
❖ **Pigments:** *Pseudomonas* produces various pigments such as:
  - Pyocyanin: It is a blue-green pigment, produced only by *P. aeruginosa*
  - Pyoverdin: It is greenish-yellow pigment, produced by most species
  - Pyorubin: This pigment imparts red color.
❖ **Alginate coat:** Mucoid strains of *Pseudomonas* have a slime layer or alginate layer which facilitates biofilm formation.
❖ **Multidrug resistance:** *Pseudomonas* is known to possess genes coding for resistance to several antimicrobial agents.
❖ **Multi-disinfectant resistance:** It helps the bacilli to grow in presence of various disinfectants; thus, spreading the infection in the hospitals.

Clinical Manifestations

Most of the infections are encountered in hospitalized patients who get colonized with the organisms either from the heavily contaminated hospital environment or from the hospital staff (through contaminated hands). Colonized patients develop the disease in the presence of underlying risk factors such as burn wounds, patients with immunosuppression, and post surgeries. The manifestations are as follows:
❖ **Healthcare-associated infections** such as—(i) ventilator-associated pneumonia (VAP), (ii) central-line associated bloodstream infection (CLABSI), (iii) catheter-associated urinary tract infection (CAUTI), (iv) surgical site infection (SSI)
❖ **Chronic respiratory tract infections:** It occurs in patients with underlying conditions that cause airway damage such as cystic fibrosis, or bronchiectasis
❖ **Bacteremia** leading to sepsis and septic shock
❖ **Infective endocarditis (native valves):** It occurs among IV drug abusers
❖ **Ear infections:** The infections are either mild, such as **swimmer's ear** (among children), or serious necrotizing form designated as **malignant otitis externa** (in elderly diabetic patients)
❖ **Eye infections** such as corneal ulcers (in contact lens wearers) and endophthalmitis secondary to bacteremia
❖ **Shanghai fever**: It is a mild febrile illness resembling typhoid fever

- **Skin and soft tissue infections** such as burns wound infection, ecthyma gangrenosum, green nail syndrome, and cellulitis with blue-green pus
- **Other infections:** Bone and joint infections such as osteomyelitis and septic arthritis and meningitis (in postoperative or post-traumatic patients).

Laboratory Diagnosis

Specimen collection depends upon the site of infection, such as—pus, blood, tracheal aspirate, sputum, wound swab, urine, etc.

- **Direct smear:** Reveals gram-negative bacilli, and pus cells
- **Culture:** Incubation at 37°C aerobically for 24 h yields the following growth
  - Nutrient agar: Opaque, irregular colonies with metallic sheen (iridescence) and blue green diffusible pigments **(Fig. 31.1)**. Mostly *Pseudomonas* colonies have a sweet ether or alcohol-like **fruity odor**.
  - Blood agar: β-hemolytic gray moist colonies
  - MacConkey agar: Non-lactose fermenting (NLF) colonies
  - Selective media such as cetrimide agar may be used.
- **Culture smear and motility:** Motile, gram-negative bacilli
- **Identification** from the colonies is made by automated ID systems such as MALDI-TOF or VITEK or by conventional biochemical tests such as:
  - Oxidase and catalase positive
  - Indole test: negative
  - Citrate test: positive
  - Urease test: negative
  - Triple sugar iron (TSI) test: The test shows alkaline slant/alkaline butt (no change), with no gas and no H_2S.
- **AST:** Antimicrobial susceptibility testing is performed by disk diffusion test (on Mueller–Hinton agar) or by automated MIC detection method (e.g. VITEK).

> **TREATMENT** *P. aeruginosa*
>
> ❏ *Pseudomonas aeruginosa* is intrinsically resistant to ceftriaxone, amoxicillin-clavulanate, ertapenem, tetracyclines, tigecycline, etc. Therefore, these drugs should not be used in the therapy
> ❏ Only limited agents have good anti-pseudomonal action such as ceftazidime, piperacillin-tazobactam, carbapenems, amikacin, quinolones (ciprofloxacin or levofloxacin), etc.

Preventive Measures

Infection control measures (contact precaution) such as hand hygiene are crucial to limit the spread of *Pseudomonas* infection in the hospitals (*see* **Chapter 15**).

ACINETOBACTER SPECIES

They are saprophytic bacilli, can cause widespread healthcare-associated infections, especially in patients with underlying diseases and immunosuppression.

- **Clinical manifestations:** *Acinetobacter baumannii* causes widespread healthcare associated infections such as:
  - Ventilator associated pneumonia
  - Central line associated bloodstream infection
  - Catheter-associated UTI
  - Wound and soft tissue infections
  - Infections in burn patients.
- **Laboratory diagnosis:** It is an obligate aerobe, grows well on ordinary medium. Specimens can be inoculated onto blood agar (non-hemolytic colonies) and MacConkey agar (lactose non-fermenting colonies with faint pink tint) **(Fig. 31.2)**. Important identification features are:
  - **Gram staining:** They are gram-negative coccobacilli
  - Oxidase negative and catalase positive
  - Non-fermenter of sugars and non-motile
  - **Biochemical (ICUT) tests:** Indole test (negative), citrate test (positive), urease test (negative) and TSI (triple sugar iron agar) test shows alkaline slant/alkaline butt with no gas and no H_2S
  - **Species identification** can also be made by automated identification systems such as MALDI-TOF or VITEK
  - **Antimicrobial susceptibility testing** is performed by disk diffusion method (on Mueller–Hinton

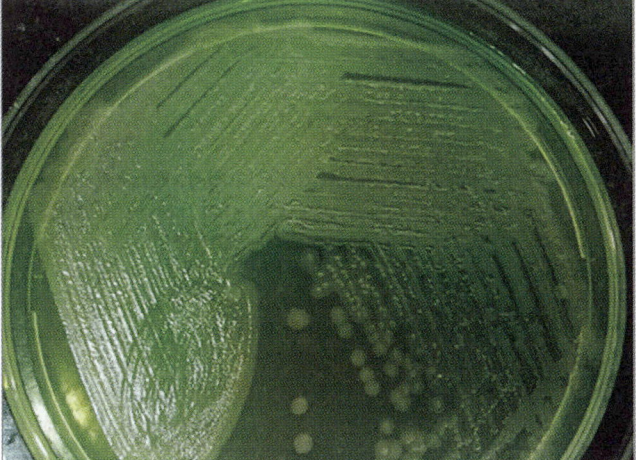

Fig. 31.1: *Pseudomonas aeruginosa* on nutrient agar showing: large irregular colonies with metallic sheen and green color pigmentation.
Source: Department of Microbiology, Pondicherry Institute of Medical Sciences, Puducherry (*with permission*).

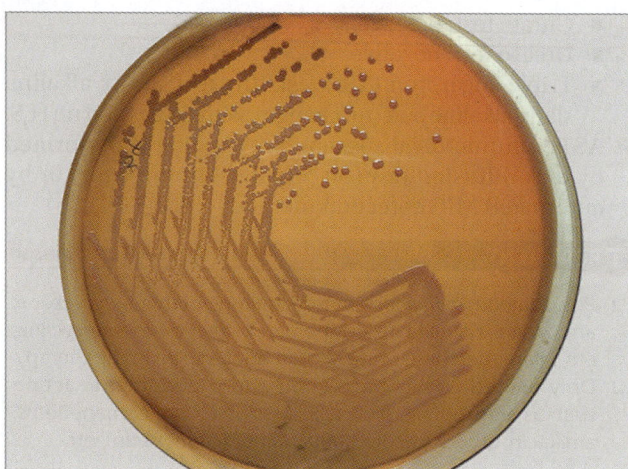

Fig. 31.2: Lactose non-fermenting colonies (with faint pink tint) of *Acinetobacter* on MacConkey agar.
Source: Department of Microbiology, JIPMER, Puducherry (with permission).

agar) or by automated MIC detection method (e.g. VITEK).
- ❖ **Treatment** for *Acinetobacter* is similar to that of *Pseudomonas*, except that it responds to certain additional agents such as minocycline or tigecycline
- ❖ **Prevention:** Infection control measures such as improved hand hygiene are essential to prevent nosocomial infections due to *Acinetobacter* (*refer* contact precaution, **Chapter 15**).

■ BURKHOLDERIA SPECIES

Burkholderia species are also oxidase positive, non-fermenters similar to *Pseudomonas*; however, they differ from the latter in being bipolar stained (safety pin appearance) and resistant to polymyxin B. Important species that are pathogenic to man include *B. cepacia* complex and *B. pseudomallei*.

Burkholderia cepacia

It is an environmental organism that inhabits moist environments and IV fluids.
- ❖ **Clinical manifestations** include:
  - Rapidly fatal respiratory infection and septicemia in patients with cystic fibrosis
  - It is an important emerging nosocomial pathogen in ICUs causing pneumonia, wound infections, etc.
- ❖ **Laboratory diagnosis:** It is an obligate aerobe, grows well on ordinary medium.
  - Specimens can be inoculated onto blood agar and MacConkey agar (lactose non-fermenting colonies)
  - Identification is done by biochemical tests or by automated identification systems
  - Antimicrobial susceptibility testing is performed by disk diffusion method or by automated MIC detection method (e.g. VITEK).
- ❖ **Treatment:** Cotrimoxazole, meropenem, and doxycycline are the most effective agents
- ❖ **Prevention:** Implementation of infection control measures is crucial to prevent nosocomial spread of infection (*refer* contact precaution, **Chapter 15**).

Burkholderia pseudomallei

- ❖ *B. pseudomallei* is a saprophyte of soil and water and have large number of animal reservoirs. Humans are infected by various routes such as inoculation, inhalation, or ingestion
- ❖ **Clinical manifestations:** It is the causative agent of **melioidosis**; which presents in various clinical forms ranging from acute localized infection, subacute pulmonary infection, bloodstream infection, and chronic suppurative infection
- ❖ **Laboratory diagnosis:** It shows bipolar staining in Gram-stained smear, intrinsically resistant to polymyxin B
  - It grows on various media, e.g. nutrient agar, blood agar and MacConkey agar. Colonies are typically rough and corrugated
  - It grows on selective media such as Ashdown's medium; produces wrinkled colonies
  - Identification is done by biochemical tests or by automated identification systems
  - Antimicrobial susceptibility testing is performed by disk diffusion method on Mueller Hinton agar
- ❖ **Treatment:** Compromises of—(i) intensive phase (2 weeks) with ceftazidime or meropenem, followed by (ii) maintenance phase (12 weeks) with oral cotrimoxazole.

■ STENOTROPHOMONAS MALTOPHILIA

S. maltophilia is a saprophyte. Infection by this organism is seen commonly among patients with immunocompromised conditions and on broad-spectrum antibiotics.
- ❖ **Clinical manifestations:** It can cause various hospital infections such as pneumonia in ventilated patients, bloodstream infections and ecthyma gangrenosum in neutropenic patients
- ❖ **Laboratory diagnosis:** Identification of *S. maltophila* is made either by conventional biochemical tests or by automated identification systems
- ❖ **Treatment:** *S. maltophilia* is intrinsically resistant to most of the β-lactams including carbapenems, polymyxins, aminoglycosides and fosfomycin. The recommended antibiotics are cotrimoxazole, minocycline, and levofloxacin.

CHAPTER 31 ❖ Pseudomonas, Acinetobacter and Other Nonfermenters

EXPECTED QUESTIONS

I. **Write short notes on:**
   1. Infections caused by *Pseudomonas*.
   3. Melioidosis.
   5. Infections caused by *Acinetobacter*.

II. **Multiple Choice Questions (MCQs):**
   1. **Which of the following drug is not active against *Stenotrophomonas maltophilia*?**
      a. Cotrimoxazole
      b. Minocycline
      c. Meropenem
      d. Levofloxacin
   2. **Melioidosis is caused by:**
      a. Burkholderia pseudomallei
      b. Burkholderia cepacia
      c. Burkholderia mallei
      d. Pseudomonas aeruginosa
   3. **Ecthyma gangrenosum is caused by:**
      a. Pseudomonas
      b. Bordetella
      c. Brucella
      d. H. influenzae
   4. **All of the following bacteria are non-fermenters, *except*:**
      a. Pseudomonas
      b. Burkholderia
      c. Acinetobacter
      d. Escherichia

Answers
1. c   2. a   3. a   4. d

Fastidious Gram-negative Bacilli: Haemophilus, Bordetella and Brucella

CHAPTER 32

CHAPTER PREVIEW
- Haemophilus
- Bordetella
- Brucella

This chapter deals with gram-negative bacilli (GNB) infections caused by the fastidious gram-negative bacilli such as *Haemophilus*, *Brucella* and *Bordetella*.

HAEMOPHILUS SPECIES

Haemophilus species are oxidase positive, capsulated pleomorphic gram-negative bacilli that require special growth factors present in blood, such as factors X and V (*Haemo* means blood, *philus* means loving). The important species include—*H. influenzae, H. ducreyi, H. aegyptius, H. parainfluenzae*, etc.

Haemophilus Influenzae

It is the most pathogenic species; causes pneumonia and meningitis in children. It requires both X and V factors for its growth.

Pathogenesis

It is capsulated, which is the main virulent factor. Based on capsular polysaccharide antigen, it can be typed into 6 serotypes (a to f)—serotype b being the most pathogenic and invasive.

Clinical Manifestations

H. influenzae type b is the most common and most invasive serotype of *H. influenzae*. It causes systemic disease by invasion and hematogenous spread from the respiratory tract to distant sites such as the meninges, bones, and joints. The spectrum of illness can be divided into:
- Common invasive infections such as pneumonia, bacteremia, meningitis, and epiglottitis
- Less common invasive infections such as otitis media, sinusitis, osteomyelitis, septic arthritis, pericarditis, etc.

Laboratory Diagnosis

Depending upon the site of infection, various specimens may be collected such as CSF, blood, sputum, pus, aspirates from joints, middle ears or sinuses. As *H. influenzae* is highly sensitive to low temperature, the specimens for culture **should never be refrigerated**. The specimens should be transported to the laboratory without any delay and processed immediately.

- **Direct examination:**
  - Gram staining reveals pleomorphic gram-negative coccobacilli **(Fig. 32.1A)**
  - Antigen detection from CSF can be done by latex agglutination test.
- **Culture:** *H. influenzae* is highly fastidious, requires two accessory growth factors (factor X and V) in blood for their growth. Factors X is a hemin, present freely in blood, where as factor V is nicotinamide adenine dinucleotide (NAD), which is present inside RBCs. It is also produced by some bacteria, such as *Staphylococcus aureus*.
  - Growth is scanty on blood agar, because only factor X is available freely in blood agar
  - Grows well on chocolate agar: While preparing chocolate agar, blood is poured into molten agar at 75°C which lyses RBCs releasing excess of factor V **(Fig. 32.1C)**
  - Grows well on blood agar with *S. aureus* streak line: Colonies of *H. influenzae* grow well adjacent to *S. aureus* streak line—a phenomenon called as **satellitism**. Factor X (hemin) is present in blood agar and factor V is released from *S. aureus*. Therefore larger colonies are formed adjacent to *S. aureus* streak line and size of the colonies decreases gradually away from the *S. aureus* streak line **(Figs. 32.1B and 32.2)**
- **Identification** is confirmed by disk test for X and V requirements or automated ID systems.
- **Antimicrobial susceptibility testing** is performed by disk diffusion method on *Haemophilus* test medium.

Treatment

Ceftriaxone is given for treatment. Alternatively ampicillin plus chloramphenicol may be used.

CHAPTER 32 ◆ Fastidious Gram-negative Bacilli: Haemophilus, Bordetella and Brucella

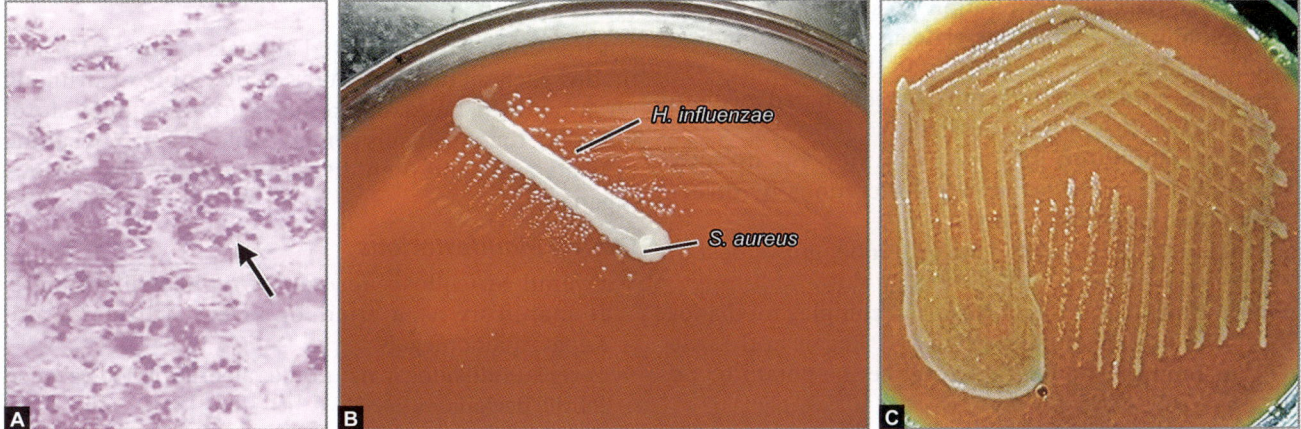

Figs. 32.1A to C: A. Gram-stained smear showing pleomorphic gram-negative bacilli; **B.** Satellitism of *H. influenzae* around *S. aureus* streak line; **C.** Colonies of *H. influenzae* on chocolate agar.
Source: A. Department of Microbiology, JIPMER, Puducherry; B and C. Department of Microbiology, Pondicherry Institute of Medical Sciences, Puducherry (*with permission*).

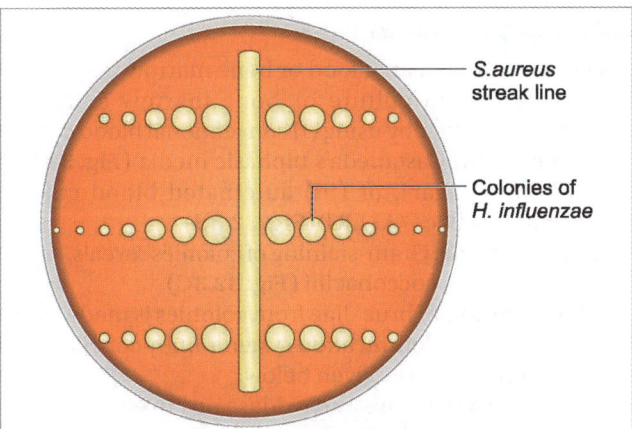

Fig. 32.2: Satellitism of *Haemophilus influenzae* (schematic diagram).

Vaccine

Hib conjugate vaccine (*H. influenzae* type b) is available for children. Under the national immunization program, it is given as a part of the pentavalent vaccine at 6, 10, and 14 weeks.

Other Haemophilus Species

Haemophilus ducreyi

It is the causative agent of soft chancre (chancroid); a sexually transmitted infection characterized by painful genital ulcers and enlarged tender inguinal lymph nodes (bubo).

HACEK Group

They represent a group of highly fastidious gram-negative bacilli, which are found as the normal commensal of the oral cavity but can cause serious infections such as endocarditis. They include—*Haemophilus* species, *Aggregatibacter* species, *Cardiobacterium hominis*, *Eikenella corrodens* and *Kingella kingae*.

■ BORDETELLA PERTUSSIS

Bordetella pertussis is the causative agent of **whooping cough**; a highly contagious toxin-mediated disease, characterized by paroxysmal cough ending in a high pitched inspiratory sound described as "whoop".

Pathogenesis

B. pertussis produces a wide array of toxins and biologically active products. Pathogenesis is mediated by the expression of several virulence factors such as pertussis toxin, tracheal cytotoxin, adhesins, etc.

Clinical Manifestations

The clinical course of whooping cough or pertussis passes through three stages following an incubation period of 7–10 days.
- **Catarrhal phase** is characterized by common cold like nonspecific symptoms, low-grade fever and malaise. It is highly infectious stage
- **Paroxysmal phase:** Patients are less infectious. It is characterized by specific symptoms, such as whooping cough and post-tussive vomiting
- **Convalescent stage:** During this frequency and severity of coughing gradually decreases.

Laboratory Diagnosis
- **Specimen collection:** Nasopharyngeal secretions are the best specimens which may be obtained by—

(i) nasopharyngeal aspiration (best method), or (ii) pernasal swab. For culture, alginate swabs are the best followed by dacron swabs.
- **Specimen transport** is done in charcoal-based medium (e.g. Amies, Regan-Lowe media)
- **Direct detection:** *B. pertussis* may be directly detected from nasopharyngeal secretions by **direct immunofluorescence test**
- **Culture:** *B. pertussis* is a strict aerobe, grows best at 35–37°C.
  - It is fastidious, requires special complex media for primary isolation, such as—(i) Regan and Lowe medium, (ii) Bordet-Gengou glycerine-potato-blood agar
  - Colonies are greyish white, convex with a shiny surface appear after 3–5 days, described as mercury drops or bisected pearls appearance
- **Culture smear:** Gram-staining of culture reveals small, coccobacilli, arranged in loose clumps, giving a **thumb print** appearance
- **Identification** from colonies can be done by automated methods such as MALDI-TOF or VITEK.
- **Molecular method:** PCR remains positive in first four weeks of onset of symptoms.

Treatment

Macrolide such as azithromycin is the drug of choice. Isolation of patient in a quiet environment may inhibit the stimulation of paroxysms.

Prevention

Two vaccines are available—(1) whole-cell pertussis vaccine and (2) acellular pertussis vaccine.
- In India whole cell (WC) pertussis vaccine is given under national immunization programme, along with diphtheria toxoid and tetanus toxoid (DPT).
- Three doses of DPT are given at 6, 10 and 14 weeks, followed by two boosters of DPT at 1½ years and 5 years.

■ BRUCELLA SPECIES

Brucella is an obligate aerobic, fastidious small gram-negative coccobacillus, responsible for a highly contagious febrile illness called **brucellosis**. It is a zoonotic febrile illness also called undulant fever or Malta fever.

Agents

Brucella melitensis is the most common species, affects sheep and goat. Other species are *B. abortus* (cattle), *B. canis* (dog), etc.

Transmission

It is transmitted from infected animals to man by various modes such as direct contact or by eating or drinking unpasteurized/raw dairy products. From the initial site of infection, the organisms spread to bloodstream resulting in bacteremia and then disseminate to involve various organs.

Clinical Manifestations

- Overall brucellosis resembles typhoid-like illness. It manifests as a triad of fever, arthralgia, and hepatosplenomegaly
- Fever is undulating in nature, i.e., afebrile period between febrile periods
- Musculoskeletal involvement is common such as vertebral osteomyelitis or septic arthritis
- Other nonspecific symptoms such as abdominal pain, headache, diarrhea, rash, weakness/fatigue, weight loss may be present.

Laboratory Diagnosis

Specimen collected are blood or bone marrow.
- **Culture:** Blood culture or bone marrow culture is performed either by using (i) conventional blood culture bottles, or (ii) Castaneda's biphasic media **(Fig. 32.3A)** (BHI broth/agar), or (iii) automated blood culture systems like BacT/ALERT **(Fig. 32.3B)**
- **Culture smear:** Gram-staining of colonies reveals, small, gram-negative coccobacilli **(Fig. 32.3C)**
- **Identification** of brucellae from colonies is made either by automated identification systems or by conventional biochemical tests as given below.
  - *Brucella* is catalase and oxidase positive
  - Urease test is rapidly positive for *B. suis* and *B. canis*.

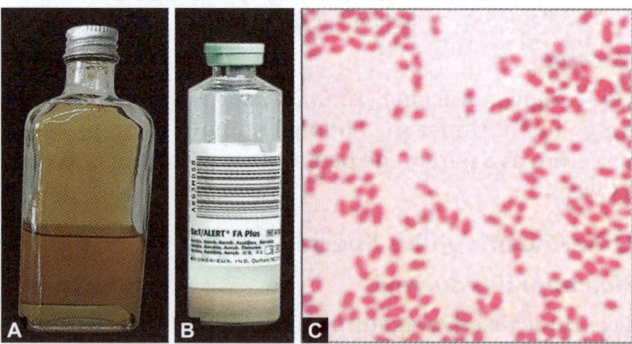

Figs. 32.3A to C: A. Castaneda's biphasic blood culture medium; **B.** BacT/ALERT bottle; **C.** Gram-stained smear of *Brucella* species showing small gram-negative coccobacilli.

Source: A and B. Department of Microbiology, JIPMER, Puducherry; C. Public Health Image Library, ID# /15243, Dr WA Clark/Centers for Disease Control and Prevention (CDC), Atlanta (*with permission*).

CHAPTER 32 ◆ Fastidious Gram-negative Bacilli: Haemophilus, Bordetella and Brucella

- ❖ **Detection of antibodies** by serological tests such as standard agglutination test (SAT) or ELISA.
- ❖ **Molecular method:** PCR assays are available; rapid, sensitive and specific. Blood and tissues are ideal samples for PCR assays.

Treatment

The treatment comprises of doxycycline, in combination with rifampicin or streptomycin, given for a longer duration (6 weeks).

EXPECTED QUESTIONS

I. Write short notes on:
   1. Laboratory diagnosis of *H. influenzae*.
   2. Laboratory diagnosis of brucellosis.
   3. Laboratory diagnosis of pertussis.

II. Multiple Choice Questions (MCQs):
   1. Satellitism is observed in culture for:
      a. *Bordetella*
      b. *H. influenzae*
      c. *Brucella*
      d. *Pseudomonas*
   2. Undulant fever is caused by:
      a. *Burkholderia*
      b. *Helicobacter*
      c. *H. influenzae*
      d. *Brucella*
   3. Mercury drop appearance colony of *B. pertussis* is seen on which of the following culture media?
      a. Blood agar
      b. Chocolate agar
      c. Regan-Lowe agar
      d. Nutrient agar

Answers
1. b   2. d   3. c

Miscellaneous Gram-negative Bacilli

CHAPTER 33

> **CHAPTER PREVIEW**
> - *Campylobacter* species
> - *Helicobacter pylori*
> - *Legionella* species
> - *Pasteurella* species
> - *Francisella tularensis*
> - *Gardnerella vaginalis*
> - Agents of Rat-bite Fever

This chapter deals with miscellaneous gram-negative bacilli such as *Campylobacter, Helicobacter, Legionella, Pasteurella, Francisella, Gardnerella vaginalis*, and agents of Rat-bite fever.

■ CAMPYLOBACTER

Campylobacter species are motile, nonsporing, microaerophilic, curved gram-negative rods. The common human pathogen is *Campylobacter jejuni;* an important agent of inflammatory diarrhea or dysentery.

- ❖ **Transmission** is mainly by ingestion of raw or undercooked food products
- ❖ **Clinical manifestations:** Characterized by inflammatory diarrhea, abdominal pain, and fever. Extraintestinal complications can also be occasionally seen (mainly due to other species such as *C. fetus*) such as bacteremia, sepsis, meningitis, etc.
- ❖ **Laboratory diagnosis:** Freshly collected stool specimen and rectal swab are the preferred specimens.
    - **Direct microscopy:** Gram stained smear of feces may show curved gram-negative bacilli, comma or S-shaped or spiral (*gull wing*) shaped **(Fig. 33.1A)**
    - **Dark ground microscopy** demonstrates the darting motility of the bacilli
    - **Stool culture:** Cary-Blair medium can be used as transport medium. Skirrow's medium **(Fig. 33.1B)**, Butzler's media, Campy BAP medium are used as selective media for isolation of the bacilli from stool specimen. The culture plates are incubated at microaerophilic condition (5% oxygen). Species identification can be performed by conventional biochemical tests or automated systems such as MALDI-TOF or VITEK.
- ❖ **Treatment:** Fluid and electrolyte replacement is the mainstay of treatment. Oral macrolides are the drug of choice (erythromycin or azithromycin).

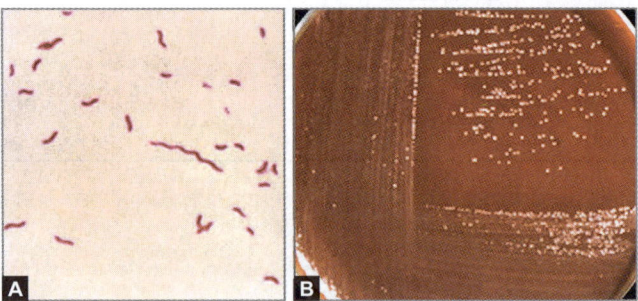

Figs. 33.1A and B: *Campylobacter:* **A.** Gram-negative spiral rods; **B.** Growth on Skirrow's media.

Source: Public Health Image Library: A. ID#: 6657; B. D#: 3918/Centers for Disease Control and Prevention (CDC), Atlanta (*with permission*).

■ HELICOBACTER PYLORI

Helicobacter pylori is curved gram-negative rod that colonizes stomach and is associated with peptic ulcer disease and gastric carcinoma.

- ❖ **Colonization of the gastric mucosa:** Man is the only important reservoir host of *H. pylori*. It colonizes the stomach of 50% of the world's human population. The colonization is favored by the the factors such as (i) highly motile bacilli, (ii) acid-resistance due to production of urease enzyme (that catalyzes urea hydrolysis to produce

ammonia which in turn buffers the gastric acid) (iii) by expressing adhesins
- **Clinical manifestations:** *H. pylori* is associated with the pathogenesis of the following conditions:
  - Acute gastritis involving the antrum region
  - Peptic ulcer disease (duodenal and gastric ulcers): It presents with epigastric pain with a burning sensation; develops either following a meal (as in duodenal ulcer) or in an empty stomach (as in gastric ulcer)
  - Adenocarcinoma of stomach
- **Laboratory diagnosis:** The diagnosis of *H. pylori* infection may be established by invasive and noninvasive methods.
  - **Invasive tests:** Endoscopy-guided multiple biopsies can be taken from gastric mucosa (antrum and corpus) and are subjected to:
    - **Histopathology** with Warthin Starry silver staining
    - **Microbiological tests** such as (i) Gram-staining showing gram-negative bacilli with seagull-shaped morphology, (ii) Culture on Skirrow's media and chocolate agar (at 37°C under microaerophilic condition), (iii) Identification by automated identification systems, and (iv) **Biopsy urease test** (also called **rapid urease test**) to detect the presence of urease activity in gastric biopsies (rapid, sensitive and cheap method)
  - **Noninvasive tests** include—(i) urea breath test, (ii) fecal antigen (coproantigen) assay, (iii) antibody (IgG) detection by ELISA.
- **Treatment** includes a triple-drug regimen, comprising omeprazole, clarithromycin, and metronidazole; given for 7–14 days.

LEGIONELLA

L. pneumophila is a fastidious, pleomorphic gram-negative short rod, associated with two clinical syndromes—(i) Pontiac fever (an acute, milder flu-like self-limited illness), and (ii) Legionnaires' disease (a severe form of interstitial pneumonia)
- **Transmission:** Aspiration of the organism from oropharyngeal colonization or directly via the drinking of contaminated water is the most common mode. Aerosols from contaminated air conditioners, nebulizers, and humidifiers are another mode of transmission
- **Laboratory diagnosis** includes—(i) direct microscopy by silver impregnation and Giemsa staining, (ii) isolation of the organism in buffered charcoal yeast extract (BCYE) agar, and (iii) urinary antigen detection
- **Treatment:** Macrolides (e.g. azithromycin) and respiratory quinolones are now the antibiotics of choice.

OTHER MISCELLANEOUS GRAM-NEGATIVE BACILLI

Other miscellaneous gram-negative bacilli are *Pasteurella*, *Francisella*, *Gardnerella vaginalis*, and agents of Rat-bite fever.

Pasteurella

Pasteurella species are primarily harbored as normal flora in the oral cavity of cats and dogs.
Pasteurella multocida is the most common species infecting man.
- **Clinical manifestations:** In humans, *P. multocida* is the most common cause of wound infections after dog or cat bites. In more serious cases, bacteremia can result, causing an osteomyelitis or endocarditis or meningitis
- **Laboratory diagnosis:** *P. multocida* is a gram-negative coccobacillus that readily grows in culture media. Identification is made biochemically or through automated methods.
- **Treatment:** Penicillin G or amoxicillin-clavulanate is considered as the drug of choice.

Francisella tularensis

Francisella tularensis is the causative agent of 'tularemia' primarily a plague-like disease of rodents and other small animals. Human infection is zoonotic and usually results from interaction with biting or blood-sucking insects.
- **Clinical manifestations:** Tularemia is characterized by various clinical syndromes such as ulceroglandular tularemia (most common form), pulmonary, oropharyngeal, oculoglandular form and typhoid-like illness
- **Agent of bioterrorism:** Because of the highly infectious nature, *F. tularensis* is currently classified as category A agent of bioterrorism
- **Laboratory diagnosis:** Ulcer scrapings and lymph node biopsy are the preferred specimens.
  - *F. tularensis* is highly fastidious; needs special media, such as BCG agar (blood cysteine glucose agar).
  - Species identification from colonies is made either by conventional biochemical tests or by automated identification systems.

SECTION 4 ◆ Systematic Bacteriology

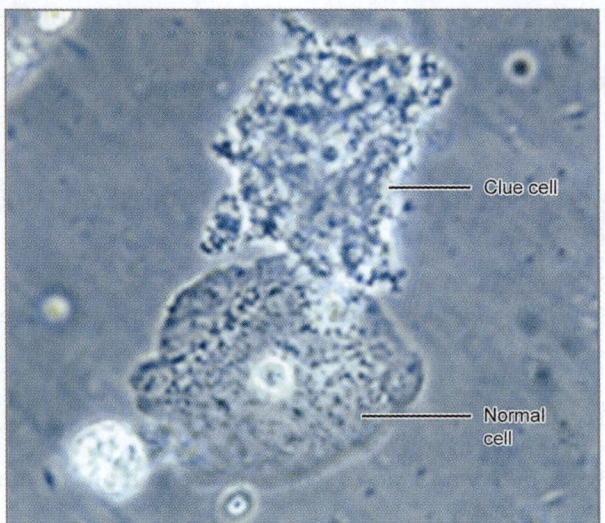

Fig. 33.2: Wet mount of vaginal secretion depicting clue cell.
Source: Public Health Image Library/ID#: 14574/ M. Rein/Centers for Disease Control and Prevention (CDC), Atlanta (*with permission*).

❖ **Treatment:** Gentamicin is the drug of choice; doxycycline or ciprofloxacin can be given as alternatives.

Gardnerella vaginalis

It causes profuse watery vaginal discharge—a condition called bacterial vaginosis. It is diagnosed if any 3 of the following 4 findings are present (Amsel's criteria):

1. **Discharge:** Thin white homogeneous vaginal discharge uniformly coated on the vaginal wall
2. **pH** of vaginal discharge more than 4.5
3. **Whiff test:** Accentuation of a distinct fishy odor of vaginal secretions, when mixed with 10% solution of KOH
4. **Clue cells:** They are vaginal epithelial cells coated with coccobacilli, which have a granular appearance and indistinct borders observed on a wet mount (Fig. 33.2).

Treatment of bacterial vaginosis involves oral metronidazole, given twice daily for 7 days.

Agents of Rat-bite Fever

Rat-bite fever (RBF) is characterized by septic fever, petechial rashes, and painful polyarthritis with frequent relapses. Transmission of infection occurs primarily by contact with rodents. It is caused by either of the two pathogens: (1) *Streptobacillus moniliformis* and (2) *Spirillum minus*.

1. ***Streptobacillus moniliformis*** is gram-negative, highly pleomorphic nonmotile bacilli, which is frequently arranged in chains. It has a tendency to form L-form. It can be isolated from blood, synovial fluid and other infected tissues.
2. ***Spirillum minus*** is rigid, spirally coiled motile bacilli. It doesn't grow in artificial media.

EXPECTED QUESTIONS

I. Write short notes on:
   1. Laboratory diagnosis of *Campylobacter*.
   2. Laboratory diagnosis of *Helicobacter pylori*.
   3. Laboratory diagnosis of bacterial vaginosis.
II. Multiple Choice Questions (MCQs):
   1. Urea breath test is done:
      a. *Campylobacter*
      b. *Burkholderia*
      c. *Helicobacter*
      d. *H. influenzae*
   2. Rat-bite fever is caused by:
      a. *Borrelia recurrentis*
      b. *Legionella pneumophila*
      c. *Streptobacillus moniliformis*
      d. *Helicobacter pylori*

Answers
1. c   2. c

Spirochetes: Treponema, Borrelia and Leptospira

CHAPTER 34

CHAPTER PREVIEW
- Treponema
- Borrelia
- Leptospira

SPIROCHETES

Spirochetes are thin, flexible, elongated spirally coiled helical bacilli; e.g. *Treponema*, *Borrelia* and *Leptospira*.

Treponema pallidum (Syphilis)

Treponema pallidum is the causative agent of a sexually transmitted infection called as syphilis. It is a genitoulcerative disease, transmitted by sexual contact, but rarely by non-venereal modes such as direct contact, blood transfusion or transplacental transmission. The incubation period is about 9-90 days.

Clinical Stages

The clinical course of syphilis passes through four clinical stages.

1. **Primary syphilis:** It is characterized by:
   - *Genital ulcer:* Painless, firm, non-suppurative genital ulcers (called hard chancre), and
   - *Lymphadenopathy* (usually inguinal): Painless firm, non-suppurative, and often bilateral.
2. **Secondary syphilis:** It usually develops 6–12 weeks after the healing of the primary lesion. It presents as:
   - *Skin rashes* on palms and soles
   - Mucosal patches
   - *Condylomata lata:* Mucocutaneous papules are seen in the perianal region, vulva, and scrotum.
3. **Latent syphilis**: It is a clinically silent phase between secondary and late syphilis. It is characterized by the absence of clinical manifestations with positive serological tests for syphilis
4. **Late syphilis:** It occurs several decades after the initial infection, and is associated with skin, CVS, and CNS manifestations
   - *Skin lesions* are called gummata: They are destructive granulomatous lesions
   - *CVS manifestations:* It is characterized by aneurysm of ascending aorta and aortic regurgitation
   - *CNS manifestations:* Common manifestations include—chronic meningitis, general paresis of the insane, and tabes dorsalis.

Congenital syphilis: Mother-to-fetus transmission can lead to the development of various congenital manifestations such as—Hutchinson's teeth (notched central incisors), mulberry-shaped molar, saddle nose, etc.

Laboratory Diagnosis

Syphilis is mainly diagnosed by the following diagnostic modalities.

Direct Microscopy

Treponemes can be demonstrated from the superficial lesions of primary, secondary, and congenital syphilis. The surface of the genital ulcer is cleaned with saline, gentle pressure is applied at the base of the lesion, and a drop of exudate is collected on a slide and examined by any of the following methods:

- Dark ground microscopy (DGM): *T. pallidum* appears as slender, flexible, spirally coiled bacilli with tapering ends, measuring 6-20 μm in length and contains 6-20 spirals **(Fig. 34.1A)**. *T. pallidum* shows typical slow to rapid *flexion-extension* type of movement with rotation around its longitudinal axis (corkscrew motility).
- The **sensitivity** of DGM approaches 80% with a detection limit of 10^4 bacilli/mL
- Direct fluorescent antibody staining for *T. pallidum* (DFA-TP): Sensitivity of DFA-TP test approaches 100% when smear made from fresh lesions are examined
- Silver impregnation staining—such as Levaditi stain and Fontana stain: *Treponema* do not take up ordinary stains as they are extremely thin and delicate. Therefore, silver impregnation methods can be used to increase their thickness **(Fig. 34.1B)**.

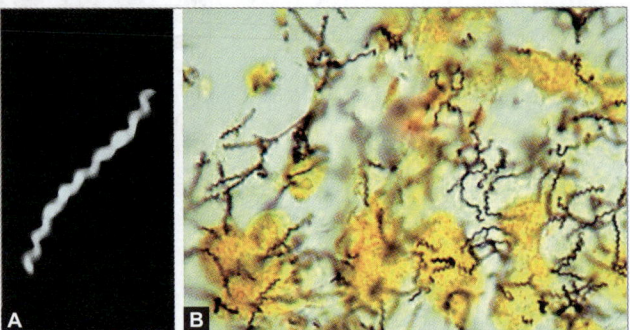

Figs. 34.1 A and B: Direct microscopy of *T. pallidum:* **A.** Dark ground microscope; **B.** Silver impregnation method.

Source: Public Health Image Library, **A.** ID# 2043; **B.** ID# 836, Centers for Disease Control and Prevention (CDC), Atlanta (*with permission*).

Cultivation

Pathogenic treponemes including *T. pallidum* cannot be grown in artificial culture media but are maintained by subcultures in susceptible animals such as rabbit testes (e.g. Nichols strain).

Serology (Antibody Detection)

As microscopy is difficult and culture methods are not available, antibody detection methods are of paramount importance in the diagnosis of syphilis. Depending upon the type of antigen used, two types of tests are available to detect antibodies in a patient's sera.

Non-treponemal Tests

These tests detect non-specific reagin antibody by using cardiolipin antigen derived from the bovine heart. The sensitivity of treponemal tests varies from 78 to 85% in primary stage, 100% in secondary stage, 94–96% in late stage and the specificity is around 97–99%. These tests work on the principle of slide flocculation (precipitation reaction).

- ❖ **Venereal disease research laboratory (VDRL) test:** 50 µL of patient's serum (heat inactivated) is mixed with a drop of VDRL antigen on a concave slide, which is then mixed by rotating the slide for 4 minutes
    - **Positive test** (i.e. reactive) is indicated by formation of medium to large clumps of antigen antibody complexes; visualized by focusing the slide under microscope (10x) **(Figs. 34.2A and B)**
    - **CSF antibodies:** VDRL test can also be performed on CSF specimen to detect antibodies
    - **Uses:** VDRL test is cheaper and preferred as a screening test and for batch testing (e.g. antenatal screening) and also to monitor treatment response.
- ❖ **Rapid plasma reagin (RPR):** It is another slide flocculation test using disposable plastic cards having

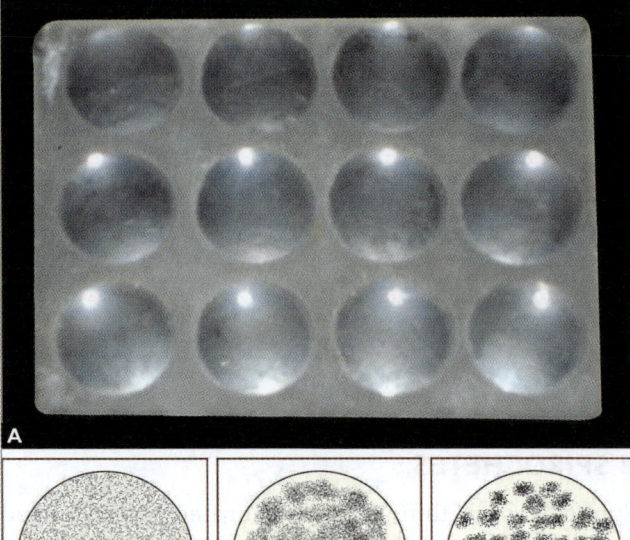
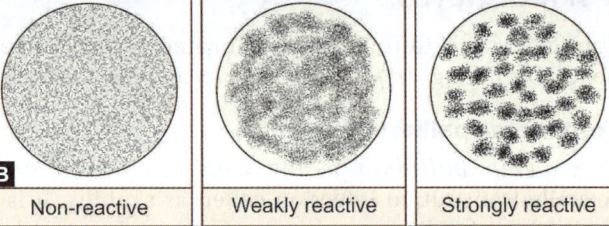

Figs. 34.2A and B: A. VDRL slide; **B.** VDRL test results.

Source: Department of Microbiology, JIPMER, Puducherry (*with permission*).

clearly defined circles. It is similar to VDRL test with some differences such as:
- RPR antigen has a prolonged shelf-life, therefore it is preferred to test individual sample (less sample load); where as VDRL is preferred for large sample load
- In RPR, finely divided carbon particles coated with cardiolipin antigens are used, hence results can be read with naked eyes, without the need of a microscope
- It can only be used for detecting antibodies in blood; not in CSF
- It is more expensive than VDRL.

Treponemal Tests

These tests detect species-specific antibody by using *T. pallidum*-specific antigen; which is polysaccharide in nature. The sensitivity of treponemal tests varies from 84 to 90% in primary stage, 100% in secondary stage, 94–96% in late stage and the specificity is around 97–99%. Various tests are:

- ❖ TPI: *T. pallidum* immobilization test
- ❖ FTA-ABS: Fluorescent treponemal antibody absorption test
- ❖ TPHA: *T. pallidum* hemagglutination test
- ❖ TPPA: *T. pallidum* particle agglutination test
- ❖ Western blot and enzyme immunoassay.

Diagnosis of Congenital Syphilis
- **Definitive diagnosis:** Demonstration of *T. pallidum* by dark ground microscopy (DGM) of umbilical cord, placenta, nasal discharge, or skin lesion material provides the definitive diagnosis
- **Presumptive diagnosis:** Infant born to a mother who had syphilis at the time of delivery regardless of findings in the infant *and* reactive treponemal test in infant *plus* clinical signs/symptoms of congenital syphilis or reactive IgM antibody test specific for syphilis (IgM FTA ABS or IgM ELISA).

Testing Algorithm
CDC recommends to use a **testing algorithm** comprising of non-treponemal test (as screening test), followed by treponemal test (for confirmation) for serodiagnosis of syphilis. Every pregnant woman should undergo a non-treponemal screening test at her first antenatal visit and, if there is high-risk of exposure, again retested at the third trimester and at delivery.

> **TREATMENT** — Syphilis
>
> Penicillin is the drug of choice for treating all stages of syphilis. Doxycycline can be used alternatively in case of penicillin allergy.

Nonvenereal Treponema species

Endemic or nonvenereal treponematoses are caused by three close relatives of *T. pallidum;* producing primary mucocutaneous lesions in non-genital sites (e.g. extremities, oral mucosa).
- *T. pertenue:* Causes yaws
- *T. endemicum*: Causes endemic syphilis
- *T. carateum:* Causes pinta.

Borrelia species

Most of the species of *Borrelia* occur as commensals on the buccal and genital mucosa. Few are pathogenic to man, such as:
- *B. recurrentis* causes epidemic relapsing fever
- *B. duttonii* and *B. hermsii* cause endemic relapsing fever
- *B. burgdorferi* is the agent of Lyme disease
- *B. vincentii* causes Vincent's angina in association with fusiform bacilli.

Relapsing Fever

Relapsing fever (RF) is characterized by recurrent episodes of fever and nonspecific symptoms following exposure to insect vector carrying *Borrelia* species. Relapsing fever is of two types:
1. **Epidemic RF:** It is caused by *B. recurrentis* and transmitted by louse
2. **Endemic RF** is caused by *B. duttonii* and *B. hermsii*. It is transmitted by tick.

Clinical Manifestations
Presence of recurrent febrile episodes lasting for 3–5 days occur intervening with afebrile periods of 4–14 days. Petechiae, epistaxis and blood-tinged sputum occur in epidemic RF.

Laboratory Diagnosis
- **Microscopy:** Various methods are available to detect *Borrelia* from blood: (i) Peripheral thick or thin smear-stained by Wright- or Giemsa-stain, (ii) Direct fluorescent antibody test and (iii) Dark ground microscopy to demonstrate motile spirochetes
- **Culture:** The confirmation is made by isolation of *Borrelia* from blood
- **Serology:** Done for detection of antibodies by ELISA and IFA (indirect fluorescence assay)
- **Molecular methods:** Multiplex real-time PCR has been developed to identify various species of *Borrelia* causing RF.

Treatment
Antibiotics such as doxycycline or erythromycin are the drug of choice for relapsing fever.

Lyme Disease

Lyme disease is caused by *Borrelia burgdorferi*. It is transmitted by **tick bite**. It presents as an annular maculopapular lesion develops at the site of the tick bite called **erythema migrans**, and later presents as disseminated and persistent infection.
- **Diagnosis** is by isolation of the bacterial agent from skin lesions, or blood in a special medium called BSK (Barbour-Stoenner-Kelly) medium or serum antibody detection by ELISA and western blot.
- **Treatment:** Oral doxycycline is the drug of choice.

Leptospira interrogans

Leptospira interrogans is the causative agent of leptospirosis; a zoonotic disease transmitted, by direct contact with the urine of infected animals such as rodents.

Leptospira interrogans is antigenically complex and comprises 26 serogroups; which are further typed into >300 serovars. The serogroups and serovars differ in their geographical distribution and severity of infection.

Clinical Manifestations

Leptospira interrogans produces two types of illnesses.
- The majority (90%) of leptospirosis cases present as mild anicteric febrile illness

Laboratory Diagnosis

Laboratory diagnosis of leptospirosis involves the following modalities. Specimens include blood and CSF (in the early stage) and urine (in the late stage).

- ❖ **Dark ground microscopy** of clinical specimens such as blood or CSF reveals 6–12 μm long, tightly and regularly coiled bacilli, with characteristic hooked ends like umbrella handle (hence the species name *interrogans*—resembling interrogation or question mark) **(Figs. 34.3A and B)**
- ❖ **Culture:** As *Leptospira* is highly fastidious, requires enriched media such as—(1) **EMJH liquid medium** (Ellinghausen, McCullough, Johnson, Harris), (2) **Korthof's** medium, and (3) **Fletcher's** semisolid medium. Cultures should be incubated at 30°C for 4–6 weeks.
- ❖ **Serology for antibody detection:** Various tests are available such as
  - *Genus specific tests:* Latex agglutination test, ELISA, and ICT (immunochromatographic test)
  - *Serovar specific test:* **Microscopic agglutination test**. It detects antibodies against specific serovars of *L. interrogans* **(Fig. 34.3A)**. It serves as the gold standard reference method for the diagnosis of leptospirosis.

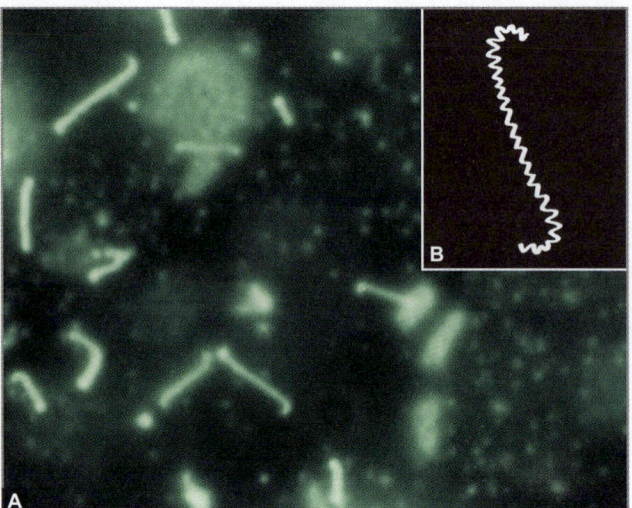

Figs. 34.3A and B: *Leptospira interrogans* (spirally coiled bacilli with hooked ends): **A.** Dark ground microscopy of the mount following microscopic agglutination test; **B.** Schematic diagram (viewed under a dark-ground microscope).
Source: **A.** Public Health Image Library/ID#: 2888/ Mrs M Gatton, Centers for Disease Control and Prevention (CDC), Atlanta (*with permission*).

- ❖ Few cases (10%) progress to severe form hepatorenal hemorrhagic syndrome or **Weil's disease**; characterized by icterus, high-grade fever, hemorrhagic manifestations, and impaired renal functions.

TREATMENT — Leptospirosis

Oral doxycycline is given for mild leptospirosis; whereas severe cases are treated with penicillin.

EXPECTED QUESTIONS

I. Write short notes on:
1. Clinical manifestations of syphilis.
2. Laboratory diagnosis of syphilis.
3. Laboratory diagnosis of borreliosis.
4. Laboratory diagnosis of leptospirosis.

II. Multiple Choice Questions (MCQs):
1. **Weil's disease is caused by:**
   a. *Leptospira interrogans*
   b. *Borrelia recurrentis*
   c. *Orientia tsutsugamushi*
   d. *Mycoplasma pneumoniae*
2. **VDRL test is done for:**
   a. Leptospirosis
   b. Lyme disease
   c. Scrub typhus
   d. Syphilis
3. **Lyme disease is caused by:**
   a. *Leptospira interrogans*
   b. *Borrelia recurrentis*
   c. *Borrelia vincenti*
   d. *Borrelia burgdorferi*
4. **All of the following are culture media recommended for isolation of *Leptospira*, except:**
   a. EMJH liquid medium
   b. Korthof's medium
   c. Fletcher's medium
   d. Potassium tellurite agar

Answers
1. a 2. d 3. d 4. d

Rickettsiae, Chlamydiae and Mycoplasma

CHAPTER 35

CHAPTER PREVIEW
- Rickettsiae
- Chlamydiae
- Mycoplasma

■ RICKETTSIAE AND RELATED GENERA

Rickettsiaceae comprise of two genera—*Rickettsia* and *Orientia*; both possess the following properties:
- They are obligate intracellular organisms
- They are not cultivable in artificial media, although they can grow in cell lines, or by animal and egg inoculation
- They are transmitted by arthropod vectors, such as tick, mite, flea, or louse.

The various members of Rickettsiae are:
- *R. prowazekii:* It is the causative agent of epidemic typhus, transmitted by louse
- *R. typhi:* It causes endemic typhus, transmitted by flea
- *R. rickettsii:* It is the causative agent of Rocky Mountain spotted fever, transmitted by tick
- *R. conorii:* It causes Indian tick typhus, transmitted by tick
- *R. akari:* It is the causative agent of rickettsialpox, transmitted by mite
- *Orientia tsutsugamushi:* It is the causative agent of scrub typhus, transmitted by mite.

Rickettsiae

Rickettsiae can be categorized into two groups based on the clinical manifestations as:
1. Typhus group
2. Spotted fever group.

Epidemic Typhus (Louse-borne)

Epidemic typhus is caused by *R. prowazekii*. The vector for epidemic typhus is human body louse. Man gets infection by rubbing or scratching of abraded skin or mucosa contaminated by louse feces.
- **Clinical manifestations:** Epidemic typhus is an acute febrile disease; accompanied by headache, myalgia, eye discharge and rashes (generalized except for the face, palms and soles).
- **Brill–Zinsser disease:** It is a recrudescent illness occurring years after acute epidemic typhus.

Endemic Typhus (Flea-borne)

Endemic (murine) typhus is caused by *R. typhi*. The vector for endemic typhus is rat flea (*Xenopsylla cheopis*). It is transmitted by rubbing or scratching on skin or inhalation of flea's dried feces. Symptoms are similar to epidemic typhus but milder and rarely fatal.

Rocky Mountain Spotted Fever

Rocky Mountain spotted fever (RMSF) is caused by *Rickettsia rickettsii*.
- It is transmitted by the bite of an infected tick. Ticks serve as vector as well as reservoir.
- RMS fever is an acute potentially fatal disease characterized by fever, headache, rash (typically on extremities), myalgia and anorexia.
- Complications such as vascular damage, disseminated intravascular coagulation, interstitial pneumonitis, and CNS involvement may occur.

Rickettsialpox

Rickettsialpox is caused by *Rickettsia akari*. Transmitted by bite of infected mites. Mice are the principal reservoir of *R. akari*. Clinical manifestations include—vesicular rashes, eschar (painless black crusted lesions) at the site of mite bite and regional lymphadenopathy.

Scrub Typhus (Orientia)

Scrub typhus is caused by *Orientia tsutsugamushi* (formerly classified under *Rickettsia*). Scrub typhus is so named because as it can occur in areas where scrub vegetations consisting of low lying trees and bushes are encountered. It is transmitted by the bite of infected trombiculid mites. The larval stage (called **chiggers**) are the only stage that feed on humans. Hence it is also called as **chiggerosis**.

- **Clinical manifestations:** The classic presentation of scrub typhus consists of triad of an eschar (at the site of bite), regional lymphadenopathy and maculopapular rash. Complications such as encephalitis and interstitial pneumonia may occur rarely in the late stage.
- **Zoonotic tetrad:** Four elements are essential to maintain *O. tsutsugamushi* in nature:
  1. Trombiculid mites
  2. Small mammals (e.g. field mice, rats, shrews)
  3. Secondary scrub vegetations or forests
  4. Wet season (when mites lay eggs).
- **Indian scenario:** Scrub typhus is a re-emerging infectious disease in India. It is the most common rickettsial disease in India; prevalent in many parts of the country such as sub-Himalayan belt, Maharashtra, Karnataka, Tamil Nadu, Pondicherry and Kerala.

The laboratory diagnosis and treatment of scrub typhus is mentioned under laboratory diagnosis and treatment of all rickettsial infections.

Other Genera related to Rickettsiae

Other genera related to *Rickettsia* are:
- ***Ehrlichia:*** It produces an acute febrile illness called ehrlichiosis, transmitted by ticks. It infects leukocytes such as granulocytes, monocytes; producing intracellular inclusions, called **morula**
- ***Coxiella burnetii:*** It causes **Q fever**, transmitted by inhalational mode; characterized by atypical pneumonia, hepatitis and on chronic stage, produces endocarditis. Rashes are typically absent
- ***Bartonella:*** It has there important species, which are associated with distinct clinical conditions
  - *B. bacilliformis* is the causative agent of a systemic disease called Carrion's disease and a local cutaneous lesion called verruga peruana
  - *B. quintana* causes trench fever
  - *B. henselae* is the agent of cat-scratch disease.

Laboratory Diagnosis

Laboratory diagnosis of rickettsial infection includes:
- **Weil Felix test:** It is a heterophile agglutination test, where rickettsial antibodies are detected by using non-specific cross-reacting *Proteus* antigens such as OX2, OX19, and OXK antigens.
  - In epidemic and endemic typhus—sera agglutinate mainly with OX19 and sometimes with OX2
  - In tick-borne spotted fever—antibodies to both OX19 and OX2 are elevated
  - In scrub typhus—antibodies to OXK are raised
  - The test is negative in rickettsialpox, Q fever, ehrlichiosis and bartonellosis.
- **Specific antibody detection:**
  - **ELISA (IgM capture ELISA):** It is useful in early diagnosis (<1 week) with excellent sensitivity and specificity
  - **Indirect immunofluorescence antibody (IFA):** It is specific, considered as the gold standard serological test.

TREATMENT — Rickettsial infections

Doxycycline is the drug of choice in the majority of rickettsial infections.

■ CHLAMYDIAE

Chlamydiae are obligate intracellular bacteria that cause a spectrum of diseases in man infecting the eye, genital organs, and lungs.

Clinical Manifestations

Chlamydiae have three pathogenic species infecting man, which are associated with various clinical manifestations.

Chlamydia trachomatis

Chlamydia trachomatis comprise of 19 serovars, which cause various infections in man such as:
- **Trachoma:** It is a type of chronic keratoconjunctivitis, caused by serotypes A, B, and C
- **Genital chlamydiasis:** Caused by serotypes D to K, presents as urethral discharge (urethritis) and mucopurulent cervicitis, etc.
- **Inclusion conjunctivitis:** Caused by serotypes D to K. It presents as mucopurulent discharge from the eyes. It can affect adults (swimming pool conjunctivitis) or neonates (ophthalmia neonatorum)
- **Infant pneumonia:** Caused by serotypes D to K, presents as interstitial pneumonia in infants
- **LGV (lymphogranuloma venerum):** It is a sexually transmitted infection, caused by serotypes L1, L2, and L3. It is characterized by painless genital ulcers and painful inguinal lymphadenopathy.

Chlamydia psittaci

It is a pathogen of birds. Infection in man can range from mild influenza-like syndrome to fatal atypical pneumonia. It comprises of several serotypes.

Chlamydia pneumoniae

C. pneumoniae is an exclusively human pathogen. It has only one serotype. It is transmitted from person to person by inhalation route. It causes various manifestations.

- Atypical pneumonia (interstitial) pneumonia; accounting for 10% of cases of community-acquired pneumonia
- Upper respiratory tract involvement is frequent, such as pharyngitis and sinusitis
- **Atherosclerosis:** There is a strong evidence of association between *C. pneumoniae* and atherosclerosis of coronary arteries
- **Asthma and COPD:** *C. pneumoniae* may cause exacerbations of bronchial asthma and COPD (chronic obstructive pulmonary disease).

Laboratory Diagnosis

Specimens collected depend upon the types of infection associated—(1) Scrapings or swabs from infected sites: Urethral swab for urethritis, endocervical swab for cervicitis, or conjunctival swabs for ocular infections, (2) Nasopharyngeal aspirate and respiratory secretions for suspected pneumonia, or (3) Bubo aspirate for LGV.

- **Microscopy:** Useful for detection of chlamydial inclusion bodies. Common staining methods used are Gram staining, Lugol's iodine, and direct immunofluorescence test
- **Antigen detection:** Enzyme immunoassays are available for the detection of LPS antigens
- **Culture:** It was the gold standard method in the past. Various culture methods available are:
  - Egg inoculation (yolk sac)
  - Mice inoculation
  - Cell line culture by using McCoy, HeLa (for *C. trachomatis*), or HEp2 (for *C. pneumoniae*).
- **Nucleic acid amplification tests (NAAT)**, e.g. PCR
  - This is considered as the most sensitive and specific method
  - Currently the diagnostic assay of choice for chlamydial infections.
- **Serology (antibody detection):** Two formats are available
  - ELISA using group-specific LPS antigen
  - Microimmunofluorescence test detects antibody against species and serovar-specific MOMP (major outer membrane protein) antigen of *C. trachomatis*.

TREATMENT — Chlamydial infections

- Azithromycin is the drug of choice
- Alternatively, doxycycline, tetracycline, erythromycin or ofloxacin can be used.

Prevention

Control measures for the prevention of chlamydial genital infections include:

- Periodic screening of high-risk groups, such as young women having multiple sex partners
- Treatment of both the sex partners
- Use of barrier methods of contraception such as condoms
- Abstain from sex till 7 days after starting the treatment.

MYCOPLASMA

Mycoplasmas are the smallest microbes capable of free-living in the environment. They were previously called as **pleuropneumonia-like organisms (PPLO)** and **Eaton's agent**. They lack rigid cell wall and therefore, are resistant to cell wall-acting antibiotics such as beta-lactams.

General Properties

- They resemble the viruses in certain properties such as: very small in size (50–350 nm), filterable by bacterial filters
- They differ from viruses as: They are **free living** in the environment and can grow on artificial cell-free culture media
- They are highly pleomorphic, exist in coccoid, bacillary or filamentous or even in helical forms
- They are poorly gram-negative, better stained by Giemsa stain
- They exhibit **gliding motility** due to their specialized tip structures
- Mycoplasmas are common contaminants of continuous cell lines, thus interfere with the growth of viruses in cell cultures
- **L-form:** As mycoplasmas lack cell wall permanently, it has been suggested that mycoplasmas may represent stable L-forms of bacteria.

Mycoplasma pneumoniae

M. pneumoniae is the pathogenic species, which is the causative agent of **primary atypical pneumonia** (community acquired pneumonia).

- **Clinical manifestations:** *M. pneumoniae* produces upper respiratory tract infection (manifests as pharyngitis,

SECTION 4 ◆ Systematic Bacteriology

tracheobronchitis), **atypical pneumonia** (community acquired interstitial pneumonia) and extrapulmonary manifestations (e.g. septic arthritis, Guillain-Barre syndrome or neurologic manifestations)

❖ **Laboratory diagnosis** include—(i) Detection of antibodies (e.g. ELISA), (ii) isolation of the organism in specific culture media such as PPLO broth [produces **fried egg appearance** colonies **(Fig. 35.1)**], (iii) accurate species identification from colonies is made by biochemical tests or by automated identification systems such as MALDI-TOF and (iv) antigenic detection by direct IF and antigen capture ELISA.

❖ **Treatment:** Macrolides are the drug of choice.

Urogenital mycoplasmas

These include *M. hominis*, *M. genitalium* and *Ureaplasma urealyticum*. They cause urethritis. Culture and PCR are the useful methods for diagnosis. Macrolides are the drug of choice.

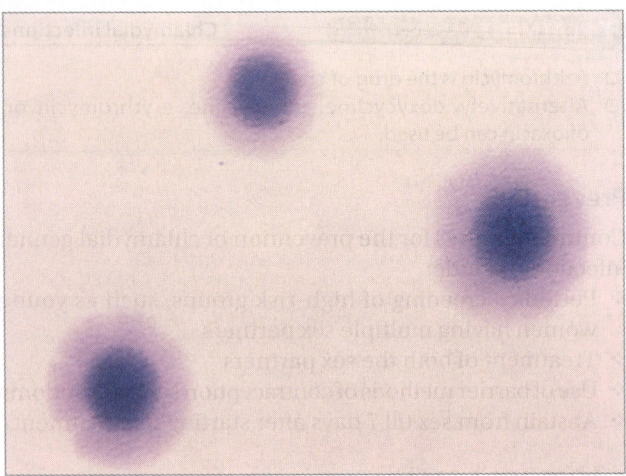

Fig. 35.1: *Mycoplasma* colonies (typical fried egg appearance).
Source: Public Health Image Library, ID# 11024/Dr E Arum; Dr N Jacobs/Centers for Disease Control and Prevention (CDC), Atlanta (*with permission*).

EXPECTED QUESTIONS

I. Write short notes on:
1. Infections produced by Chlamydiae.
2. Laboratory diagnosis of rickettsial infections.
3. *Mycoplasma* infections.

II. Multiple Choice Questions (MCQs):
1. Selective medium for isolating *Mycoplasma* is _____.
   a. Lowenstein-Jensen medium
   b. Buffered charcoal, yeast extract agar
   c. Levinthal agar
   d. PPLO medium
2. Which of the following is associated with pathogenesis of atherosclerosis?
   a. *M. pneumoniae*
   b. *C. psittaci*
   c. *C. pneumoniae*
   d. *Legionella*
3. Primary atypical pneumonia is caused by:
   a. *Leptospira interrogans*
   b. *Borrelia recurrentis*
   c. *Mycoplasma pneumoniae*
   d. *Orientia tsutsugamushi*
4. Mode of transmission of scrub typhus is by:
   a. Bite of chiggers
   b. Rubbing of tick feces into skin abrasion
   c. Bite of lice
   d. Bite of flea
5. Drug of choice of scrub typhus is:
   a. Chloramphenicol
   b. Ceftriaxone
   c. Doxycycline
   d. Ciprofloxacin

Answers
1. d   2. c   3. c   4. a   5. c

SECTION 5: Virology

SECTION OUTLINE

36. General Virology
37. Herpesviruses
38. Other DNA Viruses (including Bacteriophage)
39. Myxoviruses and Rubella Virus
40. Coronaviruses
41. Arboviruses
42. Rabies Virus
43. Picornaviruses (Poliovirus, Coxsackievirus and Rhinovirus)
44. HIV/AIDS
45. Hepatitis Viruses
46. Miscellaneous RNA Viruses: Agents of Viral Gastroenteritis, Ebola Virus, Rodent-borne Viruses, Oncogenic Viruses, Slow Viruses and Prions

General Virology

CHAPTER 36

CHAPTER PREVIEW
- Morphology of Virus
- Classification
- Viral Replication
- Pathogenesis of Viral Infections
- Laboratory Diagnosis of Viral Diseases
- Treatment
- Immunoprophylaxis

Viruses are the smallest unicellular organisms that are obligate intracellular. They differ from bacteria and other prokaryotes in many ways.
- They possess either DNA (deoxyribonucleic acid) or RNA (ribonucleic acid), but never both
- They cannot be grown on artificial cell-free media
- They do not have a cell wall or cell membrane or cellular organelles
- They lack the enzymes necessary for protein and nucleic acid synthesis
- They are not susceptible to antibacterial antibiotics.

MORPHOLOGY OF VIRUS

The virus particle comprises a **nucleic acid** surrounded by a protein coat called as **capsid**, together known as the nucleocapsid. Some viruses also have an outer **envelope** (**Figs. 36.1A and B**).
- **Nucleic acid:** Viruses have only one type of nucleic acid, either DNA or RNA but never both. Accordingly, they are classified as DNA viruses and RNA viruses. The nucleic acid may be single or double-stranded, segmented, or unsegmented
- **Capsid:** It is composed of several protein subunits called capsomeres. It protects the nucleic acid core from the external environment
- **Symmetry:** It is the arrangement of capsomeres with respect to the surrounding nucleic acid, which can be of three types:
  1. *Icosahedral symmetry:* The capsomeres are arranged surrounding the nucleic acid in a cubical shape; e.g. all DNA viruses (except poxviruses) and most of the RNA viruses (**Fig. 36.1A**)
  2. *Helical symmetry:* The capsomeres are coiled surrounding the nucleic acid in the form of a helix or spiral. Examples include—myxoviruses, rhabdoviruses, etc. (**Fig. 36.1B**)
  3. *Complex symmetry:* Poxviruses possess complex symmetry.

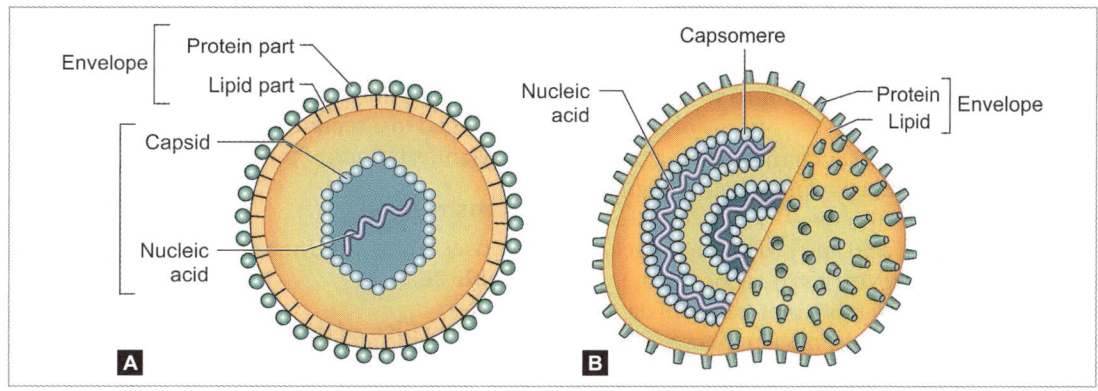

Figs. 36.1A and B: Structure and symmetry of virus: **A.** Enveloped virus with icosahedral nucleocapsid; **B.** Enveloped virus with helical nucleocapsid.

- **Envelope:** Certain viruses possess an envelope surrounding the nucleocapsid.
  - The envelope is lipoprotein in nature. The protein spikes (called peplomeres) are embedded into the lipid layer
  - Peplomers bind to specific receptors on the host cells, thus facilitating the entry of the virus
  - Peplomers are antigenic; therefore, antibodies against them are protective
  - **Examples** of enveloped viruses include—influenza virus, hepatitis B, and coronavirus.
- **Size of the viruses:** Viruses are extremely small, and vary from 20–400 nm in size. The smallest virus is parvovirus (20 nm) and the largest is poxvirus (400 nm)
- **Shape of the viruses:** Mostly animal viruses are spherical shaped, with some exceptions:
  - Rabies virus: Bullet-shaped
  - Poxvirus: Brick-shaped
  - Adenovirus: Space vehicle-shaped
  - Rotavirus: Wheel-shaped.

CLASSIFICATION

There are various DNA and RNA virus groups, which further comprise several important viruses infecting humans as enlisted in **Table 36.1**.

VIRAL REPLICATION

Viruses undergo a complex way of cell division. Replication of viruses passes through seven sequential steps:

> Attachment → Penetration → Uncoating → Biosynthesis → Assembly → Maturation → Release.

1. **Adsorption/attachment:** It is the most specific step of viral replication. It involves receptor interactions between virus and host surface receptors
2. **Penetration:** After attachment, the virus particles penetrate into the host cells
3. **Uncoating:** Lysis of capsid due to host lysozymes and release of the nucleic acid
4. **Biosynthesis** of various viral components: i) nucleic acid, ii) capsid protein, iii) enzymes iv) other regulatory proteins
5. **Assembly:** Viral nucleic acid and proteins are packaged together to form progeny viruses (nucleocapsids)
6. **Maturation:** Following assembly, maturation of daughter virions takes place either in the nucleus or cytoplasm, or membranes
7. **Release** of daughter virions occurs either by:
   - Lysis of the host cells
   - Budding through the host cell membrane.

Table 36.1: Important DNA and RNA viruses infecting humans.

DNA virus groups	DNA viruses
Herpesviruses	Herpes simplex virus 1 and 2, Varicella-zoster virus, Cytomegalovirus (CMV), Epstein-Barr virus (EBV), Human herpesvirus-6, 7 and 8
Poxviruses (largest virus in size)	Variola virus (smallpox), Molluscum contageosum virus
Papovaviruses	Human papillomavirus
Parvoviruses (smallest virus in size)	Parvovirus B19
Hepadnavirus	Hepatitis B virus
Adenoviruses	Human adenovirus
RNA virus groups	**RNA viruses**
Myxoviruses	Influenza viruses–A, B, and C Parainfluenza viruses, mumps virus, measles virus, respiratory syncytial virus, Nipah virus
Coronaviruses	Coronaviruses (SARS-CoV, MERS-CoV and SARS-CoV-2)
Arboviruses	Dengue virus, yellow fever virus, chikungunya virus, Kyasanur forest disease virus, Japanese B encephalitis virus, Zika virus
Retroviruses	HIV (human immunodeficiency virus)
Rabies virus	Rabies virus
Picornaviruses	Poliovirus, Coxsackievirus, enterovirus, rhinovirus
RNA hepatitis viruses	Hepatitis A, C, D, E viruses
RNA viruses causing gastroenteritis	Rotavirus, calicivirus, Norwalk virus, astrovirus
Miscellaneous RNA viruses	Filoviruses–Marburg virus and Ebola virus, Rubella virus

PATHOGENESIS OF VIRAL INFECTIONS

Most of the viral infections progress through the following steps inside the human body:
- Transmission (entry into the body)
- Primary site of replication
- Spread to a secondary site
- Manifestations of the disease.

Transmission

Viruses enter the human body through various routes **(Table 36.2)**.

Primary Site of Replication

- Some viruses are restricted to the portal of entry where they multiply and produce local diseases
- On the other hand, most of the viruses first multiply locally to initiate a silent local infection, which is followed

CHAPTER 36 ◆ General Virology

Table 36.2: Mode of transmission of viruses.	
Transmission	Viruses
Respiratory route (probably the most common route)	• Myxoviruses such as influenza virus • Coronaviruses such as SARS-CoV-2 • Rhinovirus • Varicella-zoster virus • Cytomegalovirus • Rubella virus • Parvovirus • Smallpox virus
Oral route	• Rotavirus and other viral agents causing gastroenteritis • Poliovirus and other enteroviruses • Hepatitis viruses—A and E
Cutaneous route	• Herpes simplex virus-1 • Human papillomavirus • Molluscum contagiosum virus
Vector bite	Arboviruses such as: • Dengue virus (*Aedes*) • Chikungunya virus (*Aedes*) • Japanese encephalitis virus (*Culex*) • Yellow fever virus and Zika virus (*Aedes*) • Kyasanur Forest disease virus (Tick)
Animal bite	Rabies virus
Sexual route	• Herpes simplex virus-2 • Human papillomavirus • Hepatitis B, C and rarely D viruses • Human immunodeficiency virus (HIV)
Blood transfusion	• Hepatitis B, C and rarely D viruses • HIV
Needlestick injury	• Hepatitis B, C and rarely D viruses • HIV
Mother-to-child transmission (including transplacental route)	• Rubella virus • Cytomegalovirus • Herpes simplex virus • Varicella-zoster virus • Parvovirus B19 • Hepatitis B and C viruses • HIV

by the spread via lymphatics to regional lymph nodes (most viruses) or via blood (e.g. poliovirus) or via neuronal spread to reach the central nervous system or CNS (e.g. rabies virus).

Spread of Virus

- **Primary viremia:** Viruses spread to the bloodstream either from the primary sites or from the lymph nodes
- **Secondary site of replication:** Viruses are then transported to the reticuloendothelial system (bone marrow, endothelial cells, spleen and liver) where further multiplication takes place
- **Secondary viremia:** From the spleen and liver, viruses spill over into the bloodstream leading to secondary viremia which results in the onset of non-specific symptoms
- **Target organs:** Via the bloodstream, they reach the target organs (lung, brain, skin, etc.). Certain viruses (e.g. rabies) affect the brain, there is no viremia. Instead, the virus reaches the target organ via neuronal spread
- **Tropism** of the viruses for specific organs determines the pattern of systemic illness; e.g. hepatitis viruses have tropism for hepatocytes and thus produce hepatitis
- **Shedding:** Following infection viruses escape the host by shedding either at the portal of entry (e.g. influenza virus in respiratory secretions) or in the blood (e.g. dengue virus) or near the target organ (e.g. salivary gland for mumps).

Manifestations of Viral Infections

- **Incubation period:** It is the time interval between the entry of the virus into the body and the appearance of the first clinical manifestation
  - The incubation period is shorter if the virus produces lesions near the site of entry, e.g. influenza virus
  - It is longer if the target organ is much far from the site of entry, e.g. poliovirus and rabies virus.
- **Clinical manifestations:** Persons infected with viruses develop either an inapparent (subclinical) infection or apparent (clinical) infection. The symptoms developed depend on the target body sites where the virus multiplies
  - Respiratory viruses such as influenza and coronaviruses produce respiratory infections
  - Gastroenteritis: Produced by rotavirus
  - Neurotropic viruses can produce meningitis (enteroviruses) or encephalitis (rabies)
  - Hepatitis viruses produce hepatitis

LABORATORY DIAGNOSIS OF VIRAL DISEASES

Laboratory diagnosis of viral infections is useful for the following purposes:

- **To start antiviral drugs** for infections caused by herpes, CMV, HIV, influenza viruses, etc.
- **Screening of blood donors** for HIV, hepatitis B, and hepatitis C helps in the prevention of transfusion-transmitted infections
- **Surveillance purpose:** To assess the disease burden in the community
- **For outbreak or epidemic investigation**: To initiate appropriate control measures
- **To start post-exposure prophylaxis** of antiretroviral drugs to the health care workers following needlestick injury **(Chapter 18)**

- **To initiate certain measures:** For example, if the newborn is diagnosed to have hepatitis B infection, then immunoglobulins (HBIG) should be started within 12 hours of birth.

Direct Demonstration of Virus

- **Electron microscopy:** Detection of viruses by electron microscopy (EM) is increasingly used nowadays. Viruses can be identified based on their distinct appearances; for example:
  - Rabies virus—bullet-shaped
  - Rotavirus—wheel-shaped
  - Coronavirus—petal-shaped peplomers
  - Adenovirus—space vehicle-shaped
  - Astrovirus—star-shaped peplomers.
- **Fluorescent microscopy:** Direct immunofluorescence (Direct-IF) technique is useful to detect viral particles in clinical samples. Its clinical applications are:
  - Diagnosis of rabies virus antigen in skin biopsies, corneal smear of infected patients
  - Rapid diagnosis of respiratory infections caused by influenza virus, rhinoviruses, and respiratory syncytial virus
- **Light microscopy:** It is useful for demonstration of inclusion bodies by histopathological staining of tissue sections, which helps in the diagnosis of certain viral infections (see highlight box below).

> **Inclusion Bodies**
> They are the aggregates of viral proteins and other products of viral replication that confer altered staining property to the host cell.
>
> *Role in Laboratory Diagnosis*
> Inclusion bodies are characteristic of specific viral infections. They have distinct size, shape, location and staining properties by which they can be demonstrated in virus infected cells under the light microscope.
>
> *Location*
> They may be present either in the host cell cytoplasm or nucleus or both
> - **Intracytoplasmic inclusion bodies:** They are seen as pink structures (acidophilic)
>   - Paschen bodies—variola virus
>   - Molluscum bodies—molluscum contagiosum virus
>   - Negri bodies— rabies
> - **Intranuclear inclusion bodies:** They are basophilic.
>   - Cowdry type A inclusions—e.g. Torres body in yellow fever
>   - Cowdry type B inclusions—in poliovirus and adenovirus
> - **Both intracytoplasmic and intranuclear inclusions**—in cytomegalovirus (owl's eye appearance) and measles.

Detection of Viral Antigens

Detection of viral antigens in serum and other samples can be done by techniques such as enzyme-linked immunosorbent assay (ELISA), immunochromatographic test (ICT), enzyme-linked fluorescence assay (ELFA), etc. Some important antigen detection tests include:
- HBsAg antigen detection for hepatitis B virus infection from serum
- SARS-CoV-2 antigen (nucleocapsid protein) detection in nasopharyngeal swabs.

Detection of Viral Antibodies

Antibody detection from serum is one of the most commonly used methods in diagnostic virology. Techniques such as ELISA, ELFA, ICT are widely used. Some important antibody detection tests include:
- Anti-hepatitis C antibodies in serum
- Antibodies against HIV antigens from serum
- Anti-dengue IgM/IgG antibodies from serum.

Molecular Methods

Molecular techniques have eased the diagnosis of viral infections. They are more sensitive, specific and yield quicker results.
- **Polymerase chain reaction (PCR)** is useful to detect viral DNA in clinical specimens
- **Reverse transcriptase-PCR (RT-PCR)** is used for the detection of RNA viruses in clinical specimens
- **Multiplex PCR** can simultaneously detect genes of common organisms responsible for a clinical syndrome; for example, multiplex PCR for respiratory infection simultaneously detects genes of many respiratory viruses in clinical specimens
- **Real time-PCR (rt-PCR):** It is considered as the gold standard method for the diagnosis of several viral infections such as influenza, COVID-19, etc. It has several advantages such as—
  - Quantifying viral nucleic acid in the samples, hence used to monitor the treatment response
  - Takes lesser time
  - More sensitive and specific than PCR.

Isolation of Virus

Viruses cannot be grown on artificial culture media. They are cultivated by animal inoculation, embryonated egg inoculation, or tissue cultures.

Animal Inoculation

Animal inoculation is largely restricted only for research purposes and for limited diagnostic purposes such as—primary isolation of arboviruses and coxsackieviruses.

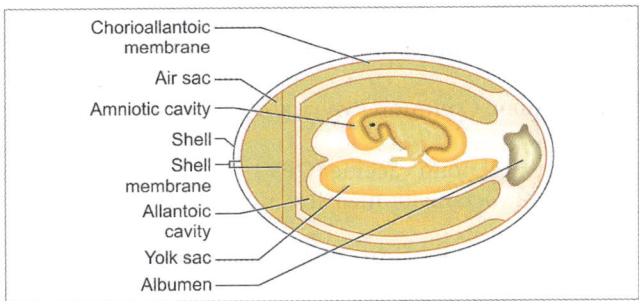

Fig. 36.2: Schematic diagram of an embryonated egg.

Egg Inoculation

Embryonated eggs were first used for viral cultivation by Goodpasture in 1931. Subsequently, this technique was widely used in the past. An embryonated hen's egg has four sites that are specific for the growth of certain viruses (Fig. 36.2).

- **Yolk sac inoculation:** Used for arboviruses (e.g. JE virus) and some bacteria such as *Rickettsia* and *Chlamydia*
- **Amniotic sac:** Used for the isolation of influenza virus
- **Allantoic sac:** It is used for the production of viral vaccines such as—influenza vaccine, yellow fever (17D) vaccine
- **Chorioallantoic membrane:** Used for the isolation of poxviruses. They produce visible lesions over the chorioallantoic membrane called pocks.

Tissue Culture

The tissue culture technique was widely used in the past in diagnostic virology. It is of three types—(i) organ culture, (ii) explant culture, and (iii) cell line culture.

Cell line culture is the only isolation method that is in use now.

Types of Cell Lines

There are three types of cell lines —(i) primary cell lines, (ii) secondary cell lines, and (iii) continuous cell lines.
1. **Primary cell lines:** They are capable of very limited growth in culture, maximum up to 5–10 divisions. Examples include—human amnion cell line and chick embryo cell line
2. **Secondary cell lines:** They can divide a maximum of up to 10–50 divisions. Examples include—human fibroblast cell line and human embryonic lung cell starin
3. **Continuous cell lines:** They are derived from cancerous cell lines, and hence are capable of indefinite growth. Examples include—
    - HeLa cell line (human carcinoma of cervix cell line)
    - Vero cell line (vervet monkey kidney cell line).

Detection of Viral Growth in Cell Cultures

The following methods are used to detect the growth of the virus in cell cultures.
- **Cytopathic effect (CPE):** It is defined as the morphological change produced by the virus in the cell line detected by a light microscope. Examples of CPE effect produced by viruses include—
    - Syncytium formation by the measles virus
    - Granular clumps (like bunches of grapes) by adenovirus
    - Rapid crenation and degeneration of entire cell sheet by enteroviruses.
- **Other methods** to detect viral growth include—
    - Detection of viral antigens by direct immunofluorescence assay
    - Viral genes detection by using PCR
    - Electron microscopy, demonstrating the viruses in infected cell lines.

TREATMENT OF VIRAL DISEASES

Only for limited viral diseases, effective antiviral drugs are available. Commonly used antiviral drugs for viral diseases are as follows:
- Acyclovir for herpes simplex virus and VZV infections
- Ganciclovir for CMV infections
- Oseltamivir for H1N1 flu
- Telbivudine, tenofovir, lamivudine for hepatitis B.

Interferons (IFNs)

IFNs-α, β have antiviral action; produced by many cell types such as macrophages (IFN-α) and fibroblasts (IFN-β). INF-γ does not have antiviral action.
- **Mechanism of action:** IFNs are part of innate immunity; the body's first line of antiviral defense. They are nonspecific in action; produced quickly following viral infection
- **Inducers:** Certain RNA viruses can induce IFN synthesis
- **Application:** IFN-α is used in the following clinical conditions:
    - Topically—used in rhinovirus infection, genital warts, and herpetic keratitis
    - Systemically—used in chronic hepatitis B, C, and D infections.

IMMUNOPROPHYLAXIS FOR VIRAL DISEASES

Viral Vaccines (Active Immunization)

Viral vaccines confer prolonged and effective immunity. Vaccines for viral infections may be available either in live, killed, or subunit forms.

Killed Viral Vaccines

Killed vaccines are available for various viral agents.
- **Preparation:** They are prepared by inactivating viruses with heat, phenol, formalin, or beta-propiolactone
- **Advantages:** They are more stable and are considered safe when given in immunodeficiency or pregnancy
- **Disadvantages:** Killed vaccines are associated with more adverse side effects due to reactogenicity
- **Examples:** Common killed viral vaccines for human use are:
  - Rabies non-neural vaccine—e.g. HDC (human diploid cell) vaccine
  - Killed injectable polio vaccine (IPV).

Subunit Vaccines

In subunit vaccines, only a particular antigen of the virus is used; prepared by DNA recombinant technology, e.g. hepatitis B vaccine.

Live Vaccines

Live vaccines are available for various viral agents.
- **Preparation:** They are prepared by attenuation by serial passages
- **Advantages:** Live vaccines provide a stronger and long-lasting immunity and are administered as a single dose (except OPV)
- **Disadvantages:** Live vaccines are risky in immuno-deficiency or pregnancy. They are less stable than killed vaccines
- **Examples:** Common live viral vaccines for human use are:
  - Live oral polio vaccine (OPV)
  - MMR vaccine for measles, mumps, and rubella.

Passive Immunization (Immunoglobulin)

Passive immunization is indicated when an individual is immunodeficient or when early protection is needed (i.e. for post-exposure prophylaxis). Currently, human immunoglobulins are available for many viral infections such as mumps, measles, hepatitis B, rabies, and varicella-zoster.

Combined Immunization

Simultaneous administration of vaccine and immunoglobulin in post-exposure prophylaxis is extremely useful. It is recommended for:
- Hepatitis B (neonates born to HBsAg positive mothers or for unvaccinated people following exposure)
- Rabies (for exposures to severe class III bites).

EXPECTED QUESTIONS

I. Write short notes on:
1. Laboratory diagnosis of viral infections.
2. Interferons.
3. Inclusion bodies.
4. Viral vaccines.

II. Multiple Choice Questions (MCQs):

1. All of the following are RNA viruses, *except*:
   a. Enterovirus
   b. Human adenoviruses
   c. Coxsackievirus
   d. Hepatitis A virus

2. All of the following viruses are transmitted by the respiratory route, *except*:
   a. Influenza virus
   b. Rotavirus
   c. Respiratory syncytial virus
   d. Rhinovirus

3. All of the following are intracytoplasmic inclusion bodies, *except*:
   a. Negri bodies
   b. Molluscum bodies
   c. Cowdry type A inclusions
   d. Guarnieri bodies

4. Which of the following vaccine is a killed vaccine?
   a. Mumps vaccine
   b. Measles vaccine
   c. Rubella vaccine
   d. IPV

5. The largest virus in size is:
   a. Herpes simplex virus
   b. Hepatitis B virus
   c. Poxvirus
   d. Adenovirus

6. The smallest virus in size is:
   a. Picornaviruses
   b. Parvovirus
   c. Hepatitis D virus
   d. Adenovirus

7. Which of the following is continuous cell line?
   a. HeLa cell line
   b. Amnion cell line
   c. Chick embryo cell line
   d. Human fibroblast cell line

8. Amniotic sac of embryonated hen's egg is used for isolation of:
   a. HIV
   b. Influenza virus
   c. Hepatitis B virus
   d. Poliovirus

Answers
1. b 2. b 3. c 4. d 5. c 6. b 7. a 8. b

Herpesviruses

CHAPTER 37

CHAPTER PREVIEW

- Herpes Simplex Viruses
- Varicella-Zoster Virus
- Cytomegalovirus
- Epstein-Barr Virus
- Less Common Herpesviruses
- Human Herpesvirus 6
- Human Herpesvirus 7
- Human Herpesvirus 8

■ HERPESVIRUSES

Herpesviruses are a group of DNA viruses that possess a unique property of establishing latent or persistent infections in their hosts and later on undergoing periodic reactivation.

Morphology

Herpesviruses are large (150–200 nm size), spherical in shape with icosahedral symmetry.
- ❖ **Nucleocapsid:** They possess a linear dsDNA, surrounded by a capsid comprising of capsomeres **(Fig. 37.1)**
- ❖ **Envelope:** The nucleocapsid is surrounded by a lipid envelope into which glycoprotein spikes are inserted; which help in viral entry by binding to the specific host cell receptors
- ❖ **Tegument:** It is the amorphous, asymmetric structure present between the capsid and envelope
- ❖ **Replication** of herpesviruses takes place in the host cell nucleus.

Classification

Based on the site of latency, they can be further grouped into three subfamilies.
1. **α-herpesviruses:** They undergo latency in neurons. Examples include—Herpes simplex viruses (HSV-1 and HSV-2), varicella-zoster virus
2. **β-herpesviruses:** They undergo latency in glands and kidneys. An example includes cytomegalovirus
3. **γ-herpesviruses:** They undergo latency in lymphoid tissues. An example includes Epstein-Barr virus.

■ HERPES SIMPLEX VIRUS

Herpes simplex viruses are extremely widespread and exhibit a broad host range. They replicate fast (12–18 hours cycle), spread fast and are cytolytic. They can cause a spectrum of diseases, involving skin, mucosa and various organs. They undergo **latency in nerve cells**; reactivate later causing recurrent lesions. Herpes simplex viruses (HSV) are of two distinct types; HSV-1 and HSV-2.

Pathogenesis

The pathogenesis of HSV-1 and HSV-2 involves the following steps:
- ❖ **Transmission:** Infection is transmitted through abraded skin or mucosa—oropharyngeal contact is common for HSV-1, whereas sexual contact is common for HSV-2
- ❖ **Primary infection:** HSV replicates at the local site of infection and can produce lesions anywhere, but more commonly in:

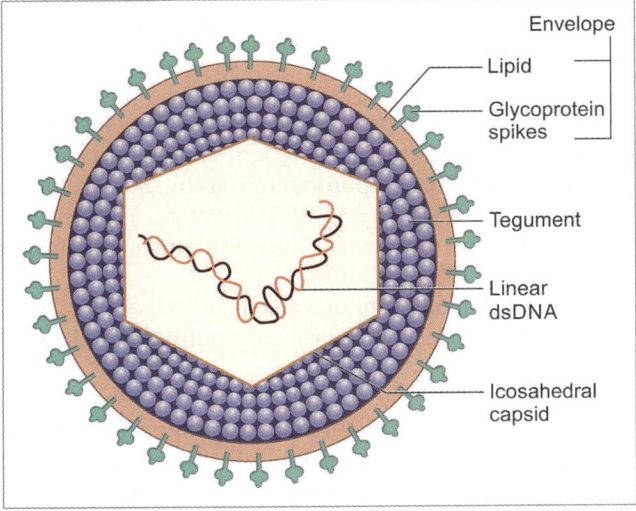

Fig. 37.1: Herpes simplex virus (schematic diagram).

- HSV-1 lesions are confined to areas above the waist (most common site—around the mouth)
- HSV-2 produces lesions below the waist (most common site—genital area).

❖ **Latency:** They invade the local nerve endings and migrate to dorsal root ganglia where they undergo latency (HSV-1 in trigeminal ganglia and HSV-2 in sacral ganglia)

❖ **Recurrent infections:** Reactivation of the latent virus can occur following various provocative stimuli, such as fever, stress, etc., which leads to the spread of the virus via the nerves back to the peripheral site (skin or mucosa or organs) producing secondary lesions. The recurrent lesions are typically less severe than the primary lesions.

Clinical Manifestations

HSV are extremely widespread and can cause a spectrum of diseases—involving skin, mucosa, and various organs.

❖ **Oral-facial mucosal lesions:** They are the most common manifestation of HSV infections, characterized by painful vesicular lesions **(Figs. 37.2A and B)**
- The most commonly affected site is buccal mucosa
- The most frequent primary lesions are gingivostomatitis and pharyngitis
- The most frequent recurrent lesion is herpes labialis (painful vesicles near lips) **(Fig. 37.2A)**.

❖ **Cutaneous lesions:** HSV usually infects abraded skin and causes various cutaneous lesions
- Herpetic whitlow: Small blisters on fingers and lips
- Febrile blisters: Fever due to any other cause can provoke HSV to cause recurrent blisters
- Herpes gladiatorum: Mucocutaneous lesions present on the body of wrestlers
- Eczematous lesion called eczema herpeticum
- Erythema multiforme.

❖ **CNS infections:** Various CNS infections such as:
- Encephalitis: HSV is the most common cause of acute sporadic viral encephalitis
- Chronic meningitis (called Mollaret meningitis).

❖ **Genital lesions:** HSV-2 is more common than HSV-1 to produce genital lesions; described as bilateral, painful, multiple, tiny vesicular ulcers

❖ **Ocular lesions:** HSV produces various ocular manifestations such as keratoconjunctivitis, corneal ulcer (called dendritic ulcers), and blindness

❖ **Neonatal herpes:** Transmission of infection during birth can lead to neonatal herpes. Transmission is more common during birth than in utero. Neonates can present with either local lesions or disseminated infection or CNS infections.

Laboratory Diagnosis

Laboratory diagnosis of HSV infections includes the following modalities.

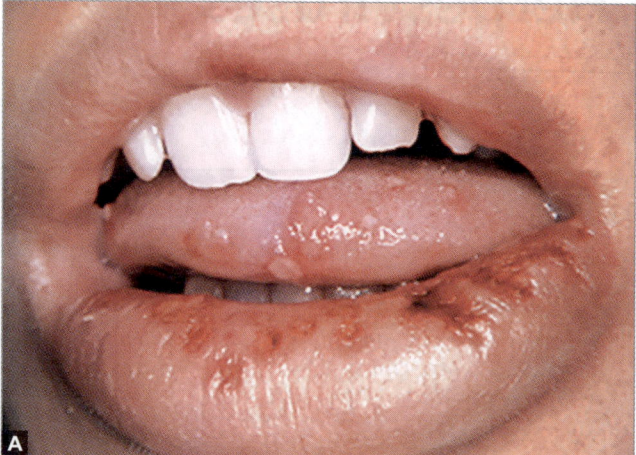
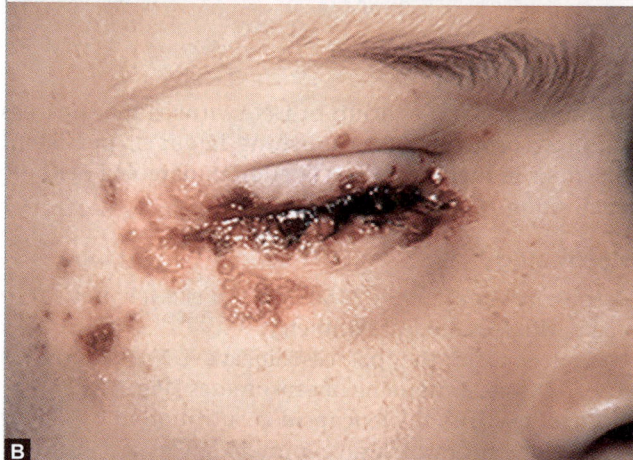

Figs. 37.2A and B: A. Vesicular lesions on lips and tongue due to HSV-1 infection; **B.** Periocular vesicular lesions due to HSV-1 infection.

Source: Public Health Image Library, **A.** ID# 12616 (Robert E Sumpter), **B.** ID# 6492 (Dr KL Hermann)/Centers for Disease Control and Prevention (CDC), Atlanta (*with permission*).

❖ **Cytopathology:** Scrapings obtained from the base of the lesion can be stained with Wright's or Giemsa (Tzanck preparation), or Papanicolaou stain. Sensitivity of staining is low (<30% for mucosal swabs).
- Production of Cowdry type A intranuclear inclusion bodies (Lipschutz body)
- Formation of multinucleated giant cells with faceted nuclei and ground-glass chromatin (Tzanck cells) **(Fig. 37.3)**.

❖ **Viral isolation** in various cell lines (e.g. McCoy cell line) to demonstrate characteristic cytopathic effect such as diffuse rounding and ballooning of cell lines. Viral antigen detection by neutralization test or immunofluorescence staining with specific antiserum

❖ **Viral antigen detection** in the specimen by direct immunofluorescence (DIF)

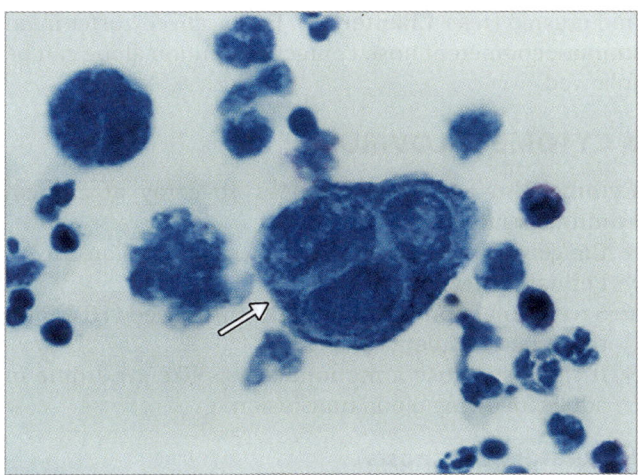

Fig. 37.3: Tzanck smear of a tissue scraping showing multi-nucleated giant cell (Tzanck cell) in the center (arrow showing).
Source: Public Health Image Library, ID# 14428/Centers for Disease Control and Prevention (CDC), Atlanta.

- ❖ **HSV DNA detection** by PCR and real-time PCR
- ❖ **Antibody detection:** Antibodies appear in 4–7 days after the infection and peak in 2–4 weeks. IgM appears first and is replaced by IgG, which persists for life.
    - ELISA based on the type-specific antigens such as glycoprotein G antigens (gG1 and gG2) can differentiate between HSV-1 and HSV-2
    - Western blot is more accurate, with 98% sensitivity and specificity.

> **TREATMENT** — HSV infections
>
> Antiviral drugs such as acyclovir are effective for HSV infections. In case of acyclovir resistance, foscarnet is the drug of choice.

Prevention

General measures can be taken such as:
- ❖ Use of condom to prevent genital herpes
- ❖ Neonatal herpes can be prevented by prior administration of acyclovir to mothers during third trimester of pregnancy or delivery by elective cesarean section.

Infection control measures: Patients with mucocutaneous herpes in hospitals, should be kept on contact precautions until lesions are dry and crusted (*refer* **Chapter 15**).

■ VARICELLA-ZOSTER VIRUS

Varicella-zoster virus (VZV) produces vesicular eruptions (rashes) on the skin and mucous membranes in the form of two clinical entities:

Chickenpox

It occurs following primary infection, usually affecting children, characterized by:
- ❖ **Rashes:** Generalized diffuse bilateral vesicular rashes, centripetal in distribution and appear in multiple crops. Rashes appear in multiple crops: Lesions in various stages of evolution, such as maculopapules, vesicles, pustules, and scabs can be found in one area at the same time **(Fig. 37.4A)**
- ❖ **Complications**: More common in adults and immunocompromised individuals
    - *The most common* complications are secondary bacterial infections of the skin and CNS involvement (encephalitis and meningitis, etc.)
    - *Most serious* complication: varicella pneumonia
    - *Reye's syndrome* can occur secondary to VZV infection. It is characterized by fatty degeneration of the liver following salicylate (aspirin) intake.
- ❖ **Epidemiology:** Chickenpox is a highly contagious disease
    - Common in children between 1 to 14 years of age
    - **Period of infectivity:** Child is infectious from 2 days before the onset of rash to 5 days thereafter, until the vesicles are crusted
    - **Source of infection:** Patients are the only source, there are no carriers.
- ❖ **Pregnancy:** Chickenpox in pregnancy can affect both mother and the fetus.
    - Mothers are at high-risk of developing varicella pneumonia
    - Fetus is at higher risk of developing **congenital varicella syndrome** (in early pregnancy); characterized by cicatricial skin lesions and limb hypoplasia.

Zoster or Shingles

Zoster usually occurs following reactivation of latent VZV present in the trigeminal ganglia that occurs mainly in old age or immunocompromised individuals.
- ❖ **Rashes:** They are unilateral and segmental, confined to the area of skin supplied by the affected nerves **(Fig. 37.4B)**. Head, neck, and trunk are the most common affected sites
- ❖ **Complications:** Zoster may present with complications such as:
    - *Zoster ophthalmicus:* Unilateral painful crops of skin rashes surrounding the eye
    - *Ramsay Hunt syndrome:* It develops when the facial nerve is involved; presents as facial paralysis, and vesicles on the face and ears

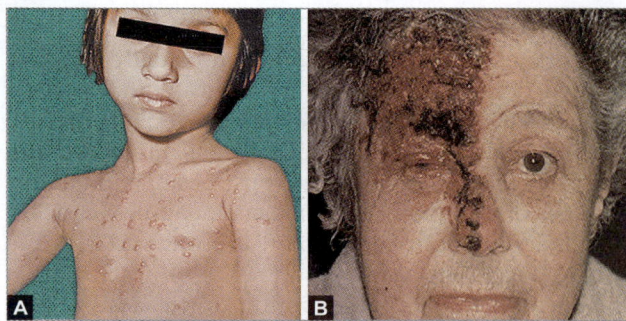

Figs. 37.4A and B: A. Rashes of chickenpox; **B.** Segmental distribution of rashes of Zoster.

Source: **A.** Public Health Image Library, ID#/2882/JD Millar/Centers for Disease Control and Prevention (CDC), Atlanta (*with permission*); **B.** Recommendations of the Advisory Committee on Immunization Practices [ACIP]. MMWR Morb Mortal Wkly Rep 2008;57[RR-5]:1 (*with permission*).

- *Post-herpetic neuralgia*: Pain at the local site lasting for months; most common complication in elderly patients.

Laboratory diagnosis and treatment of varicella-zoster virus are similar to as discussed for HSV.

Vaccine

Live attenuated vaccine using **Oka strain** of VZV is available.
- It is given to children after 1 year of age; 2 doses, first dose is given at 12–15 months and second at 4–6 years.
- The vaccine is >80% effective in preventing chickenpox in children but less so in adults (70%).
- However, it is 95% effective in preventing severe disease.

VZIG (Varicella-Zoster Immunoglobulin)

It is useful for **post-exposure prophylaxis;** preferably within 72 hours of exposure.
- As adults are at higher risk of varicella-related deaths, VZIG is recommended for adults.
- It is also indicated for **neonates born to mothers** suffering from chickenpox if the onset of chickenpox in mother is between <5 days before delivery till 48 hours after delivery.

Infection Control Measures

Patients infected with VZV should be kept in isolation. Airborne precautions (e.g. negative air-flow rooms) plus contact precautions must be followed until lesions are dry and crusted (*refer* **Chapter 15**). For localized zoster in an immunocompetent host, contact precaution alone can be followed.

CYTOMEGALOVIRUS

Cytomegalovirus (CMV) causes an array of clinical syndromes such as:
- Congenital infection called cytomegalic inclusion disease
- Perinatal infections
- Severe infection in immunocompromised (HIV) and transplant recipients
- It can also cause a mononucleosis-like syndrome in adults following blood transfusion.

Laboratory Diagnosis

Laboratory diagnosis of CMV infections include:
- **Inclusion bodies:** Detection of perinuclear inclusion bodies (with owl's eye appearance) in urine specimen
- **Virus isolation** in human fibroblasts cell line: cytopathic effect can be demonstrated after 2–3 weeks
- **Antibody detection** (by ELISA): Detects IgM and IgG antibodies against various viral antigens
- **Antigen detection** (e.g. pp65 antigen) by indirect immunofluorescence test using specific monoclonal antibody
- **Molecular methods**: Detection of various target genes by PCR.

TREATMENT — CMV infections

Drugs such as ganciclovir, valganciclovir, foscarnet and cidofovir are used for the treatment of CMV infections.

EPSTEIN-BARR VIRUS

Epstein-Barr Virus (EBV) is transmitted by oropharyngeal contact through infected salivary secretions.
- **Pathogenesis:** They infect the B-lymphocytes. The infected B cells become immortalized and produce a large number of polyclonal immunoglobulins. In response to this, the bystander CD8 T lymphocytes are stimulated and appear atypical
- **Clinical manifestations:** EBV is associated with several manifestations
  - *Infectious mononucleosis:* It is characterized by pharyngitis, cervical lymphadenopathy, and atypical lymphocytosis

- **Malignancies:** EBV is associated with the pathogenesis of several malignancies such as Burkitt's lymphoma and nasopharyngeal carcinoma, Hodgkin's, and non-Hodgkin's lymphoma.
- **Other conditions associated with EBV:** Lymphoproliferative disorder and oral hairy leukoplakia (wart-like growth of epithelial cells of the tongue developed in some HIV-infected patients and transplant recipients).

❖ **Laboratory diagnosis of EBV infections include:**
- Detection of nonspecific heterophile antibody to sheep RBC antigens (by Paul Bunnell test)
- Detection of specific anti-EBV antibodies: ELISA and indirect IF assay detect antibodies specific to viral capsid antigen, EBNA (nuclear antigen), and early antigen.

TREATMENT — EBV infections

- **Supportive measures** such as analgesics are used in the treatment of infectious mononucleosis
- **Acyclovir** is useful in the treatment of oral hairy leukoplakia, though relapse is common. It reduces EBV shedding from the oropharynx.
- **Antibody to CD20** (rituximab) has been effective in some cases.

LESS COMMON HERPESVIRUSES

❖ **HHV 6 and 7:** Human herpesvirus (HHV) 6 and 7 infect T-lymphocytes. HHV-6 produces an exanthematous disease called as sixth disease (exanthem subitum or roseola infantum)

❖ **Human herpesvirus 8:** It infects B-lymphocytes, and can cause a malignancy called Kaposi's sarcoma in HIV-infected individuals.

EXPECTED QUESTIONS

I. **Write an essay on:**
   1. Discuss the pathogenesis, clinical manifestations, and laboratory diagnosis of herpes simplex virus infections.

II. **Write short notes on:**
   1. Laboratory diagnosis of chickenpox.
   2. Cytomegalovirus infections.
   3. Laboratory diagnosis of Epstein-Barr virus infections.

III. **Multiple Choice Questions (MCQs):**
   1. Exanthem subitum is caused by:
      a. Human herpesvirus-6
      b. Parvovirus
      c. Human herpesvirus-7
      d. Adenovirus
   2. Paul-Bunnell test is done for:
      a. Toxic shock syndrome
      b. Infectious mononucleosis
      c. Chickenpox
      d. Hemorrhagic cystitis
   3. The owl's eye appearance inclusion bodies are seen in which viral infection?
      a. HSV
      b. VZV
      c. CMV
      d. EBV

Answers
1. a   2. b   3. c

Other DNA Viruses (including Bacteriophage)

CHAPTER 38

CHAPTER PREVIEW
- Parvoviruses
- Papillomaviruses
- Polyomaviruses
- Adenoviruses
- Poxviruses
- Bacteriophages

Other DNA viruses include parvoviruses, papilloma and polyomaviruses, poxviruses, adenoviruses, bacteriophages, and hepatitis B virus. The hepatitis B virus is discussed in **Chapter 45**, along with other hepatitis viruses. Other DNA viruses are discussed here.

■ PARVOVIRUSES

Parvovirus is the smallest virus infecting man and parvovirus B19 is the most common parvovirus pathogenic to man.
- ❖ **Clinical manifestations** are as follows:
  - **Erythema infectiosum** (fifth disease): It is a common childhood exanthema, characterized by rashes on the face, described as slapped cheek appearance
  - They infect RBC precursors to cause nonimmune hydrops fetalis and aplastic anemia
  - **Papular-purpuric gloves and socks syndrome:** It presents as rapidly progressive, painful, pruritic, and symmetric swelling and erythema of the distal hands and feet.
- ❖ **Laboratory diagnosis** include:
  - **Molecular methods** such as PCR, which detects viral DNA from serum, tissue or respiratory secretions
  - **IgM antibody detection** by ELISA; useful in detection of recent infection.
- ❖ **Treatment:** Symptomatic treatment is given.

■ PAPILLOMAVIRUSES

Human papillomavirus (HPV) has several serotypes, each other is associated with specific infections.
- ❖ **Benign lesions (warts):** They are small, hard, rough growth on the skin—e.g. common warts, plantar warts, anogenital warts, etc.
- ❖ **Epidermodysplasia verruciformis:** It is a benign skin condition with malignant potential. It is seen with serotypes 5, 8, 9, etc.
- ❖ **Malignant neoplasia,** e.g. carcinoma of the cervix and other genital mucosa, larynx, or esophagus
  - Serotypes 16 and 18 have high malignant potential for carcinoma cervix
  - Serotypes 6 and 11 are associated with a premalignant condition of the cervix called cervical intraepithelial neoplasia (CIN).
- ❖ **Vaccine:** It is available for the prevention of HPV infections. It is recommended for all adolescent boys and girls aged 11-12 years. Three types of vaccines are available:
  - **Nine valent vaccine** (Gardasil 9) includes nine HPV serotypes. It is given IM; at 11-12 years, as 2 doses (at least 6–12 months gap).
  - **Quadrivalent vaccine:** It includes serotypes 6, 11, 16 and 18.
  - **Bivalent vaccine** (Cervarix) includes only the high-risk serotypes 16 and 18. It is given as single dose, IM.

■ POLYOMAVIRUSES

They usually infect animals; only a few are human pathogens such as JC virus and BK virus. Both are named after the initials of the patients in whom they were described first.
- ❖ **JC virus:** Causes progressive multifocal leukoencephalopathy (PML); a slow virus disease infecting the brain
- ❖ **BK virus:** Causes nephropathy in kidney transplant recipients.

■ ADENOVIRUSES

Adenoviruses are non-enveloped DNA virus. It has icosahedral symmetry with fiber proteins projecting from each vertex, which gives a unique **space vehicle shaped** appearance **(Fig. 38.1)**.

CHAPTER 38 ◆ Other DNA Viruses (including Bacteriophage)

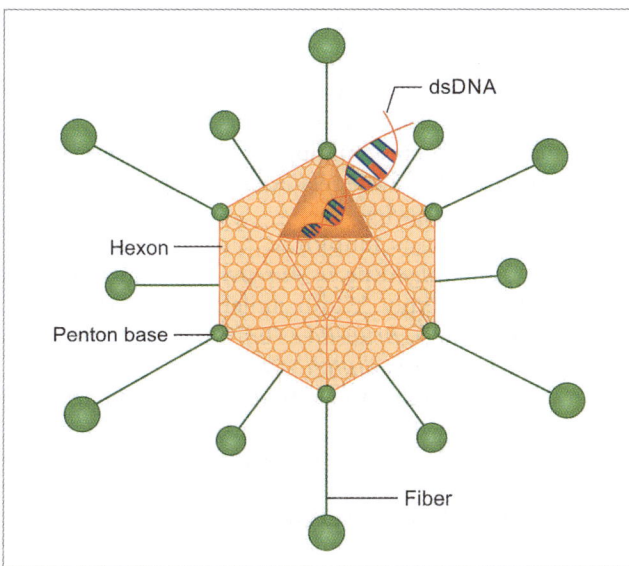

Fig. 38.1: Adenovirus (schematic diagram).

- ❖ **Clinical manifestations:** Adenoviruses infect and replicate in the epithelial cells and produce various infections such as:
  - **Respiratory infections:** Upper respiratory tract infection, pneumonia
  - **Ocular infections:** Pharyngoconjunctival fever, and epidemic keratoconjunctivitis (or shipyard eye)
  - **Infantile diarrhea:** Caused by serotypes 40 and 41
  - **Hemorrhagic cystitis:** Caused by serotypes 11 and 21
  - **Immunocompromised** patients are at higher risk of developing serious pneumonia
  - **Transplant recipients** may develop pneumonia, hepatitis, nephritis, colitis, encephalitis and hemorrhagic cystitis. Types 34 and 35 are isolated commonly from transplant recipients.
- ❖ **Laboratory diagnosis:** Depending on the manifestations, various specimens such as throat swab, conjunctival swab, stool or urine may be collected.
  - **Virus isolation** by primary human embryonic kidney cell line.
  - **Viral growth** can be detected by characteristic cytopathic effect (rounding and grape-like clustering of swollen cells)
  - **Serotyping** is done by hemagglutination test and neutralization test
  - **Direct immunofluorescence test** to detect adenoviral antigens from clinical samples such as throat or conjunctival secretions
  - **Molecular methods** such as PCR and real-time PCR are rapid and more sensitive.
- ❖ **Treatment:** Symptomatic treatment is given; only in severe cases of pneumonia cidofovir is recommended.

■ POXVIRUSES

Poxviruses are the largest (400 nm in length × 230 nm in diameter), among all the viruses infecting man. They possess single dsDNA and replicate in the cytoplasm.
- ❖ **Smallpox virus** (*Variola*): It is the agent of a highly contagious severe exanthematous disease 'smallpox'; which was the first infectious disease to be eradicated from the world
  - The rashes were typically deep-seated, appeared in one stage, and were centrifugally distributed (extremities were affected first)
  - The introduction of live-attenuated *Vaccinia* vaccine was one of the reasons for its successful eradication.
  - **Laboratory diagnosis** include—(i) Direct detection of intracytoplasmic inclusion bodies (Paschen bodies) in scrapings from rashes or by electron microscopy (brick-shaped appearance), (ii) egg inoculation into the chorioallantoic membrane (CAM) of a chick embryo showing characteristic pock formation.
  - **Treatment:** Cases used to be treated in the past with vaccinia immunoglobulins and antiviral drugs such as methisazone, or cidofovir.
- ❖ **Molluscum contagiosum virus** is another poxvirus that infects humans
  - **Lesions:** It produces pink pearly wart-like lesions, umbilicated with a characteristic dimple at the center
  - **Inclusion bodies:** Histopathological stain of skin scrapings demonstrates typical intracytoplasmic inclusions called molluscum bodies.
- ❖ **Monkeypox virus:** Can produce vesicular rash similar to smallpox but milder. Infection can be prevented by smallpox vaccination.

■ BACTERIOPHAGES

Bacteriophages are viruses that infect bacteria. They are **tadpole-shaped**; measure about 28–100 nm in size. They possess a hexagonal head (capsid) enclosing a dsDNA with a tail ending with tail fibers **(Fig. 38.2)**.

Life Cycle

Bacteriophages exhibit two different types of life cycles.
- ❖ **Lytic cycle** (or virulent cycle): After the phage infects the bacterium, the phage DNA replicates in the cytoplasm. The daughter phages produced are subsequently

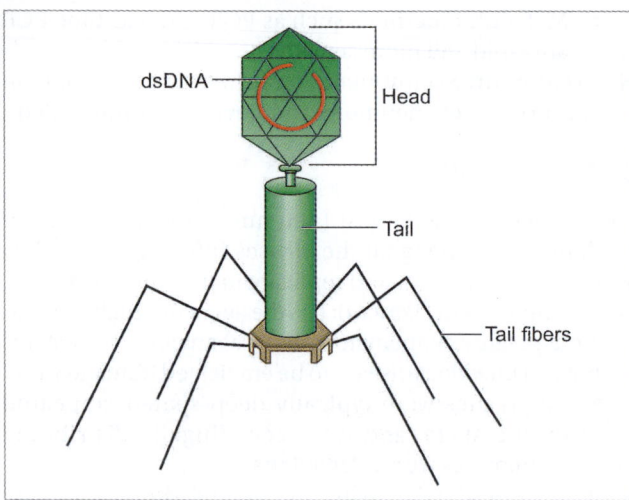

Fig. 38.2: Morphology of bacteriophage.

released from the bacteria by causing lysis of the bacterial cell
- **Lysogenic cycle** (or temperate cycle): Here, the phage DNA gets integrated into the bacterial chromosome (called lysogenic conversion). But when they want to come out, they get excised from the bacterial chromosome, then transform into lytic phages, multiply in the cytoplasm, and are released by lysis.

Significance/Uses of Bacteriophages

Bacteriophages have been used for various purposes.
- **Phage typing:** The virulent phages are useful for classifying bacteria beyond species level.
  - This helps in epidemiological investigations during outbreak to know the relatedness between the strains of the same species
  - Phage typing is employed for typing of bacteria such as: *Staphylococcus aureus*, Vi antigen typing of *Salmonella* Typhi, Vibrio cholerae (Basu Mukherjee phage typing), *Brucella* (Tbilisi phage typing) and *Corynebacterium diphtheriae*.
- **Used in treatment (phage therapy):** Lytic phages can kill the bacteria, therefore may be used for the treatment of bacterial infections such as post-burn and wound infections
- **Used as a cloning vector:** Bacteriophages have been used as cloning vectors in recombinant DNA technology
- **Transfer drug resistance:** Temperate phages can transfer bacterial genes from one bacterium to another by **transduction** (e.g. transfer of plasmids coding for β-lactamases)
- **Code for toxins:** The phage genomes code for the following bacterial toxins—diphtheria toxin, cholera toxin, Shiga toxin, etc.

EXPECTED QUESTIONS

I. **Write an essay on:**
1. Discuss the pathogenesis, clinical manifestations, and laboratory diagnosis of adenovirus infections.

II. **Write short notes on:**
1. Human papillomavirus infections.
2. Bacteriophage.

III. **Multiple Choice Questions (MCQs):**
1. Erythema infectiosum is caused by:
   a. Parvovirus
   b. Human herpesvirus-6
   c. Adenovirus
   d. Hepatitis B virus
2. Which of the following toxin is phage coded?
   a. Tetanus toxin
   b. Botulinum toxin
   c. Cholera toxin
   d. Pneumolysin
3. All of the following are clinical manifestations of HPV, *except*:
   a. Plantar and palmar warts
   b. Epidermodysplasia verruciformis
   c. Carcinoma of cervix
   d. Slapped cheek appearance
4. Which of the following adenovirus serotypes cause epidemic keratoconjunctivitis?
   a. Serotypes 3 and 7
   b. Serotypes 8, 19 and 37
   c. Serotypes 40 and 41
   d. Serotypes 11 and 21

Answers
1. a   2. c   3. d   4. b

Myxoviruses and Rubella Virus

CHAPTER 39

CHAPTER PREVIEW
- Orthomyxoviruses: Influenza Virus
- Paramyxoviruses: Parainfluenza, Measles, Mumps, RSV
- Rubella Virus

Myxoviruses are a group of viruses that bind to mucin receptors on the surface of RBCs. They are divided into two groups:
1. **Orthomyxoviruses:** They possess segmented RNA; e.g. influenza virus **(Fig. 39.1)**
2. **Paramyxoviruses:** They possess non-segmented RNA; e.g. parainfluenza virus, mumps, measles, Nipah, Hendra, and respiratory syncytial virus.

ORTHOMYXOVIRUSES

Influenza viruses are the members of Orthomyxoviridae family. They cause upper respiratory tract infections, rarely can cause pneumonia.

Influenza Virus

Influenza viruses are one of the major cause of morbidity and mortality and have been responsible for several epidemics and pandemics of respiratory diseases in the last two centuries, caused by various serotypes; of which the latest pandemic was caused by A/H1N1 serotype in 2009.

- **Morphology:** Influenza viruses are spherical in shape, measure about 80–120 nm in size **(Fig. 39.1)**
  - It comprises of a helical nucleocapsid, surrounded by an envelope
  - **Viral RNA** comprises of **multiple segments** of negative sense single stranded RNA
  - **Viral proteins:** Influenza virus contains eight structural proteins and two non-structural proteins
  - **Nucleoprotein (NP)** is the major capsid protein, associated with viral RNA to form a ribonucleoprotein (RNP)
  - **Envelope:** It consists of a lipid envelope into which two types of glycoproteins are inserted: (i) **hemagglutinin (HA)**, triangular-shaped peplomer that binds to receptors on the respiratory epithelial cells and (ii) **neuraminidase (NA)**, mushroom shaped peplomer that degrades the sialic acid receptors on the host cells
- **Types:** Based on hemagglutinin (HA) and neuraminidase (NA) antigens, influenza virus can be divided into four serotypes (A, B, C and D)
  - Influenza A virus is further divided into various subtypes, e.g. A/H1N1, H5N1, H_3N_2, etc.
  - Influenza B viruses have diverged into lineages (e.g. B/Yamagata or B/Victoria lineage)
- **Antigen variation:** Influenza virus has a unique property of undergoing frequent antigen variations; which may be either a minor genetic variation—called antigenic drift or a major genetic change—called antigen shift **(Table 39.1)**. Antigenic variation is responsible for pandemics and outbreaks of cases.

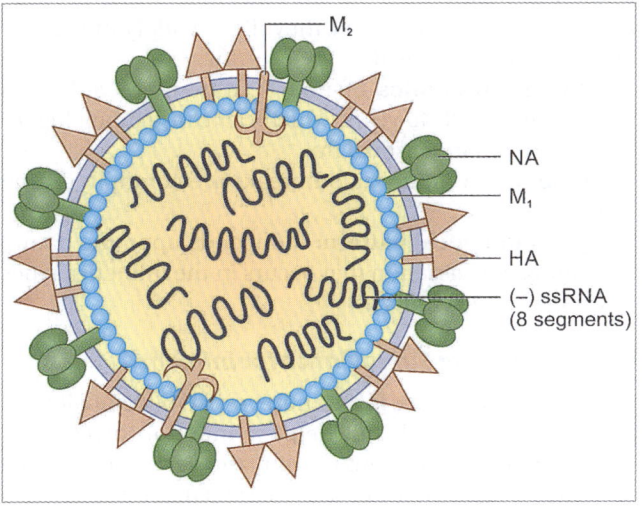

Fig. 39.1: Influenza virus (schematic diagram).

Table 39.1: Differences between antigenic drift and shift.	
Antigenic drift	**Antigenic shift**
It is a minor genetic change	It is a major genetic change
Occurs due to point mutations	Occurs due to genetic assortment between the viruses
Results in outbreaks and minor periodic epidemics	Results in pandemics and major epidemics (e.g. A/H1N1 pandemics of 2009)
Occurs more frequently, every 2–3 years	Occurs less frequently every 10–20 years
Seen in both influenza virus type—A and B	Seen only in influenza A

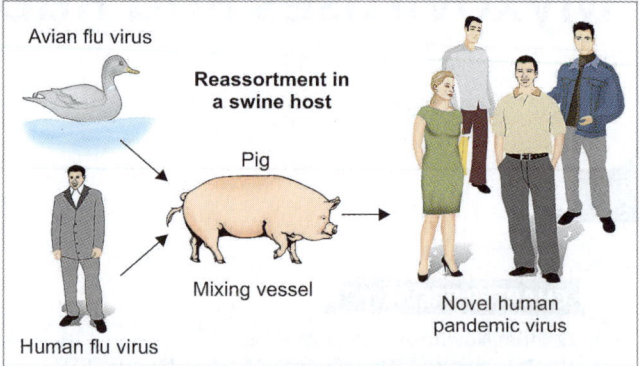

Fig. 39.2: Evolution of pandemic influenza virus.

Pathogenesis

Pathogenesis of influenza involves the transmission of the virus, followed by spread to the respiratory epithelium.

- **Transmission:** It is transmitted by (i) **inhalation of respiratory droplets** generated by coughing and sneezing, (ii) **via contact with surfaces or fomites** infected with respiratory droplets, and then touching the nose, eyes, or mouth
- **Spread:** The virus infects the respiratory epithelial cells by binding of viral HA antigens to specific sialic acid receptors on the respiratory mucosa
- **Avian flu:** Bird flu strains are highly lethal to chickens causing an economic loss in poultry
    - **A/H5N1** is the most common avian flu strain that has been endemic in the world
    - **Transmission** from birds to humans is rare. If transmitted, the disease in man is more severe than A/H1N1
    - **Less morbidity, but more mortality:** As there is no human to human transmission, morbidity is less. However, mortality rate is >60%.
    - **Clinical features:** H5N1 avian flu strains are associated with higher rates of pneumonia (>50%) and extrapulmonary manifestations such as diarrhea and CNS involvement.
- **A/H1N1 flu:** In 2009, influenza A/H1N1 caused a global pandemic affecting several countries, including India
    - A/H1N1 2009 flu originated by genetic reassortment of four strains (1 human strain + 2 swine strains + 1 avian strain) and the mixing had occurred in pigs **(Fig. 39.2)**
    - It can be transmitted from human to human, which has accounted for its rapid spread
    - Currently, it is a seasonal flu strain in India.
    - **Clinical features:** Most of the cases present with mild upper respiratory tract illness and diarrhea and **complicated/severe influenza** can occur very rarely in high-risk groups; characterized by secondary bacterial pneumonia, dehydration, CNS involvement, and multiorgan failure
- **Seasonal flu:** Influenza outbreaks are common during winters. The currently circulating strains causing seasonal flu are influenza A/H1N1, A/H3N2, and influenza B.

Clinical Manifestations

The majority of individuals develop mild flu-like symptoms such as chills, headache, and dry cough, followed by high-grade fever, myalgia, and anorexia.

- Minor cases can develop pneumonia—secondary bacterial pneumonia or rarely viral pneumonia
- Patients with risk factors such as elderly patients (≥65 years), chronic pulmonary, cardiac, renal, and hematologic diseases, and immunosuppression are more prone to develop complications.

Epidemiology

Influenza viruses cause seasonal flu epidemics worldwide almost every year, however they differ widely in severity and the extent of spread.

- **Global pandemics** of novel influenza A subtypes occur every 10–40 years, which can cause much higher mortality than seasonal flu
- **Seasonality:** Influenza outbreaks are common during winters
- **Epidemiological pattern:** It depends upon the nature of antigenic variation that occurs in the influenza types (as described earlier).

Epidemiological Surveillance for Influenza

Influenza surveillance is routinely carried out globally and also at national level. This helps to monitor the changes in the circulating influenza strain and serves as a global alert mechanism for the emergence of pandemic influenza viruses.

- **GISRS:** Influenza surveillance has been conducted globally through Global Influenza Surveillance and Response System (GISRS) under World Health Organization (WHO)
- **IDSP** (Integrated Disease Surveillance Program) under NCDC (National Center for Disease Control) conducts Influenza (H1N1) surveillance in India.

Laboratory Diagnosis

The nasopharyngeal swab is the ideal specimen, collected by dacron or polyester flocked swabs in viral transport media **(Fig. 39.3)**.

- **Molecular test:** Detection of viral RNA (HA or NA genes) in nasopharyngeal swabs by real-time reverse transcriptase PCR remains the gold standard method of diagnosis
  - It is highly sensitive and specific with a turnaround time of 2–3 hours
  - It simultaneously detects the three common seasonal flu strains (A/H1N1, A/H3N2, and type B).
- **Direct immunofluorescence test:** Viral antigens coated onto epithelial cells can be directly detected in nasal aspirates
- **Isolation of virus** in embryonated eggs and primary monkey kidney cell lines were in use in the past
- **Antibody detection** in patient serum is mainly useful for epidemiology purposes, not for clinical diagnosis.

> **TREATMENT** — Influenza
>
> Specific antiviral agents given for the treatment of influenza are neuraminidase inhibitors (e.g. oseltamivir) or matrix protein M2 inhibitors (e.g. amantadine).

Prevention

General Preventive Measures

Measures of droplet precaution (*refer* **Chapter 15**) should be followed:
- **Strict hand hygiene**
- **Isolation room:** Patients should be kept in isolation room or cohorting to be followed

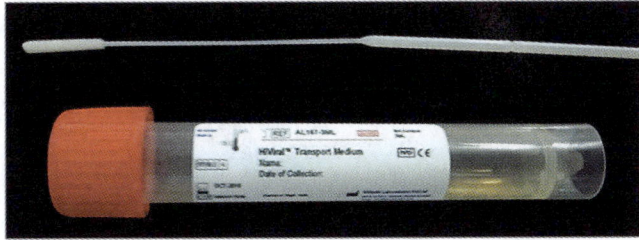

Fig. 39.3: Viral transport medium and swab.
Source: Department of Microbiology, JIPMER, Puducherry (*with permission*).

- **Containment of coughs and sneezes**
  - Respiratory hygiene and cough etiquette
  - Use of personal protective equipment (PPE) such as gloves, 3-ply masks, gown and googles for a HCW. Patient should wear a mask.
- **Work restriction:** CDC recommends that people with influenza-like illness remain at home until at least 24 hours after they are free of fever (<100°F) without the use of fever-reducing medications.

Influenza Vaccine

Both live attenuated and injectable vaccines are available for influenza.

- **Strains:** The seasonal flu strains are usually included in the vaccine such as A/H1N1, A/H3N2, and influenza B strain
- **Schedule:** It is taken as a single dose, every year before the winter season begins
- **Injectable vaccines** are the most widely used vaccines in immunization programs.
  - Single dose administered by intramuscular (IM) route
  - Routine annual influenza vaccination is recommended for all persons aged ≥6 months; except people who have history of severe allergic reaction to previous dose of vaccine
  - Injectable vaccines are of three types: (i) inactivated influenza vaccine, (ii) cell culture-based inactivated influenza vaccine and (iii) recombinant influenza vaccine.
- **Live attenuated influenza vaccine:** This vaccine is generated by reassortment between currently circulating strains of influenza A and B virus with a cold adapted attenuated master strain which is adapted to grow at 25–33°C.
  - It is administered by intranasal spray.
  - It can be given to all healthy persons of 2–49 years age (except in pregnancy), but is not given to high risk groups.

■ PARAMYXOVIRUSES

Paramyxoviridae contains a group of viruses, which are transmitted via the respiratory route following which:
- They may cause localized respiratory infection in children (e.g. respiratory syncytial virus, and parainfluenza viruses) or;
- They may disseminate throughout the body to cause mumps (parotid gland enlargement) and measles.

Paramyxoviruses are larger (100–300 nm) in size and more pleomorphic when compared to orthomyxoviruses.

Parainfluenza Viruses

Human parainfluenza viruses are one of the major cause of respiratory tract disease in young children. They have five serotypes (types 1, 2, 3, 4a and 4b); all are transmitted by the respiratory route.

- **Clinical manifestations** include—mild common cold syndrome, croup (laryngotracheobronchitis), lower respiratory tract infections (pneumonia or bronchiolitis).
- **Laboratory diagnosis** as follows:
  - **Antigen detection** in the infected exfoliated epithelial cells of the nasopharynx by direct immunofluorescence
  - **Viral isolation** from specimens such as nasal washes, bronchoalveolar lavage fluid using primary monkey kidney cell line
  - **Serum antibodies** detection by neutralization test or ELISA
  - **Reverse transcriptase PCR** is highly sensitive and specific.

Measles Virus

Measles is an acute, highly contagious exanthematous childhood disease.

Pathogenesis

Measles is transmitted via the respiratory route either by—droplets inhalation or small-particle aerosols. It multiplies locally and subsequently spreads through the bloodstream to various target sites, including the skin, respiratory tract, and conjunctiva.

Clinical Manifestations

Symptoms appear after an incubation period of about 10 days. The disease can be divided into the following stages.
1. **Prodromal stage:** This stage lasts for 4 days and is characterized by manifestations such as:
   - **Fever** is the first manifestation (appears on the 10th day), followed by Koplik's spots (i.e. on the 12th day)
   - **Koplik's spots:** They are pathognomonic of measles, characterized by the bluish white spot on buccal mucosa **(Fig. 39.4A)**
   - **Non-specific symptoms** may be present such as cough, cold, nasal discharge, redness of eye, etc.
2. **Eruptive stage:** This stage starts on the 14th day, characterized by exanthematous rashes **(Fig. 39.4B)**, which begin from behind the ears → then spread to the face, arm, trunk and legs → then fade in the same order after 4 days of onset.

> Fever (10th day) → Koplik's spot (12th day) → rashes (14th day)

Complications

Patients with risk factors such as age <5 or >20 yrs, pregnant women, and immunocompromised hosts, etc. are more prone to develop complications.
- **Secondary bacterial infections** such as otitis media and bronchopneumonia
- **Giant-cell pneumonitis** (Hecht's pneumonia) occurs due to the virus itself
- **Diarrhea** leads to malnutrition
- **CNS complications** such as subacute sclerosing panencephalitis (SSPE). This is a rare, but severe complication of measles.

Laboratory Diagnosis

Nasopharyngeal swab, conjunctival swab, respiratory secretions, etc. are the ideal specimens.
- **Antigen detection** in the infected cells by using anti-nucleoprotein antibodies (by direct IF test)
- **Virus isolation:** Using monkey or human kidney cells and demonstrating cytopathic effect such as multinucleated giant cells (Warthin-Finkeldey cells) containing both intranuclear and intracytoplasmic inclusion bodies **(Fig. 39.4C)**
- **Antibody detection:** Demonstration of raised titers of anti-measles antibody in the CSF is diagnostic of SSPE

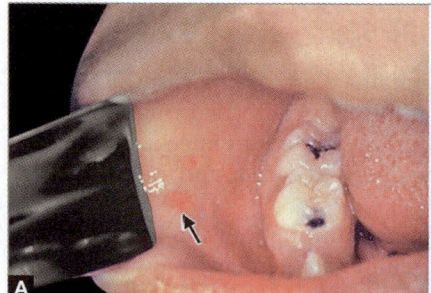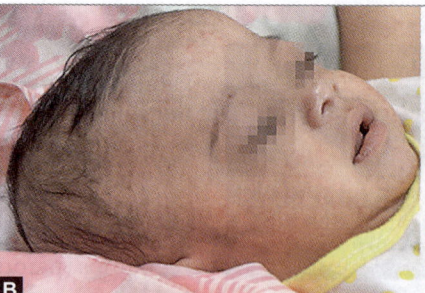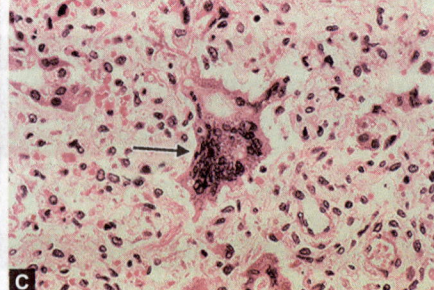

Figs. 39.4A to C: A. Koplik spot in the buccal mucosa (measles) (arrow showing); **B.** Measles rashes (on face); **C.** Multinucleated giant cell of measles infected cell lines (arrow showing).
Source: **A.** Public Health Image Library, ID# 6111; **B.** ID# 17980; **C.** ID# 859/Centers for Disease Control and Prevention (CDC), Atlanta (*with permission*).

❖ **RT-PCR** is available targeting measles-specific N gene (nucleoprotein) in the clinical specimens.

> **TREATMENT** — **Measles**
>
> ❑ There is no specific antiviral therapy available for measles
> ❑ Treatment is symptomatic and consists of general supportive measures.

Prevention

General Preventive Measures

Airborne precautions such as isolation in negative pressure room, use of PPEs such as N95 respirator, etc. must be followed while handling measles cases (**Chapter 15** for detail).

Measles Vaccine

Live attenuated vaccine is available for measles using Schwartz strain or Edmonston-Zagreb strain.

❖ It is available as a monovalent vaccine or along with mumps and rubella vaccine (MMR vaccine) or with rubella vaccine (MR vaccine)
❖ **Indication:** Under the national immunization schedule of India, the measles-rubella (MR) vaccine is given at 9 completed months to 12 months along with vitamin A supplements, and the second dose of MR vaccine at 16–24 months
❖ **Post-exposure prophylaxis:** Susceptible contacts may be protected against measles if the vaccine is given within 3 days of exposure. Measles immunoglobulin (Ig) can also be given within 3 days. However, both vaccine and Ig should not be given together.

Mumps Virus

Mumps virus is the most common cause of parotid gland enlargement in children.

❖ **Transmission:** It is transmitted through the respiratory route via droplets, saliva, and fomites
❖ **Target sites:** Mumps virus has a special affinity for glandular epithelium. The classic sites include salivary glands, testes, pancreas, ovaries, CNS, etc.
❖ **Clinical manifestations:** It causes bilateral parotitis, although it can also infect other salivary glands. In severe cases, it can cause complications such as orchitis, pancreatitis, oophoritis, and aseptic meningitis
❖ **Epidemiology:** Mumps is endemic worldwide, epidemics occur every 3–5 years; typically associated with unvaccinated people living in overcrowded areas
  ■ **Period of communicability:** Patients are infectious from 1 week before to 1 week after the onset of symptoms
  ■ **Source:** Cases (both clinical and subclinical cases) are the source of infection
  ■ **Age:** Children of **5–9 years** of age are most commonly affected.

❖ **Laboratory diagnosis:** The buccal or oral swab specimens are most ideal
  ■ Direct viral antigen detection can be done by using mumps-specific fluorescent staining
  ■ Virus isolation using monkey kidney cell line
  ■ Serum antibodies detection: ELISA
  ■ Reverse-transcription PCR is available to detect mumps specific N gene (nucleoprotein).
❖ **Vaccine:** Live attenuated vaccine using Jeryl Lynn strain is available for the prevention of mumps. It is available either as monovalent or more commonly as a part of the trivalent MMR vaccine. It is administered as two doses of MMR vaccine by subcutaneous route at 1 year (12–15 months) and 4–6 years (before starting of school).

Respiratory Syncytial Virus

Respiratory syncytial virus (RSV) is a major respiratory pathogen of young children and is the most common cause of bronchiolitis in infants. It can also cause pneumonia and tracheobronchitis in infants.

❖ **Transmission:** It is transmitted by direct contact of eyes with contaminated fingers or by droplet inhalation
❖ **Clinical manifestations:** It is the most common cause of bronchiolitis, and tracheobronchitis in infants. Infection is severe in premature infants and underlying congenital cardiac disease, bronchopulmonary dysplasia, nephrotic syndrome, or immunosuppression.
❖ **Laboratory diagnosis:** (i) Antigen detection in respiratory secretions by direct-IF, (ii) isolation of virus using HeLa and HEp-2 cell line and demonstration of typical cytopathic effect—syncytium formation (multinucleated giant cell), (iii) RT-PCR amplifying viral RNA (such as nucleoprotein N gene)
❖ **Treatment:** Ribavirin is the drug of choice.

Nipah and Hendra Viruses

They cause an emerging viral infection, affecting CNS (producing encephalitis).

❖ **Transmission:**
  ■ Hendra virus is transmitted by exposure to infected body fluids and excretions of horses
  ■ Transmission of Nipah virus to humans may occur after direct contact with infected fruit bats, pigs, or persons. Human-to-human transmission has been reported among family members and care givers of infected patients.
❖ **Clinical manifestations:** The incubation period is 4 to 14 days. Both the viruses can produce **encephalitis** in humans; patients present with fever, headache, myalgia, and CNS symptoms such as dizziness, drowsiness, altered consciousness and seizure. Severe cases progress to coma within 48 hours and death
❖ The **case-fatality rate** is very high (50-70%)

- **The latest outbreak** of Nipah encephalitis occurred in Kerala, India in 2018, which witnessed 18 cases with 16 deaths
- **Laboratory diagnosis:** Real-time PCR from the throat and nasal swabs, CSF, urine, and blood performed in the early stages of the disease confirms the diagnosis
- **Treatment:** No effective antiviral treatment is available.

■ RUBELLA

Rubella virus produces a childhood exanthema similar to that of measles. Therefore, rubella is also known as **German measles**. However, unlike measles, it is highly teratogenic; can cause congenital rubella syndrome.
- Rubella is not a Myxovirus but belongs to the Togavirus family. It is discussed here because of its clinical resemblance to measles
- Rubella may present in two clinical forms—postnatal infection and congenital infection.

Postnatal Rubella Infection

Postnatal rubella may occur during neonatal age, childhood, and adult life. The virus is acquired by respiratory droplets.
- The incubation period is about 14 days
- **Rashes** are often the first manifestations in children. Rashes start on the face, extend to the trunk and extremities, and disappear in 3 days
- **Lymphadenopathy** (occipital and postauricular) is the most striking feature
- **Forchheimer spots** may be seen in some cases. They are petechiae spots developed on the soft palate and uvula.

Congenital Rubella Syndrome

The most serious consequence of rubella virus infection is congenital rubella syndrome.

- **Triad:** Rubella is highly teratogenic; affects three primary organs
  1. *Ear:* Sensory neural deafness (most common defect)
  2. *Eyes:* Salt and pepper retinopathy and cataract, and
  3. *Heart:* Patent ductus arteriosus.
- **Severity:** The severity is maximum if the mother acquires the infection in the first trimester.

Laboratory Diagnosis

Nasopharyngeal or throat swab taken 6 days before and after the onset of rash is the ideal specimen.
- **Isolation of virus:** Monkey or rabbit origin cell lines may be used
- **Serology (antibody detection):** ELISA is the preferred method for rubella diagnosis. It detects both IgM and IgG separately. Detection of IgM antibody is useful for the diagnosis of congenital rubella
- **Molecular test:** RT-PCR is available for detecting rubella-specific RNA (nucleoprotein N gene) in clinical specimens.

Rubella Vaccine

Live attenuated vaccine is available for rubella using **RA 27/3** strain. It is available singly or in combination with mumps and measles (MMR vaccine).
- **Indication:** In India, rubella vaccine is indicated to all women of reproductive age (first priority group) followed by all children (1–14 years). Under the national immunization schedule, rubella vaccine is given along with measles (MR vaccine) at 9–12 months of age and a second dose at 16–24 months in selected states
- **Precautions:** Vaccine is contraindicated in pregnancy. If received, women should avoid pregnancy for at least 4 weeks following vaccination.

EXPECTED QUESTIONS

I. **Write an essay on:**
1. Discuss the clinical manifestations, laboratory diagnosis, and prevention of influenza.

II. **Write short notes on:**
1. Mumps parotitis.
2. Laboratory diagnosis of measles.
3. Congenital rubella syndrome.

II. **Multiple Choice Questions (MCQs):**
1. **The classical triad in congenital rubella syndrome is characterized by all, *except*:**
   a. Cataract
   b. Deafness
   c. Cardiac defect
   d. Hepatitis
2. **Avian flu strain is:**
   a. A/H5N1   b. A/H3N2
   c. A/H1N1   d. Influenza B
3. **Seasonal flu strain includes all, *except*:**
   a. A/H5N1   b. A/H3N2
   c. A/H1N1   d. Influenza B
4. **SSPE is a complication seen with:**
   a. Influenza   b. Measles
   c. Mumps   d. Rubella

Answers
1. d   2. a   3. a   4. b

Coronaviruses

CHAPTER 40

CHAPTER PREVIEW
- Epidemiology
- Pathogenesis
- Clinical Manifestations
- Laboratory Diagnosis
- Treatment
- Vaccine and Infection Control

Coronaviruses (CoV) cause respiratory tract infections in man; illness ranging from mild common cold to severe disease like pneumonia. The coronaviruses that caused explosive outbreaks of severe respiratory disease with higher mortality are as follows.
- **SARS-CoV** (Severe acute respiratory syndrome coronavirus): It has caused an explosive epidemic called 'SARS' in China in 2003
- **MERS-CoV** (Middle East respiratory syndrome coronavirus): It has caused an explosive epidemic called 'MERS' in Middle East (Saudi Arabia) in 2012
- **SARS-CoV-2** (Severe acute respiratory syndrome coronavirus-2): It is the causative agent of an explosive pandemic that affected the whole world in 2019-20; called COVID-19.

CORONAVIRUS DISEASE (COVID)-2019

Coronavirus disease-2019 (COVID-19) is an acute respiratory disease caused by severe acute respiratory syndrome coronavirus-2 (SARS-CoV-2). It has caused an explosive catastrophic pandemic that affected almost all parts of the world and produced significant loss of lives and financial crisis.

Epidemiology

SARS-CoV-2 originated from China (Wuhan city) in December 2019 and subsequently spread rapidly to affect the rest of the world over 3-4 months—pandemic was declared on 11th March 2020 by WHO.
- **Highest cases:** USA accounted for the maximum number of cases, followed by India, France, Germany and Brazil
- **Mortality rate:** It varies among the countries and also across different time spans of the pandemic—with an overall mortality rate of 1 to 1.5%
- **India:** Accounts for the second-highest number of cases. However, the pandemic had a slower growth curve to reach its peak in India. India witnessed three distinct waves of the explosive surge in cases
  - First wave was around September 2020
  - Second wave was around April 2021 (due to delta variant)
  - Third wave was around January 2022 (due to the omicron variant).
- WHO has declared an end to COVID-19 as a public health emergency on 5th May 2023.

Morphology

The SARS-CoV-2 is a RNA virus, that comprises of a nucleocapsid with a helical symmetry, surrounded by an envelope. It possesses 4 structural proteins **(Fig. 40.1)**.

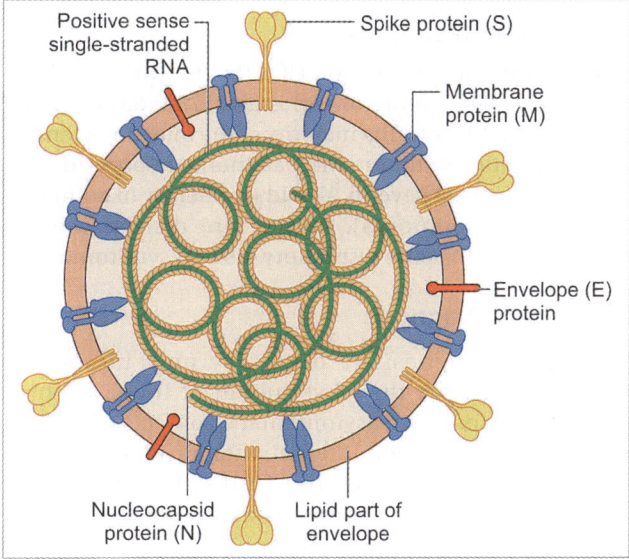

Fig. 40.1: Structure of SARS-CoV-2.

1. Nucleocapsid (N) protein
2. Spike protein (S): Helps in the attachment to the host cells
3. Membrane glycoprotein (M)
4. Envelope protein (E).

Pathogenesis

Pathogenesis of COVID-19 involves the following sequential steps.
- **Transmission**: COVID-19 virus is primarily transmitted via any of the following routes
  - *Respiratory droplets* can fall on the mouth, nose, or eyes (if present within 1 meter), and
  - *Contact routes:* (i) direct contact with infected people, or (ii) indirect contact with the surfaces or objects in the immediate environment.
  - *Aerosol transmission* can occur in specific settings in which aerosol-generating procedures are performed (e.g. endotracheal intubation).
- **Host cell entry:** The virus enters the host cell by binding of its spike (S) antigen with the host cell receptor of SARS-CoV-2 called, i.e. angiotensin-converting enzyme-2 (ACE-2). Subsequently, the virus is carried to the pharynx and then to the lungs.
- **Development of influenza-like illness (ILI):** At the initial stage, SARS-CoV-2 infects the pharyngeal epithelium, and induces inflammation; this accounts for the influenza-like illness (ILI).
- **Development of ARDS:** Certain patients with COVID-19 with comorbidity progress into acute respiratory distress syndrome (ARDS). The underlying mechanisms are due to massive release of pro-inflammatory cytokines (causes cytokine storm).

Clinical Manifestations

The incubation period for COVID-19 (time between infection and symptom onset) is about 5-6 days but can be as long as 14 days. The majority of the infections remain asymptomatic. Symptomatic patients may present with different stages of severity—mild (influenza-like illness), moderate (pneumonia), and severe disease (severe pneumonia with acute respiratory distress syndrome).

Laboratory Diagnosis

Laboratory diagnosis is necessary only in specific indications as per the Government of India, such as symptomatic patients, asymptomatic contacts with high-risk exposure, or recent international travel. Indications for testing may vary as per the COVID-19 situation.
- **Specimens:** Throat swabs and nasal swabs are the ideal specimens, collected by Dacron or polyester flocked swabs and then dipped into the viral transport media

- **Real-time RT-PCR:** Real-time reverse-transcriptase PCR testing is the gold standard method for diagnosis of COVID-19
  - *Formats:* (i) conventional real-time PCR—useful if sample load is high, takes more time (4-6h), (ii) automated real-time PCR formats (GeneXpert and Truenat)—useful in laboratories with lesser sample load, takes less time (1-2h)
  - *Gene targets:* Current guidelines recommend that the real-time PCT kits target **at least two genes** of SARS-CoV-2, among the following genes:
    - Spike protein (S)
    - Envelope protein (E)
    - Membrane protein (M)
    - Nucleocapsid protein (N)
    - RNA-dependent RNA polymerase (RdRp)
    - Open reading frames (ORF1a/b).
- **CRISPR-based assay** (clustered regularly interspaced short palindromic repeats): It is a low-cost, rapid, point-of-care test, which can identify the RNA of the SARS-CoV-2 virus
- **Antigen detection assay:** Point-of-care test; detects nucleocapsid protein antigen in nasopharyngeal swab by immunochromatographic test (ICT)
- **Antibody (IgG) detection assay:** Used for surveillance purposes in a high-risk and vulnerable group
- **Sequencing:** Useful to determine mutations in the viral genome (e.g. omicron)
- **Omicron detection:** Specific real-time PCR kit are available, which can detect the precise mutations in S gene that occurs in omicron variants
- **Viral culture:** Used for research purpose
- **Nonspecific tests** include:
  - Radiology (chest CT scan): Ground-glass appearance
  - Biomarkers: IL-6, D-dimer.

> **TREATMENT** — COVID-19
>
> COVID-19 cases can be managed either by:
> - **Home isolation:** Indicated for the asymptomatic or mild case without risk factors), or
> - **Hospitalization:** Indicated for moderate to severe cases or with risk factors like diabetes, immunosuppression, etc.
>
> **Symptomatic management:** such as
> - **Respiratory support:** (i) Supplemental oxygen to maintain SpO_2 >94%, (ii) Mechanical ventilation
> - **Others:** Steroid, anticoagulant (like heparin) to prevent coagulopathies and management of shock, etc.
> - **Antiviral drugs:** Although not very promising, but following drugs are approved for use in COVID-19
> - **Remdesivir:** Interferes with viral RNA polymerase, given in moderate to severe cases
> - **Tocilizumab:** Monoclonal antibody against IL-6 receptor, given in severe disease to reduce the cytokine storm.

Vaccine

Several vaccines are available for COVID-19. Three vaccines are licensed in India so far—Covaxin, Covishield and Sputnik V.

- **Indication:** COVID-19 vaccination is indicated for all aged ≥15 years
- **Covaxin:** It is a whole-virion inactivated vaccine, which uses spike protein as a target. It is administered in two doses (4-6 weeks apart) by IM route
- **Covishield:** It is based on a non-replicating adenovirus vector expressing spike protein. It is administered in two doses (12–16 weeks apart) by IM route
- **Sputnik V vaccine:** It is a Russian vaccine, also based on adenovirus vector. It is given in two doses (by IM route), at a gap of 3 weeks
- **Precaution dose:** A third dose of the COVID-19 vaccine is recommended to use for the high-risk groups
- **Interchangeability** between the vaccines is not permitted
- **Storage:** Covaxin and Covishield can be stored at 2–8°C, whereas Sputnik V needs to be stored at –18°C
- **Other non-COVID-19 vaccines** can be administered only after a 14 days gap of COVID vaccination
- **Efficacy:** COVID-19 vaccines induce an adequate immune response (of 70–90% efficacy) in about 2–3 weeks after the second dose.

Infection Prevention and Control

Infection prevention and control (IPC) is the most effective method for the prevention of COVID-19.

In Community-settings

The recommended IPC practices are:
- Hand hygiene after contact with other individuals, in high-touch areas, in public places, etc.
- The physical distance of at least one meter
- Use of non-medical masks in public places
- Respiratory hygiene and cough etiquette
- Quarantine of asymptomatic individuals with high-risk exposure.

In Healthcare-settings

The recommended IPC practices are:
- **Use of appropriate PPE** when giving care to COVID-19 patients (*refer* **Chapter 15**). The recommended PPE are gown, 3-ply mask, goggles, and gloves. N95 respirator may be necessary when working in places where aerosol-generating procedures are carried out such as ICUs or operation theatres
- **Environmental cleaning** of floor and surfaces, equipment, high-touch areas, etc. with appropriate disinfectants such as hypochlorite or alcohol
- **Biomedical waste management** should be carried out as per the 2016 guideline (*refer* **Chapter 17**). However, additional precautions are taken such as the use of a double bag, label as 'COVID-19 waste', and disinfecting the outer bag with hypochlorite before handing over
- **Laundry management:** Washing linens at 60-90°C with laundry detergent followed by soaking in 0.1% sodium hypochlorite.

EXPECTED QUESTIONS

I. **Write short notes on:**
  1. COVID-19 vaccines.
  2. Laboratory diagnosis of COVID-19.

II. **Multiple Choice Questions (MCQs):**
  1. While examining a stable patient with COVID-19, all the following PPE are required, *except*:
     a. N 95 mask b. Gown
     c. Goggles d. Gloves

2. Gene targets for COVID–19 detection include all, *except*:
   a. Spike protein (S)
   b. Envelope protein (E)
   c. Membrane protein (M)
   d. Reverse transcriptase gene

Answers
1. a 2. d

Arboviruses

CHAPTER 41

CHAPTER PREVIEW
- Introduction
- Dengue Virus
- Chikungunya Virus
- Kyasanur Forest Disease Virus
- Japanese B Encephalitis
- Yellow Fever Virus
- Zika Virus

INTRODUCTION

Arboviruses (arthropod-borne viruses) are diverse group of RNA viruses that are transmitted by blood-sucking arthropods (insect vectors) from one vertebrate host to another. Viruses must multiply inside the insects and establish a lifelong harmless infection in them.

Classification

Arboviruses are taxonomically diverse and belong to five different families: Togaviridae, Flaviviridae, Bunyaviridae, Reoviridae and Rhabdoviridae **(Table 41.1)**.

Individual viruses under each family are named after various features such as:

- ❖ **Clinical features:** For example, yellow fever is named after its main clinical feature—jaundice
- ❖ **Place of discovery:** For example, Kyasanur Forest disease virus
- ❖ **Multiple features:** Japanese encephalitis virus is named after the place of discovery and clinical feature.

Clinical Manifestations

Arboviruses may also be divided based on the pattern of clinical syndromes they produce **(Table 41.1)**.
- ❖ Fever and/or rash, and/or arthralgia group
- ❖ Encephalitis group
- ❖ Hemorrhagic fever group.

However, some of them may be associated with more than one clinical syndrome, e.g. dengue virus.

Epidemiology

- ❖ **Zoonotic:** Several hundred arboviruses exist in the world and all are believed to be endemic in animals
- ❖ **Transmission cycle:** Arboviruses are maintained in nature between animals and their insect vectors
- ❖ **Humans are the accidental hosts** and do not play any role in the maintenance or transmission cycle of the virus, except for urban yellow fever and dengue
- ❖ **Arthropod vector:** Most arboviruses are transmitted by mosquitoes (*Aedes*, *Culex* or *Anopheles*) followed by ticks, and other insects **(Table 41.1)**
- ❖ **Climatic variation:** Arboviruses are more prevalent in the **tropics** than in temperate climate, due to the abundance of appropriate animals and arthropods in the former
- ❖ **Geographical distribution:** Viruses that are highly endemic in one place, may not be found in other areas:
  - **Yellow fever** is highly endemic in West Africa, but not found at all in India despite its vector *Aedes aegypti* being widely distributed in India
  - Encephalitic arboviruses: Eastern, Western and Venezuelan equine encephalitis viruses are prevalent in North America whereas, in India, Japanese B encephalitis virus is the most common arbovirus causing encephalitis.
- ❖ **Arboviruses found in India:** Over 40 arboviruses have been detected in India.
  - Common arboviruses prevalent in India include—(i) hemorrhagic fever group (dengue virus, Kyasanur forest disease virus), (ii) fever with arthralgia group (chikungunya virus), and (iii) encephalitis group (Japanese B encephalitis and West Nile encephalitis viruses)
  - Rare arboviruses: Sindbis, Crimean Congo hemorrhagic fever, Ganjam, Vellore, Chandipura, Bhanja, Umbre, Sathuperi, Chittoor, Minnal, Venkatapuram, Dhori, Kaisodi, and sandfly fever viruses are among the rare arboviruses found in India, with limited geographical distribution.

CHAPTER 41 ◆ Arboviruses

Table 41.1: General features of prevalent arboviruses.			
Virus	Manifestation	Vector	Reservoir
Family: Togaviridae			
Chikungunya virus	Fever and arthritis (rarely hemorrhagic fever)	*Aedes aegypti*	Monkeys*
Eastern equine encephalitis virus	Encephalitis	*Aedes, Culex*	Birds
Western equine encephalitis virus	Encephalitis	*Culex tarsalis, Aedes*	Birds
Venezuelan equine encephalitis virus	Encephalitis	*Aedes, Culex*	Horses
Family: Flaviviridae			
Japanese B encephalitis virus	Encephalitis	*Culex tritaeniorhynchus*	Pigs, Birds
West Nile encephalitis virus	Encephalitis	*Culex, Aedes, Anopheles*	Birds
Dengue virus	Hemorrhagic fever	*Aedes aegypti*	*
Yellow fever virus	Hemorrhagic fever	*Aedes aegypti*	Monkeys
Kyasanur Forest disease virus	Hemorrhagic fever	Tick	Monkeys and rats
Zika virus	Fever and arthritis	*Aedes aegypti*	Monkeys
Family: Bunyaviridae			
Crimean Congo hemorrhagic fever virus	Hemorrhagic fever	Tick	Small mammals
Sandfly fever	Fever and myalgia	Sandfly	Small mammals
Ganjam virus	Fever	Tick	Small mammals
Family: Reoviridae			
Colorado tick fever virus	Fever, rarely encephalitis	Tick	Rodents
Family: Rhabdoviridae			
Vesicular stomatitis virus	Oral mucosal vesicles	Sandfly	*
Chandipura virus	Encephalitis	Sandfly	*

*Not yet identified.

- ❖ **Arboviruses not found in India:** There are over 100 arboviruses prevalent in various parts of the world other than India. Few of them are of global significance and hence have been discussed in this chapter (yellow fever virus and Zika virus).

■ DENGUE

Dengue virus is the most common arbovirus found in India. It has four serotypes (DEN-1 to DEN-4). *Aedes aegypti* is the principal vector followed by *Aedes albopictus*. They usually bite during the daytime.

Pathogenesis

The pathogenesis of dengue is different in the first infection from that of subsequent infections.
- ❖ **Primary dengue infection** occurs when a person is infected with the dengue virus for the first time with any one serotype
- ❖ **Secondary dengue infection:** Months to years later, a more severe form of dengue illness may appear, due to infection with another second serotype which is different from the first serotype causing primary infection

- ■ *Mechanism:* The severity of secondary infection is due to a mechanism called **antibody-dependent enhancement**. Antibodies against the first serotype combine with the second serotype and instead of neutralizing the virus, they protect the second serotype from the host immune response
- ■ *Complications:* The risk of hemorrhagic fever and shock is more in secondary dengue infection
- ■ *The sequence of infection:* Among all serotype combinations, serotype 1 followed by 2 produces the most severe disease.

Clinical Classifications

The incubation period is about 5 days. Dengue can occur in three clinical stages:
1. **Dengue fever (DF):** It is characterized by abrupt onset of high fever (also called biphasic fever, break-bone fever, or saddleback fever). Other features are rashes, headache, myalgia, joint pain, lymphadenopathy, retro-orbital pain, loss of appetite, nausea and vomiting
2. **Dengue hemorrhagic fever (DHF):** It is characterized by:

- High-grade continuous fever
- Hepatomegaly
- Thrombocytopenia (platelet count <1 lakh/mm^3)
- Raised hematocrit (packed cell volume) by 20%
- Evidence of hemorrhages can be detected by:
    - Positive tourniquet test (>20 petechial spots per square inch area in the cubital fossa
    - Spontaneous bleeding from skin, nose, mouth, and gums.
3. **Dengue shock syndrome (DSS):** Here, all the above criteria of DHF are present, and in addition manifestations of shock are present, such as:
    - Rapid and weak pulse
    - Narrow pulse pressure (<20 mm Hg) or hypotension
    - Presence of cold and clammy skin
    - Restlessness.

WHO has described a classification which grades dengue into two stages based on the severity.
1. Dengue with or without warning signs
2. Severe dengue.

Epidemiology

Globally, dengue is endemic in more than 100 countries with 2.5 billion people at risk.
- Tropical countries of Southeast Asia and the Western Pacific are at the highest risk
- **The situation in India:** Disease is prevalent throughout India affecting almost 31 states/Union territories
    - In 2023: More than 94,000 cases were reported with 91 deaths; maximum cases were reported from Kerala and Karnataka.
    - All serotypes have been reported from India, but DEN-1 and DEN-2 serotypes are widespread.

Laboratory Diagnosis

The laboratory diagnosis of dengue comprises of the following modalities.
- **NS1 Antigen detection** by ELISA and ICT formats. NS1 antigen becomes detectable from day 1 of fever and remains positive up to 7 days
- **Antibody detection** by ELISA: It detects IgM and IgG separately. For IgM, a special type of ELISA is available called IgM antibody capture (MAC) ELISA
    - *In primary infection:* IgM antibody usually appears after 5 days of fever and is suggestive of active infection
    - *In secondary infection:* Rapid rise of IgG antibody titer is suggestive of active infection.
- **Detection of specific genes of viral RNA** by real-time RT-PCR: It is the most sensitive and specific assay, and can be used for the detection of serotypes and quantification of viral load in blood. Viral RNA can be detected in blood from –1 to +5 days of onset of symptoms.

> **TREATMENT** — Dengue
>
> There is no specific antiviral therapy. Treatment is symptomatic and supportive such as:
> - Replacement of plasma losses
> - Correction of electrolyte and metabolic disturbances
> - Platelet transfusion if needed

Dengue Vaccine (CYD-TDV)

This vaccine has been licensed for human use.
- It is a live-attenuated, Chimeric Yellow Fever-Dengue-Tetravalent Dengue Vaccine (CYD-TDV); commercially available as dengvaxia
- It uses live attenuated yellow fever 17D virus as a vaccine vector in which the target genes of all four dengue serotypes are integrated by recombinant technique
- **Age:** It is indicated for 9–45 years of age
- **Schedule:** 3 doses given subcutaneously at 6-month intervals
- In India, it is not available yet because of its safety issues.

■ CHIKUNGUNYA

Chikungunya fever is a re-emerging disease characterized by acute fever with severe arthralgia.
- **Transmission:** It is transmitted by *Aedes aegypti,* which usually bites during day time
- **Clinical manifestations:** The incubation period is about 5 days (3–7 days). The most common symptoms are fever and severe joint pain (due to arthritis), worsened in the morning
    - **Arthritis** is polyarticular, migratory, and edematous (joint swelling), predominantly affecting the small joints of the wrists and ankles
    - Symptoms are often confusing with that of dengue. In general, Chikungunya is less severe, less acute, and hemorrhagic manifestations are rare compared to dengue.
- **Epidemiology:** Chikungunya is a classic example of re-emerging disease as it was clinically quiescent for a long time (1973–2005) in most parts of the world. Currently, it has been reported in India, and other Southeast Asian and African countries, where it is associated with several outbreaks
- **Laboratory diagnosis** of Chikungunya comprises of the following modalities
    - **Serum antibody detection by ELISA:** Detection of IgM or a fourfold rise in IgG titer is suggestive of infection. MAC ELISA is available for the detection of IgM antibodies

- **Reverse-transcriptase PCR** has been developed to detect specific genes in blood.

> **TREATMENT** — Chikungunya
>
> Treatment of Chikungunya is only by supportive measures; no specific antiviral drugs or vaccination are available.

■ KYASANUR FOREST DISEASE (KFD) VIRUS

KFD virus is named after the place where the disease is prevalent—Kyasanur Forest in Shimoga district of Karnataka, India.

- ❖ **Transmission:** Hard ticks are the primary vector of KFD virus; whereas monkeys are the amplifier hosts, where the virus multiplies exponentially
- ❖ **Clinical manifestations:** The incubation period varies from 3 to 8 days. The disease occurs in two stages
    - The first stage (hemorrhagic fever)
    - The second stage in the form of meningoencephalitis.
- ❖ **Epidemiology:** KFD is currently endemic in five districts of Karnataka—Shimoga, North Kannada, South Kannada, Chikkamagaluru, and Udupi
- ❖ **Laboratory diagnosis:** Diagnosis is made by detection of IgM antibody by ELISA or real-time RT-PCR has been developed to detect viral RNA
- ❖ **Treatment** of KFD is only by supportive measures; no specific antiviral drugs are available
- ❖ **Vaccine:** A formalin-inactivated killed vaccine has been developed. It is recommended in endemic areas of Karnataka (villages within 5 km of endemic foci).

■ JAPANESE B ENCEPHALITIS

Japanese B encephalitis virus is the leading cause of vaccine-preventable viral encephalitis in Asia, including India.

- ❖ **Transmission:** JE virus is transmitted by the bite of the *Culex* mosquito. *C. tritaeniorhynchus* is the primary vector, followed by *C. vishnui*
- ❖ **Host:** JE virus has several animal and bird hosts—pigs are the amplifier host; others being cattle and buffalo
- ❖ **Age:** About 85% of cases occur in children below 15 years and about 10% occur in the elderly
- ❖ **Seasonal variation:** Infection is common in rainy season which coincides with maximum mosquito activity
- ❖ **Clinical manifestations:** The clinical course of the disease can be divided into three stages:
    1. **Prodromal stage** is a febrile illness; the onset of which may be either abrupt (1–6 hours), acute (6–24 hours) or more commonly subacute (2–5 days)
    2. **Acute encephalitis stage:** JE is the most common cause of acute encephalitis syndrome (AES) in India; characterized by an acute onset of fever, mental confusion, disorientation, delirium, seizures, or coma
    3. **Late stage and sequelae:** It is the convalescent stage in which the patient may be recovered fully or retain some neurological deficits permanently (up to 50%). Case fatality rate is about 20–40%.
- ❖ **Epidemiology:** JE is endemic in several states such as Uttar Pradesh (Gorakhpur district), Assam, Manipur, etc. which account for the largest burden of cases
- ❖ **Laboratory diagnosis:** Diagnosis of JE is made by:
    - IgM antibody capture (MAC) ELISA detecting IgM antibodies
    - Real-time RT-PCR has been developed to detect JE virus-specific envelope (E) gene in blood.
- ❖ **Treatment:** Only by supportive measures; no specific antiviral drugs are available
- ❖ **Vaccine:** Live attenuated using SA 14-14-2 strain of JE virus is available
    - *Under the national immunization program*, it is given to children (1–15 years) in specific endemic districts of states such as—UP, Bihar, Assam, West Bengal, and Karnataka
    - *Schedule:* Two doses (subcutaneously); 1st at 9–12 months of age and 2nd at 16–24 months.

■ WEST NILE ENCEPHALITIS

West Nile virus (WNV) is a flavivirus related to JE virus. It is mainly transmitted by *Culex* mosquito. It is zoonotic, maintained in nature by transmission between birds and mosquitoes.

- ❖ **Clinical feature:** The incubation period is about 3–14 days. 80% of people remain asymptomatic. The rest may develop disease
    - **West Nile fever:** Common symptoms include fever, headache, tiredness, body aches, nausea, vomiting, skin rash and swollen lymph glands
    - **West Nile encephalitis** or meningitis may develop rarely. It is a severe form of disease, with a mortality of 10%.
- ❖ **India:** WNV is highly prevalent in India in various states and has caused several outbreaks in the past, such as in Kerala (2011) and Assam (2006)
- ❖ **Diagnosis:** The various laboratory tests available are:
    - IgM antibody capture ELISA detecting IgM antibodies in serum and CSF is available.
    - IgG ELISA demonstrating seroconversion in two serial specimens collected at a one-week interval is also diagnostic
    - Viral RNA detection by RT-PCR.
- ❖ **Treatment** is only by supportive measures.

YELLOW FEVER

Yellow fever is an acute, febrile illness; affecting the liver to cause jaundice (hence the name yellow fever), hemorrhage, with high mortality.

- **Vector:** Humans get the infection by the bite of *Aedes aegypti* or the tiger mosquito
- **Geographical distribution:** Yellow fever is endemic in West Africa and Central South America. It is not found in the rest of the World including India. But India has the vector (*A. aegypti*) widely distributed and therefore has the risk of getting cases in future
- **Clinical manifestations:** The incubation period is about **3–6 days**. The disease is characterized by:
    - Febrile illness: occurs in the early stage
    - Hemorrhagic manifestations
    - Platelet dysfunction
    - Features of liver involvement (hepatitis) such as jaundice.
- **Laboratory diagnosis:** Diagnosis of yellow fever is made by:
    - Antibody detection: IgM ELISA can be done after 3 days of onset of symptoms
    - RT-PCR detecting specific viral RNA (NS5 region) in blood.
- **Treatment:** Only by symptomatic care, no antiviral drugs are available. Preventive measures include vaccination and mosquito control
- **Yellow fever 17D vaccine:** It is a live attenuated vaccine
    - A strict cold chain has to be maintained during the transport (–30°C to +5°C)
    - Dosage: Single-dose, given subcutaneously
    - A certificate of vaccination is issued after 10 days of vaccination and renewed (i.e. re-immunization) every 10 years. This is the recommendation followed for international travel.

ZIKA VIRUS DISEASE

Zika virus (ZIKV) has recently gained attention due to the large outbreak that occurred in 2015–16 worldwide.

- **Transmission:** ZIKV is primarily transmitted by the *Aedes aegypti* mosquito. Other modes include—mother-to-child transmission (common in the first trimester) and rarely through sexual contact
- **Epidemiology:** The largest explosive epidemic reported was in **Brazil** (2015–2016) and then subsequently spread to other countries in America, the Caribbean, Europe, and Australia. In India, only a few cases are reported so far
- **The clinical manifestations:** The incubation period ranges from a few days to 1 week. Various clinical presentations include:
    - The majority (>80%) of infections are asymptomatic
    - Zika fever with minor symptoms
    - Congenital Zika syndrome: Characterized by microcephaly and other neurological features
    - Neurological complications.
- **Laboratory diagnosis:** The laboratory tests for confirmation of ZIKV disease include:
    - *RT-PCR* has been the investigation of choice. It can detect Zika virus RNA in blood and urine up to 7 days after onset of symptoms
    - *IgM antibody detection* by enzyme immunoassays and immunofluorescence assays.
- **Treatment:** No effective treatment and vaccine are available so far. Cases are managed only with symptomatic treatment.

EXPECTED QUESTIONS

I. **Write an essay on:**
   1. List the arboviruses that are prevalent in India. Discuss the pathogenesis, clinical presentation, and laboratory diagnosis of dengue.

II. **Write short notes on:**
   1. Chikungunya virus.
   2. Kyasanur forest disease virus.
   3. Japanese B encephalitis.

III. **Multiple Choice Questions (MCQs):**
   1. **Dengue is transmitted by:**
      a. *Aedes aegypti*   b. *Culex*
      c. Tick   d. *Anopheles*
   2. **Japanese B encephalitis is transmitted by:**
      a. *Anopheles*   b. *Aedes aegypti*
      c. *Culex*   d. Tick
   3. **Kyasanur forest disease is transmitted by:**
      a. *Aedes aegypti*   b. *Culex*
      c. Tick   d. *Anopheles*
   4. **17 D vaccine is given for:**
      a. Yellow fever
      b. Dengue
      c. Japanese encephalitis
      d. Zika virus disease

Answers
1. a   2. c   3. c   4. a

Rabies Virus

CHAPTER 42

CHAPTER PREVIEW
- Morphology
- Street and Fixed Viruses
- Pathogenesis
- Clinical Manifestations
- Laboratory Diagnosis
- Prevention of Human Rabies
- WHO Guideline of Post-exposure Prophylaxis

Rabies virus causes a rapidly progressive, acute infectious disease of the CNS in humans and animals, transmitted from another rabid animal. It is considered a major public health problem because it is almost always fatal.

MORPHOLOGY

Rabies virus is bullet-shaped and comprises a nucleocapsid (with helical symmetry), surrounded by an envelope. Rabies virus has two major antigens **(Fig. 42.1)**.

1. **Glycoprotein-G:** It is the envelope proteins embedded into the lipid part of the envelope. It is the major antigen responsible for pathogenesis (by binding to acetylcholine receptors in neural tissues). Antibodies to glycoprotein-G are protective in nature
2. **Nucleoprotein:** It is the nucleocapsid protein. It has a diagnostic role. The direct-immunofluorescence (DIF) test detects the nucleoprotein antigens in the patient's serum.

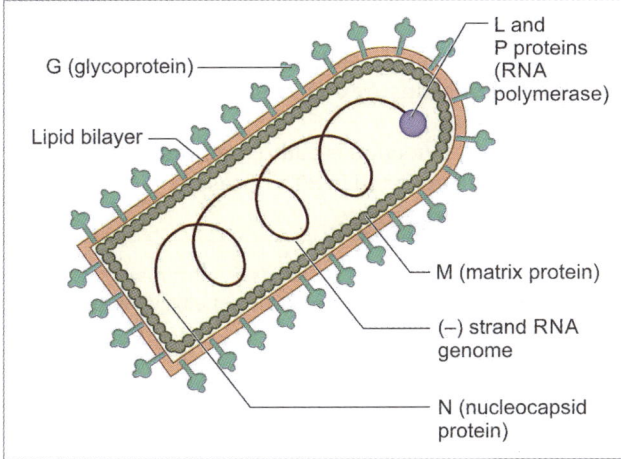

Fig. 42.1: Rabies virus (schematic diagram).

STREET AND FIXED VIRUSES

Rabies virus undergoes certain changes when it is serially propagated in animals.
- ❖ **Street viruses:** These are freshly isolated strains in the laboratory. They mimic the wild viruses; show long and variable incubation periods and produce intracytoplasmic inclusion bodies
- ❖ **Fixed viruses:** When street viruses are propagated in rabbits by serial brain-to-brain passage; they lose certain properties and become fixed strains.
    - They do not produce inclusion bodies
    - They do not multiply in extraneural tissues
    - They do not infect salivary gland
    - They multiply rapidly, and the incubation period is shortened to 4–6 days, hence these strains are best used for vaccination.

PATHOGENESIS

The pathogenesis of rabies involves the following sequential steps.
- ❖ **Transmission:** Rabies virus is usually transmitted to humans by the **bite of rabid dogs**, bats, and other wild animals such as foxes, jackals, etc. Rarely, it can also be transmitted by various non-bite exposures, e.g.—
    - Direct contact with the saliva of infected animals with mucosa or fresh skin wounds
    - Inhalation of virus-containing aerosols (important for laboratory workers)
    - Cornea or other organ transplantation.

    Transmission by human bite is not documented yet.
- ❖ **Spread to CNS:** The virus multiplies locally and spreads centripetally along the peripheral motor nerves to reach dorsal root ganglia of the spinal cord, and then ascends upward towards CNS, where it affects mainly the hippocampus and cerebellum

- **Centrifugal spread:** From CNS, the virus spreads along the sensory and autonomic nerves to various tissues such as salivary glands, cornea, and others
- **Shed in saliva:** Rabies virus is shed in the saliva of rabid animals which acts as the source of infection to other animals
- **Pathological changes:** Presence of **Negri bodies** (intracytoplasmic eosinophilic inclusions) composed of rabies virus proteins and viral RNA, in the brain parenchyma is an important pathological finding of rabies.

■ CLINICAL MANIFESTATIONS

The incubation period is prolonged and variable (20–90 days). The clinical spectrum is divided into 3 phases as follows.

Prodromal Phase

It lasts for 2–10 days, characterized by non-specific symptoms such as fever, malaise, photophobia, etc.

Acute Neurologic Phase

This may be either encephalitic type or paralytic type.
- **Encephalitic or furious rabies:** It is the most common type (80%), lasts for 2–7 days, and is characterized by:
  - *Hyperexcitability*: Anxiety, agitation, hyperactivity
  - *Autonomic (sympathetic) dysfunction* features may be seen such as ↑lacrimation, and ↑salivation
  - *Hydrophobia* (fear of water) or *aerophobia* (fear of air)—the act of swallowing precipitates an involuntary, painful spasm of the respiratory muscles.
- **Paralytic or dumb rabies:** This occurs in 20% of cases, especially in people who are partially vaccinated. It is characterized by flaccid paralysis of limbs. However, typical features of encephalitic rabies are absent.

Coma and Death

Following the acute neurological phase, the patient develops coma that eventually leads to death within 14 days.

■ LABORATORY DIAGNOSIS

- **Specimen collection:** Specimens such as saliva, CSF, serum, and skin biopsies of hair follicles at the nape of the neck are useful
- **Rabies antigen detection:** Direct fluorescent antibody (DFA) test can be performed to detect rabies nucleoprotein antigens in specimens such as hair follicle of the nape of the neck (most sensitive, best specimen) and corneal impression smear
- **Virus isolation** can be performed using suckling mice (intracerebral inoculation) or by using mouse neuroblastoma or baby hamster kidney (BHK) cell lines

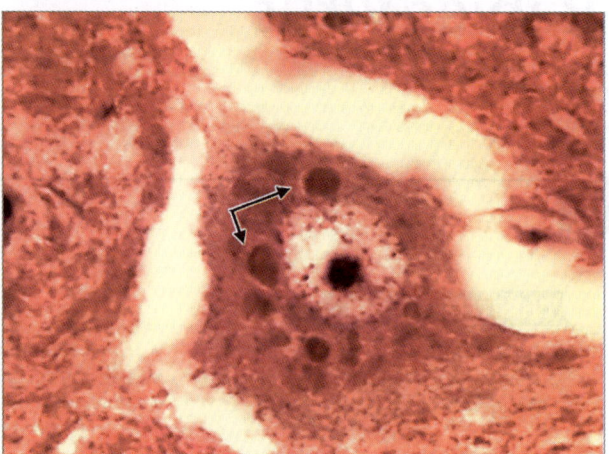

Fig. 42.2: Negri bodies in brain biopsy by H and E stain (*arrows showing*).

Source: Public Health Image Library, ID# 3377//Dr. Daniel P. Perl/Centers for Disease Control and Prevention (CDC), Atlanta (*with permission*).

- **Antibody detection:** Detection of CSF antibodies is more significant than serum antibodies, as the serum antibodies appear late and can also be present after vaccination. Several formats are available such as:
  - Mouse neutralization test (MNT)
  - Rapid fluorescent focus inhibition test (RFFIT)
  - Fluorescent antibody virus neutralization test (FAVN)
  - Indirect fluorescence assay (IFA).
- **Virus RNA detection:** Reverse transcription-PCR (RT-PCR) can be used to amplify specific genes (e.g. nucleoprotein gene). It is the most sensitive and specific assay available
- **Negri body detection:** It is useful to confirm the postmortem diagnosis of rabies **(Fig. 42.2)**
  - It is an intracytoplasmic eosinophilic inclusion body, composed of rabies virus proteins and viral RNA
  - Commonly observed in the cerebellum and hippocampus
  - **Stains:** Histological stains such as H and E **(Fig. 42.2)** and Sellers stains are commonly used to demonstrate Negri bodies.
  - Negri body detection is pathognomonic of rabies, but may not be detected in 20% of cases.

TREATMENT — Rabies

There is no specific treatment for rabies. Symptomatic treatment may prolong life, but the outcome is almost always fatal.
- Isolation of the patient
- Sedatives and anti-anxiety drugs
- Maintenance of hydration and urination.

■ PREVENTION OF HUMAN RABIES

There are three strategies available for the prevention of rabies.

Local Wound Care

Involves *physical cleansing* of all bite wounds and scratches with soap and water, followed by applying antiseptics. *Suturing should be strictly avoided* as it causes local tissue damage, which may help in the spreading of the virus.

Rabies Vaccine

Cell line-derived non-neural vaccines are recommended.
1. Purified chick embryo cell (PCEC) vaccine
2. Purified Vero cell (PVC) vaccine
3. Human diploid cell (HDC) vaccine.

Note: The neural vaccines derived from the brain of infected animals are no longer used.

Rabies Immunoglobulin (RIG)

It neutralizes the virus at the wound site within a few hours.
- RIG should be administered as soon as possible and not beyond day 7
- It is available in two forms; human RIG (hRIG) and equine RIG (eRIG)
- Recommended dose: 20 IU (for hRIG) or 40 IU (for eRIG) per kg body weight.

WHO GUIDELINE OF POST-EXPOSURE PROPHYLAXIS

WHO has provided a guideline (2018) for post-exposure prophylaxis (PEP) for rabies. The components included in PEP depend upon the type of exposure categories (Table 42.1).
- **For category I exposures:** Require only wound care. Vaccines or RIG are not required
- **For category II exposures:** Require local wound care and rabies vaccine. RIG is not required except for immunodeficient individuals who need RIG in addition
- **For category III exposures:** All three components are required—local wound care, vaccine, and RIG.

Schedule: Rabies vaccine can be administered by intradermal (ID) or intramuscular (IM). The ID regimens are cost-effective and therefore are preferred over IM regimens

Table 42.1: Risk categorization and recommended anti-rabies prophylaxis (WHO, 2018).

Category of risk	Type of exposure	Recommended prophylaxis**
Category I (No risk)	• Touching or feeding of animal • Licks on intact skin	No treatment is needed if history is reliable
Category II (Minor risk)	Minor scratches or abrasions without bleeding or nibbling of uncovered skin	• Wound management • Rabies vaccine • Observe the dog for 10 days
Category III (Major risk)	• Single or multiple transdermal bites with oozing of blood • Licks on broken skin (fresh wounds) or mucous membrane • Direct contact with bats or wild animals	• Wound management • Rabies immuno-globulin • Rabies vaccine • Observe the dog for 10 days*

*Vaccine may be discontinued if the animal is healthy after 10 days of the bite.
**In India post-exposure prophylaxis is indicated following exposure to any animal bite except rodents and bat bite.

- **ID PEP regimen (2-2-2):** 2-site ID vaccine is given on days 0, 3 and 7 (total 6 doses, 0.1 mL/dose)
- **IM PEP regimens:** A total of four doses are given (entire vial /dose). Two schedules are available
  1. 1-site IM vaccine given on days 0, 3, 7, and the fourth dose between days 14 to 28 or
  2. 2-site IM vaccine given on day 0 and 1-site IM on days 7 and 21.

PEP for Individuals Previously Vaccinated

The individuals who previously received the rabies vaccine do not need RIG regardless of exposure category. They need local wound care and an accelerated vaccine regimen (with a reduced number of doses).

Pre-exposure Prophylaxis (PrEP)

It is recommended for—individuals at higher occupational risk (e.g. animal handlers) or for people in remote endemic areas. The PrEP regimen is given in any of the schedules:
- 2-site ID vaccine given on days 0 and 7
- 1-site IM vaccine given on days 0 and 7.

EXPECTED QUESTIONS

I. Write short notes on:
1. Laboratory diagnosis of rabies.
2. Post-exposure prophylaxis of rabies.

II. Multiple Choice Questions (MCQs):
1. Rabies is transmitted by all, *except*:
   a. Dog bite
   b. Ingestion
   c. Bat bite
   d. Inhalation
2. Negri bodies are pathognomonic for:
   a. Rabies   b. Polio
   c. Dengue   d. HIV

Answers
1. b   2. a

Picornaviruses (Poliovirus, Coxsackievirus and Rhinovirus)

CHAPTER 43

CHAPTER PREVIEW

- Poliovirus
- Coxsackievirus
- Rhinovirus

Picornaviruses belong to the family Picornaviridae; which includes two major groups of human pathogens: enteroviruses and rhinoviruses.
- ❖ **Enteroviruses:** They are transmitted by feco-oral route. Though they multiply in the intestine, they do not cause any intestinal manifestations. They are associated with various systemic manifestations including *poliomyelitis* (a childhood flaccid paralysis). Enteroviruses comprise of:
    - Poliovirus (3 serotypes)
    - Coxsackieviruses—Coxsackie A (1–24 serotypes), and Coxsackie B (1–6 serotypes)
- ❖ **Rhinoviruses:** They are transmitted by respiratory route and cause common cold.

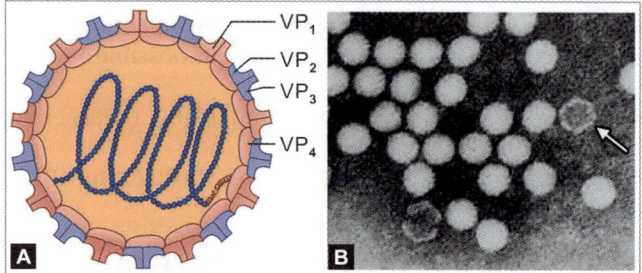

Figs. 43.1A and B: Poliovirus. **A.** Schematic diagram; **B.** Transmission electron micrograph (arrow showing).
Source: **B.** Public Health Image Library, ID#235/Dr Joseph J Esposito, Centers for Disease Control and Prevention (CDC), Atlanta (*with permission*).

■ POLIOVIRUSES

Polioviruses cause a highly infectious childhood disease called polio (or poliomyelitis)—acute flaccid paralysis due to the involvement of the nervous system. Polio is on the verge of eradication globally.

Morphology

Picornaviruses are simple in structure, very small (28–30 nm size) and nonenveloped.
- ❖ They are spherical shaped and have icosahedral symmetry **(Figs. 43.1A and B)**
- ❖ Capsid is composed of 60 subunits, each consisting of four viral proteins (VP1-VP4)
- ❖ Possess single-stranded positive sense linear RNA.

Antigenic Types

Wild polioviruses (WPV) cause natural cases of poliomyelitis. Based on the viral protein (VP1) present on the capsid, there are three types of wild strains (WPV 1-3):
- ❖ All three strains are identical, produce similar manifestations and severity of illness
- ❖ Currently, all the natural cases are caused by WPV1. It has also been the common serotype to cause poliomyelitis till now
- ❖ Both WPV2 and WPV3 are globally eradicated, in the years 1999 and 2019 respectively.

Vaccine-derived poliovirus (VDPV): They are the vaccine strains of poliovirus that have regained neurovirulence and are capable of producing disease in man (described subsequently in this chapter).

Pathogenesis

Polioviruses are transmitted by the feco-oral route. They multiply in intestinal epithelial cells, submucosal lymphoid tissues, tonsils and Peyer's patches.
- ❖ **Spread** to CNS/spinal cord occurs by:
    - Hematogenous route (most common), or
    - Rarely by direct neural route: This occurs especially following tonsillectomy.
- ❖ **Site of action:** The final target site for poliovirus is the motor nerve ending, i.e. anterior horn cells of the spinal cord which leads to muscle weakness and flaccid paralysis

- **Neuron degeneration:** Virus-infected neurons undergo degeneration. The earliest change in the neuron is the degeneration of the Nissl body (aggregates of ribosomes)
- **Pathological changes** are always more extensive than the distribution of paralysis.

Clinical Manifestations

The incubation period is usually 7–14 days. The manifestations may range from asymptomatic stage to the most severe paralytic stage.
- **Inapparent infection:** Following infection, the majority (91–96%) of cases are asymptomatic
- **Abortive infection:** About 5% of patients develop minor symptoms (e.g. fever, malaise, sore throat, etc.)
- **Nonparalytic poliomyelitis:** It is seen in 1% of patients, and presented as aseptic meningitis
- **Paralytic poliomyelitis** is the least common form (<1%), characterized by descending asymmetric acute flaccid paralysis (AFP) **(Figs. 43.2A and B)**
- **Risk factors:** Paralytic disease is more common among: (1) older children and adults, (2) pregnant women, (3) following heavy muscular exercise, (4) tonsillectomy, (5) IM injections.

Laboratory Diagnosis

Useful specimens are stool, rectal swabs, and throat swabs. Specimens should be kept frozen during transport to the laboratory.
- **Virus isolation** in primary monkey kidney cell line from specimens—viral growth is detected by demonstration of cytopathic effect (crenation and degeneration of the entire cell sheet), or detection of viral antigen or viral gene in cell line
- **Antibody detection**—by neutralization test
- **Real-time multiplex reverse-transcriptase PCR** has been developed using primers from VP1 region, which can detect and differentiate between various types of wild and vaccine polioviruses (Vaccine-associated paralytic poliomyelitis and Vaccine-derived poliovirus strains) directly from the stool specimen.

Vaccine

Both inactivated and live-attenuated polio vaccines are available; both have their unique useful properties as well as drawbacks **(Table 43.1)**.
- **Under the national immunization schedule** (India), both IPV and bivalent OPV are given
    - IPV: The fractional-dose of IPV is given by the intradermal route. It contains all three serotypes
    - Bivalent OPV is given orally. It contains serotypes 1 and 3.
- In OPV, the live-attenuated vaccine virus can undergo genetic change to regain neurovirulence and such strains are capable of causing poliomyelitis. Two types of vaccine-induced poliomyelitis have been reported
    1. **Vaccine-associated paralytic poliomyelitis (VAPP):** Caused by OPV-like strain which has a minor genetic difference (<1%) than OPV strain. They are not capable of circulating in the community and do not cause secondary cases or outbreaks
    2. **Vaccine-derived polioviruses (VDPV):** They have a genetic difference from OPV strain by >1%. They are capable of circulating in the community and therefore have a higher risk of causing outbreaks.

Epidemiology

Polio is on the verge of eradication globally.

Pulse Polio Immunization (PPI) was initiated globally to eradicate poliomyelitis. In India, it is in operation since 1995–96.
- **World:** Currently, wild polio is endemic only in two countries—Pakistan, and Afghanistan. However, vaccine-derived polio cases are still occurring in a few other countries of the world
- **India** became polio-free in 2014. No natural case has been reported since 2011

The Global Polio Eradication Initiative (GPEI) had launched 'Eradication and Endgame Strategic Plan' (2019–2023); which aims at eradication, integration, containment and certification.

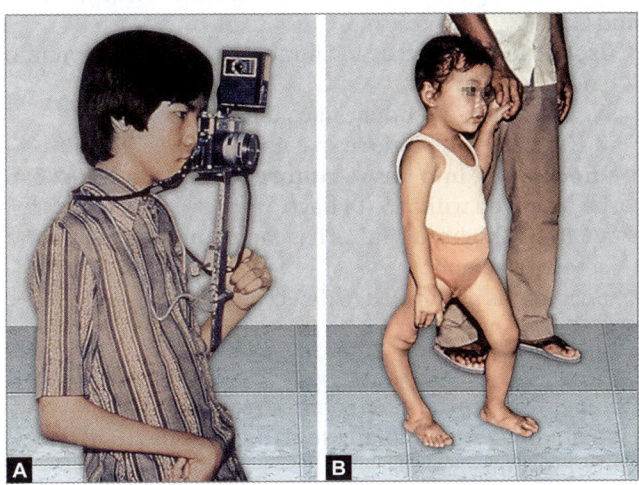

Figs. 43.2A and B: Deformities seen in poliomyelitis.
Source: Public Health Image Library, **A.** ID#: 5579; **B.** ID#: 5578, Centers for Disease Control and Prevention (CDC), Atlanta (*with permission*).

Table 43.1: Differences between injectable and oral polio vaccines.		
Polio vaccine	Injectable polio vaccine (Salk)	Oral polio vaccine (Sabin)
Developed by	Jonas Salk, in 1952	Albert Sabin, 1955
Formulations	IPV contains three serotypes 1, 2 and 3 It can be given in two doses: • Full dose IPV (0.5 mL): given by IM route • Fractional-dose (0.1 mL): given by ID route	OPV is available as: (given as 2 drops/dose, oral route) • Trivalent OPV (serotypes 1, 2 and 3) • Bivalent OPV (serotypes 1 and 3) • Monovalent OPV (any one serotype)
National Immunization Schedule (India, 2022)	Two fractional doses (intradermal route at the upper arm, 0.1 mL/dose): Given at 6th and 14th weeks of age along with bivalent OPV	Total five doses of bivalent OPV (serotype 1 and 3): • Zero dose—given at birth • 1st, 2nd, and 3rd dose —given at 6th, 10th, 14th week of age; booster dose is given at 16–24 months
Safety	Relatively safer than OPV	Safe except in immunocompromised patients, pregnancy, old age
Efficacy	A full course of IPV: produce 80–90% efficacy The immune response is developed at a slower rate than OPV	90–100% efficacy is achieved even by 1 or 2 doses of OPV efficacy decreases by: • Interference by other enteroviruses • Diarrheal diseases and breastfeeding
Economy	Relatively expensive	Economical
Duration of protection	Short, need booster doses periodically	Long-lasting
In epidemics	Can precipitate paralysis	Can be used safely
Herd immunity	Not provided	Provided due to feco-oral spread of vaccine virus
Local immunity	Weakly stimulated	Strongly stimulated (due to IgA antibody)
Storage condition	Relatively stable Does not require a stringent condition	Should be stored at (–20°C) Stabilized in $MgCl_2$, pH<7
VAPP and VDPV	Zero chance	Relatively more chance

(VAPP, vaccine-associated paralytic poliomyelitis; VDPV, vaccine-derived polioviruses)

COXSACKIEVIRUSES

Coxsackieviruses (named after the place of discovery; Coxsackie village in USA) can be divided into two groups, A and B, based on their pathogenic potentials for suckling mice. Group A coxsackieviruses are typed into serotypes 1–24 (except 15, 18 and 23) and group B are typed into serotypes 1–6.

Clinical Manifestations

Coxsackieviruses produce a variety of clinical illnesses in humans associated with different serotypes. The incubation period ranges from 2 to 9 days. Common clinical manifestations are:
- Aseptic meningitis
- Herpangina (severe febrile vesicular pharyngitis)
- Hand-foot-and-mouth disease (oral and pharyngeal ulcerations and vesicular rashes of the palms and soles)
- Pleurodynia (epidemic myalgia)
- Myocarditis and pericarditis
- Pancreatitism (common in juvenile diabetics)
- Common cold and rarely pneumonia
- Acute hemorrhagic conjunctivitis.

Laboratory Diagnosis

Specimen collection depends on the type of infection. Important specimens include throat swabs, stool and CSF
- **Isolation of the virus** by intracerebral inoculation into suckling mice
  - Coxsackie-A produce flaccid paralysis
  - Coxsackie-B produce spastic paralysis.
- **Inoculating into tissue culture:** Cytopathic effect can be observed within 5–14 days.
- **PCR:** It is highly useful as it is rapid, more sensitive and serotype-specific
- **Serology** is performed to detect neutralizing antibodies.

RHINOVIRUS

Rhinoviruses are the most common cause of common cold. Human rhinoviruses comprise of three species (A, B and C) and >150 antigen types.
- They are similar to enteroviruses in structure and properties except that: **Acid-labile** (unstable below pH 6) and transmission is by close **respiratory contact** via infected secretions

CHAPTER 43 ◆ Picornaviruses (Poliovirus, Coxsackievirus and Rhinovirus)

- Optimal temperature for growth is 33°C (in contrast to 37°C for enteroviruses)
- **Clinical manifestations:** The incubation period is about 2–4 days. Rhinoviral infection causes common cold syndrome (similar to coronaviruses, and influenza viruses). Secondary bacterial infection may produce otitis media, sinusitis, bronchitis, or pneumonitis, especially in children.
- **Laboratory diagnosis:** Rhinoviruses can be grown in human diploid cell lines such as WI-38 and MRC-5 cell lines. Most of the strains grow better at 33°C but not at 37°C
- **Treatment** is supportive (i.e. symptomatic treatment).

EXPECTED QUESTIONS

I. Write short notes on:
1. Pathogenesis of poliomyelitis.
2. Rhinovirus.
3. Polio vaccines.

II. Multiple Choice Questions (MCQs):
1. Currently, all the wild polio cases are caused by:
   a. WPV-1
   b. WPV-2
   c. WPV-3
   d. All of the above

2. National Immunization Schedule of India recommends:
   a. OPV only
   b. OPV + IPV
   c. IPV only
   d. Polio vaccines are not required

3. Not true about salk vaccine:
   a. Expensive than OPV
   b. Not useful in epidemics
   c. Provides herd immunity
   d. Booster doses are required

Answers
1. a   2. b   3. c

HIV/AIDS

CHAPTER 44

CHAPTER PREVIEW
- Morphology
- Pathogenesis
- Clinical Diagnosis
- Epidemiology
- Laboratory Diagnosis
- Post-exposure Prophylaxis

■ MORPHOLOGY

Human immunodeficiency virus (HIV) is the etiologic agent of Acquired Immunodeficiency Syndrome (AIDS)—the biggest threat to mankind in the last three decades.

❖ HIV belongs to retroviruses—a group of RNA viruses that possesses a unique enzyme called **reverse transcriptase** which converts the viral RNA into DNA inside the host cell **(Fig. 44.1)**

❖ It has a nucleocapsid surrounded by an envelope

❖ **Nucleocapsid** is icosahedral in symmetry, comprises of a capsid enclosing two copies of ssRNA and viral enzymes such as reverse transcriptase, integrase and proteases

❖ **Envelope** comprises of a lipid membrane into which the two types of protein spikes are embedded:
  - Glycoprotein 120 (gp 120): They are projected as knob-like spikes on the surface, and
  - Glycoprotein 41 (gp 41): They form anchoring transmembrane pedicles.

HIV Genome

HIV contains three structural genes—*gag, pol,* and *env*

❖ The ***gag* gene** codes for the core and shell of the virus. It is expressed as a precursor protein, p55 which is cleaved into three proteins:
  - p18—constitutes the matrix or shell antigen
  - p24 and p15—constitute the core antigens.

❖ The ***pol* gene** codes for viral enzymes such as reverse transcriptase, protease and integrase. It is expressed as a precursor protein, which is cleaved into proteins p31, p51 and p66

❖ The *env* gene codes for the envelope glycoproteins such as gp 120 and gp 41. Frequent mutations in the *env* gene account for antigenic diversity seen in HIV. This is the main reason which explains why:
  - HIV evades the host's immune response
  - Vaccination against HIV is extremely difficult.

HIV Serotyping

Based on sequence differences in the *env* gene, HIV comprises of two serotypes HIV-1 and 2.

❖ HIV-1 comprises of three distinct groups (M, N, O)
❖ 'M' is the dominant group worldwide. It comprises of eleven **subtypes** or "clades" (A-K)
❖ **Geographical distribution:** The serotypes vary from each other in geographic distribution
  - Subtype A is common in West Africa
  - Subtype B is predominant in Europe, America, Japan, and Australia
  - Subtype C is the most common form worldwide.

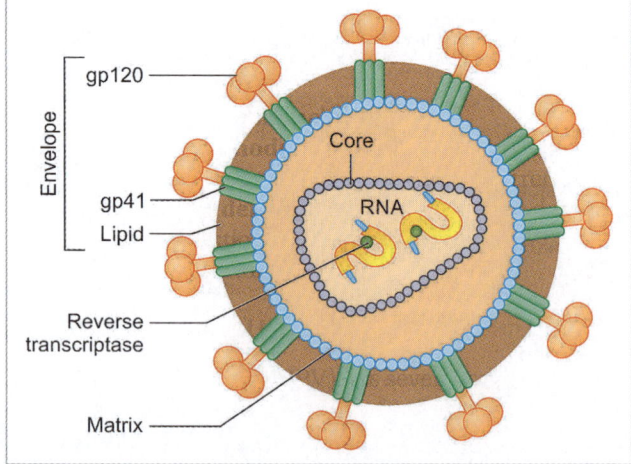

Fig. 44.1: Structure of HIV.

PATHOGENESIS

Mode of Transmission

HIV is transmitted through the following modes:
- **Sexual mode:** It is the most common mode (75%). The heterosexual route is more common, whereas anal sex has a higher risk of transmission
- **Blood transfusion** although is a less common mode (5%), the risk of transmission is maximum (90–95%)
- **Percutaneous/mucosal** transmission such as needle stick injury, splash injury on eyes, injection drug abuse, and sharing razors or tattooing
- **Mother-to-baby transmission:** Risk is maximum during delivery although transmission may occur at any time during pregnancy and breastfeeding
- **Viral load** is maximum in blood, genital secretions, and CSF; variable in breast milk and saliva; zero to minimal in other body fluids or urine.

Replication

The replication of HIV inside the host cell involves the following sequential steps.
- **Virus entry:** For the virus to enter into the host cell, the following receptor interaction is essential
  - *Main receptor:* HIV enters into the target cells by binding its gp120 to the CD4 receptor on the host cell surface (such as helper T cells and macrophages)
  - *Second co-receptor:* CXCR4 molecules of helper T cells or CCR5 molecules of macrophages.
- **Fusion:** Following receptor attachment, fusion of HIV to host cell takes place; mediated by the fusion protein gp41
- **Reverse transcription:** Inside the host cytoplasm, the ssRNA of HIV gets reversed transcribed into dsDNA
- **Integration:** The dsDNA (called proviral DNA) subsequently gets integrated into the host chromosome, mediated by viral integrase. The integrated virus is called as **provirus**
- **Latency:** In the integrated state, HIV establishes a latent infection, which lasts for a variable period.

CLINICAL STAGES (DISEASE PROGRESSION)

The clinical course of HIV infection includes the following five stages.
1. **Acute HIV disease or acute retroviral syndrome:** Initially, HIV destroys the infected T cells and spills into the bloodstream to cause primary viremia, which coincides with an initial flu-like illness that occurs in many patients (50–75%); 3–6 weeks after the primary infection. There is a significant drop in the number of circulating CD4 T cells at this stage
2. **Asymptomatic stage** (clinical latency): Restoration of adequate immune response develops within 1 month in most of the patients. It is a state of *clinical latency*, but *not microbiological latency*
3. **Persistent generalized lymphadenopathy (PGL):** It occurs as a result of HIV replication in lymph nodes
4. **Symptomatic HIV infection (AIDS-related complex):** After a variable period of clinical latency, the CD4 T cell level starts falling. Eventually, patients develop constitutional symptoms such as:
   - Unexplained diarrhea, lasting for more than 1 month
   - Weight loss (>10%), malaise, and night sweat
   - Mild opportunistic infections such as oral thrush.
5. **AIDS**: It is an advanced end-stage of HIV infection; characterized by:
   - Rapid fall in CD4 T cell count (usually <200 cells/μL)
   - High viral load
   - Lymphoid tissue is totally destroyed and replaced by fibrous tissue
   - Opportunistic infections set in secondary to profound immune suppression **(Table 44.1)**
   - Development of neoplasia **(Table 44.1)**
   - Development of direct HIV-induced manifestations such as HIV encephalopathy **(Table 44.1)**.

Table 44.1: Opportunistic infections and neoplasia associated with HIV/AIDS.

Bacterial opportunistic infections:
• Recurrent severe bacterial infections
• Extrapulmonary tuberculosis
• Disseminated non-tubercular mycobacterial infection
• Recurrent septicemia (including non-typhoidal salmonellosis)
Viral opportunistic infections:
• Chronic HSV infection
• Progressive multifocal leukoencephalopathy
• CMV (retinitis, or infection of other organs)
Fungal opportunistic infections:
• *Pneumocystis jirovecii* pneumonia
• Esophageal candidiasis
• Extrapulmonary cryptococcosis (meningitis)
• Disseminated mycoses (histoplasmosis and coccidioidomycoses)
Parasitic opportunistic infections:
• *Toxoplasma* encephalitis
• Chronic intestinal cystoisosporiasis (>1 month)
• Atypical disseminated leishmaniasis
Neoplasia:
• Kaposi's sarcoma
• Invasive cervical cancer
• Lymphoma (cerebral, B cell, and non-Hodgkin)
Other conditions (direct HIV induced):
• HIV encephalopathy
• Symptomatic HIV-associated nephropathy or cardiomyopathy

EPIDEMIOLOGY

HIV has a **global prevalence** of 0.7% in adults, whereas, in India, the prevalence is much lower (0.22%).
- **Sub-Saharan Africa** remains the most severely affected region
- **In India,** northeast states such as Mizoram, Manipur, and Nagaland have the highest prevalence. Whereas in terms of the absolute number of cases, Maharashtra is the worst affected state followed by Andhra Pradesh, Karnataka, and Telangana.

LABORATORY DIAGNOSIS

Diagnosis of HIV/AIDS is not like other infectious diseases. A number of moral, ethical, legal, and psychosocial issues are associated with a positive HIV status. The following care should be taken (3Cs) while performing the test for HIV.
- **Consent** in written format should be taken before the test is done. The patient should be explained about the nature of the test is performed
- **Confidentiality** of a positive test result is a must. The patient's name or the word "HIV positive" should not be written on the report form.
- **Counseling** should be provided to motivate the individual to tell the spouse/family and induce behavioral change.

The tests employed for laboratory diagnosis of HIV/AIDS can be grouped into specific and non-specific tests **(Table 44.2)**.

Table 44.2: Laboratory diagnosis of HIV/AIDS.
Specific Tests for HIV Infection

• **Screening tests** (antibody detection):
  ➢ ELISA (takes 2–3 hours)
  ➢ Rapid/Simple test (takes <30 minutes)
• **Supplemental tests** (antibody detection):
  ➢ Western blot assay
  ➢ Line immunoassay (LIA)
• **Confirmatory tests**
  ➢ p24 antigen detection (after 12–26 days of infection)
  ➢ Viral culture—by co-cultivation technique
  ➢ HIV RNA (best confirmatory method)—can be detected 10–14 days after infection
    ◆ Reverse transcriptase PCR (RT-PCR)
    ◆ Branched DNA assay
    ◆ NASBA (nucleic acid sequence-based amplification)
    ◆ Real time RT-PCR for estimating viral load
  ➢ HIV DNA detection: Useful for diagnosis of pediatric HIV

Non-specific Immunological Methods

• Low CD4 T cell count
• Hypergammaglobulinemia:
  ➢ Neopterin
  ➢ β2-macroglobulin
• Altered CD4: CD8 T cell ratio

Antibody Detection

Detection of anti-HIV antibodies is the mainstay of diagnosis of HIV. Tests to detect specific HIV antibodies can be classified into screening and supplemental tests.

Screening Antibody Detection Tests

Screening assays usually take less time and have high sensitivity and specificity (≥98–99%).
- **Antigens used** in most of the screening tests are:
  - HIV-1 specific antigens: p24, gp120, gp41
  - HIV-2 specific gp36.
- **Formats** available for screening tests are:
  - ELISA: It is the most commonly performed screening test at blood banks and tertiary care sites.
    - It is easy to perform, takes 2-3 hours
    - Adaptable to large number of samples
    - It is sensitive, specific, and cost effective
    - Currently available ELISA kits are of two types: (i) *3rd generation ELISA* that uses recombinant peptides to detect HIV antibodies and (ii) *4th generation ELISA* that detects both HIV antibodies and p24 antigen; thereby reducing the window period considerably.
  - Rapid/simple test: Takes less than 30 minutes. Various test formats available are:
    - Dot blot assays (or immunoconcentration or flow through method, e.g. Tridot test)
    - Immunochromatography (ICT)
    - Dipstick/Coombs tests (enzyme immune assay-based tests).
- **Should be confirmed:** Results of a single screening test should never be used as the final interpretation of HIV status as false-positive results or technical errors can occur. It is always subjected to confirmatory tests.

Supplemental Antibody Detection Tests

These assays are highly specific antibody detection methods; hence used for validation of positive results of screening tests. They are expensive, labor-intensive, need expertise to interpret, and may also give equivocal/indeterminate results. Examples include:
- Western blot assay: It works on the principle of immunoblot technique. It detects individual antibodies in serum separately against various antigenic fragments of HIV.
- Line immunoassay (LIA).

Confirmatory Tests

The following are confirmatory tests for diagnosis of HIV such as—detection of p24 antigens, HIV RNA and DNA detection, and virus isolation.

Detection of p24 Core Antigen

The p24 core antigen can be detected by various formats such as ELISA. This test is useful for:
- For confirmation of the diagnosis of HIV/AIDS
- Diagnosis of HIV during the window period
- Diagnosis of HIV in infants (not reliable)
- Monitoring the progress of HIV infection
- To resolve equivocal western blot results.

Viral RNA Detection

Detection of viral RNA is the **"gold standard"** method for confirmation of HIV diagnosis. Various formats are available targeting *pol* and *env* genes.
- Reverse transcriptase-polymerase chain reaction (RT-PCR)
- Real-time RT-PCR: For estimating viral load

Apart from the routine diagnosis of HIV, RNA detection has several other uses such as:
- It is the **most sensitive** and **specific** method and is the best method **for confirmation** of HIV
- It is the best tool for diagnosis of HIV during the **window period** and detects HIV earlier than all available methods (10–14 days post-exposure)
- **Viral load monitoring:** Real-time RT-PCR can quantify the viral load and is the most appropriate tool for monitoring the response to antiretroviral therapy
- **Typing:** To differentiate between HIV-1 and HIV-2 infections and also to determine the specific subtype
- Detection of **drug resistance** genes.

DNA PCR

PCR detecting proviral DNA is extremely useful for the diagnosis of pediatric HIV.

Non-specific Immunological Methods

Non-specific immunological methods are as follows:
- Low CD4 T cell count
- Altered CD4: CD8 T cell ratio
- Hypergammaglobulinemia, e.g. detection of neopterin and β2-macroglobulin.

NACO Strategy for HIV Diagnosis

For the resource-poor countries, it is impracticable to confirm the result of HIV screening tests by PCR or western blot as these assays are expensive and available only at limited centers.

NACO (National AIDS Control Organization, India) has formulated a strategic plan **(Fig. 44.2)** for HIV diagnosis. The guidelines are as follows:

- Depending on the situation/condition, for which the test is done, the positive result of the first screening test should be either considered as such or confirmed by another one or two screening tests
- The first screening test should be highly sensitive, whereas the second and third screening tests should have high specificity
- The three screening tests should use different principles or different antigens. The same kit should not be used again
- Supplemental or confirmatory tests should be used only when the screening test(s) results are equivocal/indeterminate.

There are four NACO Strategic Algorithms (Fig. 44.2):
1. **Strategy I:** It is done for the screening of the blood donors in blood banks. Only one test should be done. If found reactive, then the unit of blood is destroyed
2. **Strategy IIa**: It is done for sentinel surveillance of HIV infection to estimate the prevalence of infection. Positive results of the first test should be confirmed by a second test. If the second test is negative, then it is reported as negative
3. **Strategy IIb:** It is followed for the diagnosis of HIV/AIDS in symptomatic patients. A positive result of the first test should be confirmed by a second test. If the second test is negative, then a third test is done for confirmation
4. **Strategy III:** It is done for the diagnosis of asymptomatic HIV patients, antenatal screening, and screening of patients awaiting surgeries
    - **Three tests format:** All positive results in the first test should be confirmed by the second and third tests. A positive report is sent only if all three test results are found reactive
    - For indeterminate results of strategies IIB and III, (i.e. first test positive but second or third test negative), a repeat test is done after 14–28 days and the sample should be sent to the reference center for confirmation by western blot or RT-PCR.

Prognosis/Monitoring of HIV

Various tools available for monitoring the response to antiretroviral therapy include:
- CD4 T cell count: Most commonly used
- HIV RNA load: Most consistent and best tool
- p24 antigen detection
- Neopterin and β2 macroglobulin level.

Note: Viral antibody levels are inconsistent and variable during the late stage due to immune collapse; hence not reliable for prognosis.

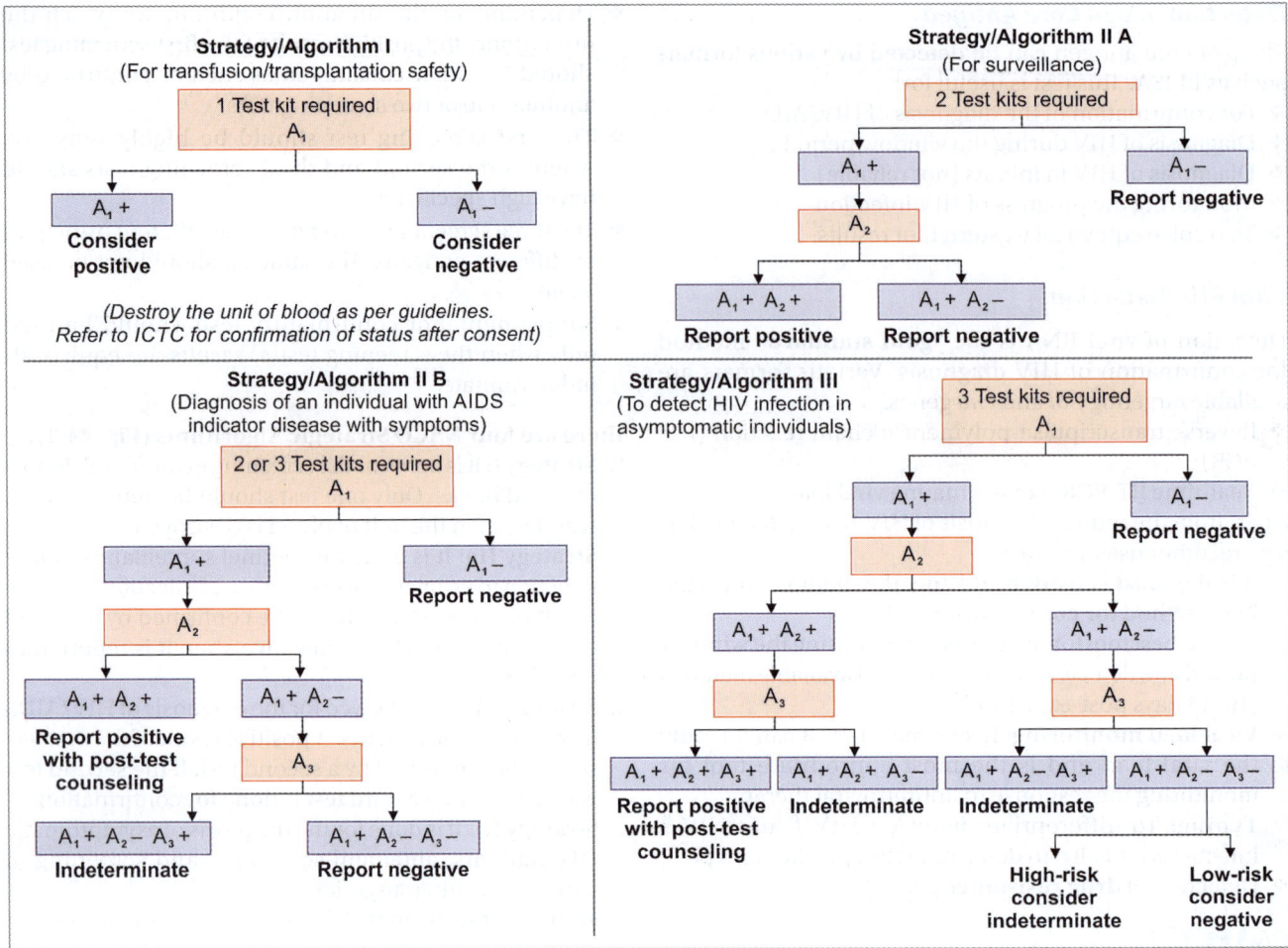

Fig. 44.2: NACO strategies/algorithms for diagnosing HIV infection.
(NACO, National AIDS Control Organization; ICTC, Integrated Counselling and Testing Centre)

Diagnosis of Pediatric HIV Infection

The routine screening methods (ELISA or rapid/simple tests) detect IgG antibodies.
- They cannot differentiate between a baby's IgG or maternally transferred IgG, hence cannot be used for the diagnosis of pediatric HIV
- As all maternal antibodies would disappear by 18 months; therefore IgG assays can be performed after 18 months of birth.

Pediatric HIV can be reliably diagnosed by methods such as:
- **HIV DNA PCR:** This is the most recommended method for the diagnosis of pediatric HIV
- **Other tests include:** HIV RNA detection and p24 antigen detection.

Diagnosis of HIV in Window Period

The window period refers to the initial time interval between the exposure and appearance of detectable levels of antibodies in the serum.
- The antibodies appear in blood within 2–8 weeks after infection but usually become detectable after 3 weeks to 12 weeks with the assays available presently. It can be as low as 22 days; when the newer third-generation antibody detection kits with high sensitivity are used
- **p24 antigen detection:** It can be detected by 12–26 days after infection
- **HIV RNA detection** (by RT-PCR) is the best method—it detects HIV RNA around 10–14 days after infection.

CHAPTER 44 ◆ HIV/AIDS

TREATMENT
HIV infection

Antiretroviral therapy (ART) Guideline, NACO 2021
Indication to start ART: TREAT ALL; i.e., antiretroviral therapy (ART) has to be started in all patients irrespective of CD4 count, clinical stage, age, population, or associated opportunistic infections (OIs)
HAART: Highly active antiretroviral therapy (HAART) refers to the use of a combination of at least three antiretroviral drugs to maximally suppress HIV and stop the progression of the disease
TLD regimen: Tenofovir + Lamivudine + Dolutegravir is the preferred first-line ART regimen for all HIV patients (HIV-1 and/or -2) in adults including pregnant women.
- It is given as as fixed dose combination in a single pill once a day
- It is also the regimen of choice for is used for post-exposure prophylaxis for healthcare workers (*refer* **Chapter 18**).

EXPECTED QUESTIONS

I. **Write an essay on:**
  1. Discuss the pathogenesis, clinical stages, and laboratory diagnosis of HIV infection.

II. **Write short notes on:**
  1. Morphology of HIV.
  2. NACO strategy for HIV diagnosis.
  3. Tests for monitoring response to treatment in AIDS patients.
  4. Tests for diagnosis of HIV in the window period.

III. **Multiple Choice Questions (MCQs):**
  1. HIV transmission: Maximum risk is associated with:
     a. Sexual transmission
     b. Mother-to-child
     c. Needlestick injury
     d. Blood transfusion

  2. The most common mode of HIV transmission is:
     a. Sexual transmission
     b. Mother-to-child
     c. Needlestick injury
     d. Blood transfusion

  3. Tests for monitoring response to treatment in HIV include all, *except*:
     a. ELISA for IgG antibody detection
     b. P24 antigen detection
     c. HIV RNA detection
     d. HIV DNA detection

  4. Tests for diagnosis of HIV in the window period include all, *except*:
     a. ELISA for IgG antibody detection
     b. P24 antigen detection
     c. HIV RNA detection
     d. HIV DNA detection

Answers
1. d   2. a   3. a   4. a

Hepatitis Viruses

CHAPTER 45

CHAPTER PREVIEW
- Hepatitis A Virus
- Hepatitis B Virus
- Hepatitis C Virus
- Hepatitis D Virus
- Hepatitis E Virus

Hepatitis viruses are a diverse group of viruses, having a common feature of being hepatotropic, and causing hepatitis. There are five major types of hepatitis viruses—A to E.

All hepatitis viruses are RNA viruses, except for hepatitis B which is a DNA virus. The features of hepatitis viruses have been depicted in **Table 45.1**.

- ❖ Hepatitis A virus (HAV) and hepatitis E virus (HEV) have similarities in various aspects such as transmission (feco-oral route), etc.
- ❖ Similarly, hepatitis B virus (HBV), hepatitis C virus (HCV), and hepatitis D virus (HDV) resemble in many properties—e.g. transmitted by blood, sexual and vertical routes.

HEPATITIS A VIRUS

Hepatitis A virus (HAV) is a non-enveloped RNA virus, that belongs to picornaviruses (Enterovirus 72).

Table 45.1: Features of hepatitis viruses.

HAV and HEV	HBV, HCV and HDV
Both HAV and HEV are RNA viruses	• HBV is a DNA virus • HCV and HDV are RNA viruses
Feco-oral transmission	Blood (common), sexual, and vertical
Incubation period: 15–50 days, onset-abrupt	Incubation period: 30– 180 days, insidious onset
No carriers	Carriers seen
No chronicity	Chronicity seen
Not oncogenic	Oncogenic
Fulminant: Rare (<1%); except HEV in pregnancy (10–20%)	Fulminant: Rare (1–2%) except HDV (10–20%)
Non-enveloped; icosahedral symmetry	Enveloped; spherical symmetry

Clinical Manifestation

HAV has an incubation period of about 15–45 days. Onset is relatively abrupt (subacute).

- ❖ **Clinically,** HAV infection is indistinguishable from other hepatitis viruses; characterized by:
  - Pre-icteric phase (mainly gastrointestinal symptoms like nausea) followed by;
  - Icteric phase or jaundice (dark urine, yellowish sclera, and mucus membrane).
- ❖ Complete recovery occurs in most (98%) cases
- ❖ **Complications** may occur such as fulminant hepatitis; characterized by severe necrosis of hepatocytes.

Epidemiology

HAV is the most common cause of acute viral hepatitis in children.
- ❖ Children and adolescents are commonly affected
- ❖ **Risk factors:** Poor personal hygiene and overcrowding are the most important risk factors.

Laboratory Diagnosis

The HAV infection is diagnosed by the following modalities.
- ❖ **Anti-HAV antibody detection** (by ELISA): IgM antibody is positive in acute HAV infection, and presence of IgG antibody indicates past infection.
- ❖ **Detection of HAV particles:** HAV appears in stool from −2 to +2 weeks of jaundice, and can be detected by electron microscopy
- ❖ **HAV antigen detection:** ELISA format is available to detect HAV antigen from a stool sample from −2 to +2 weeks of jaundice
- ❖ **Non-specific findings:** Such as elevated liver enzymes and serum bilirubin levels.

Prevention

- ❖ **General preventive measures** such as hand washing before and after using toilet, sanitary disposal of fecal matter should be followed

- **Vaccines:** The indications to administer the HAV vaccine include: all children of >1 year age, travelers to endemic countries, and patients with chronic liver disease. Two types of vaccines are available
  1. Formaldehyde inactivated vaccine
  2. Live attenuated vaccine.
- **Human immunoglobulin (HAV-Ig):** It is useful for post-exposure prophylaxis of **intimate contacts** of persons with hepatitis A or **travelers**.

TREATMENT	Hepatitis A
There is no specific antiviral drug is available.	

HEPATITIS B VIRUS

Hepatitis B virus (HBV) is the most widespread and the most important agent among hepatitis viruses. It is the only hepatitis virus, which is a DNA virus and belongs to the family Hepadnaviridae.

Morphology

HBV exits in three morphologic forms **(Figs. 45.1A and B)**:
1. **Spherical forms:** These forms are most numerous (22 nm in size) and made up of HBsAg (hepatitis B surface antigen)
2. **Tubular or filamentous forms:** They are also 22 nm in size, but 200 nm long; made up of HBsAg
3. **Complete form or Dane particles:** They are larger, 42 nm size spherical virions; made up of:
   - **Outer surface envelope:** HBsAg
   - **Inner nucleocapsid:** It consists of core antigen (HBcAg) and pre-core antigen (HBeAg) and partially double stranded DNA.

Transmission

The transmission of HBV occurs via multiple routes.
- **Parenteral route** via blood and blood products transfusion and needle prick injuries. It is considered as the most common mode in developing countries
- **Sexual transmission**
- **Vertical (perinatal) transmission:** Transmission occurs at any stage such as in-utero, during delivery (maximum risk), and during breastfeeding
- **Direct skin contact** with infected open skin lesions may transmit the virus, e.g. impetigo (especially in children).

High-risk groups which are more prone to acquire HBV infection are:
- Surgeons, technicians, phlebotomists
- Paramedical workers
- Sex workers especially homosexual males
- Recipients of blood transfusion and organ transplantation
- Drug addicts.

Clinical Manifestations

Hepatitis B has an incubation period of about 30–180 days. The onset of infection is slow and insidious.
- Patients may present with subclinical infection, acute or chronic hepatitis
- **Acute hepatitis:** Clinical presentation of HBV infection is as discussed for HAV; characterized by: preicteric phase and icteric phase or jaundice
- **The clinical outcome** of acute HBV infection may be either complete recovery (90-95%) or development of carrier state (5%) or chronic infection (5%)
- **Carriers:** There are two types of carriers:
  1. **Simple carriers:** They are capable of low infectivity (negative for HBeAg and HBV DNA)

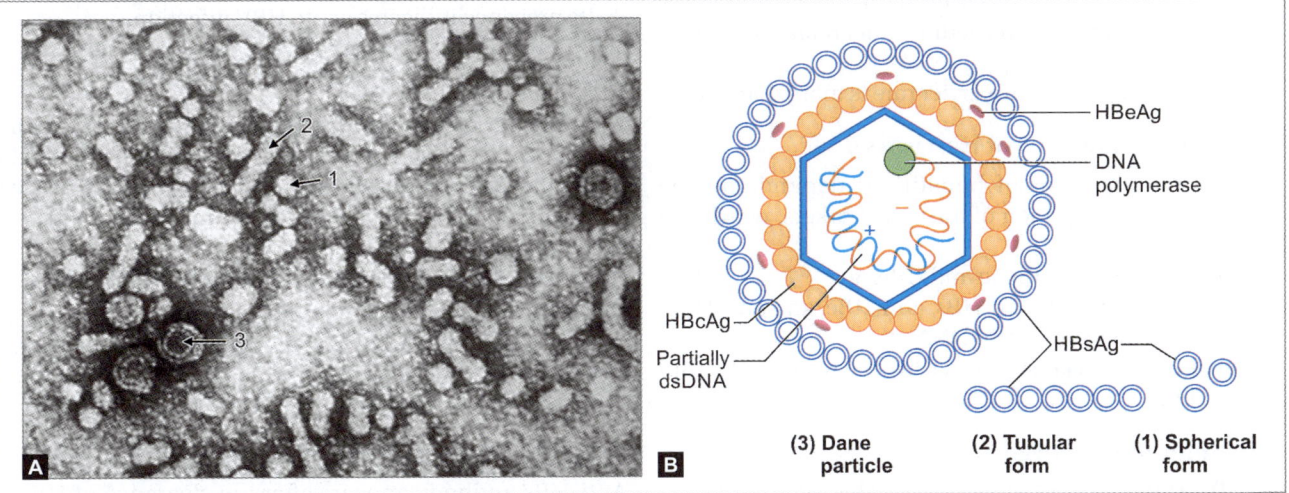

Figs. 45.1A and B: A. Electron microscopic appearance of hepatitis B virus, showing 1-spherical form, 2-tubular form, and 3-Dane particle; **B.** Schematic diagram of hepatitis B virus.

Source: **A.** ID# 5631/Public Health Image Library/Centers for Disease Control and Prevention (CDC), Atlanta (*with permission*).

2. **Supercarriers:** Here, the virus is actively multiplying and capable of high infectivity (positive for HBeAg and HBV DNA).
- **Chronic hepatitis:** This can also occur in two stages:
  1. **Chronic inactive hepatitis:** Capable of low infectivity (negative for HBeAg and HBV DNA)
  2. **Immunoreactive (chronic active) hepatitis:** Here, the virus is actively multiplying and capable of high infectivity (positive for HBeAg and HBV DNA).
- **Hepatic complications:** Rarely, it may proceed to complications such as fulminant hepatitis or cirrhosis, or hepatocellular carcinoma
- **Extrahepatic complications:** May develop in some cases due to immune complex deposition. It is characterized by arthritis, rash, angioedema, etc.

Epidemiology

Hepatitis B virus infection occurs throughout the world; usually sporadic, but occasional outbreaks can occur in hospitals.
- **Reservoir of infection:** Humans are the only reservoir of infection, who can be either cases or carriers
- **Carriers** can also be grouped into:
  - **Simple carriers:** They are of low infectivity, and transmit the virus at a lower rate. They possess a low level of HBsAg and no HBeAg
  - **Super carriers:** They are highly infectious and transmit the virus efficiently. They possess higher levels of HBsAg and HBeAg, DNA polymerase, and HBV DNA.
- **HBV prevalence:** There are three epidemiological patterns observed among various countries:
  1. *Low endemicity:* The carrier rate is less than 2%
  2. *Intermediate endemicity:* The carrier rate is between 2 and 8%. It is observed in India, China, and many countries in Eastern Mediterranean and Southeast Asian regions
  3. *High endemicity:* The carrier rate is more than 8%.

Laboratory Diagnosis of Hepatitis B

A definitive diagnosis of hepatitis B depends on the serological demonstration of the viral markers, which can be classified as:
- **Antigen markers:** HBsAg and HBeAg
- **Antibody markers:** Anti-HBs, anti-HBe, and anti-HBc
- **Molecular markers:** HBV DNA
- **Nonspecific markers:** Elevated liver enzymes and serum bilirubin.

Test Methods Employed

- **HBV antigens and antibodies:** The most common method employed is ELISA; although various rapid test formats (such as ICT) and chemiluminescence immunoassay (CLIA) are also available
- **Viral DNA** can be detected by polymerase chain reaction (PCR). Real-time PCR is very useful for the quantification of HBV DNA
- HBV does not grow in any conventional culture system.

HBsAg (Hepatitis B Surface Antigen)

It is the first marker to be elevated following infection; becomes positive within 8–12 weeks.
- It appears during the incubation period
- The presence of HBsAg indicates the onset of infectivity
- It remains elevated for the entire duration of acute hepatitis. However, it can rarely persist beyond 6 months, if the disease progresses to chronic hepatitis or in a carrier state
- It is used as an epidemiological marker of hepatitis B infection.

HBeAg (Pre-core Antigen) and HBV DNA

They appear concurrently with or shortly after the appearance of HBsAg in serum. They are the markers of active viral replication and high viral infectivity. HBV DNA load is used to monitor the response to treatment.

HBcAg (Hepatitis B Core Antigen)

Hepatitis B core antigen (HBcAg) is a hidden antigen, nonsecretory in nature; hence, it cannot be detected in the blood. However, can be detected in hepatocytes by immunofluorescence.

Anti-HBc IgM (Hepatitis B Core Antibody)

Anti-HBc IgM is the first antibody to elevate following infection:
- It appears within the first 1–2 weeks after the appearance of HBsAg and lasts for 3–6 months
- Its presence indicates acute HBV infection.

Anti-HBc IgG (Hepatitis B Core Antibody)

Anti-HBc IgG appears in the late acute stage and remains positive indefinitely whether the patient proceeds to—the chronic stage or carrier state or recovery. It can also be used as an epidemiological marker of HBV infection.

Anti-HBe Ab (Anti-Hepatitis B Precore Antibody)

Anti-HBe antibodies appear after the clearance of HBeAg and their presence signifies diminished viral replication and decreased infectivity.

Anti-HBs Ab (Anti-Hepatitis B Surface Antibody)

Anti-HBs antibody appears after the clearance of HBsAg and remains elevated indefinitely.
- Its presence indicates recovery, immunity, and noninfectivity (i.e., stoppage of transmission)

❖ It is also the marker of vaccination; if the rest of all markers are negative **(Fig. 45.2)**.

Various outcomes following HBV infection and markers for diagnosis is depicted in **Figure 45.2**.

> **TREATMENT** — Hepatitis B
>
> Treatment is indicated for chronic hepatitis, supercarriers, and associated cirrhosis. Antiviral agents include:
> - **Antiviral agents**: Nucleoside analogs such as tenofovir and telbivudine are the agent of choice currently
> - Pegylated interferon alfa: It was used previously; now not in use because of adverse effects.

Prevention (HBV)

Hepatitis B Vaccine (Active Immunization)

Hepatitis B vaccine is a recombinant subunit vaccine, made up of **HBsAg**, prepared in Baker's yeast by DNA recombinant technology.
- ❖ **Route:** Administered by intramuscular route over deltoid (in infant—anterolateral thigh)
- ❖ **Schedule:** Three doses are given at 0, 1, and 6 months. Under the National Immunization Schedule, it is given at 6, 10, and 14 weeks (along with the DPT vaccine)
- ❖ **Marker of protection:** Recipients are said to be protected if the anti-HBsAg antibody titer is above 10 mIU/mL.

Hepatitis B Immunoglobulin

Hepatitis B immunoglobulin (HBIG) is used in the following situations where an immediate protection is warranted; given at a dose of 0.06 mL/kg or 10–12 IU/kg.
- ❖ Acutely exposed to HBsAg positive blood, e.g., surgeons, nurses, laboratory workers
- ❖ Sexual partners of acute hepatitis B patients
- ❖ Neonates borne to hepatitis B carrier mothers
- ❖ Post-liver transplant patients who need protection against HBV infection
- ❖ Following accidental exposure.

The post-exposure prophylaxis for HBV is discussed in **Chapter 18**.

General Prophylactic Measures
- ❖ Screening of blood bags, semen, and organ donors
- ❖ Following safe sex practices (e.g. using condoms, avoiding multiple sex partners)
- ❖ Following safe injection practices—use of the disposable syringes and needles
- ❖ Following safe aseptic surgical practices
- ❖ Health education.

■ HEPATITIS C VIRUS

Hepatitis C virus (HCV) is a common cause of post-transfusion hepatitis in developing countries. Among

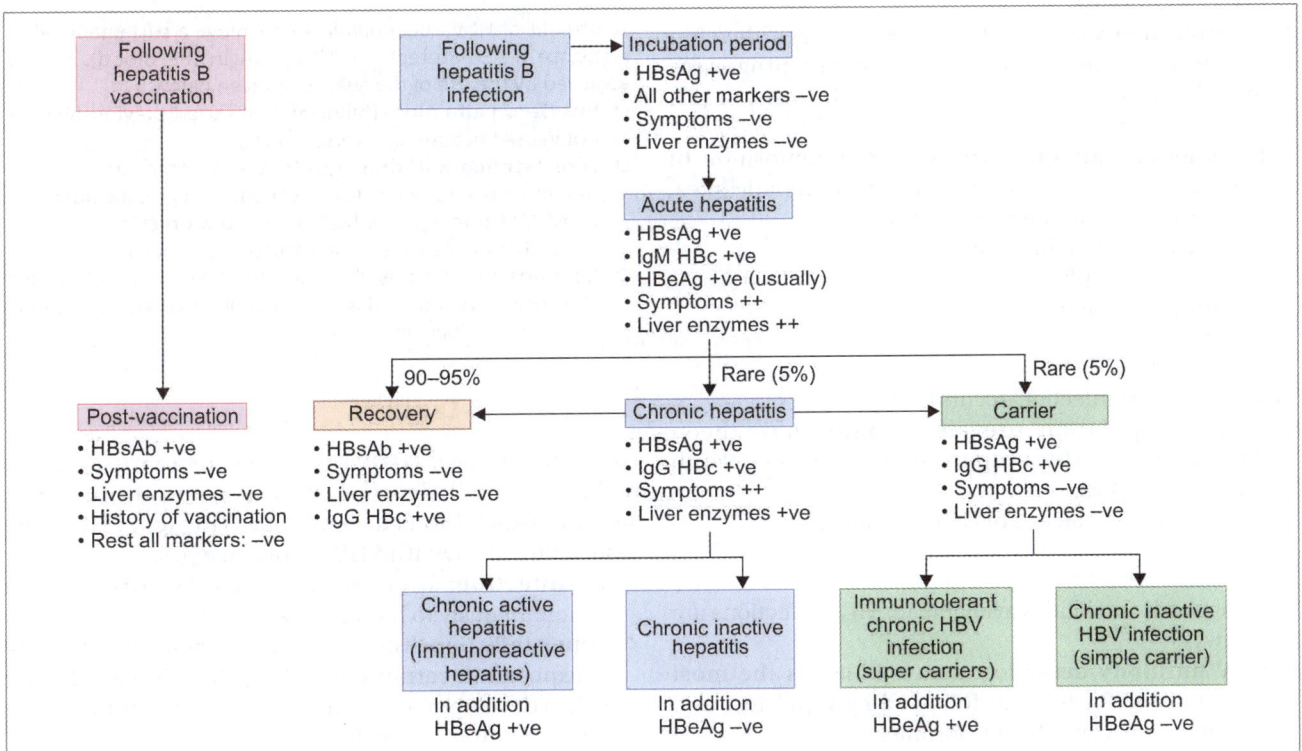

Fig. 45.2: Various outcomes following hepatitis B infection and markers for diagnosis.

hepatitis viruses, HCV has the maximum risk of developing into a chronic infection. It is a RNA virus, comprises of a nucleocapsid, surrounded by an envelope.

Genetic Diversity of HCV

Similar to HIV, the hepatitis C virus displays diversity in the RNA genome that occurs because of high rates of mutations seen in the virus. HCV is divided into six major genotypes. The genotypes also vary from each other in their epidemiological distribution and also in susceptibility to antiviral drugs.

Transmission

Various modes of transmission of HCV are as follows:
- **Parenteral:** Blood transfusions, blood products or organ transplantations, needle stick and splash injury, injection drug users
- **Vertical transmission** from infected mother to fetus
- **Sexual transmission** (rare).

Clinical Manifestations

The incubation period is about 15-160 days. Following infection with HCV:
- **Asymptomatic infection:** Seen in about >75% of cases
- **Acute hepatitis:** About 20% of people develop acute hepatitis. In about 5-15% of infections, the virus gets cleared spontaneously within 12 weeks. Rest progress to chronic disease
- **Chronic disease:** About 75-85% of cases develop the chronic disease; which subsequently progresses into either—(i) chronic hepatitis, (ii) cirrhosis, or (iii) hepatocellular carcinoma
- **Extrahepatic manifestations:** Due to deposition of circulating immune complexes in extrahepatic sites. Various manifestations can set in such as:
  - Mixed cryoglobulinemia
  - Glomerulonephritis
  - Arthritis and joint pain.

Epidemiology

Hepatitis C virus infection occurs worldwide.
- Higher population prevalence rates have been documented in Africa (up to 10%) followed by South America and Asia
- In India, the prevalence of HCV is about 1%.

Laboratory Diagnosis

The diagnostic modalities available for HCV infections are as follows:
- **HCV antibody detection assay:** ELISA is the most common platform used; followed by rapid test and chemiluminescence (CLIA) formats
  - *Third generation ELISA:* This has been the standard method for HCV serology. It employs antigens from NS5, NS3, and NS4 regions
  - *Advantages* include: (i) increased sensitivity and specificity (>99%), (ii) becomes positive within 5 weeks of infection
  - *Disadvantages*: These assays detect IgG antibodies to HCV, hence, they do not discriminate between active or past infection; for which HCV RNA test is required.
- **HCV core antigen assay:** Automated quantitative test detecting core antigen has been available recently
  - This test is less expensive and less time consuming than HCV RNA PCR
  - *Advantages:* Used for (i) diagnosis of active/ current infection, (ii) monitoring response to treatment
  - *Disadvantage:* Less sensitive than RT-PCR; hence not recommended for blood screening purposes.
- **Real-time RT-PCR** detecting HCV RNA has been the gold standard method. It is useful for:
  - Confirmation of active infection: HCV RNA can be detected in blood as early as 2-3 weeks after infection
  - Quantification of HCV RNA, which helps in monitoring the response to treatment
  - For determining HCV genotype and subtype.

> **TREATMENT** — Hepatitis C
>
> Treatment of HCV infection aims to achieve a sustainable viral response (i.e. undetectable HCV RNA in the blood). This is achieved by the use of the agents, as given below.
> - **Interferon alfa plus ribavirin:** It was used previously; now not in use because of adverse effects.
> - **Direct-acting antiviral agents (DAAs):** They are now the treatment of choice for HCV infection. Examples include:
>   - NS3/4A (proteases) inhibitors, e.g., grazoprevir
>   - NS5B (polymerases) inhibitors, e.g., sofosbuvir
> - **Combination therapy:** Currently, the treatment regimen for HCV includes combinations of different DAAs with or without PEG-IFN and ribavirin.

HEPATITIS D VIRUS

Hepatitis D virus (HDV) is a defective virus; cannot replicate by itself; depends on the hepatitis B virus for its survival, which forms the envelope (HBsAg) of HDV. The association of HDV with HBV is of two types.
- **Co-infection:** It occurs when a person is exposed simultaneously to both HDV and HBV
- **Super-infection:** It occurs when a chronic carrier of HBV is exposed to serum-containing HDV. It has a higher risk of development of complications such as fulminant disease, chronic hepatitis, and cirrhosis

- **Epidemiology:** Hepatitis D virus infection occurs worldwide, but the prevalence varies greatly. Surprisingly, HDV is not prevalent in Southeast Asia including India; where HBV carriers are maximum
- **Laboratory diagnosis:** Both co-infection and super-infection have a rise of IgM-HDV and HBsAg, but can be differentiated by anti-HBc
    - In co-infection, HBV usually occurs as an acute infection (positive for IgM anti-HBc), whereas
    - In super-infection, HBV is present as a chronic infection (positive for IgG anti-HBc).

> **TREATMENT** — Hepatitis D
>
> Patients with HDV infection can be treated with IFN-α. Treatment for HBV should be continued as described earlier.

HEPATITIS E VIRUS

Hepatitis E virus (HEV) causes an enterically transmitted (feco-oral mode) hepatitis primarily affects young adults and can cause epidemics in developing countries.

Clinical Manifestations

The incubation period is about 14–60 days.
- **Acute hepatitis:** Most of the patients present as self-limiting acute hepatitis lasting for several weeks followed by complete recovery
- **Fulminant hepatitis** may occur in 1–2% of cases; except for the **pregnant women** where the risk is higher (20%)
- There is no chronic infection or carrier state.

Epidemiology

Hepatitis E virus is a zoonotic pathogen affecting various animals such as monkeys, cats, pigs and dogs.
- **Transmission:** It is fecal-orally transmitted via sewage contamination of drinking water or food
- **Epidemics** of HEV infections have been reported primarily from Asia, Africa and Central America; HEV is the most common cause of acute hepatitis in this zone
- **In India,** HEV infection accounts for maximum (30–60%) cases of sporadic acute hepatitis and epidemic hepatitis.

Laboratory Diagnosis

The diagnostic modalities available for HEV infections are as follows:
- **HEV RNA** (by reverse transcriptase PCR) and **HEV virions** (by electron microscopy) can be detected in stool and serum even before the onset of clinical illness
- **Serum antibody** detection by ELISA:
    - **IgM anti-HEV** appears in serum simultaneously with the increased levels of liver enzymes; indicates acute infection
    - **IgG anti-HEV** replaces IgM in 2 to 4 weeks (once the symptoms resolve) and persists for years; indicates recovery or past infection.

> **TREATMENT** — Hepatitis E
>
> There is no specific antiviral drug available.

EXPECTED QUESTIONS

I. Write an essay on:
   1. Clinical manifestations, and laboratory diagnosis of HBV infection.

II. Write short notes on:
   1. Laboratory diagnosis of hepatitis A virus infection.
   2. Laboratory diagnosis of hepatitis C virus infection.

III. Multiple Choice Questions (MCQs):
   1. Which is transmitted by feco-oral mode?
      a. HBV   b. HCV
      c. HDV   d. HEV
   2. Which is a DNA virus?
      a. HBV   b. HCV
      c. HDV   d. HEV
   3. Which hepatitis virus has the maximum risk of chronicity?
      a. HBV   b. HCV
      c. HDV   d. HEV

Answers
1. d   2. a   3. b

Miscellaneous RNA Viruses

CHAPTER 46

CHAPTER PREVIEW
- Agents of Viral Gastroenteritis
- Ebola Virus
- Rodent-borne Viruses
- Oncogenic Viruses
- Slow Viruses and Prions

VIRAL GASTROENTERITIS

Viral etiology accounts for the majority of the acute infectious gastroenteritis worldwide **(Table 46.1)**.
- ❖ Viral gastroenteritis most commonly occurs among children. However, persons of all ages can be affected
- ❖ Several enteric viruses can cause acute gastroenteritis in humans, the most common being rotavirus.

Rotavirus Diarrhea

Rotaviruses are the most common cause of diarrheal illness in children.
- ❖ It has a segmented double-stranded RNA, surrounded by a triple-layered, wheel-shaped capsid
- ❖ It is typed into several serotypes and genotypes
- ❖ The **most common type** seen in the world as well as in India is **G1P[8]** type, which accounts for nearly 70% of total isolates.

Table 46.1: Viruses causing gastroenteritis.	
Virus	**Gastroenteritis features**
Rotavirus*	**Group A:** Most common cause of severe endemic diarrheal illness in children worldwide **Group B:** Causes outbreaks of diarrhea in adults in China
Norwalk virus	Causes outbreaks of vomiting and diarrheal illness in all ages (especially in older children and adults)
Sapovirus	Causes sporadic cases and occasional outbreaks of diarrheal illness in infants, young children, and in elderly
Astrovirus	
Adenovirus* (type 40 and 41)	Second most common viral agent of endemic diarrheal illness of infants and young children worldwide

*Clinical severity is maximum.

Pathogenesis and Clinical Manifestations

Rotaviruses are transmitted by fecal–oral route, then they progress further to destroy enterocytes of the small intestine.
- ❖ They multiply in the cytoplasm of enterocytes and damage their transport mechanisms resulting in secretory diarrhea
- ❖ The incubation period is about 1–3 days. It has an abrupt onset, characterized by vomiting followed by watery diarrhea, fever, and abdominal pain
- ❖ Recovery usually occurs in the majority, but a few children may suffer from severe loss of electrolytes and fluids leading to dehydration.

Laboratory Diagnosis

Feces collected early in the illness is the most ideal specimen.
- ❖ **Direct detection of virus:** Rotaviruses can be demonstrated in stool by **electron microscopy**. They have a sharp edged triple shelled capsid; look like the spokes grouped around the hub of a wheel **(Fig. 46.1)**
- ❖ **Isolation** of rotavirus is difficult. Rolling of tissue cultures may be attempted to enhance replication
- ❖ **Detection of viral antigen** in stool by ELISA and latex agglutination-based methods
- ❖ **RT-PCR** is the most sensitive detection method for detection of rotavirus from stool
- ❖ **Serologic tests** (ELISA) can be used to detect the rise of antibody titer. This may be useful for seroprevalence purposes.

TREATMENT — Viral gastroenteritis

Treatment is mainly supportive. Correct the loss of water and electrolytes such as oral or parenteral fluid replacement.

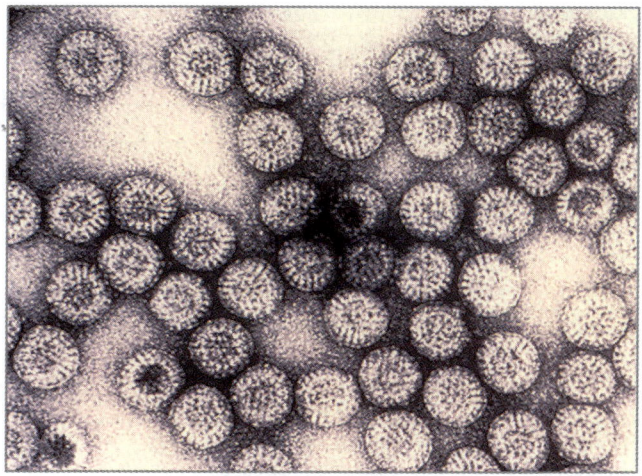

Fig. 46.1: Rotavirus (electron micrograph).
Source: Public Health Image Library, /ID# 15194/Dr Erskine L Palmer/ Centers for Disease Control and Prevention (CDC), Atlanta (*with permission*).

Vaccine

Two brands of vaccine are available: Rotavac and Rotarix.
Rotavac is introduced under the National Immunization Schedule of India (2022), in selected states:
- Three doses (5 drops/dose)
- Administered orally at 6, 10, and 14 weeks along with DPT and OPV.

General Preventive Measures

They include—(1) measures to improve hygiene and sanitation in the community, and (2) contact precautions such as strict hand hygiene to prevent transmission from infected persons **(Chapter 15)**.

Other Agents of Gastroenteritis

- **Family Caliciviridae** comprises of two important agents of human diarrhea—(1) Norwalk viruses, and (2) Sapporo-like viruses. They are icosahedral, 27–40 nm in size; possess **cup-like depressions** on the capsid surface typically observed under electron microscope.
    - **Norwalk virus** is the most important cause of epidemic viral gastroenteritis in adults.
        - It is common in winter months; therefore called as **winter vomiting disease** or gastric flu; characterized by diarrhea, abdominal pain, nausea and vomiting
        - **Common food sources** include contaminated salad, fresh fruits, shellfish (such as oysters), or water.
    - **Sapoviruses** cause sporadic cases and occasional outbreaks of diarrheal illness in infants, young children, and in elderly.
- **Adenoviruses (types 40 and 41)** are the second most common viral agents of endemic diarrheal illness of infants and young children worldwide.
- **Astroviruses** exhibit a distinctive **star-like** morphology under the electron microscope. They cause sporadic cases and occasional outbreaks of diarrhea in infants, young children and in elderly.
- **Respiratory viruses:** Diarrhea has also been reported as a part of manifestations of certain respiratory viruses such as severe acute respiratory syndrome coronaviruses (SARS-CoV and SARS-CoV-2) and influenza A/H1N1 virus (the 2009 pandemic strain).

■ EBOLA VIRUS DISEASE

Ebola and Marburg are filoviruses, known to cause hemorrhagic fever with high mortality. They have been reported from various countries in Western Africa.

The Ebola virus has become a global threat because of its explosive outbreak in 2014 in West Africa. It is named after the **Ebola River**, Africa.

- **Geographical distribution:** Most of the current Ebola outbreaks are largely seen in the Democratic Republic of the Congo and other African countries
    - *West African Epidemic (2014–16):* The largest outbreak occurred in 2014–16; reporting 28,616 cases with 11,310 deaths (40% mortality). Three primary countries affected were—Guinea, Liberia, and Sierra Leon
    - *India:* There is no confirmed case documented yet.
- **Transmission:** Ebola virus spreads among people via direct contact with blood, secretions of infected people, or indirect contact with infected surfaces and materials
- **Reservoir hosts:** Fruit bats or primates (apes and monkeys) are considered as the reservoir host
- **Risk group:** Health-care workers and close contacts/family members of infected individuals are at greater risk of contracting the infection
- **Clinical manifestations:** The incubation period is about 2–12 days. It mainly presents as hemorrhagic fever. The mortality rate is very high (50–90%)
- **Laboratory diagnosis:** Ebola virus disease is diagnosed by various modalities such as:
    - *Serum antibody detection* by ELISA: Detects both IgM and IgG separately by using recombinant nucleoprotein (NP) and glycoprotein (GP) antigens
    - *Serum antigen* is detected by capture ELISA. The target proteins are NP, VP40, and GP
    - *Molecular methods* such as RT-PCR and real-time RT-PCR assays are useful to detect specific RNA such as NP and GP gene
    - *Electron microscopy* of the specimen shows typical filamentous viruses **(Fig. 46.2)**.

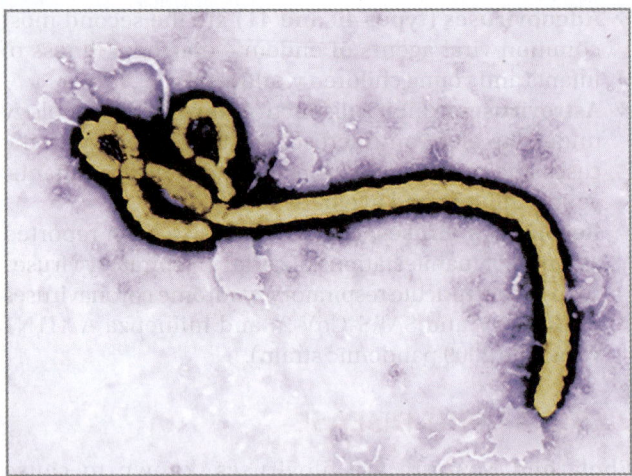

Fig. 46.2: Ebola virus, filamentous shaped (Electron micrograph).
Source: ID# 10815, Public Health Image Library/Centers for Disease Control and Prevention (CDC), Atlanta (*with permission*).

- **Treatment:** Supportive care such as rehydration and symptomatic treatment improves survival. No proven treatment or vaccine is available yet
- **Prevention:** Practice proper infection control and sterilization measures such as strict hand hygiene and personal protective equipment (PPE such as coverall and N95 respirator)
    - Isolate the patients with Ebola from other patients
    - If traveling to an Ebola outbreak area, should be monitored for 21 days after returning.

RODENT-BORNE VIRAL INFECTIONS

Rodent-borne viruses or roboviruses are transmitted from rodents to man by contact with infected body fluids or excretions. Major rodent-borne viruses include:
- **Hantaviruses:** They cause hemorrhagic fever with renal syndrome (HFRS) and hantavirus pulmonary syndrome (HPS)
- **Arenaviruses**: They are a group of segmented RNA viruses, divided into:
    - New world viruses (e.g. Junin, Machupo): They cause South American hemorrhagic fever
    - Old world viruses: e.g. Lassa viruses—cause hemorrhagic fever in Africa.

ONCOGENIC VIRUSES

Viruses account for 15% of all human malignancies. There are several oncogenic viruses found worldwide, which include the agents of two major vaccine-preventable malignancies—human papillomavirus causing carcinoma cervix and hepatitis B virus causing liver cancer **(Table 46.2)**.

Table 46.2: Human oncogenic viruses and associated malignancies.

Virus Family	Human cancer
DNA oncogenic viruses	
Human papillomaviruses	• Cervical carcinoma • Other genital tract carcinomas: anal, vulval/vaginal, penile • Esophageal carcinoma • Laryngeal carcinoma • Oropharyngeal carcinoma
Epstein-Barr virus	• Burkitt's lymphoma • Hodgkin's disease • Nasopharyngeal carcinoma • B cell lymphoma
Human herpesvirus-8	• Kaposi's sarcoma • Castleman's disease • Primary effusion lymphoma
Hepatitis B virus	Hepatocellular carcinoma
RNA oncogenic viruses	
HTLV-I	Adult T cell leukemia/lymphoma
HIV	AIDS-related malignancies
Hepatitis C virus	Hepatocellular carcinoma

(HTLV, human T cell lymphotropic virus)

SLOW VIRUS INFECTIONS

Slow virus diseases and prion diseases are a group of neurodegenerative conditions affecting both humans and animals and characterized by:
- **The long incubation period**, ranging from months to years
- Predilection for CNS
- Invariably fatal
- Strong **genetic** predisposition
- **They lack antigenicity**; hence, there is a lack of immune response against viral proteins and a lack of associated inflammation
- Does not produce a cytopathic effect in vitro.

Slow Virus Disease

Slow virus diseases are caused by a number of conventional viruses **(Table 46.3)**. They produce a chronic form of encephalitis/encephalopathy—described as chronic, progressive demyelinating disease of the CNS.

Prion Disease

Prions are infectious protein particles that lack any nucleic acid. They are filterable like viruses; but are resistant to a wide range of chemical and physical agents of sterilization.
- **Examples:** There are several prion diseases of humans and animals; *Scrapie* being the prototype **(Table 46.3)**

CHAPTER 46 ◆ Miscellaneous RNA Viruses

Table 46.3: Slow virus and prion diseases.

Slow virus disease	Hosts
Progressive multifocal leukoencephalopathy (John Cunningham virus)	Human
Subacute sclerosing panencephalitis (Measles)	Human
Progressive rubella panencephalitis	Human
Visna virus encephalitis	Sheep
Maedi virus* progressive pneumonia	Sheep
Prion disease	**Hosts**
Kuru	Humans, monkeys chimpanzees
Creutzfeldt-Jakob disease	
Scrapie	Sheep, goats
Bovine spongiform encephalopathy	Cattle
Transmissible mink encephalopathy	Mink
Chronic wasting disease	Mule deer, elk

*Does not produce CNS disease, causes progressive pneumonia.

- ❖ **Mechanism of prion diseases:** Following infection, the infectious protein particles are carried to the brain, and induce misfolding of normal cellular prion proteins (**PrP^C**) to form its disease-causing isoform (**PrP^{Sc}**)
- ❖ **Clinical manifestations:** Incubation period of prion diseases varies from months to years (longest being 30 years). But once the disease sets in, progression is fast.
  - Prodromal phase lasts for 3–5 months, followed by appearance of manifestations such as loss of muscle control, myoclonic jerks, tremors, loss of coordination and rapidly progressive dementia
  - Death occurs within 1 year of onset of disease.
- ❖ **Human prion diseases:** The various human prion diseases are as follows: Kuru and Creutzfeldt-Jakob disease (CJD), etc.
- ❖ **Laboratory diagnosis** include:
  - **Measurement of PrP^{Sc}** by conformation dependent immunoassay
  - **Neuropathological diagnosis** in brain biopsies: The pathologic hallmarks of prion diseases seen under light microscopy
  - **Sequencing the prion (PRNP) gene** to identify the mutation.
  - **Abnormal EEG** (electroencephalogram)
- ❖ **Treatment:** There is no known effective therapy for preventing or treating prion diseases.
- ❖ **Decontamination:** Prions are extremely resistant to most of the common sterilization procedures. Recommended methods for sterilization of materials contaminated with prion proteins are:
  - Autoclaving at 134°C for 1–1.5 hour
  - Treatment with 1 N NaOH for 1 hour
  - Treatment with 0.5% sodium hypochlorite for 2 hours.

EXPECTED QUESTIONS

I. **Write short notes on:**
   1. Viral gastroenteritis.
   2. Ebola virus disease.
   3. Malignancies produced by oncogenic viruses.
   4. Slow viral infections.

II. **Multiple Choice Questions (MCQs):**
   1. **The most common viral cause of gastroenteritis:**
      a. Rotavirus
      b. Norwalk virus
      c. Adenovirus 40, 41
      d. Hepadnavirus

   2. **Carcinoma cervix is caused by:**
      a. Herpes simplex virus
      b. Human papillomavirus
      c. Enterovirus
      d. Parvovirus

   3. **Viral gastroenteritis in adults is caused by:**
      a. Rotavirus
      b. Norwalk virus
      c. Adenovirus 40, 41
      d. Hepadnavirus

Answers
1. a   2. b   3. b

SECTION 6: Parasitology

SECTION OUTLINE

47. General Parasitology
48. Amoebae (*Entamoeba* and Free-living Amoebae)
49. Intestinal and Genital Flagellates: *Giardia* and *Trichomonas*
50. Hemoflagellates: *Leishmania* and *Trypanosoma*
51. Malaria Parasite and *Babesia*
52. Opportunistic Coccidian Parasites and Others
53. Cestodes: *Taenia*, *Echinococcus*, *Hymenolepis*, *Diphyllobothrium* and Others
54. Trematodes: *Schistosoma*, Hepatic Flukes, *Fasciolopsis*, and *Paragonimus*
55. Intestinal Nematodes: *Trichuris*, *Enterobius*, *Ascaris*, Hookworm, and *Strongyloides*
56. Tissue Nematodes: Filarial Nematodes, *Dracunculus*, and *Trichinella*
57. Medical Entomolgy (Ectoparasites)

General Parasitology

CHAPTER 47

CHAPTER PREVIEW
- General Parasitology
  - Life Cycle of Parasites
- Laboratory Diagnosis of Parasitic Diseases
- Treatment of Parasitic Diseases

GENERAL PARASITOLOGY

Parasite is a living organism, which lives in or upon another organism (host) and derives nutrients directly from it, without giving any benefit to the host. Medical Parasitology deals with the study of animal parasites, which infect and produce diseases in human beings. Parasites may be classified as:

- ❖ **Ectoparasites:** They inhabit the surface of the body of the host without penetrating into the tissues (e.g. fleas, mites or ticks). They serve as important vectors transmitting the pathogenic microbes. The infection produced by these parasites is called as infestation (e.g. scabies)
- ❖ **Endoparasites:** These are the parasites, that live within the body of the host (e.g., *Leishmania*). Invasion by the endoparasite is called as infection.

The endoparasites are further classified into protozoa and helminths.

- ❖ **Protozoa:** They are unicellular eukaryotic cells that perform all the physiological functions. Although like bacteria they are unicellular, they are considered as lower eukaryotes, as they possess cellular organelles and metabolic pathways, similar to that of eukaryotes
- ❖ **Helminths:** They are elongated flat or round worm-like parasites measuring few millimeters to as long as few meters. They are eukaryotic multicellular and bilaterally symmetrical. They belong to two phyla:
  1. Phylum **Platyhelminths** (flat worms)—includes cestodes (tapeworms) and trematodes (flukes)
  2. Phylum **Nemathelminths**—includes nematodes.

Medically important protozoa and helminths are listed in **Table 47.1**.

■ LIFE CYCLE OF PARASITES

The life cycle of parasites depends upon three factors: host, mode of transmission and infective form.

Table 47.1: Medically important protozoa and helminths.

Medically important protozoa
Amoeba
• *Entamoeba histolytica*
• Free-living amoebae: *Naegleria, Acanthamoeba, Balamuthia*
Flagellates
• Intestinal Flagellate: *Giardia*
• Genital Flagellate: *Trichomonas*
• Hemoflagellates: *Leishmania* and *Trypanosoma*
Apicomplexa
• Malaria parasites and *Babesia*
• Opportunistic coccidian parasites: *Toxoplasma, Cryptosporidium, Cyclospora, Cystoisospora* and *Sarcocystis*
Miscellaneous Protozoa: *Balantidium coli* and *Blastocystis*
Medically important helminths
Cestodes
Diphyllobothrium, Taenia, Echinococcus and *Hymenolepis*
Trematodes or Flukes
Schistosoma, Fasciola, Clonorchis, Opisthorchis, Fasciolopsis, Paragonimus and others
Intestinal Nematodes
Trichuris, Enterobius, hookworm, *Strongyloides, Ascaris* and others
Somatic Nematodes
Filarial nematodes, *Dracunculus* and *Trichinella*

Note: Ectoparasite infestation is discussed in **Chapter 57**.

- ❖ **Host:** It is as an organism, which harbors the parasite and provides the nourishment and shelter
  - Hosts can be classified into *definitive host* (where the parasite undergoes sexual cycle or where the adult parasite inhabits) or *intermediate host* (where the parasite undergoes asexual cycle or where the larva inhabits)
  - Depending upon the number of hosts involved, the life cycle of the parasite may be direct (simple) or indirect (complex)

- In *direct/simple life cycle,* the parasite requires only one host to complete its development
- In *indirect/complex life cycle,* the parasite requires two/three hosts (one definitive host and another one or two intermediate host/s) to complete its development.

❖ **Infective form:** It is the morphological form of the parasite which is transmitted to man

❖ **Mode of transmission:** Parasites may be transmitted by various modes such as ingestion, skin penetration, vector-borne, sexual, vertical, blood transfusion, and autoinfection.

> **Autoinfection**
> Few intestinal parasites may infect the same person by contaminated hand (external autoinfection) or by reverse peristalsis (internal autoinfection). It is observed in some parasitic infections such as *Cryptosporidium parvum, Taenia solium, Enterobius vermicularis, Strongyloides stercoralis* and *Hymenolepis nana.*

LABORATORY DIAGNOSIS OF PARASITIC DISEASES

Laboratory diagnosis plays an important role in establishing the specific diagnosis of various parasitic infections. Following are the techniques used in the diagnosis of parasitic infections.

Examination of Feces

As many parasites inhabit in the intestinal tract, stool examination is the most common diagnostic technique used for the diagnosis of parasitic infections.

Specimen Collection

Stool specimens should be collected in a wide-mouthed, clean, leak-proof, screw capped containers and should be handled carefully to avoid acquiring infection from organisms present in the stool **(Fig. 47.1)**.

❖ **Timing:** Specimen should be collected before starting anti-parasitic drugs and closer to the onset of symptoms

❖ **Frequency:** At least three stool specimens collected on alternate days (within 10 days) are adequate to make the diagnosis of intestinal parasitic diseases

❖ **When to examine:** Liquid stool specimens should be examined within 30 minutes, semisolid stools within 1hr (as on storage, trophozoites may disintegrate or become non-motile) and formed stools up to 24 hours after collection

❖ **For monitoring response to therapy:** Repeat stool examination can be done 3 to 4 weeks after the therapy for intestinal protozoan infection, and 5–6 weeks for *Taenia* infection

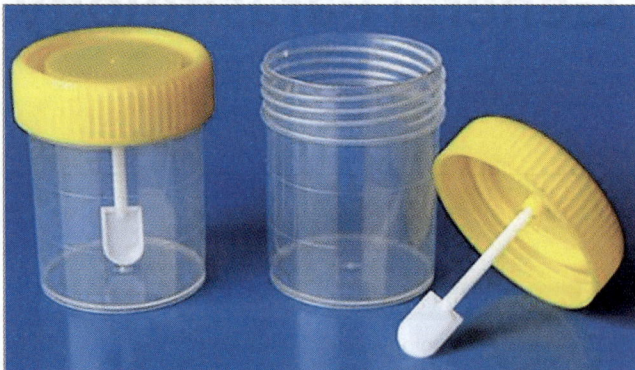

Fig. 47.1: Sample container for stool.

❖ **If delay in transport:** Fecal specimens should be kept at room temperature; preservatives (e.g. 10% formalin) can be used to maintain the morphology of the parasitic cysts and eggs

❖ **Specimens other than stool:**
- *Perianal swabs* (cellophane tape or NIH swab): Useful for detecting eggs of *Enterobius vermicularis* deposited on the surface of perianal skin
- *Duodenal contents:* It is very useful for the detection of small intestine parasites like *Giardia intestinalis* and larva of *Strongyloides stercoralis.* Duodenal fluid can be collected by endoscopy or by Entero-test.

Macroscopic Examination

Macroscopic examination of stool may provide clues about various parasitic infections.

❖ **Mucoid bloody stool:** Found in acute amoebic dysentery, intestinal schistosomiasis, and invasive balantidiasis

❖ **Color:** Dark red stool indicates upper gastrointestinal tract (GIT) bleeding and a bright red stool is suggestive of bleeding from lower GIT

❖ **Frothy pale offensive stool** (containing fat) is usually found in giardiasis

❖ **Stool consistency:** In liquid stool, trophozoites are usually found; whereas in semi-formed stool both trophozoites and cysts are found and the cysts are mainly found in formed specimens.

Microscopic Examination

The microscopic examination includes direct wet mount examination and permanent staining methods.

Direct Wet Mount (Saline and Iodine Mount)

Drops of saline and Lugol's iodine are placed on left and right halves of the slide respectively **(Fig. 47.2)**.

❖ A small amount of feces (~2 mg) is mixed with a stick to form a uniform smooth suspension

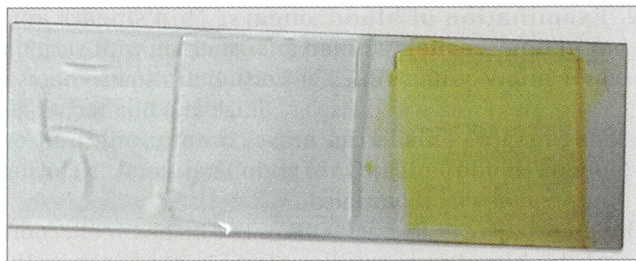

Fig. 47.2: Saline and iodine wet mount.
Source: Department of Microbiology, JIPMER, Puducherry (*with permission*).

- **Cover slip** is placed on the mount and examined under low power objective (10X) for detection of helminths eggs and larvae; followed by high power objective (40X) for protozoan cysts and trophozoites
- **Screening area:** The entire coverslip preparation should be examined in a zigzag fashion, first under low power and then under high power objective, before reporting a negative result **(Fig. 47.3)**
- **Normal constituents of stool specimen:** These include plant fiber, starch cells, muscle fibers, animal hair, pollen grains, yeast cells, bacteria, fat globules, air bubbles, etc. Some of these structures may be confused with various protozoan trophozoites, cysts or helminthic eggs and larvae.
- **Motility:** If a finding is suspected to be a trophozoite, then examination for at least 15 seconds should be allowed to detect motility. Motility can be stimulated by—the application of heat by placing a hot penny on the edge of a slide or tapping on the coverslip.

Saline Mount

The saline mount is useful in the detection of trophozoites and cysts of protozoan parasites, and eggs and larvae of helminths. It has the following advantages over iodine mount.

Fig. 47.3: Method of screening of slide during wet mount examination of stool.

- The motility of trophozoites and larvae in acute infection can be demonstrated
- Bile staining property can be appreciated—bile stained eggs appear golden brown and non-bile stained eggs appear colorless
- For stool specimens with preservatives, directly the wet mount can be prepared without using saline.

Iodine Mount

- *Advantages:* Nuclear details of protozoan cysts, helminthic eggs and larvae are better visualized, compared to saline mount
- *Disadvantages:* (i) Iodine immobilizes and kills the parasites, hence motility of the trophozoites and helminthic larvae cannot be appreciated, (ii) Bile staining property cannot be appreciated.

> **Non-bile Stained Eggs**
> Eggs of most of the intestinal parasites when they pass through intestine are stained by bile. The exceptions being *Enterobius*, hookworm and *Hymenolepis nana*; these eggs are non-bile stained.

Permanent Stained Smear

Permanent stained smears are required for accurate detection of protozoan cysts and trophozoites by staining their internal structures. Commonly used methods are:
- Iron-hematoxylin stain
- Trichrome stain
- Modified acid-fast stain—this is useful for coccidian parasites such as *Cryptosporidium*, *Cyclospora* and *Cystoisospora*.

Concentration Techniques

If the parasite output is low in feces (egg, cysts, trophozoites and larvae) and direct examination may not be able to detect the parasites, then the stool specimens need to be concentrated. The eggs, cysts and larvae are recovered after concentration procedures; however, the trophozoites get destroyed.

Commonly used concentration techniques are:
- **Sedimentation techniques:** The eggs and cysts settle down at the bottom of the tube because they have greater density than the suspending medium following centrifugation. Example includes formalin-ether concentration technique
  - The sensitivity of detecting ova or cysts increases by 8–10 folds
  - The size and shape of the parasitic structures are maintained.
- **Flotation techniques:** It involves suspending the specimen in a medium (e.g. **saturated salt solution**) of greater density, so that the helminthic eggs and

protozoan cysts float on the surface of the solution. The disadvantage is, it cannot be used for concentration of the parasites that do not float in saturated salt solution such as—unfertilized eggs of *Ascaris*, larva of *Strongyloides*, *Taenia* eggs and operculated eggs of trematodes.

Other flotation methods are:
- Zinc sulphate flotation concentration technique
- Sheather's sugar flotation technique (useful for *Cryptosporidium*, *Cystoisospora* and *Cyclospora*)

Various morphological forms of parasites seen in stool specimens are enlisted in **Table 47.2**.

Egg Counting (Egg Quantification) Methods

The intensity of intestinal helminthic infection (especially *Trichuris*, *Ascaris* and hookworm) can be estimated by egg counting in feces; which can be performed by various egg counting methods:
- Direct smear counting method of Beaver
- Kato-Katz thick film method
- Stoll's method or dilution egg counting method

Examination of Blood

Blood examination is useful in the diagnosis of infection caused by blood parasites like *Plasmodium*, *Trypanosoma*, *Leishmania*, *Babesia*, *Wuchereria bancrofti*, *Brugia malayi*, *Loa loa* and *Mansonella*.

Various methods of examination of blood include:
1. **Direct wet mount examination:** It is useful for the detection of malaria parasites and microfilariae in lymphatic filariasis
2. **Examination of blood smears:** Thin smears and thick smears are examined after staining with various Romanowsky stains such as Leishman's stain, Giemsa stain, Field's stain and Jaswant Singh and Bhattacharjee (JSB) stain. This is the most common method of microscopic examination of peripheral blood, useful for most of the blood parasites
3. **Quantitative buffy coat (QBC):** This involves collection of the blood in a capillary tube coated internally with acridine orange stain, centrifugation and then examination of the buffy coat region under fluorescence microscopy. This is extremely useful for the detection of the malaria parasites and microfilariae
4. **Concentration of blood:** This is useful for the detection of microfilariae from the blood specimen.
   Various concentration methods are:
   - Sedimentation technique
   - Cytocentrifugation (cytospin)
   - Knott concentration
   - Gradient centrifugation
   - Membrane filtration.

Microscopic Examination of Other Specimens

Microscopic examination of various specimens (other than stool) can also be performed to demonstrate different morphological forms of the parasites **(Table 47.3)**.

Immunodiagnostic Methods

Immunodiagnostic methods involve the detection of parasite-specific antibodies in serum and the detection of circulating parasitic antigens in the serum. These methods are useful when:
- Parasites are detected only during the early stages of the disease
- Parasites occur in very small numbers
- Parasites reside in the internal organs and morphological identification is not possible
- When other techniques like culture are time-consuming.

Antibody Detection Tests

Antibodies are detected in various parasitic infections; mainly from serum, sometimes from other specimens such as CSF (neurocysticercosis). The parasitic diseases where antibody detection methods are useful are:

Amoebic liver abscess, visceral leishmaniasis, toxoplasmosis, cysticercosis, hydatid disease and lymphatic filariasis. Antibodies in serum are detected by ELISA, immunochromatographic test (ICT), Western blot, and flow through assay.

Table 47.2: Morphological forms of parasites seen in stool specimens.

Morphological form	Parasites
Trophozoite and cyst	*Entamoeba histolytica* *Giardia lamblia*
Adult worm	*Ascaris lumbricoides* *Enterobius vermicularis*
Adult worm segments	*Taenia* species *Diphyllobothrium latum*
Egg	*Diphyllobothrium latum* *Taenia* species *Hymenolepis nana* *Schistosoma* species *Fasciola hepatica* *Fasciolopsis buski* *Ascaris lumbricoides* Hookworm *Enterobius vermicularis* *Trichuris trichiura*
Larva	*Strongyloides stercoralis*

CHAPTER 47 ◆ General Parasitology

Table 47.3: Various morphological forms of parasites seen in different specimens other than stool.

Specimen	Morphological form	Parasite
Peripheral blood smear	Ring form, schizont, gametocyte	*Plasmodium* spp.
	Amastigote	*Leishmania* spp.
	Trypomastigote	*Trypanosoma* spp.
	Microfilaria	Filarial nematodes*
Bone marrow, liver, lymph node, splenic aspirate	Tachyzoite	*Toxoplasma gondii*
	Amastigote	*Leishmania donovani*
Liver aspirate	Trophozoite	*Entamoeba histolytica*
Lymph node aspirate	Trypomastigote	*Trypanosoma* spp.
Lymph node biopsy	Adult worm	*Wuchereria bancrofti* *Brugia malayi*
CSF	Trophozoite	*Naegleria fowleri* *Acanthamoeba* spp.
	Trypomastigote	*Trypanosoma* spp.
Urine	Trophozoite	*Trichomonas vaginalis*
	Microfilaria	*Wuchereria bancrofti*
	Egg	*Schistosoma haematobium*
Sputum	Adult worm	*Paragonimus* spp.
	Egg	*Paragonimus* spp.
	Larva (migrating)	*Ascaris lumbricoides* *Strongyloides* spp. Hookworm
	Trophozoite	*Entamoeba histolytica*
Duodenal aspirate	Trophozoite	*Giardia lamblia*
	Larva	*Strongyloides stercoralis*
Corneal scrapings	Trophozoite	*Acanthamoeba* spp.
Skin	Amastigote	*Leishmania* spp.
	Microfilaria	*Onchocerca volvulus*
	Larva in skin ulcer fluid	*Dracunculus medinensis*
Muscle tissue	Encysted larva	*Trichinella spiralis*
	Cysticercus cellulosae	*Taenia solium*
Perianal area	Egg	*Enterobius* spp.

*Filarial nematodes found in the peripheral blood smears are *Wuchereria bancrofti, Brugia malayi, Loa loa, Mansonella* spp.

Antigen Detection Tests

Antigen detection methods are available for various parasitic diseases.
- **Amoebiasis:** ELISA, detecting lectin antigen in blood and stool
- **Triage parasite panel:** This ICT simultaneously detects antigens of *Giardia, E. histolytica/E. dispar* and *Cryptosporidium*.
- **Malaria:** ICT format available detecting:
    - Histidine rich protein-2 (Pf. HRP 2)—*P. falciparum* specific
    - Parasite lactate dehydrogenase (pLDH) and aldolase—common to all species.
- **Lymphatic filariasis:** ELISA and ICT formats are available detecting filarial antigens.

Molecular Methods

Molecular methods most frequently used in diagnostic parasitology include: Polymerase chain reaction (PCR) and real time PCR.

Other Diagnostic Modalities

- **Culture techniques:** The culture techniques have been described for amoeba, *Trichomonas,* malaria parasite, *Leishmania* and nematode larvae
- **Imaging techniques:** X-ray, ultrasound (USG), computed tomography (CT) and magnetic resonance imaging (MRI) are extensively used for parasitic infections such as amoebic liver abscess, cysticercosis and hydatid disease
- **Intradermal skin tests:** Positive intradermal skin tests are suggestive of past exposure. Skin tests are useful for hydatid disease (Casoni's test), filariasis, ascariasis, strongyloidiasis, leishmaniasis (Montenegro test), etc.

■ TREATMENT OF PARASITIC DISEASES

Treatment of parasitic diseases primarily is based on chemotherapy and in some cases by surgery.
- **Anti-parasitic drugs:** Various chemotherapeutic agents are used for the treatment and prophylaxis of parasitic infections. Commonly used anti-parasitic agents are: Metronidazole, pentamidine, amphotericin B, paromomycin, chloroquine, artemisinin derivatives, cotrimoxazole, albendazole, mebendazole, etc.
- **Surgical management:** It is useful for the management of parasitic diseases like cystic echinococcosis, neurocysticercosis, etc.

Details of treatment of some of the important human parasites have been described in **Chapters 48–57**.

EXPECTED QUESTIONS

I. **Write short notes on:**
   1. Stool concentration techniques.
   2. Serodiagnosis in parasitic diseases.

II. **Multiple Choice Questions (MCQs):**
   1. Advantages of saline mount are all, *except*:
      a. Useful in the detection of trophozoites and cysts of protozoan parasites and eggs and larvae of helminths
      b. Nuclear details of cysts and helminthic eggs and larvae are better visualized
      c. Motility of trophozoites and larvae can be seen in acute infection
      d. Bile staining property can be appreciated
   2. Flotation technique is useful for the detection of:
      a. Fertilized eggs of *Ascaris lumbricoides*
      b. Larva of *Strongyloides*
      c. *Taenia* eggs
      d. Operculated eggs of trematodes
   3. A stained peripheral blood smear is useful for the diagnosis of all of the following parasitic infections, *except*:
      a. Malaria
      b. Filaria
      c. Hookworm disease
      d. Leishmania
   4. All are non-bile stained eggs, *except*:
      a. *Enterobius*
      b. Hookworm
      c. *Ascaris*
      d. *Hymenolepis*

Answers
1. b   2. a   3. c   4. c

Amoebae

CHAPTER 48

CHAPTER PREVIEW
- Entamoeba histolytica
- Free-living Amoebae

AMOEBAE

Amoebae are classified into two groups. Based on the habitat they are of two types:
1. **Intestinal amoebae:** They reside in the human intestine. *Entamoeba histolytica* is the most important pathogenic intestinal amoeba. Most other species of *Entamoeba* are harmless commensals in the human intestine, e.g. *Entamoeba coli*
2. **Free-living amoebae:** They are small, freely living, and widely distributed in soil and water. They can cause opportunistic infections in humans, affecting the central nervous system. Important human pathogenic free-living amoebae are *Naegleria, Acanthamoeba,* and *Balamuthia*.

■ ENTAMOEBA HISTOLYTICA

Entamoeba histolytica causes amoebic dysentery and also extraintestinal amoebiasis affecting the liver (amoebic liver abscess). It is worldwide in distribution but more common in tropical and subtropical countries.

Morphology

E. histolytica exists in three morphological forms:
- **Trophozoite:** It is the invasive form as well as the feeding and replicating form of the parasite found in the feces of patients with active disease
- **Precyst:** It is the intermediate stage between trophozoite and cyst
- **Cyst:** It is the diagnostic form of the parasite found in the feces of carriers as well as patients with active disease. It exists as immature forms (uni- and bi-nucleated) and mature cyst (quadrinucleated); the latter being the infective form.

Life Cycle (Fig. 48.1)

Host: *E. histolytica* completes its life cycle in a single host, i.e. man.

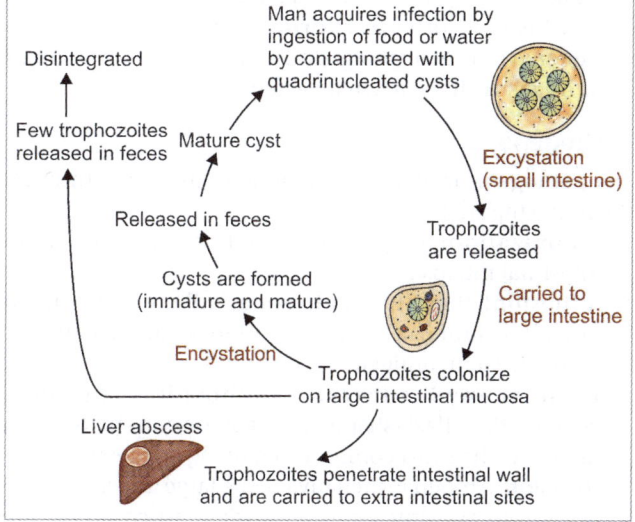

Fig. 48.1: Life cycle of *Entamoeba histolytica*.

Infective form: Mature quadrinucleated cyst is the infective form.

Mode of transmission: *E. histolytica* is transmitted by mainly by **feco-oral route** by ingestion of food or water contaminated with mature quadrinucleated cysts, which contaminate the food and water.

Development in Human Intestine

- **Small intestine:** Cysts bypass gastric juice and reach the small intestine, where they undergo **excystation**. The cyst wall gets lysed to release the trophozoites
- **Large intestine:** Trophozoites are carried to the large intestine, where they multiply actively, and then colonize on the intestinal mucosa
- After colonization, trophozoites show different courses depending on host susceptibility:

- **Asymptomatic cyst passers:** In the majority of individuals, trophozoites do not cause any lesion, transform into cysts, and are excreted in feces
- **Amoebic dysentery:** In some individuals, trophozoites adhere to intestinal mucosa producing intestinal ulcers and dysentery
- **Invasive amoebiasis**: Very rarely, trophozoites invade the intestinal mucosa, gain access to the portal veins, and migrate to extraintestinal sites, the most common site being the liver where they cause an **amoebic liver abscess**.

❖ **Encystation:** The trophozoites transform into precysts then into cysts (immature and mature), which are then liberated in feces. Encystation occurs only in the large intestine.

❖ **Cysts** released in feces can survive in the environment and become **infective form**. Trophozoites are also excreted but get disintegrated either in the environment or by gastric juice when ingested.

Pathogenesis

The pathogenesis of intestinal amoebiasis occurs through the following steps.

❖ **Colonization:** Trophozoites first colonize the large intestinal mucosa

❖ **Adhesion:** Then the trophozoites adhere to the large intestinal mucosa using a virulence factor called—amoebic lectin antigen

❖ **Flask-shaped ulcers:** Trophozoites produce characteristic flask-shaped ulcerative lesions in the large intestine, the most common site being the cecum

❖ **Invasion:** Amoebae then invade the large intestinal wall; migrate to extraintestinal sites (the most common site being the liver). The invasion is facilitated by cysteine proteases and hydrolytic enzymes secreted by *E. histolytica*

❖ **Liver abscess:** The amoebic trophozoites occlude the hepatic venules; which leads to anoxic necrosis of the hepatocytes. Inflammatory response surrounding the hepatocytes leads to the formation of an abscess

❖ A liver abscess has a **thick wall** (made up of hepatocytes invaded with amoebic trophozoites) and thick chocolate brown colored pus called **anchovy sauce pus**.

Clinical Manifestations

Intestinal Amoebiasis

The incubation period varies from one to four weeks. The majority of infections (90%) result in asymptomatic cyst passers. The remaining (10%), develop intestinal amoebiasis; characterized by:

❖ **Amoebic dysentery:** Symptoms include bloody diarrhea (up to 10 times per day) with mucus and pus cells, colicky abdominal pain, and fever

❖ **Intestinal complications:** Rarely patients develop complications such as amoebic appendicitis, amoeboma (a palpable abdominal mass), intestinal perforation, fulminant colitis, amoebic peritonitis, and amoebiasis cutis.

Amoebic Liver Abscess (ALA)

About 2–8% of patients with intestinal amoebiasis develop extraintestinal amoebiasis.

❖ The liver is the most common site; followed by lungs, brain, genitourinary tract, and spleen

❖ **The most common hepatic site** affected is the posterior-superior surface of the right lobe of the liver

❖ **Presentation:** ALA presents with tender hepatomegaly and fever along with weight loss, sweating, and weakness, very rarely jaundice, and cough

❖ **Complications:** Abscess may grow in various directions of the liver discharging the contents into the neighboring organs—leading to a subphrenic abscess, peritonitis, pericarditis, etc. Hematogenous spread can occur from the liver affecting the brain, lungs, spleen and genitourinary organs, etc.

Laboratory Diagnosis of Intestinal Amoebiasis

The stool is the specimen of choice. A minimum of three stool samples should be collected on an alternate day (within 10 days) as amoebae are shed intermittently.

Stool Macroscopy

The amoebic stool is foul-smelling, copious in amount, dark red in color mixed with blood and mucus, and is not adherent to the container. It should be differentiated from bacillary dysentery, where the stool is bright red, odorless, and adherent to the container.

Stool Microscopy

Direct examination of stool by saline and iodine mount is performed to demonstrate trophozoites and cysts (*see highlight box below*).

❖ **Stool concentration:** The sensitivity can further be improved by examining the stool samples after concentration by the formalin ether sedimentation method

❖ **Permanent staining:** Stool can also be examined by staining with permanent stains like trichrome stain

❖ **Reporting:** Cyst and trophozoite of *E. histolytica* are indistinguishable from that of *E. dispar*. So, the report should always be sent as "cyst or trophozoite of *E. histolytica/E. dispar* are found in the stool microscopy".

Trophozoites
Demonstration of trophozoite stool is considered as the gold standard microscopic test for active infection **(Figs. 48.2A and 48.3A)**. They are not found in the stool of asymptomatic carriers.
- **Measures** 15–20 µm, has cytoplasm and single nucleus
- **Motility:** They are actively motile, with finger-like pseudopodia
- **Ingested RBCs** in the cytoplasm may be found, which is a feature of *E. histolytica* (being invasive), which differentiates it from *E. dispar*
- **Nucleus:** It has a central karyosome and fine peripheral chromatin granules lining the nuclear membrane
- Trophozoites are better appreciated in saline mount than in iodine mount as iodine kills the trophozoites and motility cannot be appreciated. Therefore, trophozoites should not be reported based on iodine mount.

Quadrinucleated cysts
Cysts are found in stool specimens of both patients (with active infection) and carriers.
- The internal structure of cysts is clearly appreciated by iodine mount than saline mount and even better on permanent staining
- Cysts appear round, 12–15 µm in size containing 1–4 nuclei **(Figs. 48.2B and 48.3B)**. The appearance of the nucleus is as described for trophozoites
- Both mature cysts (contain 4 nuclei) and immature cysts (contain 1 or 2 nuclei) are found in stool.

Histology
Trophozoites can be detected in sigmoidoscopy-guided biopsies collected from the colonic mucosa and stained with Periodic acid–Schiff (PAS) or H&E stains.

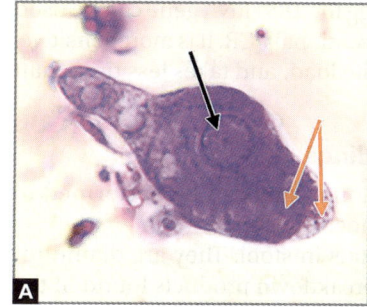
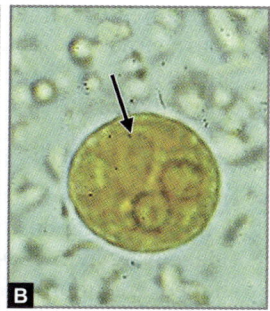

Figs. 48.3A and B: *Entamoeba histolytica*: **A.** Trophozoite (Trichrome stain); **B.** Cyst (Iodine mount).
Source: Swierczynski G, Milanesi B. Atlas of human intestinal protozoa microscopic diagnosis (*with permission*).

Stool Culture
Culture methods are not routinely used for diagnosis. They are useful in studying the pathogenicity of amoeba and for the preparation of amoebic antigens for serological tests; e.g., National Institute of Health (NIH) media.

Stool Antigen Detection (Coproantigen)
Various tests used to detect antigens in stool are:
- **ELISA** detecting 170-kDa lectin antigen: It shows >95% sensitivity and specificity. It can also differentiate pathogenic *E. histolytica* (lectin antigen-positive) from nonpathogenic *E. dispar* (lectin antigen-negative)
- **Immunochromatographic test (ICT):** It is a rapid diagnostic test, that gives results within 20-30 minutes. An example includes **Triage Parasite Panel,** which simultaneously detects three parasitic antigens in stool—*Giardia lamblia, E. histolytica/E. dispar,* and *Cryptosporidium parvum*.

Serology
- **Amoebic antigen:** ELISA is available to detect 170-kDa lectin antigen in serum.
  - Amoebic antigen in serum is found only in patients with active infection and disappears after clinical cure.
  - So its presence in serum indicates active infection.
- **Amoebic Antibody:** ELISA is available to detect serum antibodies (IgG) against lectin antigen. Antibodies appear only in the later stages of intestinal amoebiasis and therefore are not very useful in diagnosis.

Molecular Diagnosis
Molecular methods have emerged as the gold standard test for the diagnosis of amoebiasis.
- **Nested multiplex PCR** is available targeting small-subunit rRNA genes. It can differentiate *E. histolytica* and *E. dispar* with good sensitivity and specificity

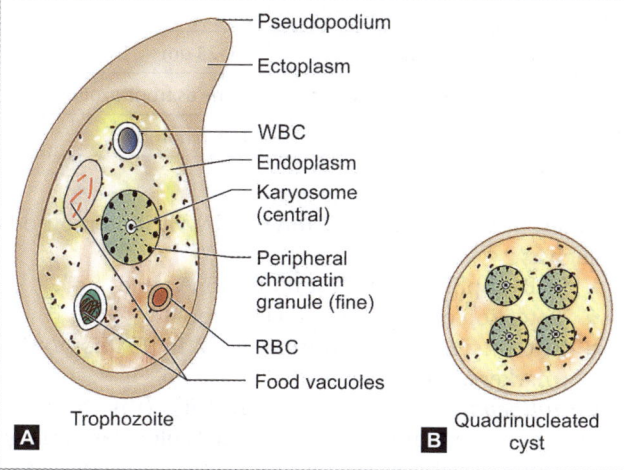

Figs. 48.2A and B: *Entamoeba histolytica* (schematic diagram): **A.** Trophozoite; **B.** Cyst.

- **Real-time PCR** targeting the 18S rRNA gene can be used as an alternative to conventional PCR. It is more sensitive, can quantify the parasite load, and takes less time than conventional PCR.

Other Nonspecific Findings
- **Imaging method:** Colonoscopy can be performed to detect flask-shaped amoebic ulcers
- **Charcot-Leyden crystals** in stool: They are diamond-shaped, eosinophilic breakdown products found in the stool in some cases
- **Moderate leukocytosis** in blood.

Laboratory Diagnosis of Amoebic Liver Abscess (ALA)

Laboratory diagnosis of ALA comprises the following modalities.
- **Microscopy of liver pus:** It can detect trophozoites, but its sensitivity is very poor (<25%). Trophozoites may be found only in the last portion of the aspirated material from the abscess wall
- **Antigen detection** (in serum, liver pus, and saliva): ELISA can be performed to detect 170-kDa of lectin antigen
- **Antibody detection:** ELISA can be performed to detect antibody to 170-kDa lectin antigen. It is much more useful in extraintestinal than intestinal amoebiasis
- **Molecular diagnosis:** Nested multiplex PCR and real-time PCR can be performed on amebic liver pus detecting 18S rRNA
- **Radiologic examination** such as ultrasonography or CT scan or MRI can detect the site of the abscess and its extension. However, they cannot differentiate ALA from a pyogenic liver abscess.

> **TREATMENT** — Amoebiasis
>
> **Asymptomatic carriage:** Treatment helps in reducing the passage of cysts in stool and thereby preventing disease transmission. Luminal agents are used for treatment.
> - Iodoquinol (for 20 days) or
> - Paromomycin (for 10 days)
>
> **Amoebic dysentery or liver abscess:** Treatment consists of:
> - **Tissue agents:** Metronidazole (for 5–10 days) or tinidazole (for 3 days) *plus*
> - **Luminal agents** as above
>
> **Other measures** include fluid and electrolyte replacement and symptomatic treatment.

Nonpathogenic Amoebae

Many nonpathogenic amoebae may be found as harmless commensals in the human intestine.
- *Entamoeba dispar:* It is morphologically (both cyst and trophozoite) similar to that of *E. histolytica*. It can be

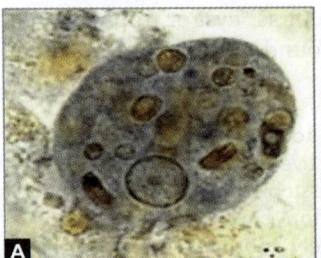 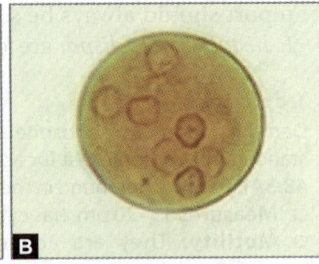

Figs. 48.4A and B: *Entamoeba coli:* **A.** Trophozoite (Iron hematoxylin stain) shows a nucleus with coarse peripheral chromatin and abundant food vacuoles in the cytoplasm containing fecal debris; **B.** Cyst (iodine mount) containing several nuclei.

Source: Swierczynski G, Milanesi B. Atlas of human intestinal protozoa microscopic diagnosis (*with permission*).

Table 48.1: Differences between *Entamoeba histolytica* and *Entamoeba coli.*

	Entamoeba histolytica	*Entamoeba coli*
Trophozoite		
Size	15–20 µm	20–25 µm
Motility	Very active motility, pseudopodia with finger-like projection	Sluggish motility, blunt pseudopodia
Cytoplasm	It is differentiated into ectoplasm and endoplasm	Not differentiated
Ingested RBCs	It may be present inside the cytoplasm	Absent
Nucleus	Karyosome is small and central. The nuclear membrane is thin and lined by fine chromatin granules	Karyosome is large and eccentric. The nuclear membrane is thick and lined by coarse chromatin granules
Cyst		
Size	12–15 µm	15–25 µm
Nucleus	Same as trophozoite	Same as trophozoite
Nuclei	1–4 in number	1–8 in number

(RBC, red blood cells)

differentiated from *E. histolytica* by various methods such as:
- PCR amplifying small subunit rRNA gene
- Detection of lectin antigen in stool
- RBC inside trophozoites—only in *E. histolytica* (marker of invasiveness)

- *Entamoeba coli* (**Figs. 48.4A and B**): It is the most common nonpathogenic amoeba that colonizes the large intestine. It is frequently found in the stool samples of healthy individuals and should be differentiated from that of *E. histolytica* (**Table 48.1**).

CHAPTER 48 ❖ Amoebae

■ FREE-LIVING AMOEBAE

Free-living amoebae are small, freely living, widely distributed in soil and water, and can cause opportunistic infections in humans. Among many free-living amoebae that exist in nature, only a few have an association with human diseases affecting CNS—*Naegleria*, *Acanthamoeba*, and *Balamuthia*.

Naegleria fowleri

It is the causative agent of primary amoebic meningoencephalitis (PAM).
- ❖ **Pathogenesis:** Man acquires infection by nasal contamination with trophozoites (infective form) while swimming in freshwater bodies. The trophozoites invade the nasal mucosa, and cribriform plate and travel along the olfactory nerve to reach the brain.
- ❖ **Laboratory diagnosis:** It is diagnosed by the following modalities.
  - ■ **Microscopy:** Demonstration of trophozoites in CSF by wet mount or direct fluorescent antibody test. Amoeboid trophozoite of *Naegleria* possesses lobular pseudopodia (called lobopodian), has granular cytoplasm and nucleus with a large central karyosome
  - ■ **Culture:** CSF sample culture on non-nutrient agar, lawn cultured with a bacterial supplement (*E. coli*). *Naegleria* feeds on bacteria and produces trails **(Trail sign)**.
- ❖ **Treatment:** No effective treatment is available. Amphotericin B has been tried. The prognosis is very poor.

Acanthamoeba species

Acanthamoeba are free-living amoebae that infect CNS, skin, and eyes.
- ❖ **Clinical manifestations:** It causes following infections:
  - ■ **GAE:** In HIV individuals, it produces a CNS infection called granulomatous amoebic encephalitis (GAE)
  - ■ **Amoebic keratitis:** In contact lens users, it can cause corneal ulcers

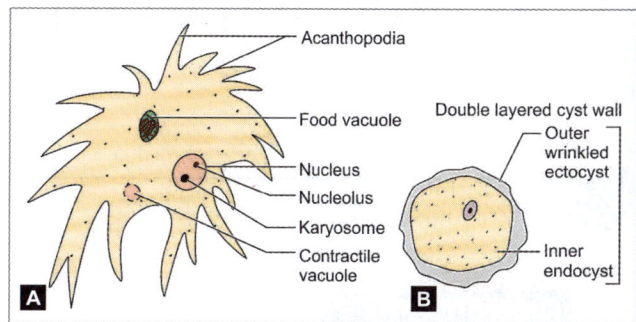

Figs. 48.5A and B: *Acanthamoeba* species (schematic diagram): **A.** Trophozoite; **B.** Cyst.

- ❖ **Pathogenesis:** Man acquires infection by inhalation of aerosol contaminated with cyst or trophozoite. The primary sites of infection are the sinuses and lungs. From the lungs, trophozoites reach the CNS by the hematogenous route
- ❖ It spreads to the cornea either by trauma or contact lens cleaning solution
- ❖ **Laboratory diagnosis:** It is diagnosed by the following modalities.
  - ■ Demonstration of trophozoites in CSF by wet mount, phase contrast microscopy, etc.
  - ■ Demonstration of trophozoites and cysts in corneal smears examination (wet mount, permanent staining)
  - ■ Trophozoite has characteristic thorn-like pseudopodia **(Fig. 48.5A)**
  - ■ The cyst is double-walled, with an outer wrinkled wall **(Fig. 48.5B)**
  - ■ Culture of CSF sample on non-nutrient agar.
- ❖ **Treatment***:* No effective treatment is available. Prognosis of GAE is very poor.

Balamuthia mandrillaris

Balamuthia mandrillaris can also cause granulomatous amoebic encephalitis (GAE), similar to that of *Acanthamoeba*. Diagnosis is made by the detection of trophozoites and cysts of *Balamuthia* in CSF and brain biopsy.

EXPECTED QUESTIONS

I. **Write an essay on:**
 1. Discuss the clinical manifestations and laboratory diagnosis of intestinal amoebiasis.
II. **Write short notes on:**
 1. Amoebic liver abscess
 2. Free-living amoebae
III. **Multiple Choice Questions (MCQs):**
 1. **Cyst of *E. histolytica*: All are true, *except*?**
    a. Infective form   b. Diagnostic form
    c. Pathogenic form   d. Has 4 nuclei
 2. **Trophozoite of *E. histolytica*: All are true, *except*?**
    a. Pathogenic form
    b. Has 4 nuclei
    c. Finger-like pseudopodia
    d. Saline mount is preferred over iodine
 3. **Primary amoebic meningoencephalitis is caused by:**
    a. *Naegleria*   b. *Acanthamoeba*
    c. *Balamuthia*   d. *E. histolytica*

Answers
1. c   2. b   3. a

Intestinal and Genital Flagellates

CHAPTER 49

CHAPTER PREVIEW
- *Giardia lamblia*
- *Trichomonas vaginalis*
- Other Intestinal Flagellates of Minor Importance

GIARDIA LAMBLIA

Giardia lamblia (also known as *G. intestinalis* or *G. duodenalis*) is an intestinal flagellate associated with diarrheal manifestations. It exists in two forms—trophozoite and cyst.
1. **Trophozoite:** It is the pathogenic form as well as the feeding and replicating form of the parasite found in the feces of patients with active disease. It bears flagella as the organ of locomotion.
2. **Cyst:** It is the diagnostic form of the parasite found in the feces of carriers as well as patients with active disease. It is also the infective form.

Life Cycle (Fig. 49.1)

Host: *Giardia* completes its life cycle in one host.

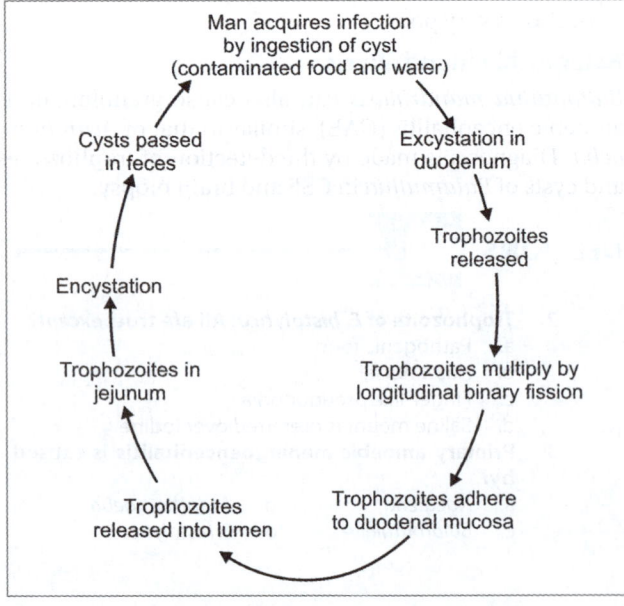

Fig. 49.1: Life cycle of *Giardia lamblia*.

Infective form: Cysts are the infective form.

Mode of transmission: Man acquires infection by ingestion of food and water contaminated with mature cysts.

Development in Man

- **Excystation:** Cysts following ingestion are carried to the duodenum, where they transform into trophozoites
- **Multiplication:** Trophozoites multiply by longitudinal binary fission in the duodenum
- **Adhesion:** Trophozoites adhere to the duodenal mucosa by the bilobed adhesive ventral disk. In active stage of the disease, the trophozoites are directly excreted in the diarrheic stool
- **Encystation:** Gradually when the trophozoites pass down to jejunum, undergo encystation to form the cysts. The cysts excreted in feces can survive in the environment and are infective to man.

Clinical Features

Most infected persons are **asymptomatic carriers**, harbor cysts in the gut, and spread the infection. The incubation period is 1–3 weeks.
- **Fatty diarrhea (steatorrhea)** is the typical presentation of giardiasis (due to the malabsorption of fat).
- **Other symptoms** include abdominal pain, bloating, belching, flatus and vomiting, and profound weight loss leading to growth retardation.

Laboratory Diagnosis

Stool Examination

Stool microscopy is considered as the gold standard for the diagnosis of giardiasis, which detects cysts and trophozoites.
- **Trophozoites** adhere firmly to the duodenal mucosa by adhesive disk leading to intermittent shedding. Hence, repeated stool examination (at least three samples collected on alternate days) should be done

❖ **Concentration techniques** like floatation or sedimentation methods are useful
❖ **Duodenal sampling:** If stool examination is negative, then direct duodenal samples like aspirates (obtained by entero-test; refer below for details) or biopsy (done by endoscopy) should be processed
❖ **Methods:** Saline and iodine mount examination is performed first to demonstrate cysts and trophozoites in the stool. Permanent stains such as trichrome stain can be used for better visualization of internal structure (refer to highlight box below).

> **Trophozoite (*Giardia lamblia*)**
> The presence of trophozoites indicates the active stage of the disease. They are better appreciated in the saline mount and permanent staining, but not in the iodine mount **(Figs. 49.2A and 49.3A).**
> ❑ **Measure** 10–20 μm in length and 5–15 μm in width.
> ❑ **Shape:** In the front view, it is pear-shaped (or teardrop or tennis racket-shaped) and laterally, it appears as a spoon or sickle-shaped **(Fig. 49.2B)**
> ❑ **Motility:** It has a falling leaf-like motility
> ❑ It is bilaterally symmetrical; bears the following structures:
>   ➢ One pair of nuclei
>   ➢ Adhesive or sucking disk (bilobed) at its ventral surface
>   ➢ Four pairs of flagella
>   ➢ Pair of axonemes (intracellular portion of flagella)
>
> **Cyst (*Giardia lamblia*)**
> *Giardia* cyst is oval-shaped, measures 11–14 μm in length and 7–10 μm in width **(Figs. 49.2C and 49.3B)**
> ❑ It contains four nuclei and axonemes
> ❑ Cysts cannot differentiate active disease from carriers, as they are passed in stool in both.

Enterotest (Fig 49.4)

It uses a gelatin capsule attached to a thread containing a weight **(Fig. 49.4)**.
❖ One end of the thread is attached to the outer aspect of the patient's cheek, and then, the capsule is swallowed. The capsule gets dissolved in the stomach releasing the thread which is carried to the duodenum, gets unfolded, and takes up the duodenal samples
❖ Four hours later, the thread is withdrawn and shaken in saline to release trophozoites which can be detected microscopically by wet mount or permanent stained smear.

Other Diagnostic Modalities

Other diagnostic modalities for giardiasis include:
❖ **Antigen detection in the stool (coproantigen):** Various test formats are available such as:
  ▪ **ELISA and direct-IF tests** can be performed to detect cyst wall protein antigen of *Giardia* in stool

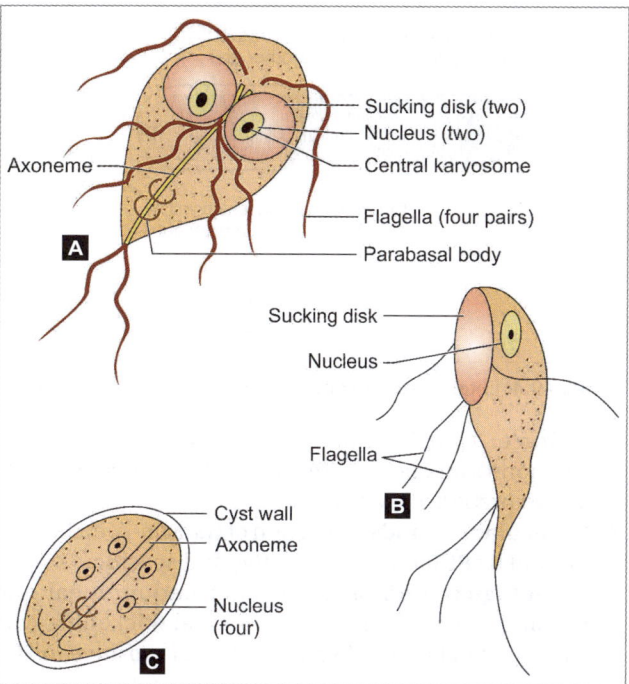

Figs. 49.2A to C: *Giardia lamblia* (schematic diagram): **A.** Trophozoite front view; **B.** Trophozoite lateral view; **C.** Cyst.

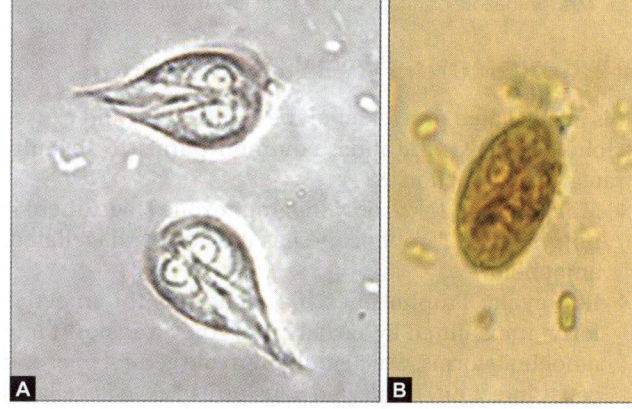

Figs. 49.3A and B: *Giardia lamblia*: **A.** Trophozoite (saline mount); **B.** Cyst (iodine mount).

  ▪ **Rapid ICT** (e.g. triage parasite panel): Detects *Giardia*, *E. histolytica*, and *Cryptosporidium*
❖ **Antibody detection:** Both indirect fluorescent antibody (IFA) and ELISA are developed to detect antibodies in the serum.
  ▪ But the presence of antibody cannot differentiate between recent and past infection
  ▪ Hence, serology is only used for the epidemiological purpose of estimating the prevalence of infection.

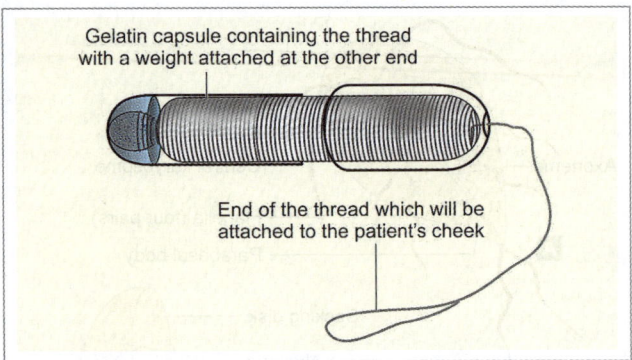

Fig. 49.4: Entero-test equipment showing duodenal capsule.

- ❖ **Culture:** *Giardia* can be cultivated in media like Diamond's media. Culture is done for research purposes and to prepare the antigens
- ❖ **Molecular methods:** Detection of *Giardia*-specific gene in stool by PCR is highly sensitive and specific
- ❖ **Radiological finding:** X-ray after barium meal may reveal non-specific irregular mucosal thickening with large dilated loops of hypotonic bowel (positive in 20% of cases).

> **TREATMENT** — Giardiasis
> - Tinidazole is the drug of choice
> - Metronidazole or nitazoxanide is given alternatively.

TRICHOMONAS VAGINALIS

It is a flagellated protozoan of the genital tract and causes trichomoniasis—the most common parasitic sexually transmitted infection (STI).

- ❖ **Morphology:** It has only the trophozoite stage; there is no cyst stage. Trophozoite has two forms: flagellated, amoeboid
- ❖ **Life cycle:** Trophozoites (flagellated) is the infective form, transmitted by sexual route. They transform into amoeboid forms, which multiply in the genital tract and cause infection. They again transform back to flagellated trophozoites that are discharged in vaginal/urethral secretions.
- ❖ **Clinical features:** In females, it causes **vulvovaginitis**, characterized by thin profuse foul-smelling purulent vaginal discharge.
  - Discharge may be frothy (10% of cases)
  - Strawberry appearance of vaginal mucosa **(Colpitis macularis)** is observed in 2% of patients due to small punctate hemorrhagic spots on vaginal and cervical mucosa
  - Other features: dysuria and lower abdominal pain
  - In males, it presents as nongonococcal urethritis.

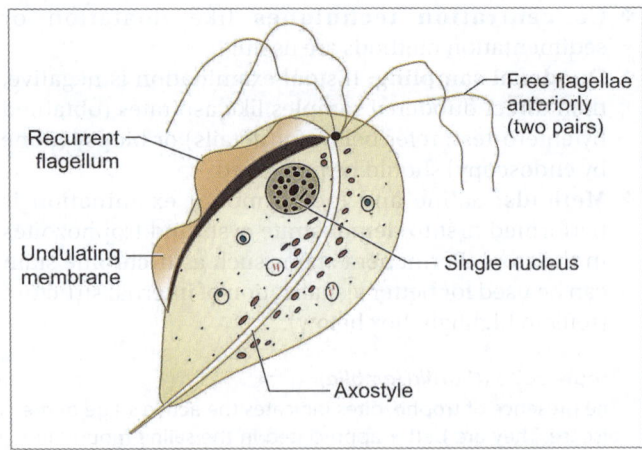

Fig. 49.5: Trophozoite (flagellated) of *Trichomonas vaginalis* (schematic diagram).

Laboratory Diagnosis

Wet (saline) mount of fresh vaginal discharge samples can demonstrate the jerky motile trophozoites and pus cells. Other staining methods include permanent stains (e.g. Giemsa), acridine orange stain, and direct fluorescent antibody test (DFA).

> **Trophozoite (*Trichomonas vaginalis*)**
> It is pear-shaped and measures 7–23 μm **(Fig. 49.5).**
> - It shows characteristic jerky or twitching motility in saline mount preparation
> - It bears five flagella—four anterior flagella and one recurrent flagellum, which traverses the parasite as an undulating membrane
> - It has a single nucleus and an axostyle (internal portion of the flagellum)
> - The cytoplasm contains a number of siderophore granules along the axostyle.

Other diagnostic modalities for trichomoniasis include:
- ❖ **Culture** using Lash's cysteine hydrolysate serum media.
- ❖ **Antigen detection** in vaginal secretion by rapid ICT and ELISA
- ❖ **Other supportive tests** include—(i) Positive whiff test (fishy odor is increased when a drop of 10% KOH is added to vaginal discharge due to the production of amine), (ii) raised vaginal pH (>4.5), and (iii) increased pus cells on wet mount examination.

> **TREATMENT** — Trichomoniasis
> - Metronidazole or tinidazole is the drug of choice
> - Both sexual partners must be treated simultaneously to prevent reinfection, especially the asymptomatic males.

OTHER INTESTINAL FLAGELLATES OF MINOR IMPORTANCE

Other intestinal flagellates of minor importance include—*Pentatrichomonas hominis, Trichomonas tenax, Chilomastix mesnili, Enteromonas hominis, Dientamoeba fragilis.*

- ❖ *Pentatrichomonas hominis*: It is a harmless commensal present in the large intestine of man. Trophozoite is pyriform shaped, similar to that of *T. vaginalis*
- ❖ *Trichomonas tenax*: It is a harmless commensal in the mouth. However, few cases of respiratory infection and thoracic abscesses are reported from patients with cancer or other underlying lung disease
- ❖ *Chilomastix mesnili*: It is a harmless commensal of caecum and colon in man. It has both trophozoite and cyst stages **(Figs. 49.6A and B)**.
    - ■ **Trophozoite:** It is pear-shaped. At the anterior end, there is a single nucleus and a distinct groove present near the nucleus called cytostome. It has four flagella and shows rotary movement
    - ■ **Cyst:** It is the infective stage. It is lemon-shaped, surrounded by a cyst wall. It has a single nucleus. It has a remnant of the curved cytostomal fibrils (called shepherd's crook).
- ❖ *Enteromonas hominis:* It is rarely found as commensal in the large intestine of man. It exists in two forms: trophozoite and cyst.
    - ■ **Trophozoite:** It is pear-shaped, smaller in size, and possesses four flagella. It shows jerky movement
    - ■ **Cyst**: It is the infective stage. It is oval shaped and possesses 1-4 nuclei.

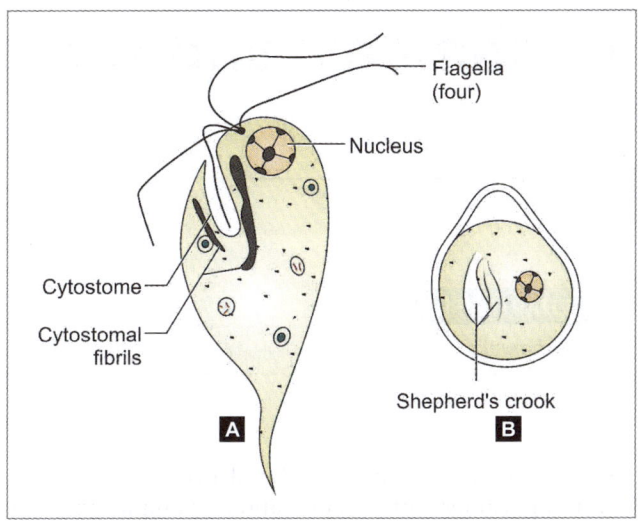

Figs. 49.6A and B: *Chilomastix mesnili* **(A and B)** trophozoite and cyst (schematic diagram).

- ❖ *Dientamoeba fragilis:* It is a common commensal in the large intestine of man.
    - ■ It is an amoebo-flagellate and flagellum is internal
    - ■ Trophozoite is the only stage found. It is amoeboid shaped; commonly having two nuclei (hence named *Dientamoeba*)
    - ■ The nuclear chromatin is usually fragmented (hence named *fragilis*)
    - ■ The organism has been reported in association with mucous diarrhea, abdominal pain and tenderness, nausea, vomiting, and low-grade fever.

EXPECTED QUESTIONS

I. **Write short notes on:**
  1. Laboratory diagnosis of giardiasis.
  2. Laboratory diagnosis of trichomoniasis.

II. **Multiple Choice Questions (MCQs):**
  1. **All are intestinal flagellates, *except*:**
      a. *Giardia*
      b. *Enteromonas*
      c. *Dientamoeba*
      d. *Trichomonas*
  2. **Enterotest is done for:**
      a. *Entamoeba histolytica*
      b. *Trichomonas vaginalis*
      c. *Enterobius vermicularis*
      d. *Giardia lamblia*

Answers
1. d   2. d

Hemoflagellates: Leishmania and Trypanosoma

CHAPTER 50

CHAPTER PREVIEW
- Leishmania
- Trypanosoma

Hemoflagellates are the flagellated protozoa that are found in peripheral blood circulation. Examples include *Leishmania* and *Trypanosoma*; both are transmitted by the bite of the insect vector.

LEISHMANIA

Leishmania is a flagellated protozoan that primarily affects the reticuloendothelial system of the host.
- **Vector:** It is transmitted by the bite of the female sandfly vector
- **Clinical forms:** Leishmaniasis presents in various clinical forms
    - *Visceral leishmaniasis* (VL) or kala-azar: It affects viscera such as spleen, liver, bone marrow, etc.
    - *PKDL* (post–kala-azar dermal leishmaniasis): It occurs a few months to years following VL
    - *Cutaneous forms:* Occurs in various forms such as cutaneous leishmaniasis (CL), diffuse cutaneous leishmaniasis (DCL), leishmaniasis recidivans (LR), and mucocutaneous leishmaniasis (MCL)
    - *Old and new world:* Depending upon the geographical distribution, leishmaniasis is classified into two groups (see highlight box).

> **Old World Leishmaniasis**
> It occurs in Asia, Africa, and less frequently in Europe; transmitted by sandfly of the genus *Phlebotomus*.
> - *L. donovani*: causes VL and PKDL
> - *L. infantum*: causes VL and PKDL
> - *L. tropica* complex: causes CL
>
> **New World Leishmaniasis**
> It occurs in Central and South America; transmitted by sandfly of the genus *Lutzomyia*.
> - *L. chagasi*: causes VL and CL
> - *L. mexicana* complex: causes CL
> - *L. braziliensis* complex: causes MCL and CL

Leishmania donovani

Leishmania donovani causes VL and also PKDL. It exists in two morphological forms **(Figs. 50.1A and B)**:
- **Amastigote:** It is the diagnostic form, found in man. It does not have a flagellum but has only the intracellular portion of the flagellum, called axoneme
- **Promastigote:** It is the infective stage to man, found in the insect vector. It possesses a single flagellum, arises anterior to the nucleus.

Epidemiology of VL

- **World:** VL has mainly been reported from three regions—(i) South-East Asia: India, Bangladesh, and Nepal; (ii) East Africa: Ethiopia, Sudan, and Kenya; (iii) Brazil
- **India:** India is one of the worst affected countries. Maximum cases were reported from Bihar, followed by Jharkhand.

Life Cycle (Fig. 50.2)

L. donovani completes its life cycle in two hosts—(i) man, and (ii) female sandfly (*Phlebotomus argentipes*).
- **Infective form:** Promastigote forms found in the alimentary canal of female sandfly serve as the infective form

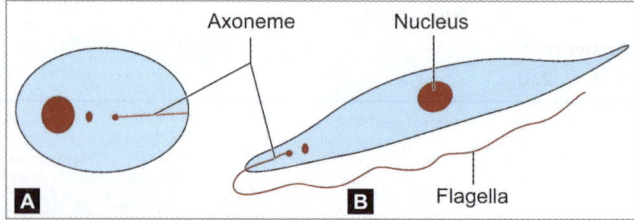

Figs. 50.1A and B: Various morphological forms of *Leishmania* (schematic diagrams): **A.** Amastigote; **B.** Promastigote.

CHAPTER 50 ◆ Hemoflagellates: Leishmania and Trypanosoma

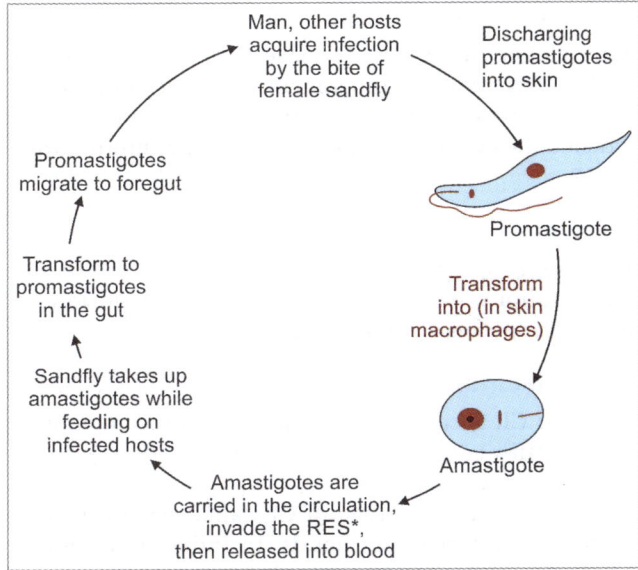

Fig. 50.2: Life cycle of *Leishmania donovani*.
*RES-Reticuloendothelial system.

- **Mode of transmission:** By the bite of an infected female sandfly, discharging the promastigotes (infective form) into the skin of a man
- **In humans:** Promastigotes are phagocytosed by the skin macrophages, where they transform into amastigote forms
    - The amastigote forms multiply inside the macrophages, causing cell rupture and are released into the circulation
    - Amastigotes are carried out in the circulation to various organs like liver, spleen, and bone marrow and invade the reticuloendothelial cells like macrophages, endothelial cells, etc.
- **In sandfly:** During the blood meal, the amastigotes are ingested and transformed into promastigote forms in the insect gut, which multiply and then migrate to their foregut. The cycle continues when this sandfly bites a new host.

Clinical Features

Visceral leishmaniasis (VL) is also called kala-azar (a Hindi term meaning 'black fever'). The incubation period ranges from 2 to 6 months. VL is characterized by:
- **Fever:** Abrupt in onset, moderate to high grade, associated with chills and rigors
- **Splenomegaly:** It is the most consistent sign. The spleen becomes enlarged and nontender **(Fig. 50.3A)**
- **Hepatomegaly** (nontender)
- **Lymphadenopathy:** Common in most of the African endemic regions (rare in the Indian subcontinent)
- **Hyperpigmentation** is observed on the face, hands, feet, and abdomen; hence the name kala-azar or black fever. This is a characteristic feature of Indian VL
- **Bone marrow dysfunction** leading to pancytopenia and hypergammaglobulinemia
- Nodular skin lesions (in African cases).

Post-kala-azar Dermal Leishmaniasis (PKDL)

PKDL is a nonulcerative lesion of the skin that occurs in 2–50% of patients of VL following treatment with antimonials. It is aggravated by exposure to sunlight.
- Mainly seen in India and East African countries
- It develops as hypopigmented macule near the mouth which spreads to the face, arms and trunk and finally becomes nodules resembling leprosy **(Fig. 50.3B)**.

Laboratory Diagnosis

Diagnosis of VL includes the following modalities.

Microscopy

Demonstration of amastigotes inside the macrophages (also known as **Leishman-Donovan bodies** or **LD bodies**) is the gold standard method for the diagnosis of VL **(Figs. 50.4A and B)**. Smears should be stained with Leishman, Giemsa, or Wright stains. The various samples include:
- Splenic aspiration: Most sensitive specimen, but less preferred because of the risk of splenic puncture
- Bone marrow aspiration: Most common specimen
- Lymph node aspiration: Useful in African patients
- Liver biopsy
- Peripheral blood from buffy coat area (after blood is centrifuged): particularly useful in HIV patients.

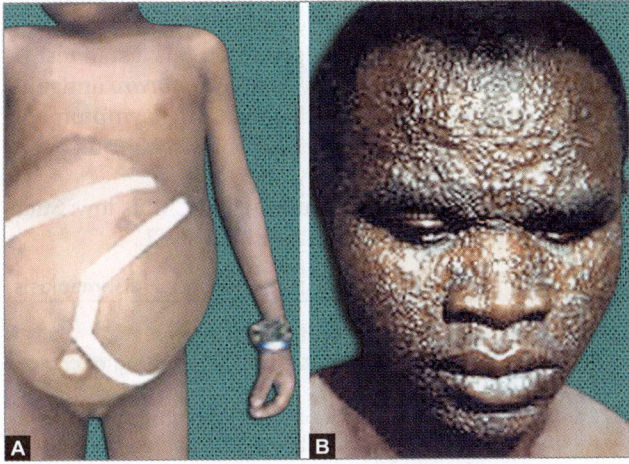

Figs. 50.3A and B: Leishmaniasis: **A.** Splenomegaly seen in visceral leishmaniasis; **B.** Extensive facial nodular lesions in PKDL.

Source: World Health Organization "Manual on visceral leishmaniasis control" Slide1/Desjeux; Slides 4 and 5/ El Hassan; Slide 6/ Bryceson (*with permission*).

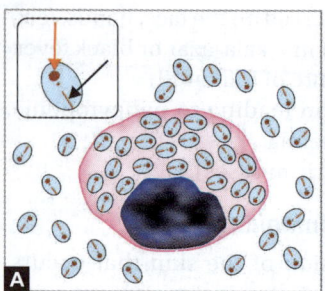
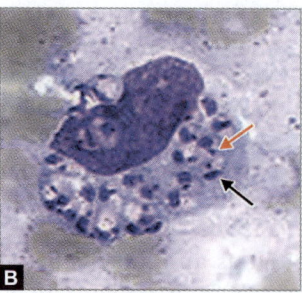

Figs. 50.4A and B: *L. donovani* amastigotes: showing a macrophage containing multiple *Leishmania* amastigotes: **A.** Schematic; **B.** In bone marrow smear stained with Giemsa. Note that each amastigote has a nucleus (red arrow) and a rod-shaped kinetoplast (black arrow).

Source: **B.** DPDx Image Library, Centers for Disease Control and Prevention (CDC), Atlanta (*with permission*).

Other Diagnostic Modalities

Other modalities for the diagnosis of VL include:
- **Culture:** Using media such as Novy-MacNeal-Nicolle (NNN) medium and Schneider's Drosophila insect medium. Amastigotes transform into **promastigotes** in the culture fluid which are detected by staining with Giemsa stain
- **Antibody detection in serum:** Sensitive, but less specific. Methods available are:
  - Direct agglutination test (DAT)
  - Others: ICT, ELISA, and indirect IF test.
- **Antigen detection:** A latex agglutination test has been available. It is more useful (i) in HIV-VL co-infection, (ii) as a prognostic marker, and (iii) in indicating active infection
- **Molecular methods:** Various formats such as PCR, nested PCR, and real-time PCR are available targeting specific kinetoplast (mitochondrial) DNA
- **Leishmanin test (Montenegro test):** It is a skin test to detect delayed hypersensitivity to *L. donovani* antigens
  - It is positive in people with good CMI: Asymptomatic individuals, cutaneous leishmaniasis, after recovery from VL
  - However, this test is negative when CMI is low: Such as in the case of active VL and diffuse CL.

TREATMENT — Visceral leishmaniasis

The various drugs used in the treatment of VL are:
- **Liposomal amphotericin B:** It is the current drug of choice for leishmaniasis
- **Pentavalent antimonials:** It has been the drug of choice in the past. However, currently, its use is restricted due to the emergence of resistance.
- **Others:** Miltefosine and paromomycin.

Prevention of VL

National Vector Borne Disease Control Programme (NVBDCP) is a national program in India that works for the control of six common vector-borne diseases in India. It has launched the **accelerated plan for kala-azar elimination** in 2017.

Cutaneous Leishmaniasis

Leishmania species can produce various cutaneous manifestations—associated with several old world and new world species of *Leishmania*.

Old World Cutaneous Leishmaniasis (CL)

Old world CL is caused by *Leishmania* tropica complex, which in turn comprises of three species—*L. tropica*, *L. aethiopica*, and *L. major*.
- *L. tropica* causes a type of CL called **oriental sore**, affecting the face and hands. In India, it is seen in Rajasthan. It is transmitted by *Phlebotomus sergenti*
- *L. aethiopica* causes diffuse cutaneous leishmaniasis. It is transmitted by *Phlebotomus longipes*.

New World Cutaneous Leishmaniasis

New World cutaneous leishmaniasis is mainly caused by:
- ***Leishmania mexicana* complex:** They cause a specific form of CL called as **chiclero ulcer**; characterized by persistent ulcerations in pinna
- ***Leishmania braziliensis* complex:** They cause mucocutaneous leishmaniasis (MCL), called **espundia**—ulcerative lesions on the nose and oral cavity
- ***Leishmania chagasi*:** It causes atypical CL and American VL.

Laboratory Diagnosis of CL

- **Microscopy:** Amastigotes can be demonstrated from punch biopsies taken from the edge of the active lesion and then stained with Giemsa
- **Culture:** Aspiration from the ulcers can be cultured in NNN (Novy, MacNeal, Nicolle) medium for the isolation of promastigote forms
- **Montenegro test:** Positive leishmanin skin test indicates delayed hypersensitivity reaction to the parasite. However, it is negative in diffuse CL.

TREATMENT — Cutaneous leishmaniasis

- **Old world CL:** Mainly treated by local therapy such as paromomycin ointment or intralesional antimonials
- **New world CL:** Systemic therapy is recommended, as the lesions are more chronic and multiple.

■ TRYPANOSOMA

Trypanosomes are hemoflagellates that reside in the peripheral blood and tissues of their host. They exist in two morphological forms—epimastigote and trypomastigote forms.

❖ In man, trypomastigotes are the diagnostic form
❖ In insect vectors, both epimastigotes and trypomastigotes are found, the latter being the infective stage to man.

Trypanosomes cause two distinct types of diseases in man.

1. **Chagas' disease:** It is caused by *Trypanosoma cruzi*, seen in America. It is transmitted by the vector reduviid bug.
   - **Various clinical stages** are as follows:
     ♦ **Early-stage disease:** It is characterized by a painful subcutaneous nodule (called chagoma) and unilateral painless edema of the eyelid (called Romana's sign).
     ♦ **Acute Chagas' disease:** About 1% of patients, progress to acute stage disease, characterized by fever, hepatosplenomegaly, and lymphadenopathy
     ♦ **Chronic Chagas' disease:** The parasite multiples in the muscles (cardiac and GIT) and nervous tissue to produce dilated cardiomyopathy, megaesophagus and megacolon.
   - **Laboratory diagnosis** is by:
     ♦ **Peripheral blood smear examination:** detecting characteristic 'C' shaped trypomastigote forms of *T. cruzi*, with a large, terminal kinetoplast, with the short blunt posterior end **(Fig. 50.5A)**
     ♦ **Other diagnostic modalities are:** Culture (blood) onto NNN medium, antibody detection, antigen detection, molecular methods, animal inoculation (mice), and xenodiagnoses.
   - **Treatment:** Benznidazole is considered as the drug of choice.

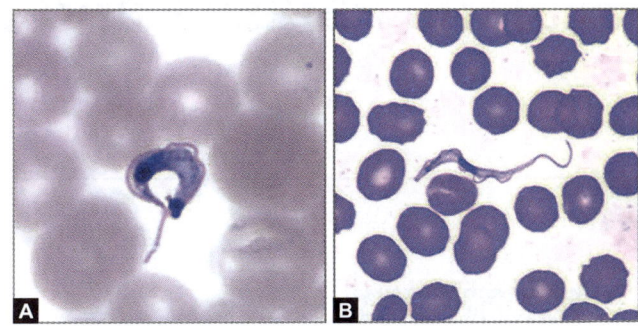

Figs. 50.5A and B: A. *Trypanosoma cruzi* (Trypomastigote form); **B.** Trypomastigote forms of *Trypanosoma brucei* in peripheral blood smear examination.

Source: **A** and **B.** DPDx Image Library, Centers for Disease Control and Prevention (CDC), Atlanta (*with permission*).

2. **African sleeping sickness:** It is caused by *Trypanosoma brucei* complex; transmitted by the vector tsetse fly. It produces progressive chronic meningoencephalitis with characteristic daytime somnolence (hence called as 'sleeping sickness'), with restlessness and insomnia at night.
   - **Clinical forms:** It occurs in two forms.
     ♦ West African sleeping sickness: It is caused by *T. brucei gambiense*
     ♦ East African sleeping sickness: It is caused by *T. brucei rhodesiense*.
   - **Laboratory diagnosis** is by:
     ♦ **Peripheral blood smear** examination: detecting characteristic elongated trypomastigote forms of *T. brucei*, having a flagellum with an undulating membrane **(Fig. 50.5B)**
     ♦ Other diagnostic modalities are same as described for *Trypanosoma cruzi*.
   - **Treatment:** Pentamidine and suramin are used for the treatment.

EXPECTED QUESTIONS

I. **Write short notes on:**
   1. Laboratory diagnosis of visceral leishmaniasis.
   2. Chagas' disease.

II. **Multiple Choice Questions (MCQs):**
   1. **Oriental sore is caused by:**
      a. *Leishmania donovani*
      b. *Leishmania mexicana*
      c. *Leishmania major*
      d. *Leishmania tropica*
   2. **African sleeping sickness is caused by:**
      a. *Leishmania donovani*
      b. *Trypanosoma cruzi*
      c. *Trypanosoma brucei*
      d. *Leishmania tropica*

Answers
1. d   2. c

Malaria Parasite and Babesia

CHAPTER 51

CHAPTER PREVIEW
- Plasmodium
- Babesia

PLASMODIUM (MALARIA PARASITE)

Malaria is a mosquito-borne febrile illness, caused by *Plasmodium*. Four different species usually infect man—*P. vivax, P. falciparum, P. malariae* and *P. ovale*.

Life Cycle (Fig. 51.1)

Host: *Plasmodium* completes its life cycle in two hosts: definitive host—female *Anopheles* mosquito (sexual cycle takes place) and intermediate host—man (asexual cycle takes place).

Transmission to Man and Infective Form

- Man acquires infection by the bite of a female *Anopheles* mosquito, transmitting the infective form—sporozoites present in its salivary gland
- Rarely, it can also be transmitted by blood transfusion or transplacental transmission—here, trophozoites (or merozoites) act as the infective form.

Human Cycle

In humans, the asexual cycle takes place through three stages: (1) pre-erythrocytic schizogony, (2) erythrocytic schizogony, and (3) gametogony.

Pre-erythrocytic schizogony: Sporozoites leave the circulation and infect the liver.
- **Trophozoites:** Inside the hepatocyte, the sporozoites transform into trophozoites
- **Schizonts:** The trophozoites multiply actively and subsequently undergo several nuclear divisions and transform into schizonts
- **Schizogony:** The schizonts undergo schizogony to release merozoites which initiate the erythrocytic cycle
- **Hypnozoites:** Some sporozoites of *P. vivax* and *P. ovale* do not develop further and may remain in the liver as hypnozoites and cause a **relapse** of malaria after many years.

Erythrocytic schizogony: Hepatic merozoites after entering into the bloodstream, infect the RBCs.
- Inside the RBCs, the hepatic merozoites transform into trophozoites
- The early trophozoites are ring-shaped (called ring forms) multiply actively and subsequently transform into late trophozoites and then into schizonts
- The schizonts undergo schizogony to release merozoites which either infect fresh RBCs to continue the erythrocytic cycle or transform into gametocytes.

Gametogony: When intended to leave the infected person, the merozoites transform into gametocytes.
- Gametocytes are of two types—male and female
- They are the sexual form; and also the infective form to the mosquito.

> **Relapse and recrudescence in malaria**
> - **Relapse:** Seen in *Plasmodium vivax* and *P. ovale* infections.
>   - Few sporozoites do not develop into schizont in the liver but remain dormant (known as **hypnozoites**) for few weeks to one year
>   - **Reactivation** of hypnozoites leads to initiation of the erythrocytic cycle and relapse of malaria
> - **Recrudescence:** Common in *P. falciparum* followed by *P. malariae*.
>   - In falciparum malaria—recrudescence is due to the persistence of drug-resistant parasites, even after the completion of treatment
>   - In *P. malariae* infection, long-term recrudescence is seen for as long as 60 years.

Mosquito Cycle

The gametocytes (male and female) are transmitted to the female *Anopheles* mosquito during the blood meal.
- **Gamete:** Inside the mosquito gut, each male gametocyte undergoes exflagellation and transforms into eight male gametes. Whereas the female gametocyte directly transforms into a single female gamete

CHAPTER 51 ◆ Malaria Parasite and Babesia

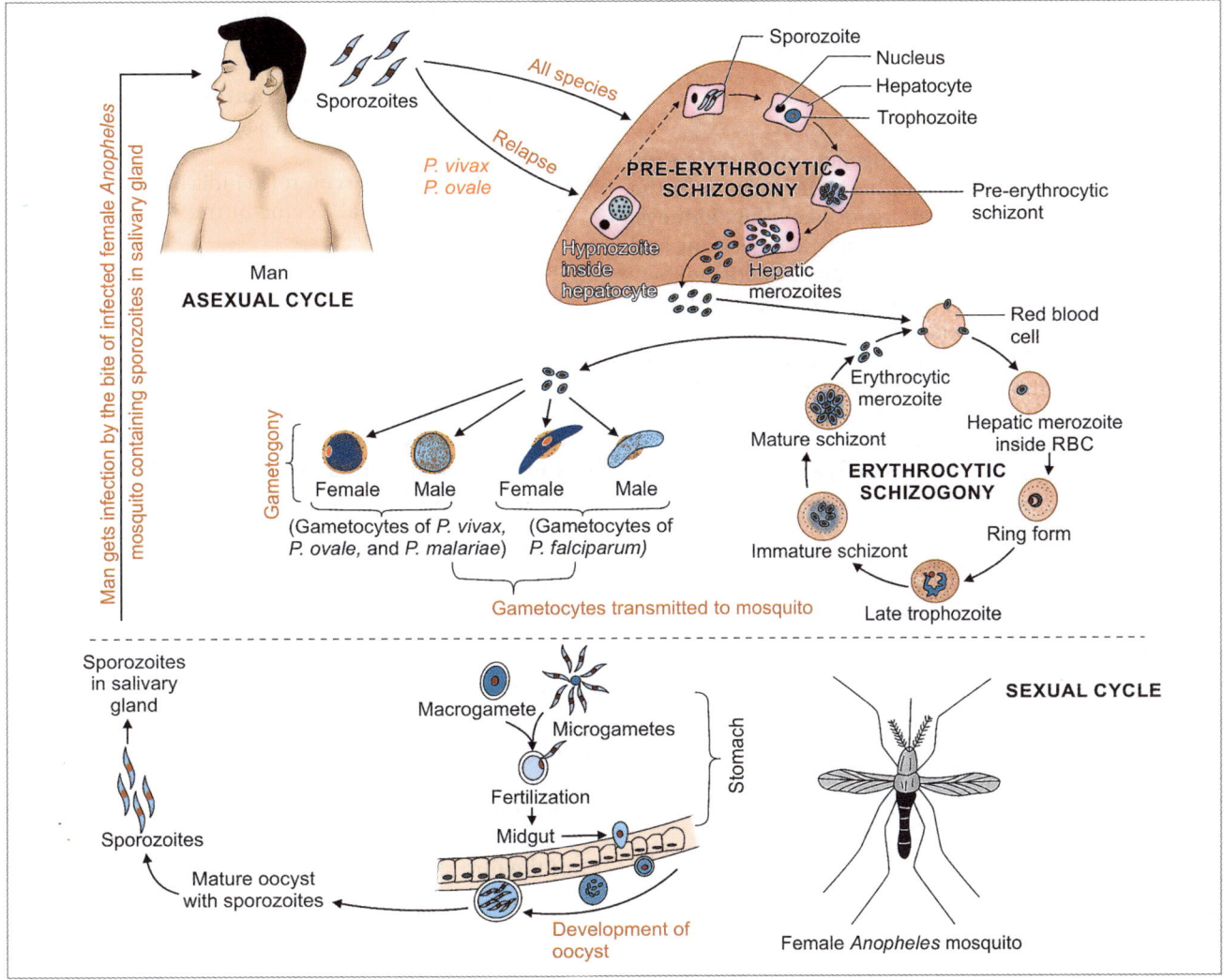

Fig. 51.1: Life cycle of the malaria parasite.

- ❖ **Fertilization:** The male gamete fertilizes with the female gamete to form a **zygote**, which subsequently transforms into a motile form called **ookinete**
- ❖ **Oocyst:** The ookinete penetrates the stomach wall of the mosquito, where it transforms into oocyst
- ❖ **Sporogony:** Each oocyst undergoes sporogony to produce four spindle-shaped sporozoites
- ❖ **Sporozoites:** On rupture of the mature oocyst, the sporozoites are released and migrate to the salivary gland of the mosquito and the cycle is repeated.

Pathogenesis and Clinical Feature

Benign Malaria

Benign malaria is milder in nature and can be caused by all four species. It is characterized by a triad of febrile paroxysm, anemia, and splenomegaly.

- ❖ **Febrile paroxysm:** Fever comes intermittently depending on the species
  - It occurs every fourth day (72-hour cycle for *P. malariae*) and every third day (48-hour cycle for other three species)
  - Paroxysm corresponds to the release of the successive broods of merozoites into the bloodstream, at the end of the RBC cycle.
- ❖ **Anemia:** Results from lysis of RBC due to release of merozoites
  - Anemia is severe in most cases of *P. falciparum* as it infects RBCs of all age groups
  - *P. vivax* and *P. ovale* infect the young RBCs and reticulocytes, whereas *P. malariae* infects the old RBCs.
- ❖ **Splenomegaly** is due to the massive proliferation of macrophages inside the spleen to remove the parasitized RBCs.

Falciparum Malaria (Malignant Tertian Malaria)

The pathogenesis of *P. falciparum* is different from other species.

Sequestration of the Parasites

An important feature of the pathogenesis of *P. falciparum* is its ability to sequester (holding back) the parasites in the blood vessels of deep visceral organs like brain, kidneys, etc. This leads to blockage of vessels, congestion, and hypoxia of internal organs. Sequestration is mediated by:
- **Cytoadherence:** It refers to the binding of infected erythrocytes to endothelial cells
- It is mediated by a specialized antigen called as *P. falciparum* erythrocyte membrane protein-1 **(PfEMP-1)**, which binds to specific receptors present on the vascular endothelium of deep organs
- Since the parasites are sequestrated back in deep vessels, they can avoid frequent spleen passage, and hence can escape splenic clearance.

Complications

Complications of Falciparum Malaria

P. falciparum infection is more acute and severe with more complications than benign malaria.
- **Cerebral malaria:** This is the most serious complication seen in falciparum malaria. It results due to the plugging of brain capillaries by the sequestered parasitized RBCs
- **Pernicious malaria:** It is characterized by blackwater fever, algid malaria, and septicemic malaria
- **Blackwater fever:** This syndrome is characterized by sudden intravascular hemolysis followed by fever, hemoglobinuria, and dark urine
- **Algid malaria:** Characterized by cold clammy skin, hypotension, peripheral circulatory failure, and profound shock
- **Others:** Pulmonary edema and adult respiratory distress syndrome, hypoglycemia, renal failure, bleeding/disseminated intravascular coagulation, severe jaundice, severe normochromic and normocytic anemia.

Chronic Complications of Malaria

Chronic complications of malaria are:
- Tropical splenomegaly syndrome
- Quartan malarial nephropathy: It is seen with *P. malariae*, characterized by nephrotic syndrome.
- Promotes Burkitt's lymphoma: Malaria-induced severe immunosuppression in African children provokes Epstein-Barr virus infection to develop Burkitt's lymphoma.

Epidemiology of Malaria

Malaria is the most lethal parasitic disease of humans.

- ***P. falciparum*** is the most common species worldwide; accounting for 99.7% of malaria cases in Africa, 50% in Southeast Asia including India
- In India, **Eastern Indian states** such as Odisha, Chhattisgarh, and Jharkhand account for the maximum cases
- **NVBDCP:** The malaria control in India has been operated through the National Vector-borne Disease Control Programme (NVBDCP)
- The national framework for malaria elimination (NFME) has been in operation in India with the vision of malaria elimination by 2030.

Laboratory Diagnosis

The diagnostic tests for malaria can be divided into:
- **Microscopic test:** Peripheral blood smear and QBC
- **Non-microscopic tests:** Rapid diagnostic test (antigen detection) and molecular test.

Peripheral Blood Smear Examination

Peripheral smear study still remains the simple and gold standard confirmatory test for detection of malarial parasites.

Types of Peripheral Blood Smear

It is of two types—(1) Thin and (2) Thick smears. Both the smears are made at the same time from capillary blood either on the same or different slides **(Fig. 51.2)**.
- **For thick smear**, a big drop of blood is spread over 1–2 cm square area on a clean glass slide. The thickness of the film should be such that it allows newsprint to be read
- **For thin smear**, a small drop of blood is taken on a corner of a slide. It is spread by another spreader slide at an angle

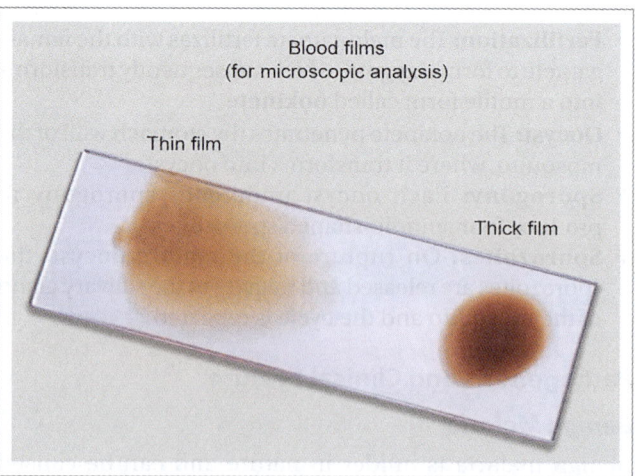

Fig. 51.2: Glass slide showing thin and thick blood smear.

of 45° and then is lowered to an angle of 30° and is pushed gently to the left, till the blood is exhausted
- ❖ The **surface of a good thin** film is: (i) even and uniform, (ii) consists of a single layer of RBCs, (iii) forms a "feathery tail end" near the center of the slide, and (iv) margins of the film do not touch the sides of the slide
- ❖ **Stains:** They are stained with one of the Romanowsky stains such as Leishman's, Giemsa and Field's, Wright's, or JSB (Jaswant Singh and Bhattacharya) stain
- ❖ **Examination:** Both the smears are examined under oil immersion objective (100x). The thin smear is screened near the feathery tail end. At least 200–300 oil immersion fields should be examined before the smears are considered as negative
- ❖ **Advantages:** Peripheral smear is simple, rapid, and cheap
    - ▪ A thick smear is useful in— (1) Detecting the parasites: It is 40 times more sensitive than a thin smear; (2) Quantification of parasitemia; (3) Demonstrating the malaria pigments
    - ▪ A thin smear is useful in the speciation of malaria parasites (see the highlight box).
- ❖ **Disadvantages:** It is labor-intensive and requires an experienced microscopist.

Speciation of Malaria Parasites

The speciation by thin smear is based on the detection of the ring forms, schizonts, gametocytes, type of pigments produced, and RBC size **(Fig. 51.3)**.
- ❏ **Parasitized RBC size:** Differ among species
    - ➤ Normal in size and shape for *P. falciparum* and *P. malariae*
    - ➤ Enlarged in size for *P. vivax*, whereas
    - ➤ Enlarged with fimbriated margin: for *P. ovale*

Contd...

Contd...

- ❏ **Ring forms:** It is the most important form that helps in accurate speciation. It comprises of a vacuole in the center, a peripheral thin rim of blue cytoplasm, surrounding the red nucleus.
    - ➤ *P. vivax*: Rings occupies 1/3rd of the RBC size **(Fig. 51.4A)**.
    - ➤ *P. falciparum*: Rings are smaller (occupy 1/6th of the RBC size) and occur in three forms **(Fig. 51.5A)**:
        - ♦ Multiple ring forms (inside the same RBC)
        - ♦ Accole form: Ring form attached to RBC membrane
        - ♦ Double dot/headphone shaped ring form: Ring form with a fragmented nucleus
    - ➤ *P. ovale*: Ring forms are similar to that of *P. vivax*, but present inside oval-shaped RBC **(Fig. 51.3)**.
    - ➤ *P. malariae*: Early trophozoite is similar to that of *P. vivax*, but late trophozoite is band-shaped (called band forms) **(Fig. 51.3)**.
- ❏ **Schizonts:** Speciation is made based on the number of merozoites present per schizont. Schizonts are not seen in the peripheral smear for *P. falciparum*
- ❏ **Gametocytes:** In *P. falciparum*, the gametocyte is crescentic or banana-shaped and larger than RBCs, whereas, for other species, it is spherical and almost occupies the RBC **(Figs. 51.4B and 51.5B)**.

Note: In falciparum malaria, only the gametocytes and ring forms are demonstrated in peripheral blood but not schizonts and late trophozoites (as the later stages of the erythrocytic cycle occur in deep vessels, not in peripheral blood).

Quantitative Buffy Coat Examination

The quantitative buffy coat (QBC) is an advanced microscopic technique for malaria diagnosis.
It consists of following basic steps:
- ❖ **Procedure:** Blood is collected in a capillary tube coated internally with acridine orange **(Fig. 51.6A)** and then centrifuged. The capillary tube is then examined at the buffy coat region under an ultraviolet (UV) light source **(Figs. 51.6B and C)**
- ❖ **Interpretation:** Parasitized RBCs appear as brilliant green dots **(Figs. 51.6C)**
- ❖ **Advantage:** QBC is faster, more sensitive and quantification is possible
- ❖ **Disadvantage:** It is expensive, less specific and speciation is difficult.

Rapid Diagnostic Tests

Rapid diagnostic tests (RDTs) have revolutionized the diagnosis of malaria.
- ❖ **Principle:** Malaria RDT kits are based on the principle of immunochromatographic test (ICT)
- ❖ **Antigens:** Malaria RDT kits are designed to detect several antigens of *Plasmodium* species such as:
    - ▪ Lactate dehydrogenase (LDH) and aldolase: Produced by all *Plasmodium* species

Plasmodium	P. vivax	P. falciparum	P. malariae	P. ovale
Early trophozoite	Nucleus, Vacuole, Cytoplasm, Ring	Accole form, Double dot ring form, Multiple ring form		
Late trophozoite		Not seen in peripheral blood	Band form	
Schizont		Not seen in peripheral blood		
Gametocyte				

Fig. 51.3: Morphological forms of malaria parasites seen in the peripheral smear.

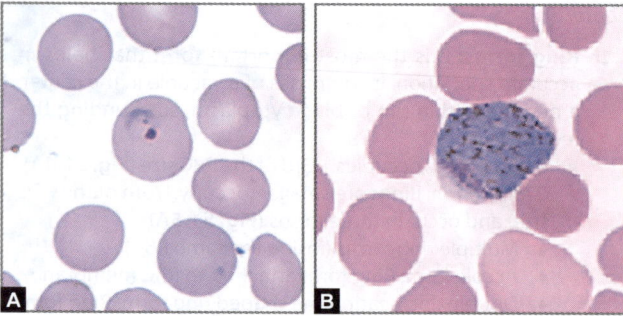

Figs. 51.4A and B: Thin blood smear *Plasmodium vivax*: **A.** Ring form; **B.** Gametocyte.

Source: DPDx Image Library, Centers for Disease Control and Prevention (CDC), Atlanta (*with permission*).

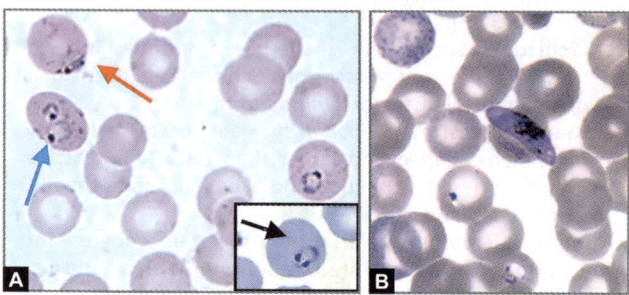

Figs. 51.5A and B: Thin blood smear *Plasmodium falciparum*: **A.** Ring forms such as multiple rings (blue arrow), accole form (red arrow), and head phone-shaped ring form (black arrow); **B.** Banana-shaped gametocyte.

Source: DPDx Image Library, Centers for Disease Control and Prevention (CDC), Atlanta (*with permission*).

- Histidine rich protein-2 (HRP-II): It is produced only by *P. falciparum*.
❖ **Advantages:** RDTs are simple to perform, and do not need extra equipment or trained microscopist
❖ **Disadvantages:** RDTs cannot differentiate between the non-falciparum malaria species. The sensitivity of RDTs is low compared to microscopy.

Molecular Methods

Various molecular tests have recently gained attention for malaria diagnosis.
❖ Nested multiplex PCR targeting 18S rDNA has been developed for speciation of malaria parasite
❖ PCR can also be used to detect drug-resistant genes
❖ Real-time PCR is useful for quantification.

Other Nonspecific Tests

Other nonspecific tests include:
❖ Normochromic and normocytic hemolytic anemia
❖ Leukopenia
❖ Raised erythrocyte sedimentation rate (ESR)

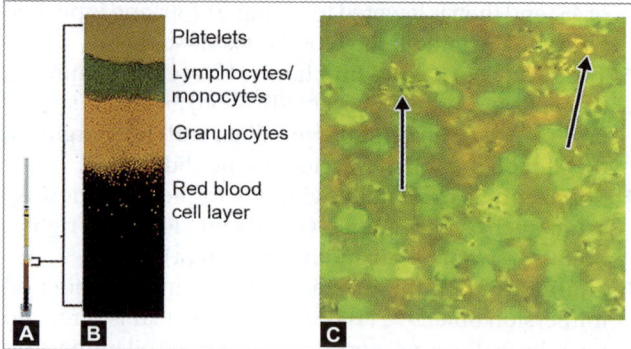

Figs. 51.6A to C: A. QBC capillary tube; **B.** Magnified view of QBC capillary tube after centrifugation; **C.** Crescent-shaped gametocyte of *Plasmodium falciparum*.

Source: **C.** Department of Microbiology, Sri Siddhartha Medical College, Tumkur, Karnataka (*with permission*).

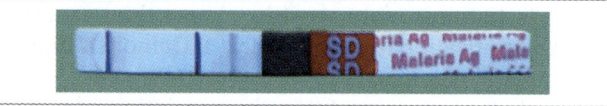

Fig. 51.7: Rapid diagnostic test kit positive for *Plasmodium falciparum*.

Source: Department of Microbiology, Sri Siddhartha Medical College, Tumkur, Karnataka (*with permission*).

❖ Hypoglycemia
❖ Severe falciparum malaria is also associated with high levels of lactate, creatinine, muscle and liver enzymes, and conjugated and unconjugated bilirubin
❖ **Human lysozyme** is a potential biomarker for detection of severity of malaria.

> **TREATMENT** — Malaria
>
> The treatment regimen given for malaria is as per guidelines provided by NVBDCP, India.
> **Vivax malaria:** Chloroquine (for three days) plus primaquine (for 14 days) is the regimen recommended
> **Falciparum malaria:** State-specific regimens are recommended
> ❑ **Northeast states:** Artemether-lumefantrine (for 3 days) plus primaquine (single dose) is given
> ❑ **Other states:** Artesunate for 3 days plus sulfadoxine-pyrimethamine (single dose, on 1st day) plus primaquine (single dose, on the second day)
> **Severe malaria:** The drug of choice includes IV artemisinin derivatives (such as artesunate, artemether, arteether) or IV quinine
> **Chloroquine resistance** in *P. falciparum* has been reported in India, especially from the northeast states.

Prophylaxis against Malaria

Prophylaxis against malaria includes chemoprophylaxis, vector control strategies, and vaccine prophylaxis.

- ❖ **Chemoprophylaxis:** It is recommended for travelers going to highly endemic areas of malaria. Agents such as doxycycline or mefloquine are recommended
- ❖ **Vector control strategies:** Include spraying with insecticides like malathion, environmental sanitation, and improvement of the drainage system
- ❖ **Vaccination:** RTS, S/AS01 is the only vaccine candidate that has been approved by WHO, for use in children living in regions with moderate to high transmission (e.g. sub-Saharan Africa).

BABESIA

Babesia is another protozoan infecting the bloodstream, similar to the malaria parasite. **Hard tick** is the definitive host.
- ❖ **Mode of transmission:** Man acquires infection by the bite of ticks where the sporozoites enter through the site of bite and are discharged into circulation.
- ❖ **Clinical features** are similar to malaria, except that it is less severe, with no cerebral involvement

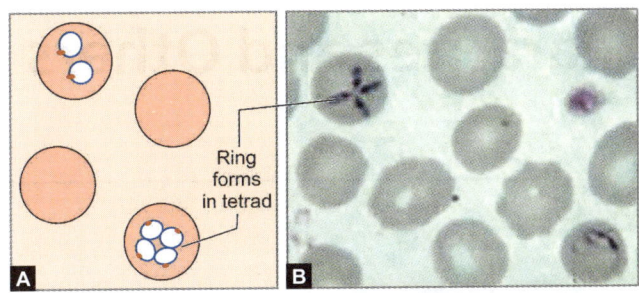

Figs. 51.8A and B: Giemsa stained blood smear showing Maltese cross form: **A.** Schematic diagram; **B.** Peripheral blood smear.
Source: **B.** DPDx Image Library, Centers for Disease Control and Prevention (CDC), Atlanta (*with permission*).

- ❖ **Diagnosis:** Peripheral blood smear examination reveals two or four rings of 1–5 μm size inside the RBCs (called as **Maltese cross forms**); characteristic feature seen in babesiosis (**Figs. 51.8A and B**)
- ❖ **Treatment:** Atovaquone plus azithromycin is given for treatment.

EXPECTED QUESTIONS

I. Write an essay on:
1. Discuss the pathogenesis and laboratory diagnosis of falciparum malaria.

II. Write short notes on:
1. The life cycle of malaria parasite.
2. Laboratory diagnosis of vivax malaria.

III. Multiple Choice Questions (MCQs):
1. Cerebral malaria is caused by:
    a. *Plasmodium falciparum*
    b. *Plasmodium vivax*
    c. *Plasmodium ovale*
    d. *Plasmodium malariae*
2. Banana-shaped gametocyte is seen for:
    a. *Plasmodium vivax*
    b. *Plasmodium falciparum*
    c. *Plasmodium ovale*
    d. *Plasmodium malariae*
3. Which of the laboratory diagnostic test is best for the speciation of malaria parasites?
    a. Thick smear examination
    b. Thin smear examination
    c. Rapid diagnostic tests
    d. QBC
4. Schizonts in peripheral blood can be seen in all, *except*:
    a. *Plasmodium vivax*
    b. *Plasmodium falciparum*
    c. *Plasmodium ovale*
    d. *Plasmodium malariae*
5. Band forms are seen for:
    a. *Plasmodium vivax*
    b. *Plasmodium falciparum*
    c. *Plasmodium ovale*
    d. *Plasmodium malariae*

Answers
1. a   2. b   3. b   4. b   5. d

Opportunistic Coccidian Parasites and Others

CHAPTER 52

CHAPTER PREVIEW
- **Opportunistic coccidian parasites**
  - Toxoplasma gondii
  - Cryptosporidium parvum
- Cyclospora cayetanensis
- Cystoisospora belli
- **Others**
  - Balantidium coli
  - Blastocystis hominis

Coccidian parasites can cause opportunistic infections in HIV-infected patients. They can be grouped into:
- ❖ *Toxoplasma gondii:* It can cause encephalitis in HIV infected patients and can also infect fetus to cause congenital infection
- ❖ **Intestinal coccidian parasites:** *Cryptosporidium, Cyclospora,* and *Cystoisospora*: They produce profuse watery diarrhea in HIV-infected patients.

■ TOXOPLASMA GONDII

Toxoplasma gondii is an obligate intracellular parasite affecting a wide range of mammals and birds including humans.
- ❖ **Disease:** Though human infection is common; very few progress to disease, mostly restricted to immunocompromised persons such as with HIV/AIDS (developing encephalitis) and congenital infection in the fetus.
- ❖ **Morphology:** It exists in three morphological forms—two asexual forms (tachyzoite and tissue cyst) and one sexual form (oocyst, containing four sporozoites).

Life Cycle (Fig. 52.1)

Host: The life cycle involves two hosts:
1. **Definitive hosts** are cats and other felines; where the sexual cycle takes place
2. **Intermediate hosts** are man and other mammals (e.g. rodents); where the asexual cycle takes place.

Human (Asexual) Cycle

- ❖ **Transmission:** *T. gondii* is unique among the protozoa as all the three morphological forms can transmit the infection. Transmission to man occurs (in the decreasing order of frequency):
  - ■ Ingestion of tissue cyst from undercooked meat (most common route)
  - ■ Ingestion of sporulated oocysts from contaminated soil, food, or water
  - ■ By blood transfusion, organ transplantation, or mother-to-fetus: Tachyzoites are the infective form
- ❖ **Transform into tachyzoites:** In the intestine, sporozoites are released from sporulated oocyst, and bradyzoites are released from the tissue cyst. They invade the intestinal epithelium and transform into tachyzoites
- ❖ **Transform into tissue cyst:** Tachyzoites multiply actively in blood and spread to extraintestinal organs like brain, muscles, eye, liver, etc. where they transform

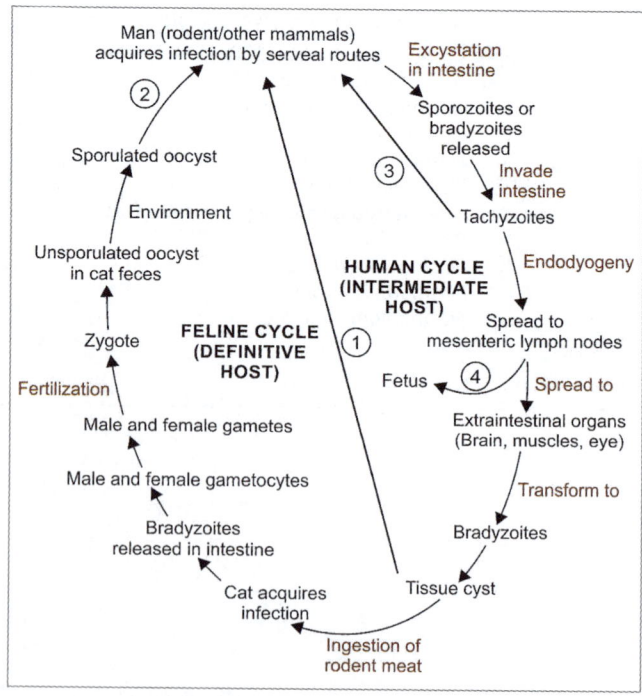

Fig. 52.1: Life cycle of *Toxoplasma gondii*.

into bradyzoites which subsequently encysted to form tissue cysts.

Sexual Cycle (The Feline Cycle)

Cat and other felines (definitive host) acquire infection by ingestion of tissue cysts present in the rodent meat.
- ❖ Bradyzoites are released from the tissue cysts in the intestine, which transform into gametocytes and then into gametes
- ❖ The male and female gametes then fertilize to form zygotes, which subsequently transform into oocysts that are excreted in the cat's feces
- ❖ Freshly passed oocysts become sporulated in a humid environment and become infectious to man.

Clinical Manifestations

The clinical manifestations of toxoplasmosis can vary depending upon the patient population affected.
- ❖ **Immunocompetent host:** The infection usually remains asymptomatic and self-limited. Rarely progresses to acute toxoplasmosis, characterized by lymphadenopathy (e.g. cervical)
- ❖ **Immunocompromised hosts** such as patients infected with HIV, transplant recipients, and malignancies, the clinical manifestations are more severe due to the lack of the immune system to control the infection. Encephalitis is the most common presentation
- ❖ **Congenital toxoplasmosis:** Mother-to-fetus transmission of *T. gondii* can occur at any time during pregnancy, maximum being in the third trimester. However, the risk of fetal damage is maximum in the first trimester, producing various congenital malformations such as chorioretinitis, hydrocephalus, and intracranial calcifications, etc.

Laboratory Diagnosis

Direct Microscopy

The specimens such as peripheral blood, bone marrow aspirate, and biopsy material from muscle and brain, etc. are stained with Giemsa, hematoxylin and eosin stain, and Periodic acid–Schiff (PAS).
- ❖ **Comma-shaped tachyzoites** are detected in the smear made from blood, body fluids, and tissue; their presence indicates acute infection **(Fig. 52.2A)**
- ❖ Tissue cysts containing strongly PAS-positive **bradyzoites** can be detected in various tissues like the brain or muscle **(Fig. 52.2B)**. This denotes the presence of infection but cannot differentiate between acute and chronic infection.

Antibody Detection

Antibody detection is useful in immunocompetent individuals. In immunocompromised patients, antibodies

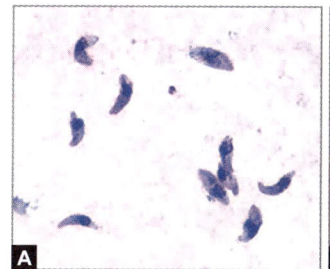 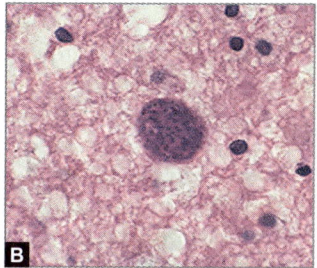

Figs. 52.2A and B: *Toxoplasma gondii*: **A.** Giemsa stain showing comma-shaped tachyzoites in the blood smear; **B.** Tissue cyst containing bradyzoites (section of the brain).
Source: **A and B**. DPDx Image Library; Centers for Disease Control and Prevention (CDC), Atlanta (*with permission*).

are produced at a very low level and therefore are not useful. Various methods available are—
- ❖ **Capture ELISA:** It can detect specific antibodies such as IgM, IgG, and IgA.
  - ■ Acute toxoplasmosis can be diagnosed by the presence of IgM or a four-fold rise of IgG
  - ■ In congenital toxoplasmosis, detection of IgM or IgA is useful for diagnosis
- ❖ **ISGA:** Immunosorbent agglutination assay
- ❖ **Sabin-Feldman Dye test:** It is the gold standard antibody detection method. But its use is limited to only the reference laboratories, because of its cumbersome procedure and inability to differentiate between IgM and IgG.

Molecular Diagnosis

Polymerase chain reaction (PCR) can be employed to detect *Toxoplasma*-specific DNA from various clinical samples like blood, CSF, or amniotic fluid.

Other Methods

- ❖ **Animal inoculation:** *T. gondii* can be isolated from mice by intraperitoneal inoculation of the clinical samples
- ❖ **Tissue culture:** *T. gondii* can be isolated by inoculating into cell lines such as HeLa and Vero cell lines
- ❖ **Imaging methods:** CT or MRI scan of the brain can be done to demonstrate lesions in encephalitis patients.

> **TREATMENT** — Toxoplasmosis
>
> **Immunocompetent patients** with only lymphadenopathy do not require any treatment
> **AIDS patients** with *Toxoplasma* infection: Treatment is essential, as it may progress to encephalitis.
> ❑ Cotrimoxazole is the drug of choice
> ❑ Indication: Patients with CD4 T cell <100/µL should receive cotrimoxazole prophylaxis to prevent encephalitis
> **Neonates with congenital toxoplasmosis** are treated with daily oral pyrimethamine and sulfadiazine with folinic acid.

Prevention

The various methods recommended to prevent toxoplasmosis include:
- Consumption of thoroughly cooked meat
- Proper hygiene maintenance and hand cleaning of people handling cats and other felines
- Regular prenatal and antenatal screening to detect *Toxoplasma* infection in women of childbearing age
- Screening of blood banks or organ donors for antibodies to *T. gondii*.

INTESTINAL COCCIDIAN PARASITES

The intestinal coccidian parasites can cause opportunistic infections in HIV-infected patients producing profuse watery diarrhea.
- *Cryptosporidium*: *C. parvum* is zoonotic, common in rural areas, whereas *C. hominis* is mainly a human parasite, more commonly seen in an urban setting
- *Cyclospora cayetanensis*: Usually infects humans, zoonotic potential is uncertain
- *Cystoisospora belli*: Humans are the only host.

Morphology (Oocyst)

Intestinal coccidian parasites exist in various morphological forms, out of which **oocysts** are the most important form, as they are the infective form as well as the diagnostic form.
- They are acid-fast, round to oval, surrounded by a cyst wall, and bear sporozoites
- They are extremely resistant to routine chlorination, heat, and other disinfectants
- In *Cryptosporidium*, two types of oocysts are demonstrated—(1) thick-walled, and (2) thin-walled; whereas *Cyclospora* and *Cystoisospora* have only one type of oocyst (i.e. thick-walled) (**Figs. 52.3A to C**).

Life Cycle

The life cycle of *Cryptosporidium* is discussed first. It completes its life cycle in a single host (man or animal).
- **Infective stage:** Sporulated oocysts (both thick-walled and thin-walled) are the infective form of the parasite

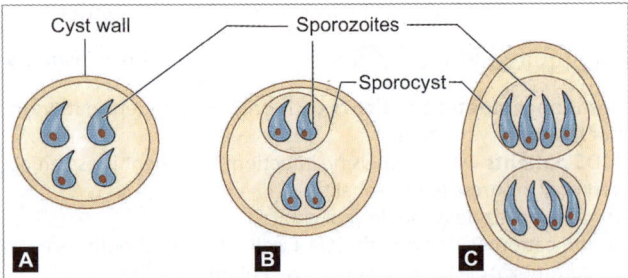

Figs. 52.3A to C: Sporulated oocysts (schematic diagram) of **A.** *Cryptosporidium*; **B.** *Cyclospora*; **C.** *Cystoisospora*.

- **Mode of Transmission:** Man acquires infection by:
  - *Ingestion* of food and water contaminated with feces containing thick-walled oocysts
  - *By autoinfection:* Thin-walled oocysts can infect the same host through contaminated fingers.
- **Development in man:** In the intestine, *Cryptosporidium* passes through a series of morphological forms in sequential order:

> Sporulated oocysts undergo excystation in the small intestine to form sporozoites → invade the small intestine and differentiate into trophozoites → schizonts (meronts) → merozoites → zygote → unsporulated oocyst (thin-walled and thick-walled) → undergoes sporulation to form a sporulated oocyst

- Sporulated oocysts are excreted in the feces; which are now infective to the same person (thin-walled) and other individuals (thick-walled).

The life cycle of *Cyclospora* and *Cystoisospora* are similar to *Cryptosporidium*, with the following differences (**Table 52.1**).
- Autoinfection is not observed
- The oocysts released in the human feces are unsporulated

Table 52.1: Differences between *Cryptosporidium*, *Cyclospora* and *Cystoisospora*.

Property	*Cryptosporidium*	*Cyclospora*	*Cystoisospora*
Infective form	Sporulated oocyst	Sporulated oocyst	Sporulated oocyst
Diagnostic form	Sporulated oocyst	Unsporulated oocyst	Unsporulated oocyst
Outbreaks	Frequent, large	Common, large	Occasional, small
Zoonotic potential	Yes	Uncertain	No
Oocyst size	4–6 µm	8–10 µm	20–33 µm
Oocyst shape	Round	Round	Oval
Sporulated oocyst contains	Four sporozoites	Two sporocysts, each having two sporozoites	Two sporocysts, each having four sporozoites
Acid-fastness	Uniformly acid-fast	Variably acid-fast	Uniformly acid-fast
Autofluorescence	No, but can be stained with fluorescent dye	Autofluorescence ++	Autofluorescence +/−
Sporulation of the oocyst	Occurs inside the host cells (enterocytes)	Occurs in soil (environment)	Occurs in soil (environment)
Treatment	Nitazoxanide	Cotrimoxazole	Cotrimoxazole

❖ The sporulation of oocyst takes place in the soil (environment); whereas, in *Cryptosporidium*, the sporulation of oocyst takes place in the human intestine.

Clinical Features

In immunocompetent hosts: The majority of infections remain asymptomatic. Some individuals develop self-limiting diarrhea.

In immunocompromised hosts (e.g. AIDS): They produce **chronic, persistent profuse diarrhea**, leading to significant fluid and electrolyte loss, and weight loss (resembling cholera).
- ❖ **Extraintestinal manifestations** are common such as biliary tract infection (sclerosing cholangitis), respiratory tract infection, and pancreatitis
- ❖ The disease is more severe in *Cryptosporidium* than in *Cyclospora* and *Cystoisospora,* which is attributed to auto-infection seen in the former—a key factor for maintaining the infection, resulting in chronic persistent diarrhea.

Laboratory Diagnosis

Direct Microscopy (Stool Examination)

Stool microscopy remains the most common method employed for diagnosis, to demonstrate the diagnostic form—oocyst.
- ❖ Based on the oocyst morphology, the coccidian parasites can be differentiated (refer to highlight box given below)
- ❖ **Methods:** Various methods employed are direct wet mount, acid-fast staining, direct fluorescent antibody staining, and epifluorescence microscopy (to demonstrate autofluorescence), and phase contrast microscopy
- ❖ **Stool concentration techniques** like Sheather's sugar floatation technique may be performed before stool microscopy, to improve the chance of detection.

Oocyst

The oocysts of intestinal coccidian parasites are highly refractile, double-walled, and acid-fast.
- ❑ *Cryptosporidium:* The oocyst is round, measures 4–6 μm in size, and contains four sporozoites **(Figs. 52.3A and 52.4A)**
- ❑ *Cyclospora:* The oocyst is round, measures 8–10 μm size, contains two sporocysts, each comprising two sporozoites **(Figs. 52.3B)**
    - ➢ The oocysts are variably acid fast (i.e. 50% of oocysts are acid-fast and the rest are nonacid fast) **(Figs. 52.4B and C)**
    - ➢ Oocysts also exhibit autofluorescence
- ❑ *Cystoisospora:* The oocyst is oval and larger, measuring 20–33 μm length; contains two sporocysts, each comprising four sporozoites **(Figs. 52.3C, 52.4D)**.

Antigen Detection from Stool

It is available for cryptosporidiosis.
- ❖ **ELISA** has been developed to detect *C. parvum*-specific coproantigen (oocyst antigen) from stool
- ❖ **ICT** is also available, e.g. Triage parasite panel for simultaneous detection of antigens of *Cryptosporidium, Giardia,* and *E. histolytica.*

Antibody Detection

Methods such as ELISA are available to detect antibodies in the patient's serum against oocyst antigens of *Cryptosporidium* or *Cyclospora*. This is useful for epidemiological purpose.

Molecular Diagnosis

Molecular methods such as PCR or real-time PCR can be performed to detect specific genes. They are more sensitive, take less time, and can differentiate *Cryptosporidium, Cyclospora,* and *Cystoisospora.*

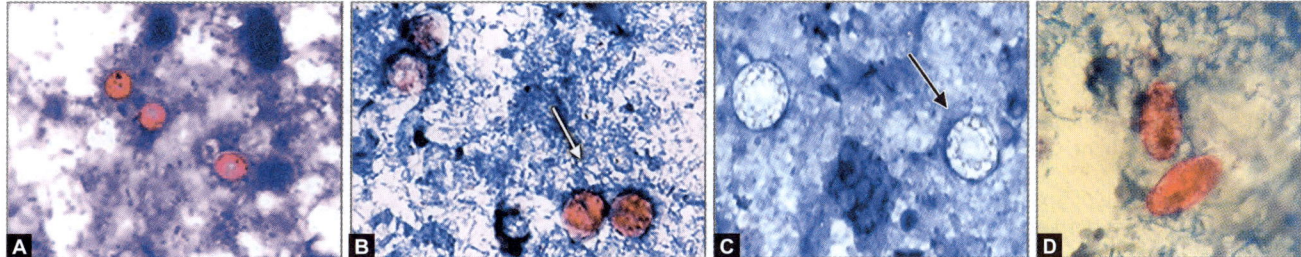

Figs. 52.4A to D: Acid-fast staining of stool specimen demonstrating oocysts of: **A.** *Cryptosporidium parvum* (acid-fast, round, 4–6 μm); **B.** *Cyclospora cayetanensis* (acid-fast, round, 8–10 μm); **C.** *Cyclospora cayetanensis* (non-acid-fast, round, 8–10 μm); **D.** *Cystoisospora belli* (acid-fast, oval, 20–33 μm).

Source: **A to C:** Swierczynski G, Milanesi B. Atlas of human intestinal protozoa Microscopic diagnosis (*with permission*); **D:** Dr Anand Janagond, Department of Microbiology, S Nijalingappa Medical College, Bagalkot, Karnataka (*with permission*).

> **TREATMENT** — Intestinal coccidian infections
>
> **Mild cases:** Self-limiting, requires fluid replacement like ORS.
> **Severe cases**
> - Cryptosporidiosis: Nitazoxanide is given to adults.
> - Cyclosporiasis and cystoisosporiasis: Treated with cotrimoxazole.

■ BALANTIDIUM COLI

Balantidium coli is the largest protozoan and the only ciliated parasite of humans. It produces intestinal disease similar to amoebic dysentery.

- ❖ **Habitat:** It resides in the large intestine, similar to *E. histolytica*
- ❖ **Host:** Pig (main reservoir) and other animals are the primary hosts. Man is an accidental host
- ❖ **Life cycle:** Man gets infection by ingestion of food and water contaminated with cysts (infective form)
- ❖ **Clinical features:** The majority of infected individuals become asymptomatic carriers. A small number of people develop acute dysenteric disease, similar to amoebic dysentery except that, it is less severe and extraintestinal involvement is very rare
- ❖ **Laboratory diagnosis:** Stool examination reveals characteristic trophozoite and cyst
  - Trophozoite is oval-shaped (50–100 μm), ciliated, and found in the dysenteric stool **(Fig. 52.5A)**
  - Cyst is round-shaped (50–70 μm), found in carriers and chronic cases **(Fig. 52.5B)**

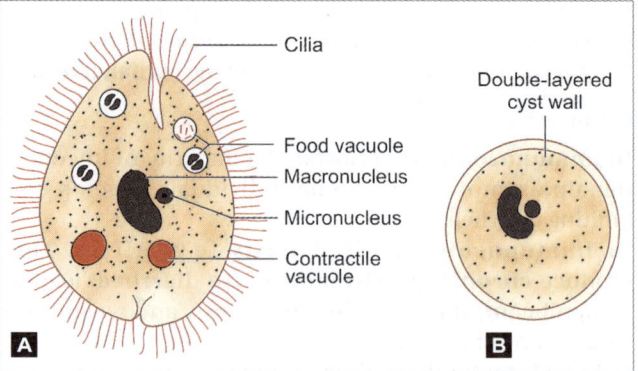

Figs. 52.5A and B: Morphology of *Balantidium coli* (schematic diagram): **A.** Trophozoite; **B.** Cyst.

- Both forms are bi-nucleated having a large kidney-shaped macronucleus and a small micronucleus
- ❖ **Treatment:** Tetracycline is the drug of choice.

■ BLASTOCYSTIS HOMINIS

Blastocystis hominis is a protozoan parasite resides in the intestine of humans and many animals as commensal; however, recently its pathogenic role has been described. Few present with symptoms of irritable bowel syndrome.

- ❖ **Morphology:** It occurs in various forms—**cysts** are the infective form, transmitted by feco-oral route; whereas **vacuolar forms** are the most common form seen in stool microscopy
- ❖ **Treatment:** Metronidazole is found to be effective.

EXPECTED QUESTIONS

I. Write an essay on:
1. Discuss the clinical manifestations and laboratory diagnosis of toxoplasmosis.

II. Write short notes on:
1. Differences between *Cryptosporidium*, *Cyclospora*, and *Cystoisospora*
2. Congenital toxoplasmosis

III. Multiple Choice Questions (MCQs):
1. Which of the following oocyst is variably acid-fast?
   a. *Cryptosporidium*
   b. *Cyclospora*
   c. *Cystoisospora*
   d. All of the above
2. Autoinfection is seen with:
   a. *Cryptosporidium*
   b. *Cyclospora*
   c. *Cystoisospora*
   d. All of the above
3. Most common infective form, for *Toxoplasma*:
   a. Oocyst
   b. Tissue cyst
   c. Tachyzoite
   d. All of the above

Answers
1. b   **2.** a   **3.** b

Cestodes

CHAPTER 53

CHAPTER PREVIEW
- *Taenia saginata* and *Taenia solium*
- *Echinococcus granulosus*
- *Hymenolepis nana*
- *Diphyllobothrium latum*
- *Spirometra* species

■ INTRODUCTION

Cestodes are long, segmented, flattened, tape-like worms, therefore also called tapeworms. Based on habitat, they are classified into two groups:
1. **Intestinal cestodes:** Here, the adult worms inhabit in human intestine. Examples include:
   - *Diphyllobothrium* species
   - *Taenia solium* and *Taenia saginata* causing intestinal taeniasis
   - *Hymenolepis nana.*
2. **Somatic/tissue cestodes:** Here, the larvae are found in the human muscles or organs. Examples include:
   - *Taenia solium*—causes cysticercosis affecting CNS, muscle, and eye
   - *Echinococcus granulosus*—the agent of hydatid disease affecting the liver.

Morphology

In general, cestodes exist in three morphological forms.
- ❖ **Adult worm:** It is long, segmented, and varies in length from a few mm to several meters. It consists of—the head (or scolex), neck, and body (strobila). The strobila further comprises of a number of segments (or proglottids) **(Fig. 53.1)**
- ❖ **Eggs:** They are formed following fertilization, fill the proglottids, and are subsequently released in feces—considered as the diagnostic form
- ❖ **Larva:** Embryonated eggs undergo further development to form larvae. The larval form is called with different names for different cestodes
  - *Taenia saginata*: Cysticercus bovis
  - *Taenia solium* Cysticercus cellulosae
  - *Echinococcus*: Hydatid cyst
  - *Hymenolepis* species: Cysticercoid larva
  - *Diphyllobothrium* species: It has 3 larval stages—coracidium, procercoid, and plerocercoid.

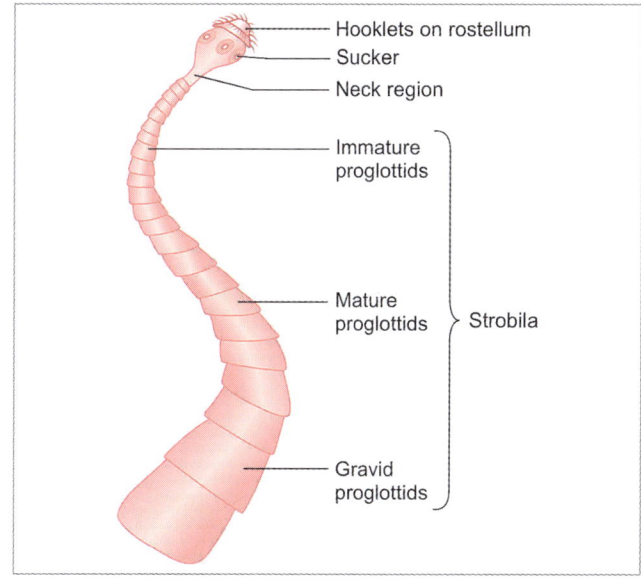

Fig. 53.1: Adult worm of cestode (schematic diagram).

The life cycle of cestodes pathogenic to man has been discussed in **Table 53.1**.

■ TAENIA SAGINATA AND T. SOLIUM

Taenia saginata and *T. solium* cause two types of manifestations in humans.
- ❖ **Intestinal taeniasis**—caused by both *T. saginata* and *T. solium*
- ❖ **Cysticercosis**—caused by only *T. solium*. It infects various tissues such as CNS, eyes, and muscles.

Intestinal Taeniasis

Life Cycle

The life cycle of *Taenia* passes through two hosts **(Fig. 53.2)**. Man is the definitive host; whereas the

Table 53.1: Life cycle of various cestodes.

Cestodes	Host Definitive	Host Intermediate	Mode of transmission	Infective form	Diagnostic form	Organs affected
Taenia saginata	Man	Cattle	Ingestion	Cysticercus bovis	Embryonated eggs	GIT
Taenia solium (intestinal taeniasis)	Man	Pig	Ingestion	Cysticercus cellulosae	Embryonated eggs	GIT
Taenia solium (cysticercosis)	Man	Man	Ingestion, autoinfection	Embryonated eggs	Cysticercus larvae	CNS, muscle, eye
Echinococcus granulosus	Dog	Man	Ingestion	Embryonated eggs	Hydatid cyst (larva)	Liver
Hymenolepis nana	Man	-	Ingestion, autoinfection	Embryonated eggs	Embryonated eggs	GIT
Diphyllobothrium latum	Man	1st Cyclops 2nd Fish	Ingestion	Plerocercoid larvae	Operculated eggs	GIT

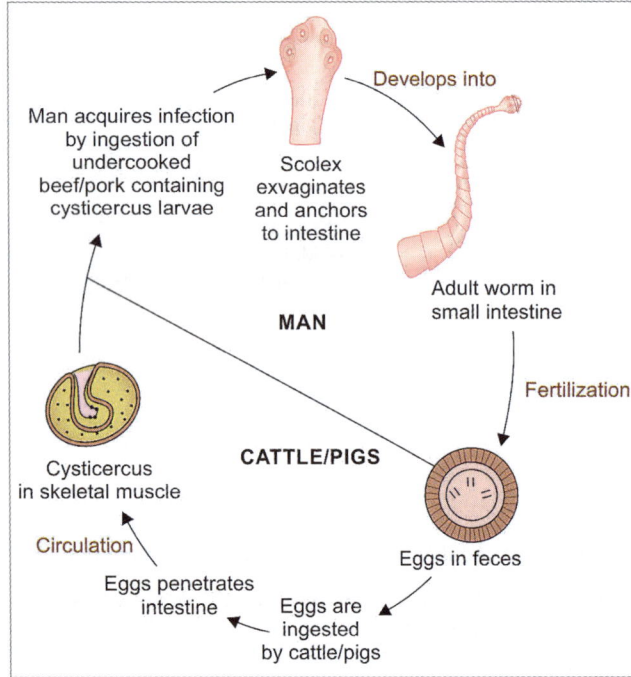

Fig. 53.2: Life cycle of *Taenia saginata* and *T. solium* causing intestinal taeniasis.

intermediate host is cattle for *T. saginata* (hence called beef tapeworm) and pigs for *T. solium* (hence called pork tapeworm).

- ❖ **Transmission:** Man acquires infection by ingestion of contaminated undercooked beef or pork containing the larvae (infective form)—i.e. cysticercus bovis (for *T. saginata*) or cysticercus cellulosae (for *T. solium*)
- ❖ **Human GIT:** The larvae develop into adult worms in the intestine, which undergo fertilization to produce eggs, that are released into feces (diagnostic form)

- ❖ **Intermediate hosts (cattle or pigs):** Eggs are ingested by cattle or pigs while grazing the field. Eggs penetrate the intestinal wall and migrate to skeletal muscles via blood, where they transform into larvae (cysticercus) that get encysted and deposited as cysts. This is the infective form to man and the cycle is repeated.

Note: T. solium has an additional part of the life cycle in man, which causes cysticercosis (discussed subsequently).

Clinical Manifestations

The majority of cases are asymptomatic. Common symptoms include mild abdominal pain, nausea, loss of appetite, and change in bowel habits and perianal pruritus may be felt (when proglottids are discharged).

Laboratory Diagnosis

Laboratory diagnosis of intestinal taeniasis includes:
- ❖ **Stool examination:** Wet mount (saline or iodine) examination of stool can demonstrate the characteristic eggs and less often proglottids of *Taenia* species
    - ■ **Eggs:** Round (31–43 μm size) and consist of an embryo with six hooklets surrounded by an embryophore. Eggs are bile-stained; do not float in the saturated salt solution **(Fig. 53.3)**
    - ■ **Proglottids** of *T. saginata* and *T. solium* can be differentiated by various features.
- ❖ **Antigen detection in stool:** Detection of *Taenia*-specific antigen (coproantigen) in the stool by ELISA
- ❖ **Molecular detection by** PCR; which can distinguish between *Taenia* species.

TREATMENT — Intestinal taeniasis

Praziquantel is the drug of choice for intestinal taeniasis. Niclosamide is also effective but is not widely available.

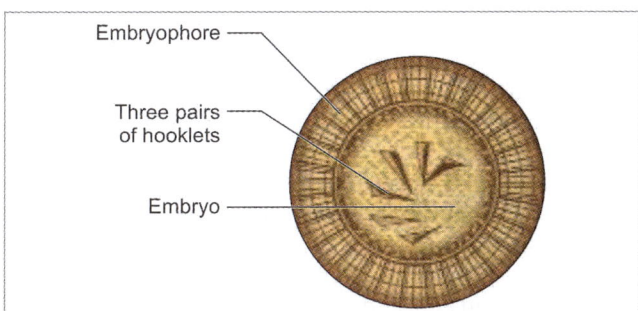

Fig. 53.3: Egg of *Taenia solium* or *T. saginata*.

Cysticercosis

Cysticercosis is caused by the larval stage of the tapeworm *Taenia solium*, affecting CNS, muscles, and the eye.
* It is a major public health problem, especially in the developing world
* In India, it is highly prevalent in the northern states such as Bihar, Odisha, Uttar Pradesh, Punjab, etc.

Life Cycle of Taenia solium causing Cysticercosis

The life cycle of *T. solium* causing cysticercosis is different than its life cycle when it causes intestinal taeniasis.
* **Host:** Man acts as both definitive and intermediate host
* **Infective stage:** Eggs of *T. solium*
* **Mode of transmission:** Firstly man acquires the infection by—(1) ingestion of contaminated food or water containing eggs of *T. solium*, and (2) autoinfection, i.e. eggs excreted in the feces re-infect the same individual
* **Human cycle:** In the gut, the egg ruptures to release the embryo, which penetrates the intestine and enters the circulation to reach various organs like subcutaneous tissue, muscle, eye, and brain where it is transformed into the larval stage.

Clinical Manifestations (Cysticercosis)

Clinical spectra of the disease depend upon the localization of the cyst—common sites are CNS, subcutaneous tissue, skeletal muscle, and eyes.

Neurocysticercosis

Neurocysticercosis (NCC) is the most common form of cysticercosis; accounts for 60–90% of cases of cysticercosis.
* **Site:** NCC occurs most commonly in the brain parenchyma, followed by subarachnoid space
* **Clinical manifestations** include **seizure** (most common), hydrocephalus, increased intracranial pressure, chronic meningitis, etc.
* The clinical presentation is variable and depends on the number, location, and size of the cyst, and the host immune response
* **NCC and HIV:** Patients with HIV have a higher risk of NCC co-infection.

Other Forms of Cysticercosis

* **Subcutaneous cysticercosis:** It may manifest as palpable nodules
* **Muscular cysticercosis:** Manifest as muscular pain, weakness, or pseudohypertrophy
* **Ocular cysticercosis:** Can involve the eyelids, conjunctiva, and sclera.

Laboratory Diagnosis

Cysticercosis is diagnosed by the following modalities.
* **Radiodiagnosis:** CT scan and MRI are the two important imaging methods used to detect cysticerci in the brain. They are useful for detecting the number, location, size of the cysticerci, and stage of the disease **(Fig. 53.4)**
* **Antibody detection** in serum or CSF by ELISA or Western blot
* **Antigen detection** in serum or CSF by ELISA. Antigen disappears following treatment hence, can be used for monitoring
* **Histopathology** of muscles, eyes, subcutaneous tissues, or brain biopsies—can detect cysticerci
* **FNAC** of the cyst and then staining with Giemsa stain
* **Fundoscopy** of the eye: can detect larvae if present.

> **TREATMENT** — Cysticercosis
>
> * **Antiparasitic agents:** Albendazole or praziquantel are the drugs of choice
> * **Symptomatic treatment** is necessary for seizures or hydrocephalus, etc.
> * **Surgery:** Surgery is indicated for ocular, spinal and ventricular lesions.

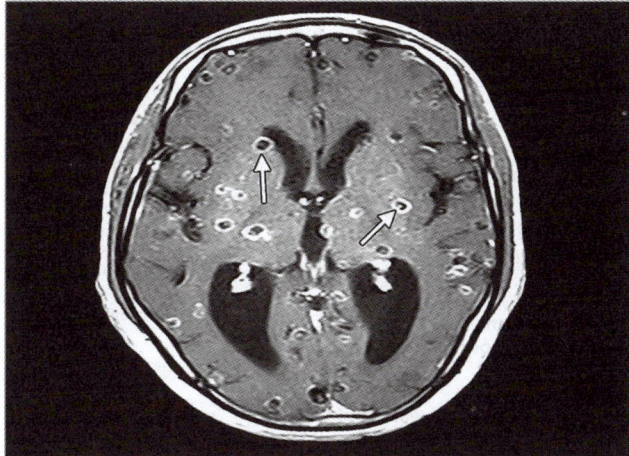

Fig. 53.4: CT scan of the brain showing multiple ring-enhancing lesions with eccentric scolex (neurocysticercosis).

Source: Dr A Subathra. Department of Radiodiagnosis, JIPMER, Puducherry (*with permission*).

ECHINOCOCCUS GRANULOSUS

Echinococcus granulosus is the causative agent of cystic echinococcosis, also known as hydatid disease.

Morphology

Echinococcus granulosus is a tissue cestode, exits in three morphological forms—adult, larva (called hydatid cyst), and egg.
- **Adult worm** resides in dog's intestine.
- **Larval form** is called as hydatid cyst. It is the pathogenic form, forms cystic lesions in liver and other viscera of man.
- **Eggs:** *E. granulosus* eggs are morphologically similar to *Taenia* eggs.

Life Cycle (Fig. 53.5)

Host: *E. granulosus* passes its life cycle through two hosts:
1. Definitive host: Dogs and other canine animals
2. Intermediate hosts: Sheep and other herbivores are the usual intermediate host. Man acts as an accidental intermediate host (dead end).

Infective form: Eggs are the infective form.

Mode of transmission: Man (and other intermediate hosts) acquires the infection by ingestion of food contaminated with dog's feces containing *E. granulosus* eggs.

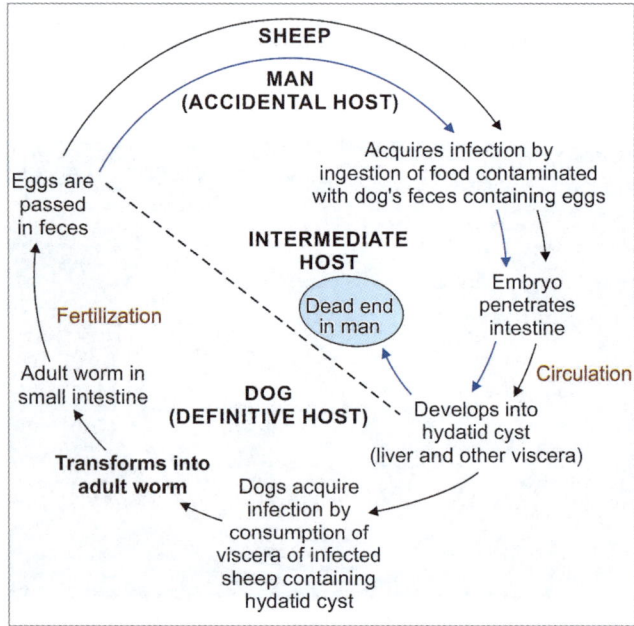

Fig. 53.5: Life cycle of *Echinococcus granulosus.*

Development in Man/Sheep

- In the duodenum, the embryo is released, which penetrates the intestinal wall, enters the portal circulation, and is carried to the liver or rarely to other organs
- The embryo develops into a fluid-filled bladder-like cyst called as **hydatid cyst,** which undergoes maturation and increases in size
- This stage is infective to dog and other definitive hosts
- Man is a dead end, as dogs do not feed on human viscera and therefore the cycle stops there.

Development in Dog

They acquire infection by consumption of the contaminated viscera of intermediate hosts (sheep) containing hydatid cysts.
- The hydatid cyst (larva) transforms into adult worm in the dog's intestine
- The adult worms sexually mature, and fertilize to produce eggs which are passed in feces and are infective to man.

Clinical Features

The manifestations are related to the deposition of the hydatid cysts in various organs—the most common site being the liver (60–70%, right lobe) or lung (20%), followed by other viscera.
- **Pressure effect of enlarging cyst:** Leads to palpable abdominal mass, hepatomegaly, abdominal tenderness, portal hypertension, and ascites
- **Obstruction:** Daughter cysts may erode into the biliary tree or a bronchus and enter into the lumen to cause cholestasis, cholangitis, and dyspnea
- **Secondary bacterial infection,** causing pyogenic abscess in the liver
- **Anaphylactic reactions** may occur due to cyst leakage or rupture.

> **Hydatid Cyst**
>
> It is a fluid-filled bladder-like cyst; the average size measures 5–8 cm **(Figs. 53.6 and 53.7)**.
> - **Cyst wall** consists of three layers: outer pericyst (host-derived), middle ectocyst, and inner endocyst
> - **Brood capsule:** The inner side of the endocyst gives rise to brood capsule which contains a number of protoscolices (future head)
> - **Hydatid fluid:** It is clear, pale yellow colored fluid, which is antigenic, and anaphylactic
> - **Hydatid sand** is formed by deposition of some of the brood capsules and protoscolices at the bottom
> - **Fate:** The hydatid cyst may undergo—(i) spontaneous resolution, or (ii) rupture of the cyst, which may lead to the formation of secondary cysts.

CHAPTER 53 ❖ Cestodes

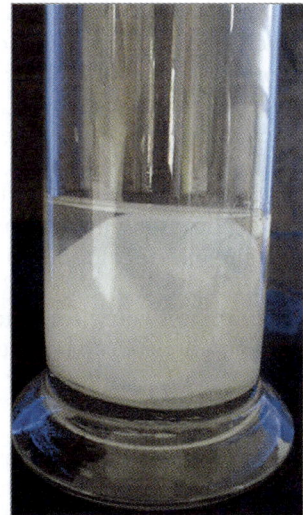

Fig. 53.6: Hydatid cyst, gross specimen.
Source: Head, Department of Microbiology, Sri Siddhartha Medical College, Tumkur, Karnataka (*with permission*).

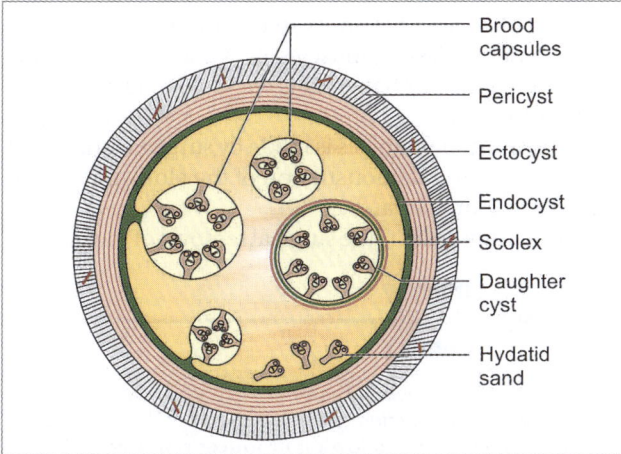

Fig. 53.7: Microscopy of hydatid cyst (schematic).

Laboratory Diagnosis

Hydatid disease is diagnosed by the following modalities.
❖ **Hydatid fluid microscopy:** Fluid aspirated from a surgically removed hydatid cyst can be subjected to direct mount—detects brood capsules and protoscolices
❖ **Histological examination:** Hematoxylin and eosin (H & E) staining demonstrates the three layers of the cyst wall and attached brood capsules
❖ **Antibody detection:** It is done by a screening test (ELISA or immunogold filtration assay) and confirmatory test by western blot
❖ **Imaging methods** such as X-ray, USG, CT scan, MRI, etc. can be performed. USG is the imaging method of choice for the diagnosis of hydatid disease

- USG helps in determining the exact location of the cyst, size of cyst, number of cysts, activity (active or dormant)
- The membranes may be detached; floating within the cyst cavity (known as the **water-lily sign**).

❖ **Molecular methods:** PCR targeting mitochondrial DNA has been developed
❖ **Skin test: Casoni test** is an immediate hypersensitivity reaction, that develops following injection of hydatid fluid antigens.

> **TREATMENT** — Hydatid disease
>
> The following are the treatment strategies for hydatid disease.
> ❑ **PAIR** (puncture, aspiration, injection, and re-aspiration): It is a semiconservative method, indicated for a single uncomplicated hepatic cyst
> ❑ **Surgical removal** of the cyst is indicated for an inaccessible cyst or extrahepatic cysts
> ❑ **Antiparasitic agents:** Albendazole is the drug of choice, given to prevent recurrence and to reduce the size of the cyst before surgery or PAIR.

■ HYMENOLEPIS NANA

Hymenolepis nana, which is the smallest cestode infecting man, hence also called as dwarf tapeworm.
❖ **Transmission:** Man is the only host. Eggs are the infective form. Man acquires the infection by ingestion of food and water contaminated with eggs or by autoinfection (with the eggs released in their small intestine)
❖ **Clinical manifestations:** Patients develop symptoms like anorexia, abdominal pain, headache, dizziness, and diarrhea with mucus
❖ **Laboratory diagnosis:** Stool microscopy detecting the characteristic eggs confirms the diagnosis **(Fig. 53.8A)**
- The egg is round to oval in shape, 30–47 μm in size
- It has two membranes that surround an embryo with six hooklets
- Polar filaments at both the poles
- Non-bile stained (colorless in saline mount)
- Eggs are the infective form as well as the diagnostic form of the parasite.
❖ **Treatment:** Praziquantel is the treatment of choice.

■ DIPHYLLOBOTHRIUM LATUM

Diphyllobothrium latum, also known as fish tapeworm—is the largest known parasite found in the human intestine.
❖ **Morphology:** It includes three forms:
- **Adult worm:** It consists of head, neck and body (strobila). It is spoon-shaped, bears two longitudinal grooves called as **bothria**
- **Eggs:** Fertilized eggs are oval and operculated at one end and bear a knob at the other end **(Fig. 53.8B)**

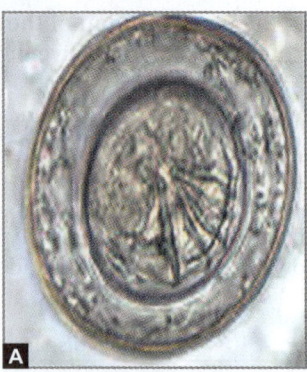 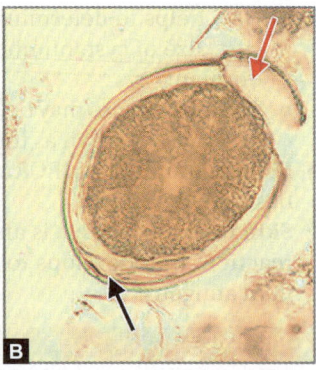

Figs. 53.8A and B: A. Egg of *Hymenolepis nana* (non-bile stained); **B.** Egg of *Diphyllobothrium latum*—note the operculum (red arrow).
Source: DPDx Image Library, Centers for Disease Control and Prevention (CDC), Atlanta (*with permission*).

- **Larva:** There are three larval stages: (i) First stage larva (coracidium), (ii) second stage larva (procercoid) and third stage larva (plerocercoid).
❖ **Life cycle:**
  - **Hosts:** Humans are the definitive host. There are two intermediate hosts: (i) **First intermediate hosts** are *Cyclops* and *Diaptomus* and (ii) **second intermediate hosts** are fresh or marine water fishes
  - **Infective form:** Third stage plerocercoid larvae
  - **Mode of transmission:** Humans get infection by ingestion of undercooked fresh water fish or marine fish containing third stage plerocercoid larva.

❖ **Manifestation:** The adult worm causes malabsorption of vitamin B12, which leads to vitamin B12 deficiency and **megaloblastic anemia**
❖ **Diagnosis** is made by:
  - Detection of characteristic bile stained egg with an operculum at one end and a knob at the other end **(Fig. 53.8B)** in stool microscopy
  - Detection of proglottids in the stool sample
  - Blood smear shows megaloblastic anemia with enlarged RBCs.
❖ **Treatment:** Praziquantel is the treatment of choice. Vitamin B12 supplement needs to be given.

■ SPIROMETRA SPECIES

❖ *Spirometra* and *Diphyllobothrium* species other than *D. latum* and few other species, can accidentally infect man and cause a disease called as **sparganosis**. This disease is caused by the plerocercoid larva (L3 stage) of these parasites which is called as **sparganum**
❖ **Life cycle:** It is similar to *D. latum*
❖ **Clinical manifestations:** The sparganum (L3 larva) penetrates the intestinal wall and migrates to subcutaneous tissues, muscles, eyes and visceral organs like brain and lymphatics; gets encysted to form painful fibrous nodule
❖ **Diagnosis** of sparganosis is made by surgical removal of the nodules and demonstration of the elongated worm like sparganum larva.
❖ **Definite treatment** is the surgical removal of the nodule.

EXPECTED QUESTIONS

I. Write short notes on:
1. Discuss the clinical manifestations and laboratory diagnosis of cysticercosis.
2. Discuss the life cycle, clinical manifestations, and laboratory diagnosis of *Echinococcus granulosus*.

II. Write short notes on:
1. Laboratory diagnosis of intestinal taeniasis.
2. *Hymenolepis nana*.
3. *Diphyllobothrium latum*.

III. Multiple Choice Questions (MCQs):
1. **Which is a somatic cestode?**
   a. *Echinococcus granulosus*
   b. *Hymenolepis nana*
   c. *Diphyllobothrium latum*
   d. *Taenia saginata*
2. **Which causes megaloblastic anemia?**
   a. *Echinococcus granulosus*
   b. *Hymenolepis nana*
   c. *Diphyllobothrium latum*
   d. *Taenia saginata*
3. **Which of the following produces non-bile stained egg?**
   a. *Echinococcus granulosus*
   b. *Hymenolepis nana*
   c. *Diphyllobothrium latum*
   d. *Taenia saginata*
4. **The causative agent of hydatid disease:**
   a. *Echinococcus granulosus*
   b. *Hymenolepis nana*
   c. *Diphyllobothrium latum*
   d. *Taenia saginata*
5. **Definitive host for Echinococcosis is:**
   a. Man   b. Dog
   c. Sheep   d. Pig

Answers
1. a   **2.** c   **3.** b   **4.** a   **5.** b

Trematodes

CHAPTER 54

CHAPTER PREVIEW
- Schistosomes
- *Fasciolopsis buski*
- Hepatic flukes
- *Paragonimus westermani*

■ INTRODUCTION

Trematodes (or flukes) are unsegmented, leaf-like, and flatworms. Based on the habitat, trematodes are classified as follows:
- **Intestinal flukes**—e.g. *Fasciolopsis buski*. It resides in the intestine and may cause various GI symptoms
- **Blood flukes**—e.g. *Schistosoma*. They reside in the venous plexus of various viscera
- **Hepatic flukes**—e.g. *Fasciola hepatica* in the liver, *Clonorchis sinensis,* and *Opisthorchis viverrini* in the bile duct
- **Lung flukes**—e.g. *Paragonimus westermani*. It resides in the lungs and may produce endemic hemoptysis.

Morphology

Trematodes exist in three morphological forms—adult worm, egg, and larva.
- **Adult worm:** The adult worms are unsegmented and flattened dorsoventrally **(Fig. 54.1A)**, but some have thick fleshy bodies (schistosomes) **(Fig. 54.1B)**
- **Eggs:** Trematodes are oviparous, i.e. they lay eggs
  - The eggs of all the trematodes except for schistosomes are characteristically operculated
  - *Schistosoma* eggs are non-operculated and bear a spine.
- **Larvae:** Most trematodes have five larval forms such as miracidium, sporocyst, redia, cercaria, and metacercaria. Schistosomes have only three larval stages miracidium, sporocyst, and cercaria.

Life Cycle

The life cycle of most trematodes is similar except for *Schistosoma* which has a different life cycle **(Table 54.1)**.

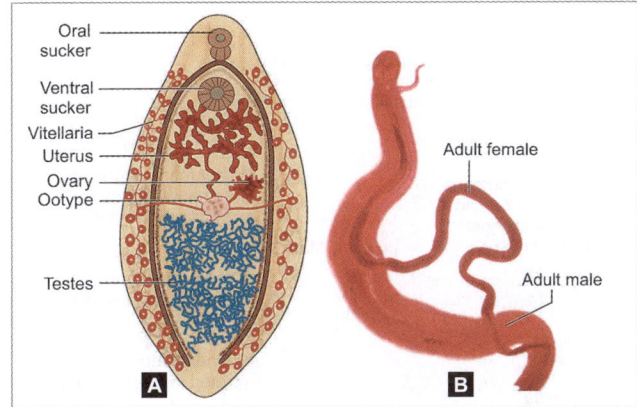

Figs. 54.1A and B: Adult worm of: **A.** *Fasciolopsis buski* (schematic); **B.** *Schistosoma* (The thin female worm resides in the gynecophoric canal of the thicker male worm).

Source: **B.** DPDx Image Library, Centers for Disease Control and Prevention (CDC), Atlanta (*with permission*).

Life Cycle of All Trematodes except Schistosomes (Fig. 54.2)

Host: Most trematodes (except *Schistosoma*) complete their life cycle in three different hosts, one definitive host (man), and two intermediate hosts.
- The first intermediate host is a fresh water snail
- The second intermediate host is either an aquatic plant or fish
  - Aquatic plant: for *Fasciola* and *Fasciolopsis*
  - Crayfish or crab: for *Clonorchis, Opisthorchis,* and *Paragonimus.*
- **Infective form:** Metacercaria larva is the infective from for all trematodes (except *Schistosoma*)

Table 54.1: Life cycle of various trematodes.						
Trematodes*	Organ affected	Host		Mode of transmission	Infective form	Diagnostic form
		Definitive	Intermediate			
Schistosoma		Man	Snail	Skin penetration	Cercaria larvae	Non-operculated eggs with spine **Figs. 54.4A to C**
S. haematobium	Bladder					
S. mansoni	Intestine					
S. japonicum	Intestine					
Fasciolopsis buski	Intestine	Man	1st Snail 2nd Aquatic plants	Ingestion	Metacercaria larvae	Operculated eggs
Fasciola hepatica	Liver					
Clonorchis spp., *Opisthorchis* spp.	Bile duct	Man	1st Snail 2nd Fish	Ingestion	Metacercaria larvae	Operculated eggs
Paragonimus spp.	Lungs	Man	1st Snail 2nd Crab	Ingestion	Metacercaria larvae	Operculated eggs

*Trematodes are hermaphrodites (male and female organs present in same worm), except schistosomes which are diecious (sexes are separate).

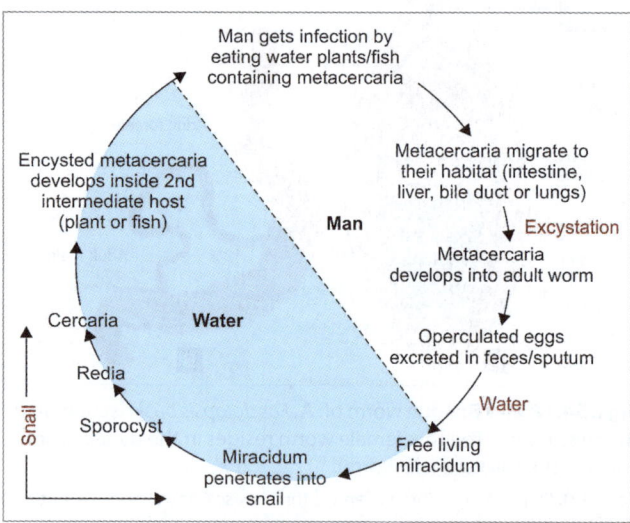

Fig. 54.2: Life cycle of all trematodes (except schistosomes).

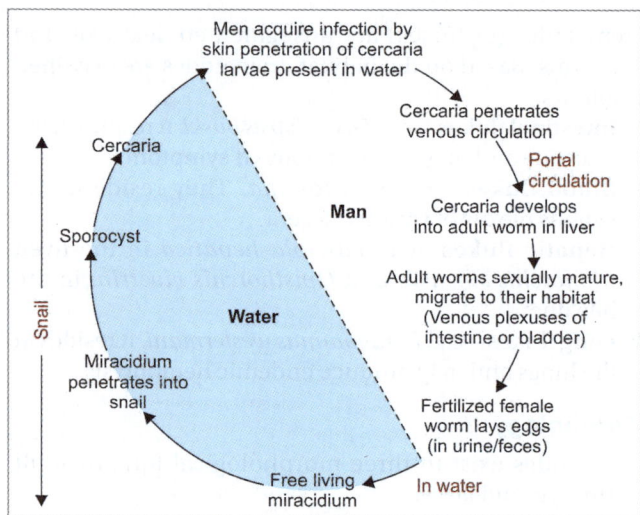

Fig. 54.3: Life cycle of schistosomes.

- **Modes of transmission:** Humans acquire infection by eating the second intermediate host (water plant or crayfish or crab), carrying the infective form, the metacercaria larvae
- **In man (migrate to habitat):** Larvae migrate to their respective habitat
  - Intestine (for *Fasciolopsis buski*) or
  - Liver (for *Fasciola hepatica*), bile duct (for *Clonorchis* and *Opisthorchis*) or
  - Lungs (for *Paragonimus*).
- **In man (produce eggs):** Larvae develop into adult worms, sexually mature, and produce eggs (diagnostic form) that are passed either in sputum (for *Paragonimus*) or feces (for other trematodes, i.e. *Fasciola*, *Fasciolopsis*, *Clonorchis* and *Opisthorchis*)
- **In water:** The eggs mature and hatch to release miracidium larvae which infect the snails

- **In the first intermediate host (snails):** The miracidium larvae undergo various larval stages of development such as sporocysts → redia → finally into cercaria larvae
- **In the second intermediate host:** The cercaria larvae escape from snails and infect the second intermediate hosts such as plants or fish/crab, where they develop into metacercaria larvae, which are infective form to man, and thus the life cycle continues.

Life Cycle of Schistosomes (Fig. 54.3)

Schistosomes are higher trematodes, their life cycle differs considerably from other trematodes **(Table 54.1)**.
- **Host:** Schistosomes complete their life cycle in two different hosts—one definitive host (man) and one intermediate host (freshwater snail). There is no second intermediate host

- **Infective form:** Cercaria larvae are the infective form, which are present freely in water
- **Mode of transmission:** Humans acquire infection by skin penetration of cercaria larvae (infective form) present freely in water
- **In man (develop into adult worms):** After penetrating the intact epidermis, cercariae travel via systemic circulation to reach the liver. In liver sinusoids, they develop into adult worms. Adult worms sexually mature (as male and female) and migrate to their habitat (venous plexuses of the intestine or urinary bladder)
  - Intestine (for *S. mansoni* and *S. japonicum*)
  - Kidney and bladder (for *S. haematobium*).
- **In man (produce eggs):** Fertilized female worms lay eggs in these venous plexuses. Eggs are the diagnostic form; passed either in feces (for *S. mansoni* and *S. japonicum*) or urine (for *S. haematobium*)
- **In water:** The eggs mature and hatch to release miracidium larvae which infect the snails
- **In intermediate host (snails):** The miracidium larvae develop into sporocyst larvae → finally into cercaria larvae, which are infective form to man, and thus the life cycle continues.

> **TREATMENT** — Trematode infections
>
> Praziquantel is the drug of choice for all trematode infections except for *Fasciola*, where triclabendazole is recommended.

SCHISTOSOMES

Schistosomes are known as **blood flukes** as they live in the vascular system of humans and other vertebrate hosts. The important schistosomes that parasitize humans are:
- *S. mansoni* and *S. japonicum*—reside in the rectal venous plexus and portal venous plexus, and cause various gastrointestinal symptoms including dysentery
- *S. haematobium*—resides in the venous plexus of the bladder; causes urinary schistosomiasis and carcinoma of the bladder.

Schistosoma mansoni

S. mansoni produces intestinal schistosomiasis in humans. The manifestations appear in three stages.
1. **Acute schistosomiasis:** It is characterized by:
   - *Cercarial dermatitis*—an itchy maculopapular rash develops at the site of skin perpetration of cercaria larvae (also called swimmer's itch)
   - *Katayama fever*—a serum sickness-like illness, due to the deposition of immune complexes, formed by binding of parasitic antigens to its antibodies.
2. **Chronic schistosomiasis:** Eggs are trapped in the small venules and carried from the intestine through portal circulation into the liver and other parts of the body.
   - The eggs are deposited in the intestinal wall and other sites such as the liver, lungs, brain, etc.
   - Soluble antigens liberated from eggs induce inflammatory reactions that lead to granuloma formation around the eggs
   - Intestinal followed by hepatosplenic disease are the most common forms.

Laboratory Diagnosis

- **Stool microscopy:** In acute cases, eggs can be detected in stool by microscopy. Eggs of *S. mansoni* are oval and elongated, non-operculated, and have characteristic lateral spine **(Fig. 54.4B)**
- **Antigen detection** by ELISA or dipstick tests to detect circulating cathodic (CCA) and circulating anodic antigens (CAA) in the serum
- **Antibody detection:** Less useful.

Schistosoma japonicum

- The clinical features of *S. japonicum* infection are almost similar to that caused by *S. mansoni*, except that in *S. japonicum*, the disease is—
  - More severe because of the higher egg production and smaller size of the eggs (easy dissemination)
  - CNS involvement is more marked
  - Both colorectal carcinoma and liver carcinoma (and cirrhosis) have been reported
- **Diagnosis:** Eggs of *S. japonicum* are relatively smaller, more spherical, and have a rudimentary lateral spine **(Fig. 54.4C)**.

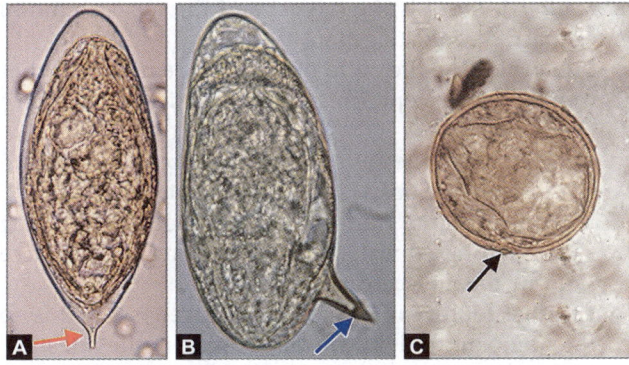

Figs. 54.4A to C: *Schistosoma* eggs: **A.** *S. haematobium*; **B.** *S. mansoni*; **C.** *S. japonicum*.

Source: **A.** ID# 4843, **B.** ID# 4841, **C.** ID#4842. Public Health Image Library, Centers for Disease Control and Prevention (CDC), Atlanta (*with permission*).

Schistosoma haematobium

S. haematobium is the causative agent of urinary schistosomiasis (also called Bilharziasis).

Clinical Manifestations

Bilharziasis is characterized by:
- **Acute schistosomiasis** presents as cercarial dermatitis
- **Chronic schistosomiasis** is due to the deposition of eggs in the urinary tract to form egg granuloma.
  - *Urogenital disease:* The eggs have terminal spines that cause damage to the bladder mucosa leading to dysuria and hematuria
  - *Obstructive uropathies:* Fibrosis of lower end of the ureters result in hydroureter and hydronephrosis
  - *Bladder carcinoma:* The metaplastic changes in urinary mucosa may lead to squamous cell carcinoma of the bladder.

Laboratory Diagnosis

- **Urine microscopy** may demonstrate *S. haematobium* eggs; oval-shaped, elongated, non-operculated with a terminal spine **(Fig. 54.4A)**
- **Detection of antibody** in serum against *S. haematobium* adult worm microsomal antigen (HAMA) by ELISA or HAMA-EITB (enzyme-linked immunotransfer blot)
- **Antigen detection** by ELISA or dipstick tests to detect circulating cathodic (CCA) and circulating anodic antigens (CAA) in the serum and urine.

> **TREATMENT** — Schistosomiasis
> **Praziquantel** is the drug of choice.

Fasciolopsis buski (Intestinal Fluke)

Fasciolopsis buski is the largest and the most common intestinal fluke infecting man.
- **Life cycle:** The life cycle of *F. buski* is similar to other trematodes (except *Schistosoma*); as described above **(Fig. 54.2)**.
  - **Host:** It has one definitive host (pig or man) and two intermediate hosts (snail and aquatic plants)
  - **Transmission:** Humans acquire infection by eating contaminated water plants, carrying the infective form, the metacercaria larvae.
- **Clinical features:** The main pathogenesis is due to the traumatic and obstructive damage to the intestine. Malabsorption may be seen with profuse yellowish-green stool
- **Laboratory diagnosis:** Stool microscopy reveals characteristic large operculated eggs **(Fig. 54.5A)**.

HEPATIC FLUKES

Fasciola hepatica, Clonorchis sinensis, and *Opisthorchis viverrini* are together called liver flukes. *Fasciola* infects the liver and bile duct, whereas the others infect only the bile duct.

Life Cycle

The life cycle of liver flukes is similar to as described for other trematodes, except for schistosomes **(Fig. 54.2)**. They have three hosts:
- **Definitive host:** Humans (or other animals like sheep for *F. hepatica*)
- **Intermediate hosts:** Snails are the first intermediate host, whereas the second intermediate host is aquatic plant (for *Fasciola*) and crayfish (for *Clonorchis* and *Opisthorchis*).

Fasciola hepatica

Fascioliasis (caused by *F. hepatica*) is reported worldwide, but in India, it is extremely rare.
- **Clinical features:** The metacercaria larvae migrate to the liver causing right upper quadrant pain, hepatomegaly and subsequently to the bile duct causing bile duct obstruction and biliary cirrhosis. It does not cause malignancies
- **Stool microscopy** reveals characteristic large operculated eggs, similar to *F. buski* **(Fig. 54.5A)**.

Clonorchis sinensis and Opisthorchis viverrini

Clonorchis sinensis is found primarily in Eastern Asia like China. *Opisthorchis viverrini* has been reported from Southeast Asia.

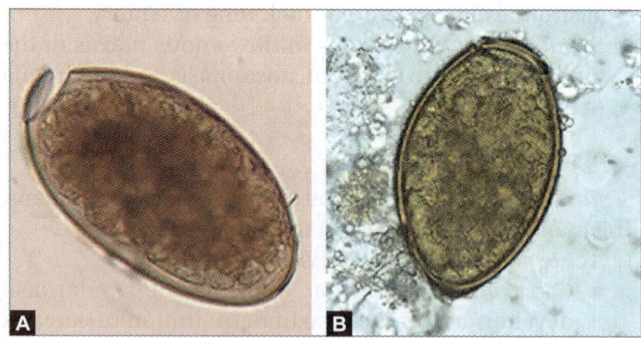

Figs. 54.5A and B: Operculated egg of: **A.** *Fasciolopsis buski/ Fasciola hepatica*; **B.** *Paragonimus westermani*.
Source: **A and B.** DPDx Image Library, Centers for Disease Control and Prevention (CDC), Atlanta (*with permission*).

- **Clinical features:** In chronic infection with heavy worm burden, they cause mechanical obstruction of the bile duct leading to
  - Cholangitis, dilatation, and fibrosis of the bile duct
  - Cholangiocarcinoma (bile duct carcinoma)
  - In addition, *O. viverrini* can also cause hepatocellular carcinoma
- **Stool microscopy:** Reveals the characteristic flask-shaped eggs. Eggs of *Clonorchis* and *Opisthorchis* are morphologically indistinguishable.

Paragonimus (Lung fluke)

Paragonimus westermani is endemic in Northeast states of India like Manipur.
- **Life cycle** of *Paragonimus* is similar to other trematodes, except for schistosomes **(Fig. 54.2)**. Humans are the definitive host. Intermediate hosts are snails (first), and crabs (second).
- **Clinical features:** Pathogenesis is due to the multiplication of the adult worm in the lungs (most common) or occasionally at other extrapulmonary sites such as the brain, skin, etc.
- **Pulmonary paragonimiasis** also called as **endemic hemoptysis**. The common presenting features are productive cough with brownish blood-tinged rusty sputum with an offensive fishy odor
- **Laboratory diagnosis** is by:
  - **Sputum microscopy** reveals the characteristic operculated eggs **(Fig. 54.5B)**. Early morning, deeply coughed sputum (multiple) samples are collected for better yield
  - **ELISA** is also available for antigen detection (which indicates active infection) or for antibody detection (used for the epidemiological purpose).
- **Treatment:** Praziquantel is the drug of choice.

EXPECTED QUESTIONS

I. Write short notes on:
   1. Schistosomiasis
   2. Paragonimiasis

II. Multiple Choice Questions (MCQs):
   1. Eggs with lateral-spine are produced by:
      a. *Schistosoma haematobium*
      b. *Schistosoma mansoni*
      c. *Schistosoma japonicum*
      d. *Fasciola hepatica*
   2. Operculated eggs are produced by:
      a. *Schistosoma haematobium*
      b. *Schistosoma mansoni*
      c. *Schistosoma japonicum*
      d. *Fasciola hepatica*
   3. The causative agent of swimmer's itch:
      a. *Paragonimus westermani*
      b. *Fasciola hepatica*
      c. *Schistosoma mansoni*
      d. *Fasciolopsis buski*

Answers
1. a   2. d   3. c

Intestinal Nematodes

CHAPTER 55

CHAPTER PREVIEW
- *Trichuris trichiura*
- *Enterobius vermicularis*
- *Ascaris lumbricoides*
- Hookworm
- *Strongyloides stercoralis*

■ NEMATODES

Nematodes are developmentally higher helminths, probably the most widespread helminths occurring in the world.

Classification based on Habitat

Based on their habitat, nematodes infecting humans are classified into two groups.

Intestinal nematodes: Include five common parasites
- Small intestinal nematodes—*Ascaris,* hookworm, and *Strongyloides*
- Large intestinal nematodes—*Trichuris* and *Enterobius.*

Somatic or tissue nematodes: They reside in various tissues or organs.
- Filarial nematodes: They comprise of several vector-borne parasites
  - *Wuchereria bancrofti* and *Brugia malayi* cause lymphatic filariasis
  - *Loa loa, Onchocerca volvulus* and *Mansonella* cause cutaneous filariasis
- *Dracunculus medinensis*: Causes Guinea-worm disease; presents as painful cutaneous blisters
- *Trichinella spiralis*: Produces profuse watery diarrhea and myalgia.

Apart from the above list, there are several nematodes of lower animals that rarely cause intestinal and somatic disease in man (described later in this chapter).

Classification based on they Lay Egg or Larva

Nematodes can be classified into three groups based on whether they lay eggs or larvae after fertilization of male and female worms.

- ❖ **Oviparous:** Here following fertilization, eggs are produced that are released in feces. Most of the intestinal nematodes are oviparous except for *Strongyloides*. Here, eggs are the diagnostic form in the stool
- ❖ **Viviparous:** Female worms directly give birth to larvae; there is no egg stage. All somatic nematodes are viviparous. Here, the diagnosis is made by the detection of larvae in tissues or blood
- ❖ **Ovoviviparous:** Here following fertilization, eggs are produced, from which the larvae immediately hatch out—e.g. *Strongyloides* species. The larvae are excreted in stool and are the diagnostic form.

Morphology

Nematodes have three morphological forms—adult worm (male and female), egg, and four larval stages (L_1–L_4). The life cycle passes through the six stages in sequential order **(Fig. 55.1)**.

- ❖ The adult form of nematodes is elongated, cylindrical in shape, and vary in size from a few mm (hookworm,

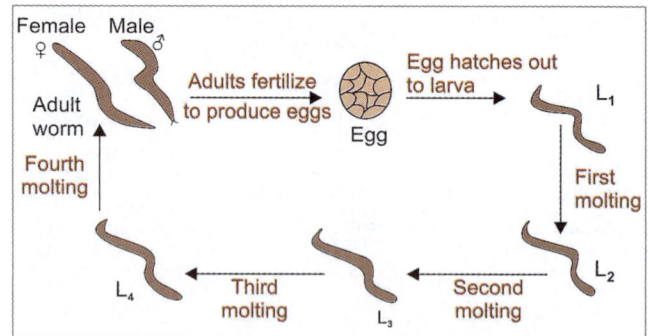

Fig. 55.1: Developmental stages of nematodes.

Trichinella, and *Strongyloides*) to as long as one meter (*Dracunculus*).
- ❖ The body is bilaterally symmetrical, containing a body cavity and various organs such as alimentary canal, nervous system, excretory system, and reproductive organs.

■ TRICHURIS TRICHIURA

Trichuris trichiura is a soil-transmitted helminth (STH), that commonly affects children. It is also called **whipworm** (as the adult worm resembles a handle of a whip).
- ❖ **Life cycle (Fig. 55.2):** Humans are the only host, acquire infection by ingestion of contaminated food and water containing embryonated egg (infective form)
    - **In the large intestine**: Eggs hatch out to form L_2 larva→L_3 larva→L_4 larva→ adult worms→ fertilize to produce eggs → are excreted in feces
    - **Environment:** The eggs become embryonated (L_2 larvae) in the environment and the cycle continues.
- ❖ **Clinical manifestations:** Adult female worms get buried in the large intestinal mucosa, which leads to abdominal pain, dysentery, iron deficiency anemia, recurrent rectal prolapse, malnutrition leading to growth retardation
- ❖ **Laboratory diagnosis:** Stool microscopy reveals characteristic eggs—barrel-shaped with mucus plugs at the ends. Eggs measure 50 × 22 μm in size, are bile-stained, and float in saturated salt solution **(Fig. 55.3A)**
- ❖ **Treatment:** Mebendazole or albendazole is the drug of choice.

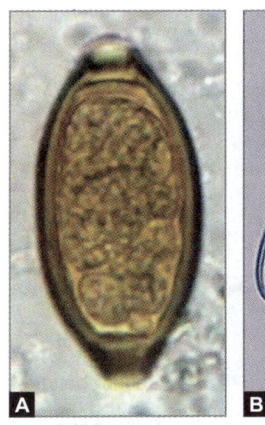 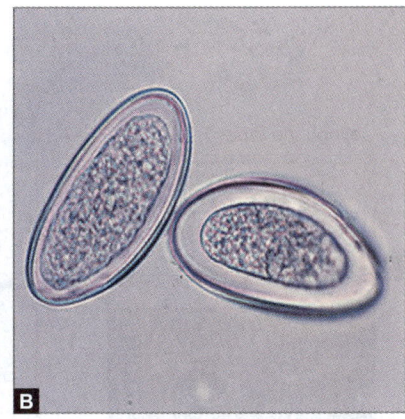

Figs. 55.3A and B: Saline mount of stool showing: **A.** Egg of *Trichuris trichiura* (bile stained); **B.** Egg of *Enterobius vermicularis* (non-bile stained).

Source: DPDx Image Library, Centers for Disease Control and Prevention (CDC), Atlanta (*with permission*).

■ ENTEROBIUS VERMICULARIS

E. vermicularis is a common large intestinal nematode affecting children. It is also called **pinworm** or **threadworm** (as the adult worm of *Enterobius* is small, white, and thread-like).

Life Cycle (Fig. 55.2)

Humans are the only host. Embryonated eggs are infective to man.
- ❖ **Transmission:** Infection occurs by:
    - Ingestion of eggs in the environment (e.g. surfaces, clothes, bed linens, etc.) or
    - By autoinfection—it occurs either by retrograde migration of the larva hatched from the eggs in the perianal skin or through contaminated finger (nail biting habit)
- ❖ Larvae hatch out from eggs in the cecum and then develop into adult worms
- ❖ After fertilization, the gravid female worms migrate to the large intestine (rectum, colon) and start laying eggs on the perianal skin
- ❖ The eggs are embryonated (carrying L_2 larvae) and are the infective stage to man.

Pathogenicity and Clinical Features

Children are commonly affected. The most cardinal symptom is **perianal pruritus,** which often gets worse at night as a result of the nocturnal migration of the female worm.
- ❖ The worms may be found in undergarments and lying in the buttock area of infected children
- ❖ Repeated scratching is the main reason of contaminated fingers; which causes autoinfection.

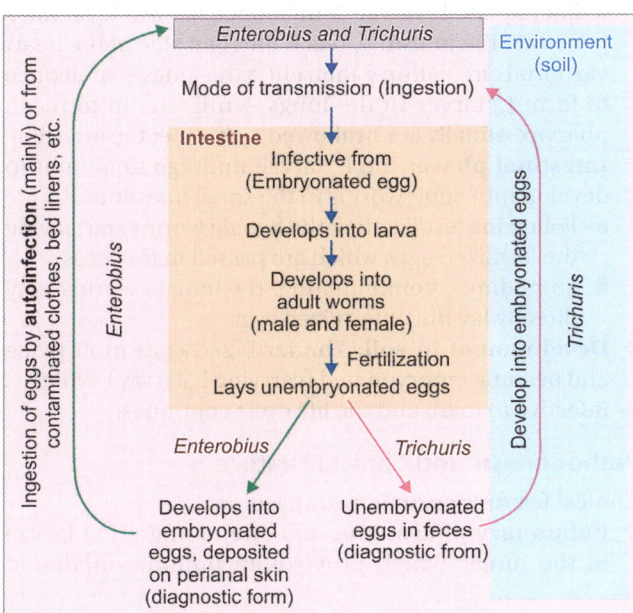

Fig. 55.2: Life cycles of *Trichuris* and *Enterobius*.

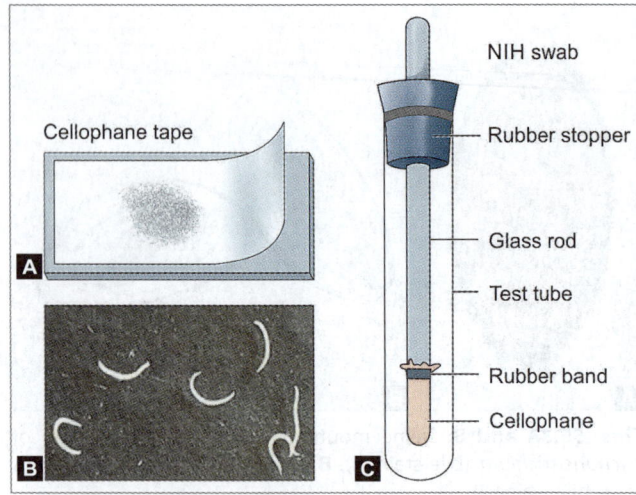

Figs. 55.4A to C: *Enterobius vermicularis*: **A.** Cellophane tape; **B.** Adult worms (actual size); **C.** NIH swab (schematic diagram).

Source: **B.** Head, Department of Microbiology, Meenakshi Medical College, Chennai (*with permission*).

Laboratory Diagnosis

Microscopy of the perianal skin samples is the test of choice which detects characteristic eggs.
- **Methods:** Specimen is collected by two methods—cellophane tape or by NIH swab (developed by National Institute of Health, USA).
  - Cellophane tape is applied onto the perianal region and then the tape is mounted with a drop of saline on a clear glass slide **(Fig. 55.4A)**
  - NIH swab: It consists of a glass rod attached to a cellophane tape by a rubber band. The cellophane part of the glass rod is rolled over the perineal skin area to collect the sample **(Fig. 55.4C)**
- **Number of specimens:** A series of 4–6 consecutive tapes may be necessary as the female worms migrate intermittently **(Fig. 55.4B)**
- **Timing:** Samples should be collected when the chance of egg deposition is more such as late evening, or early morning.

> **Eggs of *Enterobius***
> Eggs are planoconvex (one side is convex and the other side is flat), and measure 50–60 μm long **(Fig. 55.3B)**.
> ❑ Embryonated egg when freshly passed contains a tadpole-shaped larva inside
> ❑ Non-bile-stained, colorless in saline mount
> ❑ Floats in a saturated salt solution.

TREATMENT — Enterobiasis

The recommended drugs are mebendazole or albendazole or pyrantel pamoate.
❑ The same treatment should be repeated after 2 weeks
❑ Treatment of household members is advocated to eliminate asymptomatic reservoirs.

Prevention

Improving personal hygiene such as proper washing of bedclothes, keeping nails short and clean, and frequent hand washing are the key measures to contain the transmission.

ASCARIS LUMBRICOIDES

Ascaris lumbricoides is the largest nematode parasitizing the human intestine. It is commonly called as **roundworm**. It is a soil-transmitted helminth.

Morphology

Similar to other nematodes, *Ascaris* exists in three forms: adult, larvae (four stages), and egg. The adult worm is cylindrical and measures 15–31 cm. The female worms liberate two types of eggs—(1) fertilized eggs, and (2) unfertilized eggs.

Life Cycle (Fig. 55.5)

Ascaris involves only one host (man). Embryonated eggs containing the L_2 larvae are the infective form.
- **Mode of transmission:** Ingestion of embryonated eggs from the contaminated soil, food, and water
- **Migratory phase:** Following ingestion, the eggs hatch out to liberate the L_2 larvae → molt once to form L_3 larvae → penetrate the intestine, reach the right side of the heart via portal circulation → then enter the lungs → molt once to form L_4 larvae in the lungs → migrate up to reach pharynx → finally are swallowed to re-enter the intestine.
- **Intestinal phase:** The L_4 larvae undergo final molt to develop into adult worms in the small intestine
  - Following fertilization, the female worms start laying the fertilized eggs which are passed in the feces
  - Sometimes, before mating, the female worms may directly lay the unfertilized eggs
- **Development in soil:** The fertilized eggs molt twice and become embryonated (carrying L_2 larvae), which is infective to man, and the life cycle continues.

Pathogenesis and Clinical Feature

Clinical features occur in two stages.
- **Pulmonary phase:** It occurs due to migrating larvae in the lungs, which provoke an immune-mediated

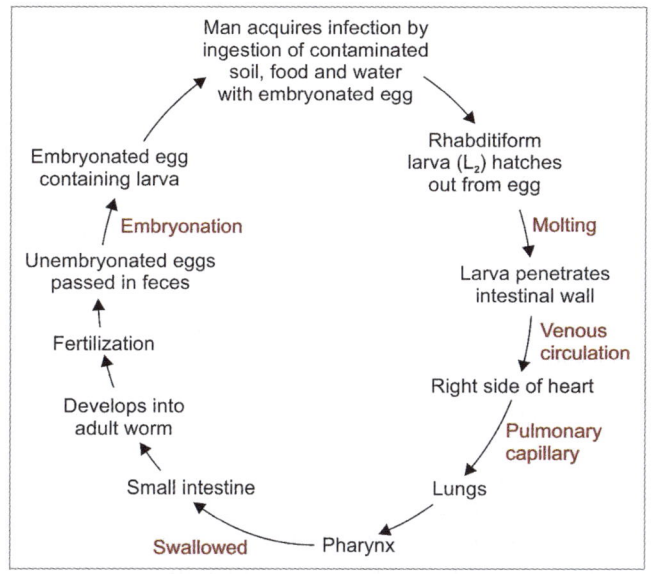

Fig. 55.5: Life cycle of *Ascaris lumbricoides*.

hypersensitivity response—called eosinophilic pneumonia (**Loeffler's syndrome**). Common symptoms are non-productive cough, chest discomfort, fever, dyspnea, and transient patchy infiltrates seen in the chest X-ray along with transient peripheral eosinophilia

- **Intestinal phase:** It results due to the effect of adult worm in the intestine; characterized by:
  - *Malnutrition and growth retardation:* Due to robbing of the nutrition from the host by the adult worm. It is often associated with impairment of the educational performance, language learning, gross motor, and fine motor skills in children
  - *Intestinal complications:* Intestinal obstruction, intestinal perforation, intussusception, or volvulus.

Laboratory Diagnosis

Stool examination: Detecting both fertilized and unfertilized eggs in saline and iodine wet mount.

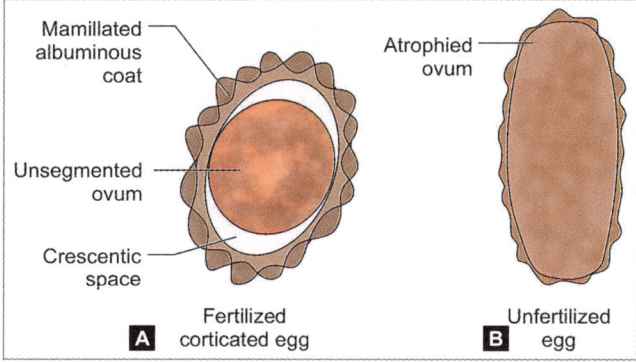

Figs. 55.6A to B: Eggs of *Ascaris lumbricoides*: **A.** Fertilized eggs; **B.** Unfertilized eggs (*schematic diagram*).

- Sedimentation method of stool concentration techniques is preferred to improve the detection
- The flotation method is not preferred as unfertilized eggs do not float on a saturated salt solution.

Eggs of *Ascaris*

Fertilized eggs (Figs. 55.6A and 55.7A)
Round to oval, measure 45–75 μm × 35–50 μm
- Surrounded by a thick mamillated, albuminous coat
- Contains a large, unsegmented ovum with clear crescentic space at both the poles
- Bile-stained, appear golden brown in saline mount
- Floats in saturated salt solution

Unfertilized eggs (Figs. 55.6B and 55.7B)
Elongated, measure 85–95 μm × 43–47 μm
- Albuminous coat is thin, distorted and scanty
- Contains an unsegmented, small atrophied ovum
- Bile-stained, appear golden brown in saline mount
- Do not float in the saturated salt solution.

Other diagnostic modalities include:

- **Adult worms** may be detected occasionally in the stool or sputum of the patients
- **Larvae** can be found in sputum or gastric aspirates during the early pulmonary migratory phase
- **Antibody detection** by ELISA
- **PCR** assay has been developed targeting *Ascaris*-specific genes in the stool.
- **Eosinophilia** is prominent during the early lung stage
- Presence of **Charcot-Leyden crystals** in sputum and stool.

TREATMENT — Ascariasis

Albendazole or mebendazole is the drug of choice. It effectively kills the adult worm but has a limited effect on the larval migration phase.

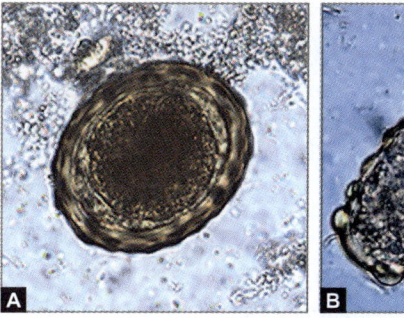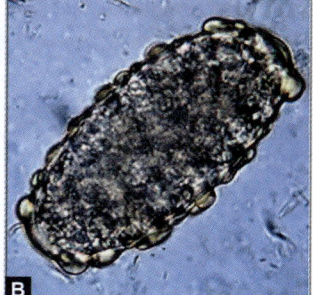

Figs. 55.7A to B: Eggs of *Ascaris lumbricoides*: **A.** Fertilized eggs; **B.** Unfertilized eggs.

Source: DPDx Image Library, Centers for Disease Control and Prevention (CDC), Atlanta (*with permission*).

HOOKWORM

Hookworm is a soil-transmitted helminth, one of the important causes of iron deficiency anemia.

* **Pathogens:** Two species are human pathogens: (i) *Ancylostoma duodenale* and (ii) *Necator americanus*
* **Epidemiology:** Hookworm infection is widespread in the world and also in India
* **Endemic index:** *Chandler's index* is used to estimate the morbidity and mortality in the community due to hookworm infection (which depends much upon the worm load)
* **Morphology:** Similar to other nematodes, hookworm exist as an adult worm, larvae (four stages), and egg.
    * The adult worm is small in size and has a bent in the anterior end (hence called as hookworm)
    * L_1 larva is called as rhabditiform larva whereas L_3 stage larva is called as filariform larva
    * *Ancylostoma* and *Necator* can be differentiated by the morphology of adult worm and third stage larva. Eggs and first-stage larvae of both are morphologically indistinguishable.

Life Cycle (Fig. 55.8)

Hookworm involves only one host (man). Third stage filariform (L_3) larva is the infective form.

* **Mode of transmission:** Through penetration of the skin by the L_3 larva; during walking barefoot in dampened soil
* **Migratory phase:** Following penetration, the L_3 larvae are carried to the lungs through venous circulation. From the lungs, they migrate up to the pharynx, and finally, by swallowing sputum, they enter the GIT
* **Intestinal phase:** The L_3 larvae molt twice in the small intestine to develop into adult worms, which attach to the intestinal mucosa by their teeth in the buccal capsule. Following fertilization, female worms lay eggs, which are excreted in the feces
* **Development in soil:** Eggs released in feces become embryonated in soil and subsequently the L_1 (rhabditiform) larvae hatch out from eggs which molt

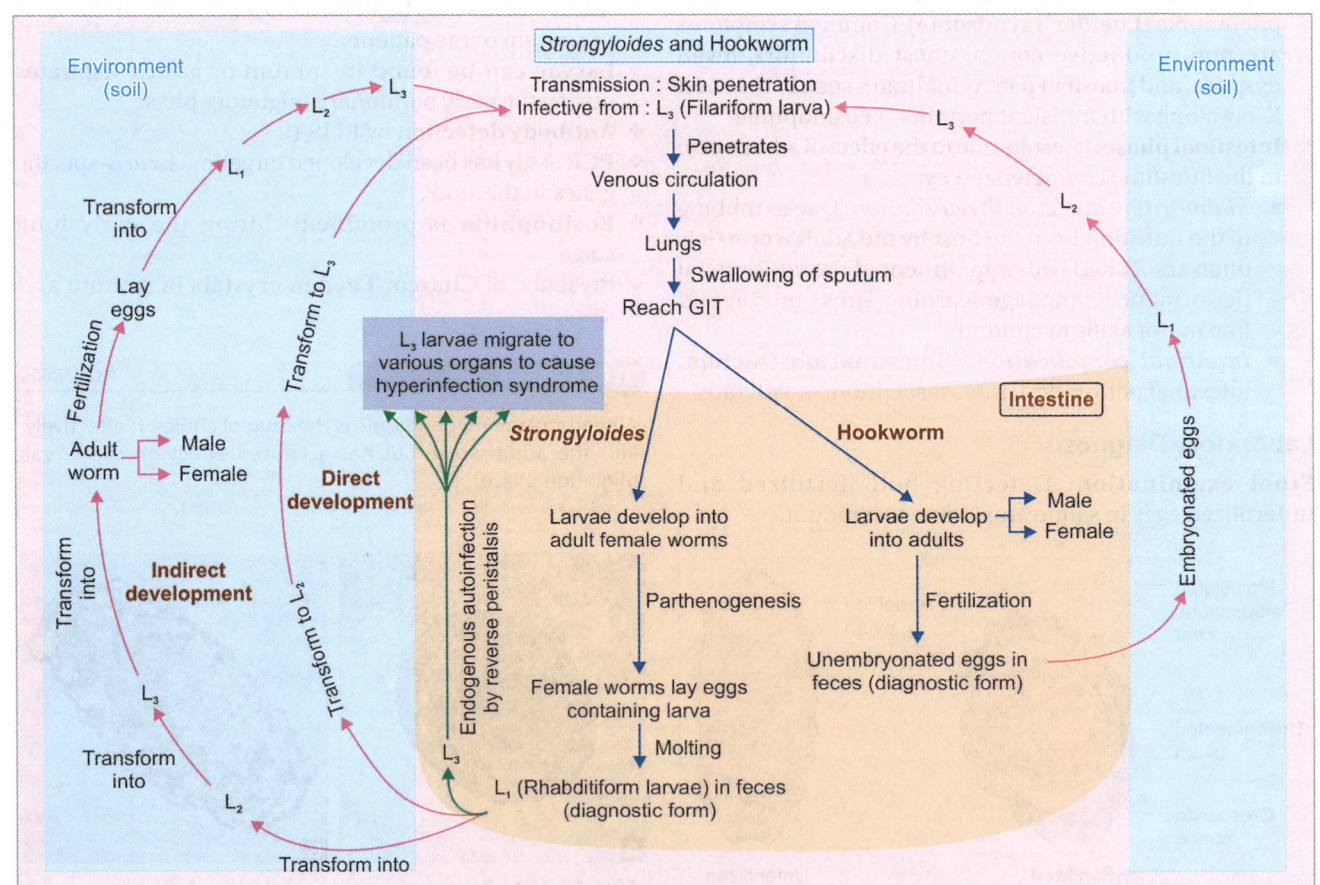

Fig. 55.8: Life cycles of Hookworm and *Strongyloides*.

twice to develop into L_3 larvae (infective form). Thus, the life cycle is continued.

Clinical Features

Affect due to Migrating Larva

- Cutaneous lesions: (i) **ground itch:** pruritic maculopapular rashes at the site of skin penetration; (ii) **serpiginous tracks** may be formed due to subcutaneous migration of the larva
- Mild transient pneumonitis due to the passage of migrating larvae through the lungs.

Affect due to Adult Worm in Intestine

- **Early intestinal phase (less worm load):** Infected persons may develop epigastric pain, inflammatory diarrhea, etc. accompanied by eosinophilia
- **Late intestinal phase (chronic infection with heavy worm load):** Patients develop iron deficiency anemia and protein-energy malnutrition resulting from blood loss. *Ancylostoma* is more pathogenic, and sucks more blood than *Necator*.

Laboratory Diagnosis

Stool Microscopy

The diagnosis is established by finding characteristic eggs in the feces.

- Stool concentration procedures may be required to detect eggs in case of lighter infections
- **Egg counting:** The number of eggs per gram of stool can be counted (by the Kato Katz technique) to estimate the disease burden.

> **Eggs of Hookworm (Fig. 55.9)**
> Hookworm eggs are oval, measure 60 × 40 μm, surrounded by thin eggshell.
> - Not bile stained, appear colorless in saline mount
> - Ovum is segmented; comprises of four blastomeres
> - Clear space between the eggshell and the embryo
> - Eggs float in saturated salt solution
> - Eggs of both *A. duodenale* and *N. americanus* are morphologically indistinguishable.

Stool Culture

The freshly passed stool samples can be cultured (so that the eggs hatch out to develop into L_3 stage filariform larvae) by Harada-Mori filter paper tube method or agar plate technique (more sensitive).

Molecular Diagnosis

PCR-based assays can differentiate between *Ancylostoma* and *Necator*.

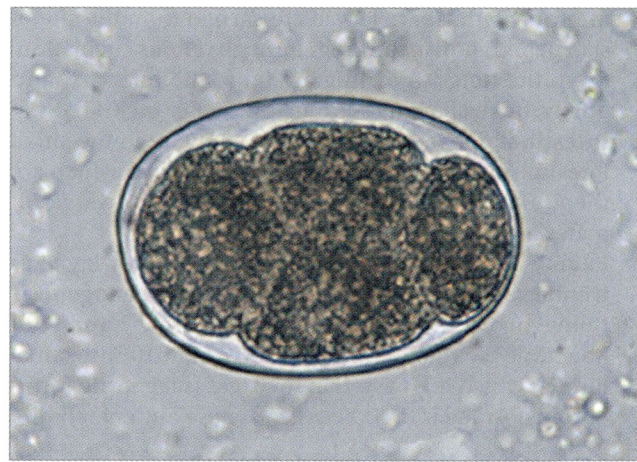

Fig. 55.9: Hookworm egg with four blastomeres.
Source: DPDx Image Library, Centers for Disease Control and Prevention (CDC), Atlanta (*with permission*).

Other Findings

Other findings include: (i) hypochromic microcytic anemia and (ii) eosinophilia.

> **TREATMENT** — Hookworm infections
> Albendazole is the drug of choice.
> **Symptomatic treatment**
> - Iron-deficiency anemia with oral iron and folic acid
> - Malabsorption warrants nutritional support.

■ STRONGYLOIDES STERCORALIS

Strongyloides stercoralis is a small intestinal nematode that causes strongyloidiasis. The disease is particularly common in Southeast Asia (including India).

Morphology

S. stercoralis exists in three forms: adult, larvae (four stages), and egg.

- **Adult worm:** Only female worms are seen in the small intestine of man, and measure 2–3 mm long. Male worms are free-living in the environment, but not in the human intestine
- **Eggs:** *Strongyloides* are ovoviviparous, i.e. eggs once laid, immediately hatch out to larvae.

Life Cycle (Fig. 55.8)

S. stercoralis involves only one host (man). L_3 larva (filariform) is the infective form.

- **Mode of transmission:** (1) Penetration of skin by the L_3 larva (by walking barefoot); (2) Autoinfection (internal autoinfection)

❖ **Migratory phase**: L_3 larvae are carried from the site of skin penetration to the lungs through venous circulation. From the lungs, they migrate up to the pharynx, and finally, by swallowing sputum, they enter the GIT
❖ **Intestinal phase:** The L_3 larvae molt twice in the small intestine to develop into adult female worms, which are then buried in the intestinal mucosa. However, adult males are not found in the human intestine
❖ **Laying eggs:** The female worms can directly lay eggs without fertilization, by a process called **parthenogenesis**
❖ Being ovoviviparous, eggs immediately hatch out liberating the rhabditiform (L_1) larvae into the intestinal lumen, which are passed in the feces (diagnostic form) or transformed into (L_3) larvae to cause autoinfection.

> **Autoinfection:** Sometimes, the L_1 larvae released in the human intestine do not pass in the feces but develop into filariform (L_3) larvae that eventually penetrate the intestinal wall or perianal skin, enter the venous circulation and reach the lungs. Autoinfection is responsible for disseminated infection.

❖ **Development in the environment:** The L_1 larvae molt twice to form the L_3 larvae. Then two types of development take place:
  ■ **Direct cycle:** The L_3 larvae act as the infective form to man. This cycle usually occurs in the temperate climate
  ■ **Indirect development:** The L_3 larvae develop into adult worms (male and female) → fertilize to produce eggs → L_1 larvae hatch out → molt twice to form the infective L_3 larvae. This cycle usually occurs in the tropical climate.

Pathogenesis and Clinical Feature
Effect due to Migrating Larva
❖ **Cutaneous larva migrans:** Migrating larvae may produce the pathognomonic serpiginous urticarial rash (commonly on the thigh) called **larva currens**
❖ **Pulmonary symptoms** are uncommon.

Effect due to Adult Worm and Filariform Larva
❖ **Mild to moderate worm load:** May produce epigastric pain, nausea, diarrhea, constipation, and blood loss
❖ **Heavy larva load:** Hyperinfection syndrome and disseminated strongyloidiasis are the important complications, observed in heavy larva load **(Table 55.1)**.

Laboratory Diagnosis
Stool Microscopy
Stool microscopy reveals the characteristic rhabditiform larvae (diagnostic form) **(Fig. 55.10)**.
❖ Repeated stool examination and concentration techniques can be performed to increase the yield

Table 55.1: Complications of strongyloidiasis.

Hyperinfection syndrome
The underlying cause is the repeated autoinfection cycles; which lead to the generation of a large number of filariform larvae.
- **Risk factors:** Impaired host immunity, e.g. glucocorticoid therapy, transplant recipients, co-infection with HTLV-1 or rarely HIV
- **Features:** Colitis, enteritis, or malabsorption, and in severe cases disseminated strongyloidiasis may develop.

Disseminated strongyloidiasis
Larvae may invade the GIT and migrate to various organs
- **CNS invasion:** leads to brain abscess and meningitis
- **Passage of enteric flora** through disrupted mucosa leads to gram-negative bacterial sepsis/meningitis
- **The mortality rate** is very high if left untreated.

(HTLV-1, human T cell lymphotropic virus)

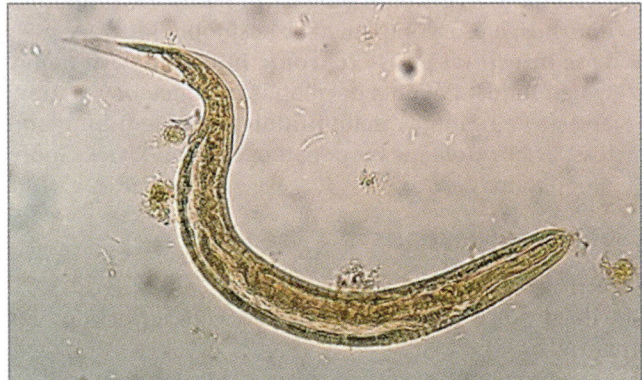

Fig. 55.10: Rhabditiform larva of *Strongyloides stercoralis* (Iodine mount).
Source: Department of Microbiology, Meenakshi Medical College, Chennai (*with permission*).

❖ Sometimes, the hookworm eggs may hatch in the stool releasing the rhabditiform larva which has to be differentiated from that of *S. stercoralis*.

Stool Culture
Various stool culture techniques used are: Harada-Mori filter paper tube method and agar plate technique. It is useful to differentiate rhabditiform larvae of *Strongyloides* from hookworm.

Other Diagnostic tests
❖ **Serology** by ELISA using crude larval antigens has a greater sensitivity.
❖ **Coproantigen** detection in stool is useful.
❖ Molecular diagnosis by real-time PCR assays has high sensitivity.

> **TREATMENT** — Strongyloidiasis
> Ivermectin is the drug of choice and is more effective than albendazole.

CHAPTER 55 ◆ Intestinal Nematodes

■ LARVA MIGRANS

Larva migrans refer to the lesions produced by nematodes of lower animals when they accidentally infect man.

Arrested Life Cycle and Pathogenesis

There are a number of nematodes of lower animals for which humans are an abnormal accidental host.

- Larvae of these lower animal nematodes when accidentally infect man, they are not able to complete their normal development (because humans are the unusual host for them) and their life cycle gets arrested. The larvae wander around aimlessly in the body. This is called larva migrans (LM).
- In some cases, transmission to man occurs through ingestion of embryonated eggs (infective form) contaminated in soil. Larvae hatch out and then wander aimlessly.

Larva migrans occur in—cutaneous and visceral forms.

Cutaneous Larva Migrans

It is also called **creeping eruption**. Larva migration occurs in the skin and subcutaneous tissue, following which the life cycle gets arrested.

- It is mainly caused by nonhuman hookworm species such as *Ancylostoma brasiliensis, A. caninum,* and *A. ceylanicum.*
- Rarely, can be caused by human nematodes such as *Strongyloides stercoralis* (larva currens), *Ancylostoma duodenale,* and *Necator americanus* (ground itch).
- **Diagnosis** made mainly by clinical feature (presence of the linear tracks) and history of exposure. Larvae are usually not detected in skin biopsy. Elevated eosinophilia may be seen in peripheral blood or sputum.

Table 55.2: Etiology of larva migrans (LM).

Causes of cutaneous larva migrans (CLM)	
Important causes (nonhuman *Ancylostoma* species): • *A. brasiliensis* • *A. caninum* • *A. ceylanicum*	**Rare causes:** Occasionally human nematodes may cause LM: • *Strongyloides stercoralis* • *Ancylostoma duodenale* • *Necator americanus*
Other rare nematodes: • *Gnathostoma spinigerum* • *Uncinaria stenocephala* • *Bunostomum phlebotomum*	**Due to non-helminthic agents:** • *Hypoderma* species • *Gasterophilus* species
Causes of visceral larva migrans (VLM)	
Important causes: *Toxocara* species (*T. canis* and *T. cati*)	
Other agents: • *Angiostrongylus* species • *Gnathostoma spinigerum* • *Anisakis* species	• *Baylisascaris procyonis* • *Hexametra leidyi* • *Lagochilascaris minor*

A list of agents causing cutaneous larva migrans is given in **Table 55.2**.

Visceral Larva Migrans

Larva migrates to viscera, following which the life cycle gets arrested. It is caused by various nematodes of lower animals such as:

- *Toxocara canis*: Infects the liver (hepatomegaly) and other organs. It can also infect eyes (ocular larva migrans) causing painless chorioretinal granuloma
- *Angiostrongylus cantonensis:* Infects CNS and causes eosinophilic meningitis.

A list of agents causing visceral larva migrans is given in **Table 55.2**.

EXPECTED QUESTIONS

I. **Write essays on:**
 1. Discuss the life cycle, clinical manifestations and laboratory diagnosis of *Ascaris lumbricoides* infection.
 2. Discuss the life cycle, clinical manifestations, and laboratory diagnosis of hookworm infection.
 3. Discuss the life cycle, clinical manifestations, and laboratory diagnosis of *Strongyloides stercoralis* infection.

II. **Write short notes on:**
 1. Laboratory diagnosis of *Enterobius vermicularis* infection
 2. Laboratory diagnosis of *Trichuris trichiura* infection
 3. Larva migrans

III. **Multiple Choice Questions (MCQs):**
 1. **All of the following intestinal nematodes are oviparous,** *except***:**
    a. Roundworm b. *Strongyloides*
    c. Hookworm d. *Enterobius*
 2. **Barrel-shaped eggs are seen for:**
    a. Pinworm b. Roundworm
    c. Hookworm d. Whipworm
 3. **Nocturnal anal pruritus is seen for:**
    a. Pinworm b. Roundworm
    c. Hookworm d. Whipworm
 4. **Hyperinfection syndrome is seen for:**
    a. Roundworm b. *Strongyloides*
    c. Hookworm d. *Enterobius*

Answers
1. b 2. d 3. a 4. b

Tissue Nematodes

CHAPTER 56

CHAPTER PREVIEW

- Filarial nematodes
- *Dracunculus medinensis*
- *Trichinella spiralis*

Somatic or tissue nematodes are the group of nematodes that reside in various tissues or organs.
- **Filarial nematodes:** They comprise several vector-borne parasites (described below)
- ***Dracunculus medinensis*:** Causes Guinea-worm disease; presents as painful cutaneous blisters
- ***Trichinella spiralis*:** Produces profuse watery diarrhea and myalgia.

■ FILARIAL NEMATODES

Filarial nematodes are vector-borne parasites that reside in the lymphatic system, skin, subcutaneous tissue, and rarely in body cavities. Accordingly, they cause various types of clinical manifestations in humans **(Table 56.1)**.
- **Lymphatic filariasis:** Filarial worms reside in the lymphatics; and produce chronic obstruction and fibrosis of lymphatics. Agents include:
    - *Wuchereria bancrofti*
    - *Brugia malayi* and *Brugia timori*
- **Cutaneous and ocular filariasis:** The agents include *Loa loa*, *Onchocerca volvulus* and *Mansonella* species. They reside in the skin, subcutaneous tissues, and some in the eyes and serous cavity. They produce various cutaneous and ocular manifestations.

Morphology

Filarial nematodes are viviparous; exist in two morphological forms: adult worm and larvae (four stages). There is no egg stage.
- **Filariform larva:** It is the third stage larva; which is the infective form to man
- **Microfilariae:** They are the first-stage larvae and also the diagnostic form in the blood. They usually reside in pulmonary blood vessels and occasionally come to the peripheral blood at a specific time, according to the '*periodicity of the parasite*'.
    - **Nocturnal:** peak at night (9 pm to 4 am), e.g. *Wuchereria* and *Brugia*
    - **Diurnal:** peaks at mid-day (12 noon–2.00 pm), e.g. *Loa loa*
    - **Subperiodic:** Peaks in the afternoon (3–5 pm), or late evening (7–9 pm), e.g. *Wuchereria* transmitted through *Aedes* mosquito
    - **Non-periodic:** No periodicity is noticed, e.g. *Onchocerca* and *Mansonella*.

■ WUCHERERIA BANCROFTI

W. bancrofti, is the most widely distributed filarial parasite of humans; accounts for >90% of cases of lymphatic

Table 56.1: Differences between various filarial nematodes causing lymphatic filariasis.

Parasite/Disease	Location of adult	Location of microfilaria	Microfilaria periodicity	Vector
Wuchereria bancrofti (bancroftian filariasis)	Lymphatic tissue	Blood, rarely hydrocele fluid and chylous urine	Nocturnal (mostly)	*Culex*—Worldwide *Anopheles* in rural Africa
			Subperiodic (rare)	*Aedes*
Brugia malayi (brugian filariasis)	Lymphatic tissue	Blood	Nocturnal (mostly)	*Mansonia* *Anopheles*
			Subperiodic (rare)	*Coquillettidia* and *Mansonia*
Brugia timori	Lymphatic tissue	Blood	Nocturnal	*Anopheles barbirostris*

filariasis. In general, *W. bancrofti* is nocturnally periodic, except in Pacific Islands; where it is subperiodic.

Life Cycle (Fig. 56.1)

W. bancrofti completes its life cycle in two hosts—(i) man (definitive host), and (ii) intermediate host (mosquito).
* *Culex quinquefasciatus* is the principal vector worldwide
* Rarely, *Anopheles* (in rural Africa) or *Aedes* (in Pacific Island) can serve as a vector. Subperiodic *W. bancrofti* is transmitted by *Aedes* mosquito.

Human Cycle

L_3 filariform larvae (infective form) get deposited in the skin by the mosquito bite.
* **Develop into adults:** Larvae penetrate the skin, enter into lymphatic vessels, and migrate to the local lymph nodes where they molt twice to develop into adult worms
* **Adults lay L_1 larvae:** Adult worms reside in the lymphatics or lymph nodes where undergo fertilization to produce L_1 larvae (**microfilariae**). Male worms die after mating, whereas female worms live long (pathogenic form).

Mosquito Cycle

When the mosquito bites an infected man, the microfilariae are ingested. *Culex* bites at night, whereas *Aedes* bites in the daytime. Inside the mosquito, the microfilariae molt twice to develop into L_3 larvae (infective stage to man).

Clinical Features

The incubation period is about 8–16 months. Clinical manifestations can be categorized into: (1) lymphatic filariasis and (2) tropical pulmonary eosinophilia.

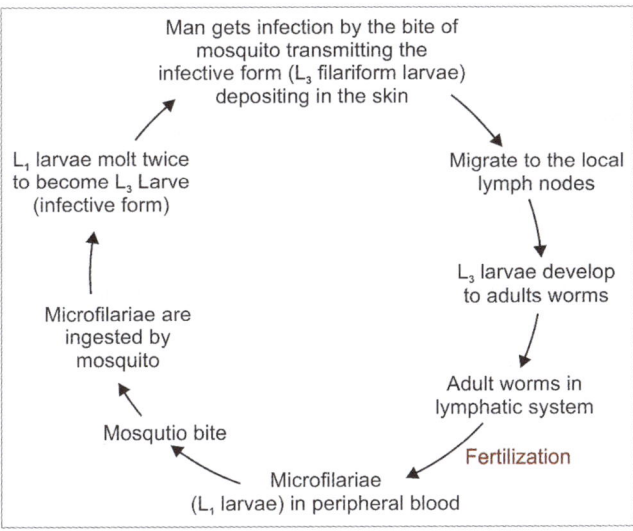

Fig. 56.1: Life cycle of *Wuchereria bancrofti*.

Lymphatic Filariasis

Lymphatic filariasis passes through four stages.
* **Endemic normal:** These are the normal people residing in an endemic area. They are not infected by the parasite due to various reasons insufficient exposure, immunological resistance
* **Asymptomatic microfilaremia:** In the endemic area, many infected individuals do not exhibit any symptoms of filarial infection, but microfilariae can be demonstrated in their peripheral blood
* **Acute filariasis** (acute adenolymphangitis): It is characterized by recurrent episodes of:
  * Filarial fever (high-grade fever)
  * Lymphatic inflammation (lymphangitis and lymphadenitis)
  * Transient local edema: Early pitting edema; reversible on limb elevation
  * Dermatolymphangitis: A plaque-like lesion is formed over the affected skin with fever, chill, and lymphatic inflammation
* **Chronic filariasis:** It develops 10–15 years after infection. Chronic host immune response against the dead worms leads to granuloma formation and fibrosis of the lymph vessels leading to severe lymphatic obstruction and pedal edema. The common manifestations are:
  * Elephantiasis: Swelling of the lower limb or less commonly arm, vulva, or breast **(Fig. 56.2A)**
  * Hydrocele: Fluid collection in testes **(Fig. 56.2B)**
  * Chronic funiculitis and epididymitis
  * Chyluria: Excretion of a milky white fluid (chyle) in urine, due to rupture of lymph vessels into the urinary system.

Tropical Pulmonary Eosinophilia (TPE)

TPE is also called **occult filariasis**, represents a hypersensitivity reaction to microfilaria antigen.

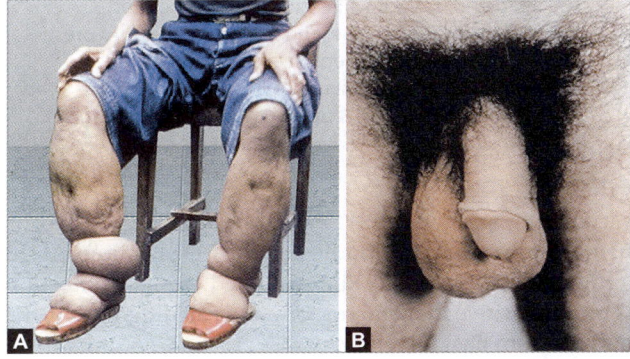

Figs. 56.2A and B: Clinical features of filariasis: **A.** Elephantiasis; **B.** Hydrocele of scrotum.

Source: **A.** ID#-373; **B.** ID# 354, Public Health Image Library, Centers for Disease Control and Prevention (CDC), Atlanta (*with permission*).

Microfilariae are rapidly cleared from the bloodstream and filtered, lodged, and destroyed in the lungs initiating an allergic response. Hence, microfilariae are not detected in the peripheral blood.
- **Common features** include nocturnal paroxysmal cough and wheezing weight loss, and low-grade fever.
- **Diagnosis:** Occult filariasis is diagnosed by blood eosinophilia, diffuse infiltration (chest X-ray), and elevated serum IgE levels
- **Treatment:** It responds well to diethylcarbamazine (DEC).

Laboratory Diagnosis

Microscopy (To Detect Microfilariae)

Microfilariae can be found in blood, and occasionally in hydrocele fluid, urine, or other body fluids.
- **Methods:** Include (i) direct wet mount, (ii) peripheral blood smear (thick and thin), and (iii) quantitative buffy coat examination (QBC)
- **Collection time:** Should be as per the periodicity of the microfilariae—e.g. for nocturnal periodicity, blood should be collected between 9 pm and 4 am
- **DEC provocation test:** This test is done to collect the blood in the daytime.
    - The patient takes a DEC tablet orally so that the nocturnal microfilariae are stimulated and come to peripheral blood within 30 min
    - Contraindicated for *Onchocerca* and *Loa loa*
- **False-negative:** Microfilariae may not be found in blood for many reasons such as:
    - Occult filariasis
    - Chronic filariasis and endemic normal people
    - Wrong time of blood collection.

> **Microfilaria (*W. bancrofti*)**
> Detection of microfilariae in peripheral blood is diagnostic of filariasis **(Figs. 56.4A and B)**.
> ❑ It measures 260 μm long, covered by a long hyaline sheath
> ❑ The head end is blunt while the tail end is pointed
> ❑ The nuclei are large, coarse, and well-separated and present throughout the body except near the tail end
> ❑ It differs from the microfilaria of *Brugia malayi* in the head and tail region **(Figs. 56.3 and 56.4)**.

Antigen Detection

Circulating antigens of *W. bancrofti* can be detected by using monoclonal antibodies against Og4C3 and AD12 antigens by methods like ELISA and ICT. Antigen detection is more sensitive than microscopy and can differentiate the current from past infection.

Antibody Detection

In the endemic area, antibody detection tests are useful only for epidemiologic purposes.

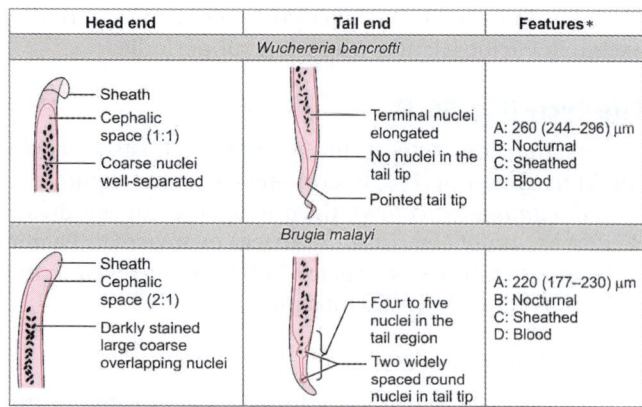

Fig. 56.3: Differences between the microfilaria of *Wuchereria bancrofti* and *Brugia malayi*.

Imaging Methods

Imaging methods are useful for the following purposes.
- **Ultrasound:** Serpentine movement of adult worms within the lymphatic vessels of the scrotum, called **filarial dance sign**—is positive in 80% of cases
- **Lymphoscintigraphy** of the limbs demonstrates the functional abnormalities of lymphatics.

Molecular Methods

Molecular methods such as PCR and real-time PCR are useful; have several advantages such as: (i) Can detect low levels of parasitemia and (ii) useful for monitoring treatment response.

Other Methods

- Eosinophilia
- Elevated serum concentrations of IgE
- Urine examination reveals microscopic hematuria and proteinuria.

> **TREATMENT** Lymphatic filariasis
> ❑ **Diethylcarbamazine (DEC):** It is the drug of choice. It can kill both adult worms and microfilariae
> ❑ **Albendazole:** It is active against both adult worms and microfilariae
> ❑ **Ivermectin:** It can kill microfilariae but does not affect adult worms.

■ BRUGIA MALAYI

Brugia malayi accounts for 10% of lymphatic filariasis.
- It occurs primarily in Eastern India and Kerala
- **The life cycle** of *B. malayi* is similar to *W. bancrofti* except that *Mansonia* is the main vector followed by *Anopheles* and *Aedes*

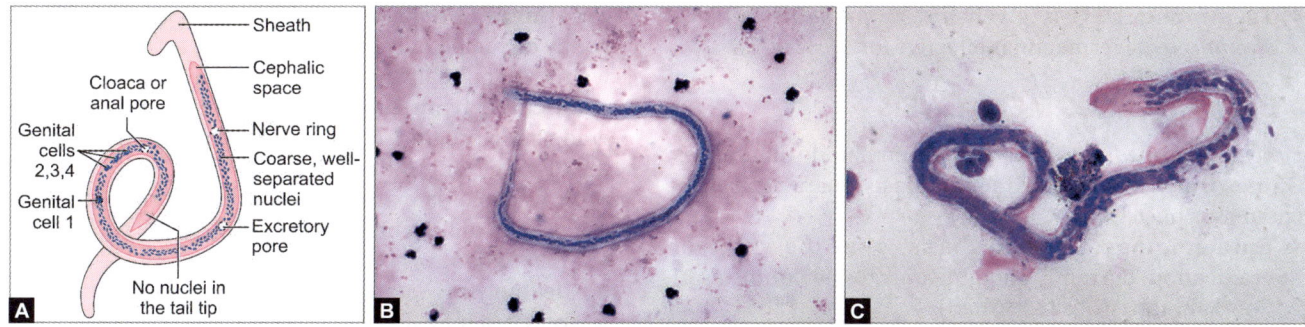

Figs. 56.4A to C: A. Microfilaria of *Wuchereria bancrofti* (schematic); **B and C.** Thick blood smear stained with Giemsa stain showing microfilariae of (B) *Wuchereria bancrofti*; (C) *Brugia* species.
Source: **B.** ID# 3009/; **C.** ID# 3003; Dr. Mae Melvin, Public Health Image Library, Centers for Disease Control and Prevention (CDC), Atlanta.

- ❖ **Clinical features** are similar to bancroftian filariasis except:
  - Frequent episodes of acute adenolymphangitis, and filarial abscesses
  - Chronic manifestations (lymphedema and elephantiasis) occur less frequently
  - The genital involvement is not seen
  - Elephantiasis: Swelling is limited to the leg below the knee
  - Chyluria does not occur.
- ❖ **Detection of microfilaria** of *B. malayi* in peripheral blood confirms the diagnosis **(Fig. 56.4C)**.
  - Measures 220 μm long, covered by a sheath
  - Nuclei are large, coarse, darkly stained, overlapping, and present throughout the body, extending till the tail region
  - The tail tip is blunt and contains two-widely spaced nuclei
- ❖ **Antibody detection** methods include—(i) ***Brugia* rapid** (ICT), and (ii) **Bm14 ELISA** employing recombinant *B. malayi* antigen (Bm14) is available
- ❖ **Prevention** by removal of pistia plants: Mosquito breeding is best controlled by removing/destroying the supporting pistia plants.

Brugia timori

B. timori can also cause lymphatic filariasis. It is limited to the Timor islands of Indonesia. It is transmitted by *Anopheles barbirostris*. Clinical features, laboratory diagnosis, and treatment are similar to *B. malayi*.

■ CUTANEOUS FILARIASIS

There are many other filarial nematodes which reside in skin and subcutaneous tissues producing several cutaneous manifestations—*Loa loa, Onchocerca volvulus,* and *Mansonella* species.

Loa loa

Loa loa (also called as African eye worm), causes infection of subcutaneous tissue and eyes. Infection is restricted to West and Central Africa.

- ❖ **Transmission:** By the bite of *Chrysops* species (deer flies, or tabanid flies)
- ❖ **Clinical features:** It produces subcutaneous swelling of the knee or wrist (called **Calabar swelling**) or also affects the eyes (conjunctival granuloma)
- ❖ **Peripheral blood smear:** Blood is collected in the daytime (12–2pm) as microfilaria shows diurnal periodicity. Microfilariae are sheathed and bear a column of nuclei extending till the tail tip.
- ❖ **Treatment:** DEC is the drug of choice.

Onchocerca volvulus

Onchocerca volvulus is endemic in West Africa and also in South and Central America.
- ❖ **Transmission:** By the bite of *Simulium* (black flies).
- ❖ **Clinical features:** It affects skin, eyes, and lymph nodes
  - Skin: produces dermatitis (pruritic rashes) and subcutaneous nodules (called **onchocercoma**)
  - Eyes: bilateral blindness (**river blindness**)
  - Lymphadenopathy: enlarged inguinal nodes may hang down (**'hanging groin'**)
- ❖ **Diagnosis:** Microfilariae are detected in a skin snip smear. They have a pointed tail tip without any nuclei. They are unsheathed and non-periodic
- ❖ **Mazzotti skin test:** Topical application of DEC on the skin leads to local reaction (erythema and itching) to the dead worm. It is also called as DEC patch test
- ❖ **Treatment:** Ivermectin is the drug of choice.

Mansonella Species

There are three species of *Mansonella*, affecting various regions of Africa and in Central and South America—*M. perstans, M. streptocerca,* and *M. ozzardi*.
- ❖ **Transmission:** By the bite of *Culicoides* (midges)
- ❖ **Clinical feature:** Most infections are asymptomatic. Rarely can produce skin lesions like pruritic rashes, subcutaneous swelling, etc.
- ❖ **Laboratory diagnosis:** Detection of characteristic microfilariae in blood or skin snips confirms the diagnosis. They are unsheathed and non-periodic.

❖ **Treatment:** DEC is given for *M. perstans* and *M. streptocerca*. Ivermectin is effective for *M. ozzardi*.

DRACUNCULUS MEDINENSIS

Dracunculus medinensis is a somatic nematode that causes **Guinea worm disease** or **dracunculiasis**, characterized by cutaneous blisters.

❖ **Epidemiology:** Dracunculiasis is on the verge of eradication, currently endemic only to 3-4 countries in Sub-Saharan Africa (e.g. Chad)
❖ **Hosts**: Involves two hosts—definitive host (man) and intermediate host (*Cyclops*)
❖ **Transmission:** Man gets infection by drinking water from stagnant pools containing minute freshwater *Cyclops* infected with third-stage L_3 larvae (infective form)
❖ **Clinical features:** After the L_3 larvae become adults, the female worms migrate to the skin, particularly over the ankles, feet, and lower legs, and induce a local painful blister **(Fig. 56.5A)**
❖ **Diagnosis:** When the skin comes in contact with water, the blister eventually ruptures, releasing large numbers of adult worms and L_1 larvae into the water **(Fig. 56.5B)**.

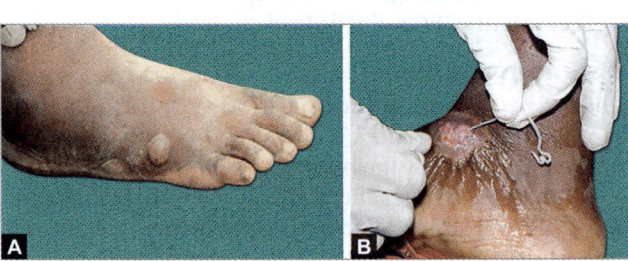

Figs. 56.5A and B: Dracunculiasis: **A.** Blister formed; **B.** Adult female worm of *Dracunculus medinensis* emerging from the blister.
Source: DPDx Image Library, Centers for Disease Control and Prevention (CDC), Atlanta (*with permission*).

❖ **Treatment (worm removal):** Worms are slowly and gently extracted over 15–20 days using a small stick and wounding out daily with small traction
❖ **Eradicated from India:** The national guinea worm eradication program had initiated measures to eradicate the disease from India such as
  ▪ Provision of safe drinking water: Filtration of drinking water, installing hand pumps and pipes
  ▪ *Cyclops* control
  ▪ Cleaning the water of boreholes or wells (was a major source of infection).

TRICHINELLA SPIRALIS

Trichinella spiralis causes trichinellosis, which is a zoonotic infection from pigs or other carnivores.

❖ **Host:** Pigs are the usual host; man is an accidental host and acts as a dead end
❖ **Transmission:** By ingestion of raw or uncooked pork containing infective form L_1 larvae
❖ **Clinical features:** Ingested L_1 larvae are released from pig meat in the intestine and are carried to skeletal muscles, where they become encysted (*muscle encystment*). Common symptoms are myositis, muscle edema, and weakness (myalgia)
❖ **A definite diagnosis** is made by the demonstration of larvae in muscle biopsy; obtained from gastrocnemius, deltoid, and biceps
❖ **Other diagnostic modalities** include antibody detection (by ELISA), coproantigen detection in the stool (by ELISA), and a skin test called **Bachman intradermal test**
❖ **Treatment:** Mebendazole and albendazole are active against enteric stages of the parasite, but their efficacy against encysted larvae has not been conclusively demonstrated.

EXPECTED QUESTIONS

I. Write an essay on:
1. Discuss the etiological agents, clinical manifestations, and laboratory diagnosis of lymphatic filariasis.

II. Write short notes on:
1. Brugian filariasis.
2. Cutaneous filariasis
3. *Dracunculus medinensis*

III. Multiple Choice Questions (MCQs):
1. **Microfilaria of *Brugia malayi* differs from that of *Wuchereria bancrofti* by all, *except*:**
   a. Nuclei are large, coarse, darkly stained
   b. Nuclei are overlapping and present throughout the body
   c. The tail tip is blunt
   d. The tail tip free from nuclei
2. **Which of the following microfilaria comes to peripheral blood in the daytime?**
   a. *Brugia malayi*   b. *Wuchereria bancrofti*
   c. *Loa loa*   d. *Brugia timori*

Answers
1. d   2. c

Medical Entomology

CHAPTER 57

CHAPTER PREVIEW
- Medical entomology
- Vector
- Class insecta
- Class arachnida
- Class crustacea
- Control of arthropods

MEDICAL ENTOMOLOGY

A study of the arthropods of medical importance is known as **medical entomology**. Arthropods act as important vectors in disease transmission of many parasitic diseases which are of human concern. Arthropods are invertebrates, consisting of a segmented body, several pairs of jointed legs, rigid exoskeleton, internal organs and body divided into head, thorax, and abdomen.

Phylum Arthropoda is divided into five classes, out of which Class Insecta, Class Arachnida, and Class Crustacea are of medical importance **(Tables 57.1 and 57.2)**.

Ectoparasites inhabit the surface of the body of the host without penetrating into the tissues. They are important vectors transmitting the pathogenic microbes. The infection by these parasites is called as infestation. Examples include louse, fleas, mites, ticks etc. Some of these ectoparasites may penetrate into the host causing disease; examples include myasis and scabies (described later in this chapter).

VECTOR

It is an arthropod that transmits infection. Transmission of infection to the host is by biting or by deposition of the infective material near the bite, on food or other objects. Biological transmission are of three types (see highlight box).

> **Biological transmission**
> - **Propagative:** Only multiplication of the parasite takes place inside the vector, e.g. *Yersinia pestis* in rat fleas
> - **Cyclodevelopmental:** Only development of the parasite takes place inside the vector, e.g. *Wuchereria bancrofti* in mosquitoes
> - **Cyclopropagative:** Multiplication and development (both) takes place inside the vector, e.g. *Plasmodium* species in mosquitoes.

CLASS INSECTA

Mosquitoes

Anopheles, *Culex*, *Aedes* and *Mansonia* are the common mosquitoes which transmit infection to man.

Identification Features

Body of mosquito consists of three parts:
- ❖ **Head:** It is semi-globular, bears a pair of compound eyes, a long proboscis, a pair of palpi and a pair of antennae (bushy in males). The proboscis is used by the mosquito for biting during the feed
- ❖ **Thorax:** It is large and rounded. It bears a pair of wings dorsally and three pairs of legs ventrally
- ❖ **Abdomen:** It is long, narrow and has ten segments. The last two segments are modified to form external genitalia. General identification features and diseases transmitted by *Anopheles*, *Culex* and *Aedes* mosquitoes are described in **Tables 57.2 and 57.3**.

Flies

Housefly

Musca domestica is the most common house frequenting fly. It is non-biting in nature. They act as mechanical vector for transmission of many diseases (*see* **Fig. 57.1A**).

Table 57.1: Classification of arthropods (Phylum Arthropoda).

Class	Common names
Insecta	Mosquitoes, black flies, sand flies, deer flies, house flies, tsetse flies, fleas, cockroaches, lice, bugs, etc.
Arachnida	Hard ticks, soft ticks, itch mites, chiggers, etc.
Myriapoda	Centipedes, millipedes, etc.
Pentastomida	Tongue worms, etc.
Crustacea	*Cyclops*, crabs, crayfish, etc.

SECTION 6 ❖ Parasitology

Table 57.2: Arthropods acting as vectors in transmission of medically important human diseases.

Arthropods	Diseases transmitted		
	Parasitic	**Viral**	**Bacterial**
Mosquito	Malaria (*Anopheles*) Bancroftian filariasis (*Culex, Aedes* and *Anopheles*) Malayan filariasis (*Mansonia, Anopheles*)	Yellow fever (*Aedes*) Dengue fever (*Aedes*) Chikungunya (*Aedes*) Japanese encephalitis (*Culex*) O'Nyong-Nyong (*Anopheles*)	–
Sandfly	Kala-azar Oriental sore	Sandfly fever (Papatasi fever)	Oroya fever (Carrion's disease)
Tsetse fly	Sleeping sickness	–	–
Housefly (mechanical vector)	Amoebiasis Intestinal helminthiasis	Poliomyelitis Enterically transmitted hepatitis (hepatitis A and E)	Typhoid fever Paratyphoid fever Cholera Trachoma Yaws
Blackfly (*Simulium* species)	Onchocerciasis	–	–
Deer fly	Loiasis	–	–
Rat flea (*Xenopsylla cheopis*)	*Hymenolepis diminuta* and *Hymenolepis nana*	–	Bubonic plague Endemic typhus
Cockroach (mechanical vector)	Amoebiasis Helminthiasis	Hepatitis Poliomyelitis	Enteric pathogens
Reduviid bug	Chagas' disease	–	–
Louse	Ectoparasitic infection	–	Relapsing fever Epidemic typhus Trench fever
Hard tick	Babesiosis	Viral encephalitis Viral fever Viral hemorrhagic fever	Tularemia Tick typhus
Soft tick	–	–	Q-fever Relapsing fever
Trombiculid mite	–	–	Scrub typhus Rickettsial pox
Itch mite	Scabies	–	–
Cyclops	Dracunculiasis Diphyllobothriasis Gnathostomiasis	–	–
Crabs and crayfish	Paragonimiasis	–	–

Identification features
- **Head:** It has a pair of compound eyes, a pair of antennae and a single proboscis on its head
- **Thorax:** Has pair of wings and three pairs of legs
- **Abdomen:** Segmented and shows dark and light markings.

Diseases transmitted by housefly—refer **Table 57.2**.

Sandfly

Identification features
Sandflies are light or dark brown flies, smaller than mosquitoes **(Fig. 57.1B)**.

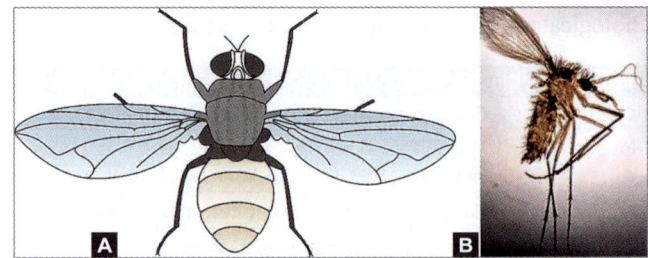

Figs. 57.1A and B: A. Housefly (schematic diagram); **B.** Sandfly (real image).
Source: **B.** Public Health Image Library, ID# 6273/Centers for Disease Control and Prevention (CDC), Atlanta (*with permission*).

CHAPTER 57 ◆ Medical Entomology

Table 57.3: Identification features of *Anopheles*, *Culex*, and *Aedes* mosquitoes.

Identification features	Anopheles mosquito	*Culex* mosquito	Aedes mosquito
Body	Body is slender and rests with an angle to the surface	Body rests parallel to the surface	Head is slightly bent downward and body shows a hunch back at rest
Wings	Have dark spots	Unspotted	Unspotted and has white markings on legs and abdomen (hence named as tiger mosquito)
Hind legs	Held outstretched	Curled up over the back	Held curled upward
Proboscis and body	Proboscis and body is in same straight line	Proboscis and body at an angle to one another	Proboscis and body at an angle to one another
Maxillary palpi	Maxillary palpi are as long as proboscis (both sexes)	Maxillary palpi are shorter than proboscis (females)	Maxillary palpi are shorter than proboscis (females)
Tip of the abdomen	-	Blunt	Pointed
Biting time	Each species has specific peak biting hours	Midnight	Day time
Important species	A. culicifacies A. fluviatilis A. stephensi	C. fatigans C. tritaeniorhynchus C. tarsalis	A. aegypti A. albopictus
Vector for diseases	Malaria Encephalitis	Bancroftian filariasis West Nile fever Japanese encephalitis	Yellow fever Chikungunya fever Dengue
Schematic diagram and real images of *Anopheles*; *Culex* and *Aedes* mosquitoes			

Source: DPDx Image Library, Centers for Disease Control and Prevention (CDC), Atlanta (*with permission*).

- Their body and wings are covered by dense hair
- Head contains pair of long, slender and hairy antennae, palpi and a proboscis
- Thorax contains pair of wings and three pairs of legs
- Abdomen has ten segments
- Though winged, they **only hop** about and do not fly
- The legs are longer as compared to the size of the body
- They bite during night and only females bite; the males live on fruit juices
- **Important species:** *Phlebotomus argentipes* (vector of kala-azar).

Diseases transmitted by sandfly—refer **Table 57.2**.

Tsetse Fly (Fig. 57.2A)

Tsetse flies belong to the genus *Glossina*, and family, Glossinidae. They are found only in tropical Africa.

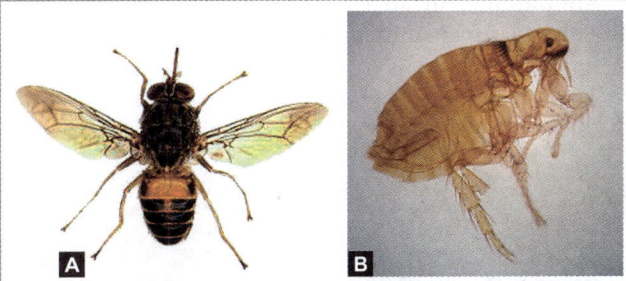

Figs. 57.2A and B: A. Tsetse fly (real image); **B.** Male rat flea (mounted specimen).

Source: **A.** DPDx Image Library, Centers for Disease Control and Prevention (CDC), Atlanta (*with permission*); **B.** Head of Deptartment, Microbiology, Meenakshi Medical College, Chennai.

- They are yellowish or dark brown, medium-sized flies
- They can be distinguished from other large biting insects by their forward pointing mouthparts

- They bite only in daytime
- They are biological vectors of trypanosomes; can transmit an infectious disease called as sleeping sickness.

Flea

Rat Flea (Fig. 57.2B)

Identification features

Fleas are small, bilaterally compressed, wingless insects.
- Important species of rat fleas are *Xenopsylla cheopis* and *X. astia*
- Contains a hard chitinous exoskeleton and their body is covered by backward pointing spines
- **Head:** Conical and attached to the thorax without neck
- **Thorax:** Contains three segments and three pairs of legs; hind legs are well developed for jumping
- Abdomen is divided into ten segments. The male contains a coiled structure, the penis, and female contains a short, stumpy structure, the spermatheca, in the abdomen. The shape of spermatheca helps in distinguishing the species.

Diseases transmitted by rat flea—*refer* **Table 57.2**.

Louse (Fig. 57.3)

Identification features

Louse is a small wingless human ectoparasite.
- Human lice are of three types—(1) head lice (*Pediculus humanus capitis*), (2) body lice (*P. humanus corporis*) and (3) pubic or crab lice (*Pthirus pubis*)
- **Head:** Pointed in front and contains a pair of five jointed antennae. Mouth parts are adapted for blood sucking and they bite severely
- **Thorax:** Square-shaped, with three pairs of legs attached ventrally. The legs are provided with claws
- **Abdomen:** Elongated in shape and has nine segments.

The diseases transmitted by louse are:
- Epidemic typhus
- Trench fever
- Epidemic relapsing fever.

CLASS ARACHNIDA

Mites

Trombiculid Mite (Fig. 57.4A)

It contains four pairs of legs (first pair of legs is the largest).
- The body is not well demarcated into three parts (head, thorax and abdomen)
- Disease transmitted—scrub typhus.

Itch Mite/Sarcoptes scabei (Fig. 57.4B)

Scabies is caused by itch Mite or *Sarcoptes scabei*. It has four stages: egg, larva, nymph and adult. Transmission to man is through transfer of impregnated female mites during person to person and skin to skin contact.

Clinical manifestations

Initial infestation is asymptomatic for two months although the person can still transmit scabies during this time.

In case of reinfection, symptoms appear much earlier in 1–4 days.
- **Primary infection:** The mites burrow into the upper layer of the skin but never below the stratum corneum. Mites burrowing under the skin cause a **rash**, which is most frequently found on the hands, particularly the finger **web spaces**; wrist folds, elbow or knee; penis and breast. **Severe itching** is the most common presentation, especially at night
- **Crusted (Norwegian) scabies**: This is a severe form of scabies, seen among persons who are immunocompromised, elderly, or institutionalized. It is characterized by vesicles and formation of thick crusts over the skin, accompanied by abundant mites but only slight itching. Secondary bacterial infections are common.

Laboratory diagnosis

Suspicion of scabies is made based upon the appearance and distribution of the rash and the presence of burrows.

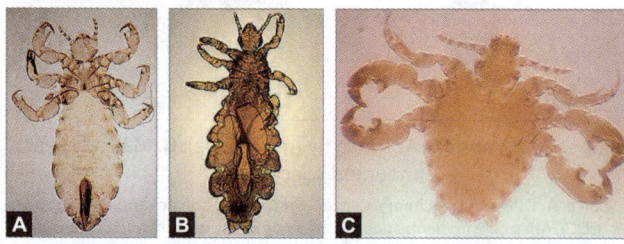

Figs. 57.3A to C: Louse (mounted specimens): **A.** Body louse; **B.** Head louse; **C.** Pubic louse (mounted specimen).

Source: DPDx Image Library, Centers for Disease Control and Prevention (CDC), Atlanta (*with permission*).

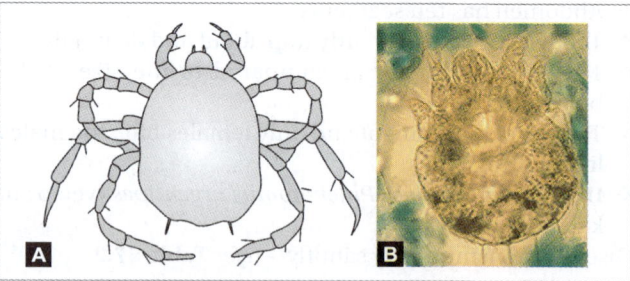

Figs. 57.4A and B: A. Trombiculid mite (schematic diagram); **B.** *Sarcoptes scabiei* (Itch mite).

Source: **B.** DPDx Image Library, Centers for Disease Control and Prevention (CDC), Atlanta (with permission).

It is confirmed by isolating the mites, ova or feces in a skin scraping at the burrows, especially on the finger webspace and wrist folds.

- ❖ **Skin scrapping:**
  - ■ Scrapings are best performed at the end of the burrows in non-excoriated and non-inflamed areas using a sterile scalpel blade containing a drop of mineral oil. The mineral oil enhances the adherence of the mites to the blade and can then be transferred to a glass slide
  - ■ An additional 1–2 drops of mineral oil can be added to the slide, followed by a coverslip for microscopic examination. Skin scrapings should be screened at 4× or 10× magnification and then evaluated at 40× magnification for confirmation.
- ❖ **Identification:** *S. scabies* is very small in size, just visible to naked eyes. Adult female mites measure 0.30–0.45 mm long; males are smaller at 0.20–0.24 mm long
  - ■ Body is rounded above and flattened below
  - ■ The body surface is covered with short bristles
  - ■ It has two pairs of legs in front, and two pairs behind
  - ■ The front legs have suckers at the end and the hind legs have long bristles.

Treatment

Scabies is treated with any of the following: (i) permethrin cream 5%, (ii) crotamiton lotion 10%, (iii) sulfur ointment 5%–10%, (iv) lindane lotion 1%, (v) oral ivermectin-two doses (200 µg/kg/dose), one week apart (vi) benzyl benzoate 25%, this is mainly for crusted scabies.

Ticks

Hard Tick (Ixodid Tick) (Fig. 57.5A)

Identification features

Hard tick has a hard, chitinous shield (scutum) covers the dorsum.
- ❖ Body cannot be distinctly separated into head, thorax and abdomen
- ❖ They have four pairs of legs, no antennae
- ❖ When viewed from above its head is visible
- ❖ They are dark/bright colored
- ❖ Both sexes suck blood and feed both day and night, cannot withstand starvation
- ❖ Medically important species:
  - ■ *Haemaphysalis* species
  - ■ *Amblyomma* species.

Diseases transmitted by hard tick—*refer* **Table 57.2**.

Soft Tick (Argasid Tick) (Fig. 57.5B)

Identification features

Ornithodoros species is a medically important soft tick
- ❖ Length of adult soft tick 5 mm
- ❖ They are oval in shape
- ❖ They have four pairs of short legs
- ❖ When viewed from above head is not visible
- ❖ They can survive without blood meals for long periods
- ❖ Both sexes suck blood
- ❖ They bite only at night time and their bite is very painful.

Diseases transmitted by soft tick—*refer* **Table 57.2**.

CLASS CRUSTACEA

Cyclops (Fig. 57.6C)

Identification Features

Cyclops are also called as **water fleas.**
- ❖ They measure less than 1mm in length and pear-shaped
- ❖ Their tail is forked
- ❖ They have two pairs of antennae, five pairs of legs and a pigmented eye
- ❖ They swim in water with typical jerky movements.

Diseases transmitted by cyclops—*refer* **Table 57.2**.

CONTROL OF ARTHROPODS

Physical Control Methods

- ❖ Proper disposal of sewage, garbage, manure and elimination of stagnant water
- ❖ Use of door and window screens and bed nets.

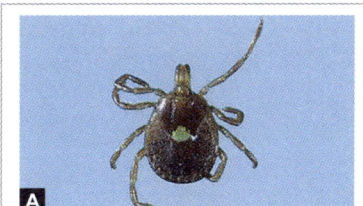 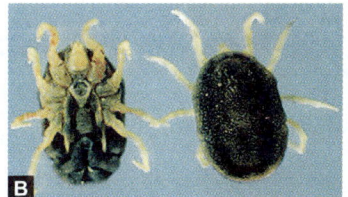 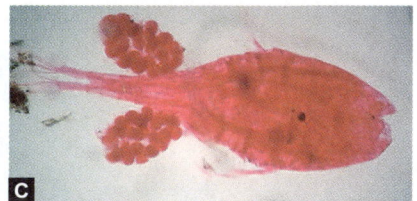

Figs. 57.5A to C: A. Female hard tick (*Amblyomma* species); **B.** Dorsal and ventral view of soft tick; **C.** Cyclops (mounted specimen).
Source: DPDx Image Library, Centers for Disease Control and Prevention (CDC), Atlanta (*with permission*).

Biological Control Methods

❖ Use of specific viruses, bacteria, protozoa, fungi which are pathogenic to various morphological forms of arthropods
❖ Use of Gambusia fish that feed on larvae of mosquitoes
❖ Barbell fish and Gambusia fish have been successfully used for control of cyclops.

Chemical Control

Insecticides can be used such as dichlorophenyl-trichloroethane (DDT), baygon and pyrethrum flowers, and arsenical compounds.

EXPECTED QUESTIONS

I. **Write short notes on:**
  1. Role of mosquitoes in transmission of infectious diseases.
  2. Role of ticks in transmission of infectious diseases.

II. **Multiple choice questions (MCQs):**
  1. **Mosquito acts as vector for transmission of all the parasitic infections,** *except*:
     a. Malaria
     b. Bancroftian filariasis
     c. Malayan filariasis
     d. Leishmaniasis
  2. **Housefly acts as mechanical vector for transmission of all the following infections,** *except*:
     a. Amoebiasis
     b. Typhoid fever
     c. Malaria
     d. Cholera
  3. **Hard tick acts as vector for transmission for which of the following parasitic infection:**
     a. Babesiosis
     b. Diphyllobothriasis
     c. Dracunculiasis
     d. Leishmaniasis
  4. **Cyclops acts as vector for transmission for all the following parasitic infections,** *except*:
     a. Diphyllobothriasis
     b. Dracunculiasis
     c. Gnathostomiasis
     d. Malaria

Answers
1. d   2. c   3. a   4. d

SECTION 7

Mycology

SECTION OUTLINE

58. Medical Mycology

Medical Mycology

CHAPTER 58

CHAPTER PREVIEW

- General Mycology
- Classification of Fungi
- Laboratory Diagnosis of Fungal Infections
- Superficial Mycoses
  - Tinea versicolor
  - Tinea nigra
  - Piedra
  - Dermatophytoses
- Subcutaneous Mycoses
- Mycetoma
- Sporotrichosis
- Chromoblastomycosis
- Phaeohyphomycosis
- Rhinosporidiosis
- Systemic Mycoses
  - Histoplasmosis
  - Blastomycosis
  - Coccidioidomycosis
  - Paracoccidioidomycosis
- Opportunistic Mycoses
  - Candidiasis
  - Cryptococcosis
  - Zygomycosis
  - Aspergillosis
  - Penicilliosis
  - Pneumocystis pneumonia
  - Fusariosis
- Mycotoxicoses

GENERAL MYCOLOGY

Medical mycology is the branch of medical science that deals with the study of medically important fungi. The name 'fungus' is derived from Greek '*mykes*' meaning mushroom (a type of edible fungus). Some of the important properties of fungi are:

- Fungi are eukaryotic and they possess all the eukaryotic cell organelles
- They possess a rigid cell wall, composed of chitin, β-glucans, and other polysaccharides
- The fungal cell membrane contains ergosterol instead of the cholesterol
- They divide by asexual and/or sexual means by producing spores.

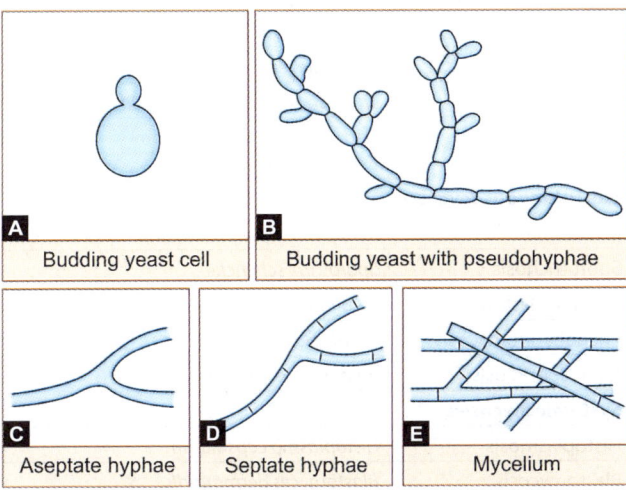

Figs. 58.1A to E: Morphological forms of fungi.

CLASSIFICATION OF FUNGI

Morphological Classification

Based on the morphological appearance, there are four main groups of fungi as follows **(Figs. 58.1A to E)**:

1. **Yeast:** They grow as round to oval cells that reproduce by an asexual process called **budding** in which cells form protuberances that enlarge and eventually separate from the parent cells. An example includes—*Cryptococcus neoformans*
2. **Yeast-like:** In some yeasts (e.g. *Candida*), the bud remains attached to the mother cell, elongates, and undergoes repeated budding to form chains of elongated cells known as **pseudohyphae**. They can be differentiated from true hyphae as they have constrictions at the septa
3. **Molds:** They grow as long branching filaments of 2–10 µm width called **hyphae**.
   - Hyphae are either septate (i.e. form transverse walls) or nonseptate (there are no transverse walls)
   - Hyphae grow continuously and form a branching tangled mass of growth called **mycelium**
   - Molds reproduce by formation of different types of sexual and asexual spores

- Examples of true molds include—Dermatophytes, *Aspergillus, Penicillium, Rhizopus, Mucor*, etc.
4. **Dimorphic fungi:** They exist as molds (hyphal form) at 25°C and as yeasts in human tissues at body temperature (37°C). Several medically important fungi are thermally dimorphic such as:
    - *Histoplasma capsulatum*
    - *Blastomyces dermatitidis*
    - *Coccidioides immitis*
    - *Paracoccidioides brasiliensis*
    - *Penicillium marneffei*
    - *Sporothrix schenckii*

Clinical Classification of Fungal Diseases

Fungal infections can be classified into four groups based on the organ/system involved and clinical manifestations produced—superficial mycoses, subcutaneous mycoses, systemic (deep) mycoses, and opportunistic mycoses **(Table 58.1)**.

Table 58.1: Classification of fungal diseases.	
Fungal disease	**Agents**
Superficial mycoses	
Tinea versicolor	*Malassezia furfur*
Tinea nigra	*Hortaea werneckii*
Piedra	*Trichosporon beigelii, Piedraia hortae*
Dermatophytosis	*Trichophyton, Microsporum, Epidermophyton*
Subcutaneous mycoses	
Mycetoma	*Madurella mycetomatis* and others
Sporotrichosis	*Sporothrix schenckii*
Chromoblastomycosis	*Phialophora* and others
Phaeohyphomycosis	*Exophiala* and others
Rhinosporidiosis	*Rhinosporidium seeberi*
Systemic mycoses	
Histoplasmosis	*Histoplasma capsulatum*
Blastomycosis	*Blastomyces dermatitidis*
Coccidioidomycosis	*Coccidioides immitis*
Paracoccidioidomycosis	*Paracoccidioides brasiliensis*
Opportunistic mycoses	
Candidiasis	*Candida albicans* and other species
Cryptococcosis	*Cryptococcus neoformans*
Zygomycosis	*Rhizopus, Mucor*
Aspergillosis	*Aspergillus flavus, Aspergillus fumigatus, Aspergillus niger*
Penicilliosis	*Penicillium marneffei*
Pneumocystosis	*Pneumocystis jirovecii*
Fusariosis	*Fusarium* species

LABORATORY DIAGNOSIS OF FUNGAL INFECTIONS

The laboratory diagnosis of fungal diseases comprises the following:

Specimen Collection

It depends on the site of infection such as skin scraping, hair, nail, sputum, etc. For systemic mycoses, blood sample may also be collected. Cerebrospinal fluid (CSF) is collected for cryptococcal meningitis.

Microscopy

Microscopy is useful to demonstrate fungal elements in clinical specimens. Following microscopy techniques are used:

- **Potassium hydroxide (KOH) preparation**: Keratinized tissue specimens such as skin scrapings and plucked hair samples are treated with 10% KOH which digests the keratin material so that the fungal hyphae will be seen under the microscope **(Fig. 58.2A)**
- **Gram stain:** It is useful in identifying the yeasts (e.g. *Cryptococcus*) and yeast-like fungi (e.g. *Candida*). They appear as gram-positive budding yeast cells **(Fig. 58.9A)**
- **India ink and nigrosin stains:** They are used as negative stains for demonstration of capsule of *Cryptococcus neoformans* **(Fig. 58.10A)**
- **Calcofluor white stain:** It is more sensitive than other stains; fungal elements fluoresce under UV light **(Fig. 58.2B)**
- **Histopathological stains:** They are useful for demonstrating fungal elements from biopsy tissues. This is useful for detecting invasive fungal infection
    - Periodic acid Schiff (PAS) stain

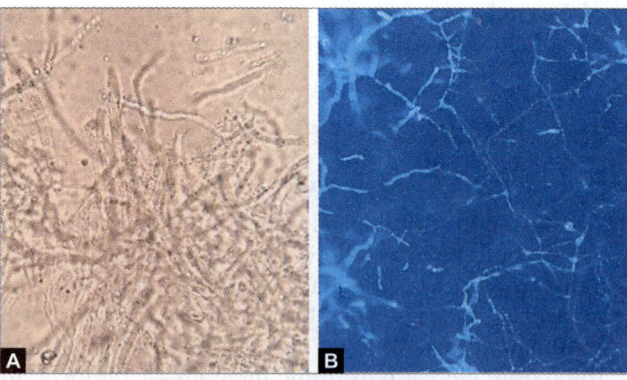

Figs. 58.2A and B: Fungal hyphae in: **A.** KOH mount; **B.** Calcofluor white stain mount.

Source: **A.** Dr Sherly Antony, Pushpagiri Institute Medical Sciences and Research Centre, Kerala; **B.** Department of Microbiology, JIPMER, Puducherry (*with permission*).

- Gomori methenamine silver (GMS) stain
- Hematoxylin and Eosin (H and E) stain.

❖ **Lactophenol cotton blue (LPCB):** It is used to study the microscopic appearance of the fungal isolates grown in culture. It contains:
- Phenol acts as disinfectant
- Lactic acid preserves the morphology of fungi
- Glycerol prevents drying
- Cotton blue stains the fungal elements blue.

Culture

A fungal culture is frequently performed for isolation and correct identification of the fungi.

Culture Media

❖ **Sabouraud's dextrose agar (SDA):** It is the most commonly used medium in diagnostic mycology. It contains peptone (1%), dextrose (4%) and has a pH of 5.6
❖ **Neutral SDA** (Emmons' modification): It differs from the original SDA in having neopeptone (1%) and dextrose (2%) and pH of 7.2
❖ **Corn meal agar and rice starch agar:** They are the nutritionally deficient media used for stimulation of chlamydospore production
❖ **Brain heart infusion (BHI) agar and blood agar:** They are the enriched media, used for growing fastidious fungi like *Cryptococcus* and *Histoplasma*
❖ **Niger seed agar** and **bird seed agar:** They are used for the selective growth of *Cryptococcus*
❖ **CHROMagar *Candida* medium:** It is used for isolation as well as a differential medium for speciation of *Candida*.

Culture Condition

❖ **Temperature:** Most of the fungi grow well at 25–30°C except the dimorphic fungi that grow at both 25°C and 37°C
❖ **Incubation:** A special incubator called as **BOD incubators** (biological oxygen demand) are used for fungal culture and culture plates should be incubated for 2–3 weeks
❖ **Antibiotics** such as cycloheximide, and chloramphenicol can be added to the culture media to inhibit bacterial growth.

Culture Identification

The correct identification of the fungus is based on the macroscopic appearance of the colonies grown on culture and microscopic appearance (LPCB mount of colonies).
❖ **Macroscopic appearance of the colony:**
- **Rate of growth** can be either (i) rapid (<5 days), as seen in yeasts and agents of opportunistic mycoses or (ii) slow growth (1–4 weeks) as observed in dermatophytes, agents of subcutaneous and systemic mycoses
- **Pigmentation:** It can be seen on the reverse side of the culture media
- **Texture:** It refers to how the colony would have felt if allowed to touch. It may be of various types such as—glabrous (waxy/leathery), velvety, yeast-like, cottony or granular/powdery
- **Colony topography:** Colony surface may be rugose (radial grooves), folded, verrucous or cerebriform (brain-like).

❖ **Microscopic appearance of fungi:** Microscopic examination of the fungi can be done by:
- **LPCB teased mount:** A bit of fungal colony is teased out from the culture tube and the LPCB mount is prepared. Fungal identification is based on the following: (i) nature of hyphae (such as septate or aseptate, hyaline or phaeoid, narrow or wide) and (ii) type of sporulation (conidia or sporangiospores)
- **Slide culture:** Though this is a tedious procedure, it gives the most accurate *in situ* microscopic appearance of the fungal colony. A sterile slide is placed on a bent glass rod in a sterile petri dish. Two square agar blocks are placed on the slide. Bit of the fungal colony is inoculated onto the margins (at the center) of the agar block. Then the coverslip is placed on the agar block and the petri dish is incubated at 25°C. After sufficient growth occurs, LPCB mounts are made both from the coverslip and the underneath slide **(Fig. 58.3)**.

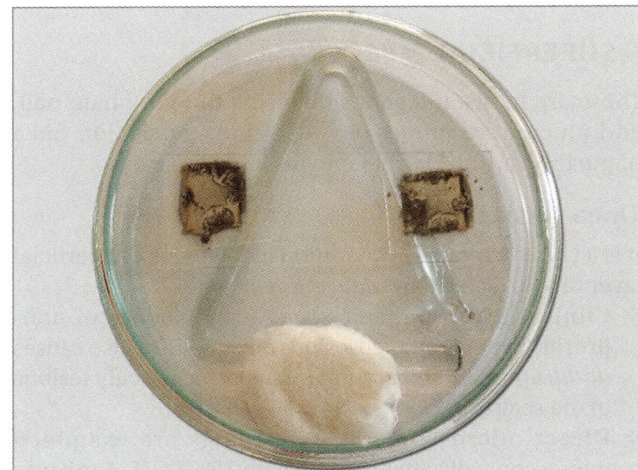

Fig. 58.3: Slide culture technique.
Source: Department of Microbiology, Pondicherry Institute of Medical Sciences, Puducherry (*with permission*).

Immunological Methods

These tests are available to detect the antibody or antigen from serum and/or other body fluids.
- **Antibody detection** can be done by ELISA and agglutination test
- **Antigen detection:** Various fungal antigens can be detected in clinical specimens such as blood, CSF, urine, etc.
  - **Cryptococcal capsular antigen** from CSF by latex agglutination test
  - Detection of *Aspergillus* specific **galactomannan antigen** in patient's sera or urine (by ELISA)
  - **β-d-Glucan assay** by ELISA: It is a marker of all invasive fungal infections.

Automation

Automated identification systems such as MALDI-TOF and VITEK are revolutionary in the accurate identification of yeasts and to some extent molds.

Molecular Methods

Molecular methods useful in the diagnosis of fungal infections include—polymerase chain reaction (PCR), real-time PCR, and DNA sequencing methods.

■ TREATMENT OF FUNGAL INFECTIONS

Some of the commonly used antifungal agents include—amphotericin B, caspofungin, griseofulvin, fluconazole and voriconazole.

Treatment of the important human fungal infections has been described in under respective fungal agents later in this chapter.

■ SUPERFICIAL MYCOSES

These are fungal infections involving the skin, hair, nail, and mucosa. Examples include—tinea versicolor, tinea nigra, Piedra, and Dermatophytosis.

Tinea Versicolor

It is a chronic recurrent condition involving the superficial layer of skin, caused by *Malassezia furfur*.
- **Clinical feature:** Manifests as scaly patches of non-pruritic hypopigmented lesions on the skin. It also causes **dandruff** in adults (erythematous pruritic scaly lesions of the scalp)
- **Direct microscopy:** Skin scrapings are examined microscopically after treating with 10% KOH. A mixture of budding yeasts and short septate hyphae are seen, described as **spaghetti and meatballs** appearance
- **Culture:** On Sabouraud dextrose agar (SDA), *Malassezia furfur* typically produces '**fried egg**' colonies
- **Treatment:** Topical lotions like selenium sulfide shampoo, ketoconazole shampoo or cream, and terbinafine cream should be used for 2 weeks.

Tinea Nigra

It is characterized by painless, black, non-scaly patches present on the palm and sole. It is caused by *Hortaea werneckii*. It is a black-colored yeast-like fungus.

Piedra

Piedra is characterized by nodule formation on the hair shaft, which may be either black or white. Accordingly, piedra is of two types.
- White piedra: caused by *Trichosporon beigelii*
- Black piedra: caused by *Piedraia hortae*

Dermatophytoses

Dermatophytoses (or tinea or ringworm) are the most common superficial mycoses affecting skin, hair, and nail; caused by a group of related fungi called **dermatophytes**. These include:
- *Trichophyton* species: Infect skin, hair, and nail
- *Microsporum* species: Infect skin and hair
- *Epidermophyton* species: Infect skin and nail.

Depending on the habitat, dermatophytes are classified as anthropophilic (humans), or zoophilic (animals) or geophilic (soil).

Pathogenesis and Clinical Types

Dermatophyte infection is acquired by direct contact with soil, animals, or humans infected with fungal spores.
- **Predisposing factors** include moist humid skin and tight ill-fitting underclothing
- **Spread:** The spores are carried to different areas (skin, hair, or nail) due to scratching of the inoculated site
- **Skin:** Dermatophytes produce well-demarcated annular- or ring-shaped pruritic scaly skin lesions
- **Nails:** They invade the nails and then spread throughout the nails
- **Hair shafts:** They can invade within the hair shaft (called endothrix) or may be found surrounding it (called ectothrix). Hair becomes brittle and areas of alopecia may appear
- **Clinical types:** Depending on the site of involvement, various clinical types of ringworm infections are produced (**Table 58.2**).

CHAPTER 58 ◆ Medical Mycology

Table 58.2: Clinical types of dermatophytoses.

Clinical types	Area involved
Tinea capitis (Fig. 58.4A)	Infection of the scalp, producing scaly patches on the scalp, and broken hair shafts (alopecia)
Tinea faciei	Infection of the non-bearded area of the face (Fig. 58.4B)
Tinea pedis	Infection of the web space between the toes, (also called athlete's foot) (Fig. 58.4C)
Tinea corporis	Infection of the non-hairy skin of the body (trunk and limbs) (Fig. 58.4D)
Tinea cruris	Infection of the groin area (called jock itch)
Tinea barbae	Infection of the beard area of the face
Tinea unguium	Infection of nail beds

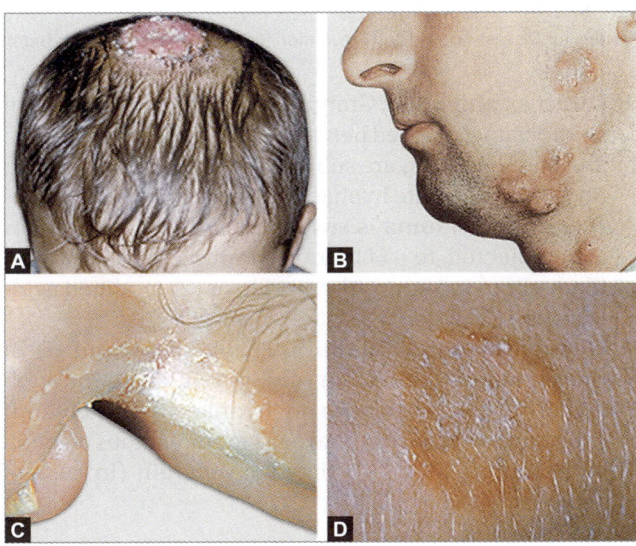

Figs. 58.4A to D: Ring worm infections (Tinea): **A.** Tinea capitis; **B.** Tinea faciei; **C.** Tinea pedis; **D.** Tinea corporis.

Source: Public Health Image Library: **A.** ID#: 2936; **B.** ID#: 4807; **C.** ID#: 2939; **D.** ID#: 2938, Centers for Disease Control and Prevention (CDC), Atlanta (*with permission*).

Laboratory Diagnosis

Specimen Collection

Skin scrapings, hair pluckings, and nail clippings are obtained from the active margin of the lesions and are kept in folded black paper. Hair should be plucked, but not cut.

Culture

Specimens should be inoculated onto SDA and incubated at 26–28°C for 4 weeks. Identification is made by:
* Macroscopic appearance of the colonies
* Microscopic appearance: The colonies are teased and subjected to lactophenol cotton blue (LPCB) mount to demonstrate the hyphae and spores. Spores are of two types—macroconidia and macroconidia, which help in identification (**Figs. 58.5A to C and Table 58.3**).

Other Methods of Diagnosis

Apart from culture, there are several other methods available for the identification of dermatophytes such as:
* Hair perforation test
* Urease test
* Dermatophyte test medium
* Dermatophyte identification medium
* Molecular methods such as PCR
* Woods lamp examination

> **TREATMENT** — **Dermatophytoses**
>
> ❏ **Oral terbinafine or itraconazole** are the drugs of choice for the treatment of dermatophytosis:
> ❏ Alternative: Oral griseofulvin and ketoconazole
> ❏ Topical lotions such as Whitfield ointment or tolnaftate can be applied.

■ SUBCUTANEOUS MYCOSES

The agents of subcutaneous mycoses usually inhabit the soil. They enter the skin by traumatic inoculation with contaminated material.

Mycetoma

Mycetoma is a chronic, slowly progressive granulomatous infection of the skin and subcutaneous tissues.
* Mycetoma is also known as **Maduramycosis** or **Madura foot,** as it was first described in Madurai
* **Types**: Mycetoma can be classified into two types.
  * **Eumycetoma:** Caused by fungal agents, that may produce black or white granules. Black granules are produced by *Madurella mycetomatis, Madurella grisea,* etc. White granules are produced by *Pseudallescheria boydii, Aspergillus nidulans,* etc.
  * **Actinomycetoma:** Caused by bacteria such as *Nocardia* or *Actinomadura madurae.* They produce white to yellow granules.

Table 58.3: Distribution of conidia of dermatophytes.

Dermatophytes	Macroconidia	Microconidia
Trichophyton (Fig. 58.5A)	Rare, thin-walled, smooth, pencil-shaped	Abundant
Microsporum (Fig. 58.5B)	Numerous, thick-walled, rough, spindle-shaped	Rare
Epidermophyton (Fig. 58.5C)	Numerous, smooth-walled, club-shaped	Absent

SECTION 7 ❖ Mycology

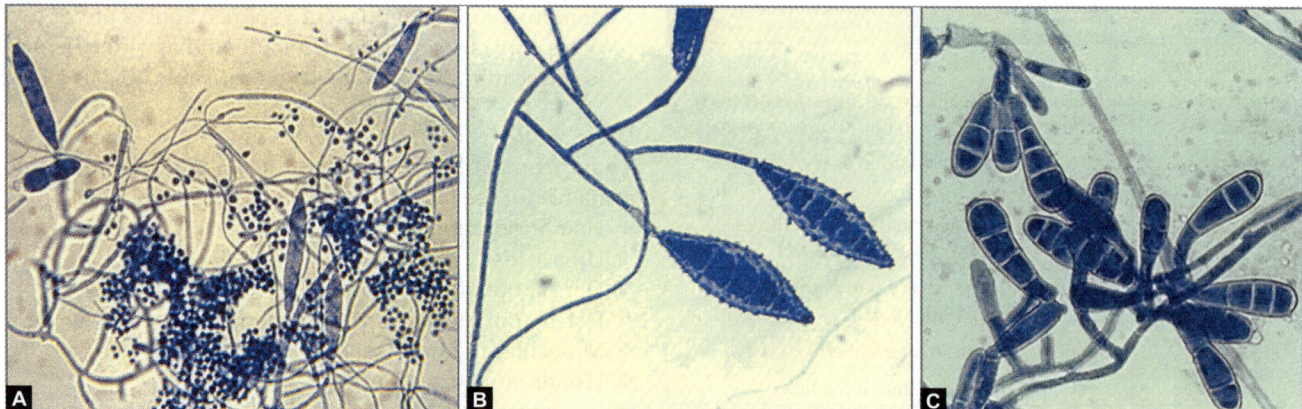

Figs. 58.5A to C: Microscopic appearance of various dermatophyte species (LPCB mount): **A.** *Trichophyton mentagrophytes*; **B.** *Microsporum canis*; **C.** *Epidermophyton floccosum*.
Source: Public Health Image Library/**A.** ID#: 15105; **B.** ID#: 15472; **C.** ID#: 14588, Centers for Disease Control and Prevention (CDC), Atlanta (*with permission*).

- ❖ **Clinical feature:** It manifests as a triad of painless subcutaneous swelling, discharging sinuses, and discharge oozing from the sinuses containing granules
  - Eumycetoma produces a single swelling with serous discharge, whereas in actinomycetoma the swellings are multiple with purulent discharge
  - Feet are the most common site affected, although any site can be involved
  - Can invade underlying fascia and bones, producing osteolytic or osteosclerotic bony lesions.
- ❖ **Specimen collection:** The lesions should be cleaned with antiseptics and the grains should be collected on sterile gauze by pressing the sinuses from the periphery or by using a loop
- ❖ **Direct examination:** Granules are thoroughly washed in sterile saline; crushed between the slides and examined. The black granules are subjected to KOH mount, which reveals thin septate hyphae of 2–6 μm width
- ❖ **If actinomycetoma is suspected:** The white granules are subjected to—(1) Gram staining which reveals filamentous gram-positive bacilli; or (2) modified acid-fast stain (*Nocardia* is partially acid-fast)
- ❖ **Histopathological staining (Figs. 58.6A and B)** of the granules reveals a granulomatous reaction with a palisade arrangement of hyphae in the cement substance (in eumycetoma) or a granulomatous reaction with filamentous bacteria at the margin (in case of actinomycetoma)

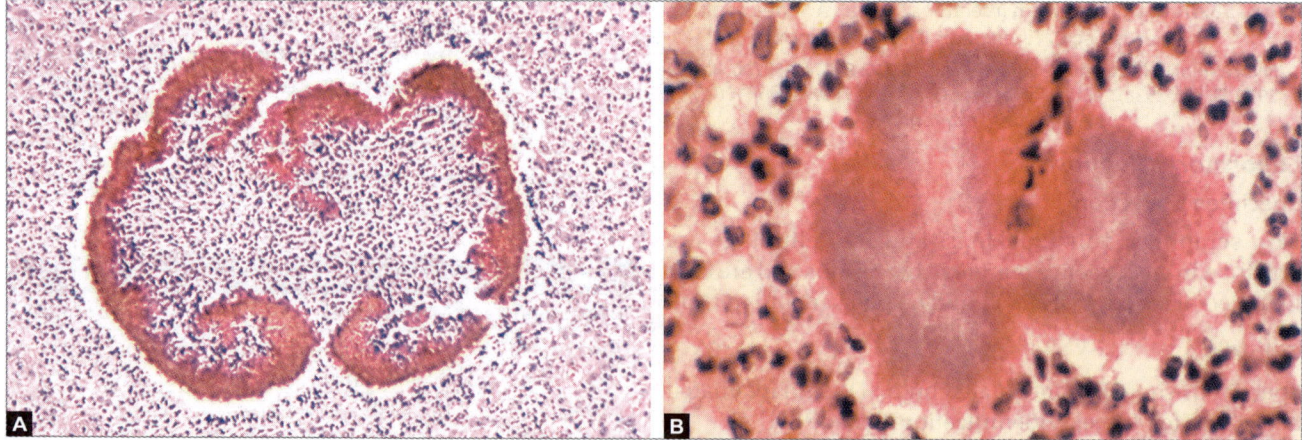

Figs. 58.6A and B: A. Eumycetoma (black grain and cement-like substance); **B.** Actinomycetoma (hematoxylin-eosin staining).
Source: PHIL/**A.** ID#: 4331; **B.** ID#: 15055/Centers for Disease Control and Prevention (CDC), Atlanta (*with permission*).

- **Culture:** Granules obtained from deep biopsies are the best specimens for culture as they contain live organisms. Both fungal (e.g. SDA) and bacteriological media (such as Lowenstein-Jensen media) should be included in the panel.

> **TREATMENT** — Mycetoma
>
> Consists of surgical removal of the lesion followed by use of:
> - For eumycetoma: Antifungal agents such as itraconazole or amphotericin B or
> - For actinomycetoma: Antibiotics such as Welsh regimen (amikacin plus cotrimoxazole).

Sporotrichosis

Sporotrichosis or Rose Gardner's disease is presented as a subcutaneous granulomatous disease; caused by *Sporothrix schenckii*.
- **Transmission:** Spores are introduced into the skin following minor trauma such as thorn prick, etc.
- **Clinical features:** It presents as noduloulcerative lesions (painless), which spread along the lymphatics
- **Diagnosis:** *S. schenckii* is a dimorphic fungus, that presents in two forms (**Figs. 58.7A and B**):
    - Yeast form at 37°C: described as cigar-shaped asteroid bodies in tissue sections stained by histopathological stains and
    - Mold form at 25°C: LPCB mount of SDA culture shows thin septate hyphae with flower-like sporulation
- **Treatment:** Itraconazole is the drug of choice, except for the disseminated form where amphotericin B is recommended.

Chromoblastomycosis

It refers to slow-growing chronic subcutaneous lesions caused by a group of dematiaceous or phaeoid fungi (i.e. darkly pigmented fungi) that produce a characteristic morphology called **sclerotic body**. Common agents include: *Fonsecaea, Phialophora, Cladosporium*, etc.

Phaeohyphomycosis

It refers to chronic subcutaneous lesions, caused by phaeoid fungi other than that are described in chromoblastomycosis. Common agents include *Alternaria, Bipolaris, Curvularia*, etc.

Rhinosporidiosis

It is characterized by large friable polyps in the nose.
- Caused by *Rhinosporidium seeberi*
- Stagnant water is the main source of infection
- **Diagnosis** is made by histopathology of the polyps that demonstrates **spherules** (large sporangia containing numerous endospores). It is not cultivable and does not grow in culture
- **Treatment:** Radical surgery with cauterization is the mainstay of treatment.

SYSTEMIC (DEEP) MYCOSES

Systemic mycoses include the four important fungal diseases that involve multiple organs.
1. Histoplasmosis, caused by *Histoplasma capsulatum*
2. Blastomycosis, caused by *Blastomyces dermatitidis*
3. Coccidioidomycosis, caused by *Coccidioides immitis*
4. Paracoccidioidomycosis, caused by *Paracoccidioides braziliensis*.

All four agents are **dimorphic fungi**, which exist as yeast at 37°C (inside the human body) and mold at 25°C (in the environment).
- **Transmission:** They are saprophytic fungi, spread by inhalation of spores leading to pulmonary infection.
- **Spread:** In the lungs, the mold form transforms into the yeast form. Then the yeast form disseminates to cause various systemic manifestations.

Histoplasmosis

Histoplasma capsulatum is widely prevalent, but particularly endemic in USA.
- **Clinical manifestations** are:
    - Pulmonary histoplasmosis (common form)
    - Mucocutaneous histoplasmosis
    - Disseminated histoplasmosis may occur in patients with low immunity. The common sites are bone marrow, spleen, liver, eyes, etc.
- **Laboratory diagnosis:** Useful specimens include sputum, bone marrow aspirate, blood, etc.
    - Histopathological staining of the specimens reveals tiny oval yeast cells (2–4 μm size) with narrow-based budding

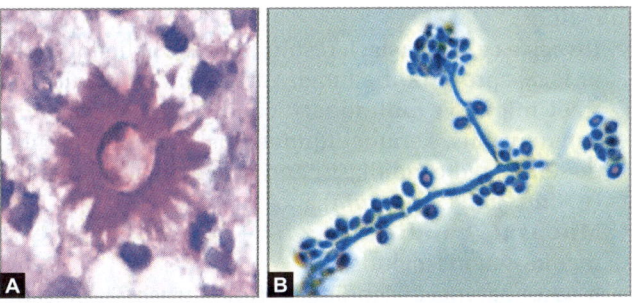

Figs. 58.7A and B: *Sporothrix schenckii:* **A.** Yeast form (asteroid body); **B.** Mold form showing thin septate hyphae with flower-like sporulation.
Source: **A.** Dr Manoj Singh and Dr M Ramam, AIIMS, New Delhi; **B.** PHIL/Dr Libero Ajello B. ID#: 4208/Centers for Disease Control and Prevention (CDC), Atlanta (*with permission*).

- Culture on SDA yields mycelial forms at 25°C (described as tuberculate macroconidia) and yeast form (creamy white colonies) at 37°C
- **Treatment:** Amphotericin B is the drug of choice.

Blastomycosis

Blastomycosis is also endemic in North America, caused by *Blastomyces dermatitidis*.
- **Clinical manifestations:** Acute pulmonary blastomycosis is the most common form. Other sites involved are skin, bone (osteomyelitis), CNS (brain abscess)
- **Histopathological staining** of the tissue biopsy specimens reveals thick-walled round yeast cells of 8–15 μm size with single broad-based budding (**Figure of 8 appearance**)
- **Culture media** such as SDA, yields mycelial form at 25°C and yeast at 37°C (dimorphic fungi)
- **Treatment:** Amphotericin B is the drug of choice.

Coccidioidomycosis

It is also called desert rheumatism or Valley fever, caused by a dimorphic fungus, *Coccidioides immitis*.
- **Clinical manifestations:** Pulmonary infection is the most common form. Rarely disseminated form may be seen involving skin, bone, joints, soft tissues, and meninges.
- **Histopathological staining** of sputum or tissue biopsy specimens demonstrates **spherules** which are large sac-like structures (20–80 μm size), filled with endospores
- **Cultures** on SDA produce mycelial growth, described as fragmented hyphae consisting of **barrel-shaped arthrospores**
- **Treatment:** Azoles such as itraconazole are the drug of choice to treat most cases.

Paracoccidioidomycosis

It is a systemic disease caused by the dimorphic fungus—*Paracoccidioides brasiliensis*. It is endemic in South America.
- **Clinical manifestations:** It occurs in two major forms.
  - Acute form (or juvenile type): It affects young adults under 30 years of age. It is a less common variety, but manifests as disseminated infection and is refractory to treatment
  - Chronic form (or adult form): It accounts for 90% of cases and predominantly affects older men. It results from the reactivation of quiescent lung lesions
- **Histopathological staining** of pus, tissue biopsies, or sputum reveals round thick-walled yeasts, with multiple narrow-necked buds attached circumferentially giving rise to **Mickey Mouse or pilot wheel** appearance
- **Culture** on SDA yields mycelial form at 25°C which converts into yeast phase at 37°C when grown in BHI agar supplemented with blood and glutamine
- **Treatment:** Amphotericin B is the drug of choice.

OPPORTUNISTIC MYCOSES

Opportunistic mycoses include the fungal infections that usually occur in immunocompromised patients, such as:
- Candidiasis
- Cryptococcal meningitis
- Zygomycoses
- Aspergillosis
- Penicillosis
- *Pneumocystis jirovecii* pneumonia

Candidiasis

Candidiasis is the most common fungal disease in humans; caused by *Candida*, a yeast-like fungus that produces pseudohyphae. Various species of *Candida* include:
- *Candida albicans:* It is the most pathogenic species of *Candida* infecting humans
- Other *Candida* species that can also cause infection are *C. tropicalis, C. glabrata, C. krusei, C. parapsilosis,* and *C. auris*.

Predisposing Factors

Predisposing factors that are associated with increased risk of infection with *Candida* include:
- **Physiological state:** Extremes of age, pregnancy
- **Low immunity:** Patients on steroid or immunosuppressive drugs, post-transplantation, malignancy, HIV-infected people
- Patients on **broad-spectrum antibiotics**—suppress the normal flora
- **Others:** Diabetes mellitus, febrile neutropenia, and zinc or iron deficiency.

Clinical Manifestations

Candida species produce a spectrum of infections ranging from skin and mucosal infections to invasive infections.
- **Invasive candidiasis:** It results from the hematogenous or local spread of the fungi. Various forms are urinary tract infection, pulmonary candidiasis, septicemia, osteomyelitis, keratoconjunctivitis, endophthalmitis, disseminated candidiasis, and nosocomial candidiasis (*C. auris* and *C. glabrata*).
- **Mucosal candidiasis:** The various mucosal manifestations include
  - Oropharyngeal candidiasis (oral thrush): It presents as white, adherent, painless patches in the mouth (**Fig. 58.8A**)
  - Vulvovaginitis: It is characterized by pruritus, pain, and vaginal discharge that is usually thin, but may become whitish curd like in severe cases

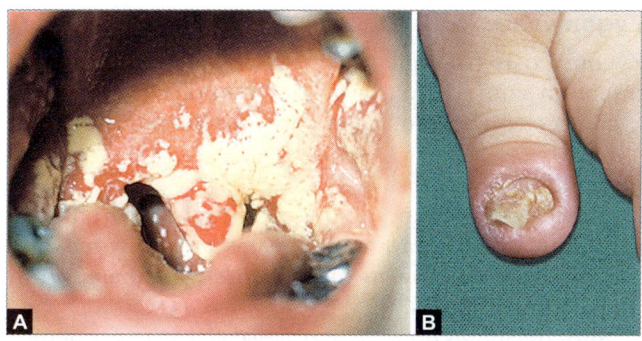

Figs. 58.8A and B: Candidiasis: **A.** Oral thrush; **B.** Onychomycosis.
Source: Public Health Image Library/**A.** ID#: 1217; **B.** Mr Gust, ID#: 15669/ Centers for Disease Control and Prevention (CDC), Atlanta *(with permission)*.

- Esophageal candidiasis: common in HIV-infected persons
- **Cutaneous candidiasis:** The cutaneous manifestations seen in candidiasis are intertrigo (pustules in the skin folds) and nail infections such as paronychia and onychomycosis **(Fig. 58.8B)**

Laboratory Diagnosis

- **Direct microscopy:** Gram-positive oval budding yeast cells with pseudohyphae **(Fig. 58.9A)**
- **Culture on SDA:** Produces creamy white and pasty colonies **(Fig. 58.9B)**
- **Tests for species identification:**
  - Germ tube test (positive for *C. albicans*) **(Fig. 58.9D)**
  - Dalmau plate culture for chlamydospore production **(Fig. 58.9E)**
  - CHROMagar: Different *Candida* species produce different colored colonies on CHROMagar **(Fig. 58.9C)**
  - Growth at 45°C (positive for *C. albicans*)
  - Carbohydrate assimilation and fermentation tests
  - Automated identification systems, e.g. MALDI-TOF and VITEK

- Molecular methods such as PCR detecting genes specific to various *Candida* species.
- **Immunodiagnosis:**
  - Antibody detection against cell wall mannan antigen
  - Antigen detection such as cell wall mannan antigen
  - Enzyme detection, e.g. enolase
  - Detection of metabolites, e.g. mannitol, arabinitol
  - β-d-Glucan assay: It is a marker of invasive fungal infections, raised in most invasive fungal infections (including invasive candidiasis).

> **TREATMENT** — Candidiasis
>
> - Cutaneous candidiasis: the drug of choice is a topical azole
> - Systemic candidiasis: drugs given are oral fluconazole, voriconazole or caspofungin or amphotericin B
>
> *C. glabrata, C. krusei* and *C. auris* exhibit resistance to azoles; therefore should be treated with caspofungin or amphotericin B.

Cryptococcal Meningitis

Cryptococcal meningitis is potentially fatal meningitis, caused by a capsulated yeast called *Cryptococcus neoformans*.

Pathogenesis

Infection is acquired by inhalation of yeast cells.
- **Spread:** First, it infects the lungs and subsequently disseminates through the blood to various organs such as CNS, bones, and skin.
- **Virulence factor:** Polysaccharide capsule is the principal virulence factor of the fungus. It is antiphagocytic
  - **Risk factors:** Individuals at high risk for cryptococcosis include—patients with advanced HIV infection, hematologic malignancies, transplant recipients, or immunosuppressive therapy.

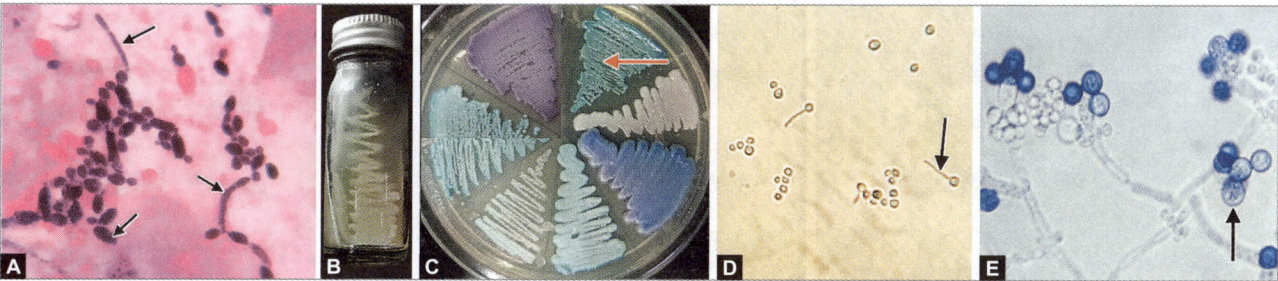

Figs. 58.9A to E: A. *Candida albicans*—gram-positive oval budding yeast cells with pseudohyphae; **B.** SDA shows creamy white colonies; **C.** CHROMagar showing colonies of various *Candida* species producing different colors; **D.** Positive germ tube test (arrow); **E.** Chlamydospore (arrow).
Source: **A to D.** Department of Microbiology, Pondicherry Institute of Medical Sciences, Puducherry; **E.** ID#:2917/Centers for Disease Control and Prevention (CDC), Atlanta *(with permission)*.

Clinical Manifestations

Various clinical manifestations of cryptococcosis include:
- **Pulmonary cryptococcosis**: It is the first and the most common presentation
- **Cryptococcal meningitis**: It presents as chronic meningitis with headache, fever, sensory and memory loss, cranial nerve paresis, and loss of vision (due to optic nerve involvement)
- **Others**: Skin lesions and osteolytic bone lesions.

Laboratory Diagnosis

Specimens such as CSF, blood, or skin scrapings can be collected.
- **Negative staining:** Modified India ink stain is used to demonstrate the capsule, which appears as refractile delineated clear space surrounding the round budding yeast cells against a black background **(Fig. 58.10A)**
- **Gram staining** may show gram-positive round budding yeast cells
- **Antigen detection:** The capsular antigens can be detected from CSF or serum by latex agglutination test. It is a rapid and sensitive and specific method
- **Culture:** CSF is inoculated onto SDA, blood agar, or chocolate agar and incubated at 37°C. Blood culture is also performed in addition. Colonies appear as mucoid creamy white and yeast-like **(Fig. 58.10B)**.

> **TREATMENT — Cryptococcosis**
>
> Treatment depends upon the type of cryptococcosis.
> - Cryptococcosis without CNS involvement: Fluconazole is the drug of choice
> - HIV-infected patients with CNS involvement: The regimen is an induction phase (amphotericin B ± flucytosine) followed by oral fluconazole therapy.

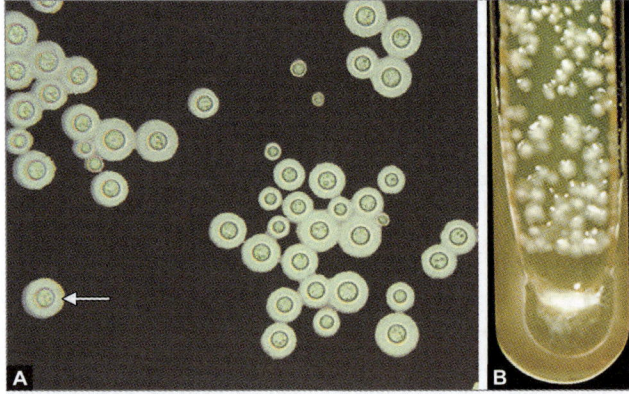

Figs. 58.10A and B: *Cryptococcus neoformans:* **A.** India ink staining shows clear refractile capsules surrounding round budding yeast cells (arrow showing); **B.** Growth on SDA at 37°C—shows creamy white mucoid colonies.

Source: Public Health Image Library/**A.** Dr. Leanor Haley, ID#:3771; **B.** Dr. William Kaplan, ID#:3199/Centers for Disease Control and Prevention (CDC), Atlanta (*with permission*).

Zygomycosis

Zygomycosis (or mucormycosis) is a life-threatening infection caused by a group of aseptate fungi called zygomycetes. Common agents are *Rhizopus* and *Mucor*.

Pathogenesis

Zygomycetes are found ubiquitously in the environment. Common human pathogen species are *Rhizopus* and *Mucor*. Transmission to man occurs via inhalation or inoculation of spores.
- **Spread**: Spores develop into a mycelial form containing wide aseptate hyphae. The hyphae are angioinvasive resulting in the spread of infection
- **Predisposing factors:** Common conditions that increase the risk of mucormycosis include **diabetic ketoacidosis** (most common), end-stage renal disease, and patients taking iron therapy, etc.

Clinical Manifestations

Mucormycosis manifests in various clinical forms.
- **Rhinocerebral mucormycosis**: It is the most common form; presents as orbital cellulitis, proptosis, and vision loss
- Pulmonary mucormycosis
- Other forms: Cutaneous, gastrointestinal, and disseminated mucormycosis.

Laboratory Diagnosis

- **Histopathological staining** of tissue biopsies shows broad aseptate hyaline hyphae
- **Culture on SDA at 25°C:** Reveals characteristic white cottony woolly colonies which become brown-black later, due to sporulation giving rise to **salt and pepper** appearance **(Fig. 58.11A)**
- **Microscopic appearance:** LPCB mount of the colonies reveals broad aseptate hyaline hyphae, sporangiophore

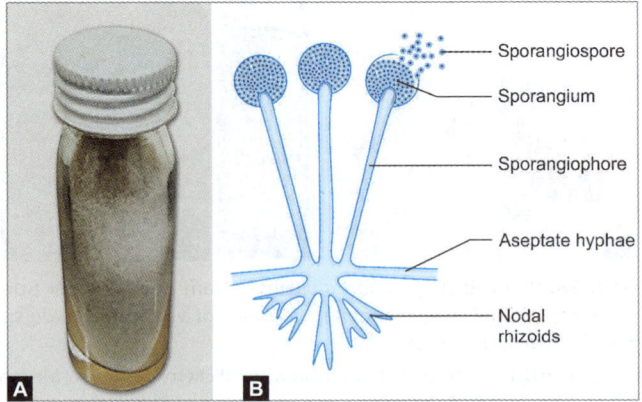

Figs. 58.11A and B: *Rhizopus:* **A.** Colonies on SDA show white cottony woolly colonies with black spores (salt and pepper appearance); **B.** Microscopic schematic diagram.

ending at sporangium, and a root-like growth arising from hyphae, called rhizoids **(Fig. 58.11B)**. In *Mucor*, rhizoids are absent.

> **TREATMENT** — **Zygomycosis**
>
> Amphotericin B remains the drug of choice for mucormycosis. Posaconazole can be given alternatively.

Aspergillosis

Aspergillosis is a group of invasive fungal diseases caused by a hyaline mold named *Aspergillus*. The important pathogens are—*A. fumigatus, A. flavus* and *A. niger*.

Pathogenesis

Aspergillus is widely distributed in nature. Transmission to man occurs by inhalation of airborne conidia. **Risk factors** for invasive aspergillosis are glucocorticoid use, profound neutropenia, underlying pneumonia, chronic obstructive pulmonary disease, tuberculosis or sarcoidosis and transplant recipients.

Clinical Manifestations

Depending upon the site of involvement, *Aspergillus* produces various clinical manifestations such as:
- **Pulmonary aspergillosis:** It is the most common form of aspergillosis; includes various manifestations like:
  - Allergic bronchopulmonary aspergillosis (ABPA)
  - Severe bronchial asthma
  - Aspergilloma (fungal ball) in the lungs
  - Invasive pulmonary aspergillosis
- **Other forms** of aspergillosis include:
  - Invasive sinusitis
  - Systemic infection: Endocarditis, brain abscess
  - Ocular infection: Keratitis and endophthalmitis
  - Ear infection: Otitis externa
  - Cutaneous aspergillosis
  - Nail bed infection: Onychomycosis
  - Mycotoxicosis: *A. flavus* produces aflatoxin, which causes liver carcinoma. Mycotoxicosis has been discussed later in this chapter.

Laboratory Diagnosis

Useful specimens such as sputum and tissue biopsies, etc.
- **Direct microscopy:** KOH (10%) mount or histopathological staining of specimens reveals characteristic narrow septate hyaline hyphae with acute angle branching.
- **Culture:** Specimens are inoculated onto SDA and incubated at 25°C. Species identification is done based on the macroscopic and microscopic (LPCB mount) appearance of the colonies **(Table 58.4 and Figs. 58.12A to D)**.
- **Antigen detection:** Enzyme immunoassays are available to detect antigens such as:
  - β-d-Glucan antigen assay: Raised in invasive fungal infections including aspergillosis
  - Galactomannan antigen: Specific for *Aspergillus*.

> **TREATMENT** — **Aspergillosis**
>
> ☐ For invasive aspergillosis—voriconazole is the drug of choice
> ☐ For ABPA—itraconazole is the drug of choice

Penicilliosis

Penicilliosis denotes the group of infections caused by pathogenic *Penicillium* species.
- *Penicillium marneffei*: It is a dimorphic fungus, that produces wart-like skin lesions (discussed below)
- Other *Penicillium* species are usually found in the environment and are isolated as common laboratory contaminants. Rarely they are associated with human diseases such as:
  - Invasive penicilliosis: e.g. endophthalmitis and endocarditis
  - Superficial disease: e.g. otomycosis, keratitis, and onychomycosis
  - Allergic disease: e.g. asthma and allergic pneumonitis.

Laboratory Diagnosis

Except for *P. marneffei*, which is a dimorphic fungus, all other *Penicillium* species occur only as molds and grow easily on SDA at 25°C.
- **Colonies** are rapidly growing, flat with velvety to powdery texture, and greenish **(Fig. 58.13A)**

Table 58.4: Identification features of *Aspergillus* species.

Aspergillus species	Macroscopic appearance of colony	Microscopic appearance of colony (LPCB mount)
A. fumigatus (Figs. 58.12A and C)	Colonies—smoky green, velvety to powdery, reverse is white	• Vesicle is conical-shaped • Phialides are arranged in single row • Conidia arise from upper third of vesicle • Conidia are hyaline
A. flavus (Figs. 58.12B and D)	Colonies—yellow green, velvety, reverse is white	• Vesicle is globular-shaped • Phialides in one or two rows • Conidia arise from upper two-third to entire vesicle • Conidia are hyaline
A. niger	Colonies—black, cottony type, reverse is white	• Vesicle is globular-shaped • Phialides in two rows • Conidia arise from entire vesicle • Conidia are black in color

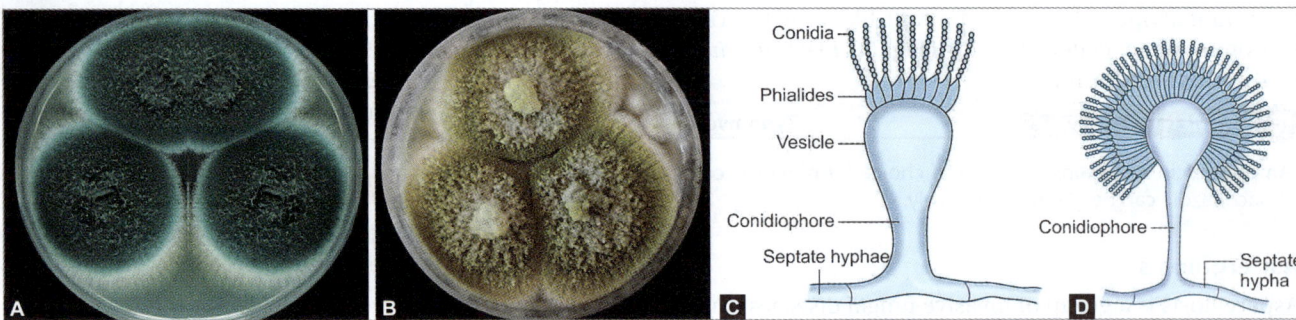

Figs. 58.12A to D: A and B: *Aspergillus* (colonies on SDA): **A.** *Aspergillus fumigatus*; **B.** *Aspergillus flavus*; **C and D:** Conidiation of various *Aspergillus* species: **C.** *A. fumigatus*; **D.** *A. flavus* (schematic diagram).
Source: **A and B.** Department of Microbiology, Pondicherry Institute of Medical Sciences, Puducherry (*with permission*).

- **Microscopic appearance:** LPCB mount of the colonies reveals hyaline thin septate hyphae. The conidiophore gives rise to elongated metulae, from which flask-shaped phialides originate which bear a chain of conidia. Such an arrangement is called **brush border appearance** (Fig. 58.13B).

Penicillium marneffei

Penicillium marneffei is a dimorphic fungus that causes opportunistic infection in HIV-infected patients.
- **Clinical features:** It produces both systemic infection and skin lesions (described as warty lesions mimicking molluscum contagiosum)
- **Histopathological staining** of tissue sections and skin scrapings shows oval yeast cells with central septation
- **Culture:** *P. marneffei* being dimorphic; produces yeast-like colonies at 37°C and mold form at 25°C. The mold form has a characteristic **brick-red pigment**
- **Treatment:** AIDS patients with severe penicilliosis are treated with amphotericin B.

Pneumocystis Pneumonia

Pneumocystis pneumonia is a clinical condition caused by the fungi *Pneumocystis jirovecii*. This infection has been increasingly reported after the discovery of HIV/AIDS.
- **Pathogenesis:** Once inhaled, the cysts are carried to the lungs where they transform into the trophozoite stage. The trophozoites induce an inflammatory response that recruits plasma cells to induce **frothy exudate** filling the alveoli. Hence, this condition is also called **plasma cell pneumonia**.
- **Laboratory diagnosis:** Useful specimens include bronchoalveolar lavage (BAL), open lung biopsy, etc.
  - Gomori's methenamine silver (GMS) staining demonstrates the cysts of *P. jirovecii*. The cysts resemble black-colored **crushed ping-pong balls**, against a green background
  - *Pneumocystis* is not cultivable
  - PCR assay is useful
  - Detection of 1, 3 β-D-glucan in serum
- **Radiology:** Chest X-ray depicts the classical finding of bilateral diffuse infiltrates. CT of the lung may reveal **ground-glass opacities**.

> **TREATMENT — Pneumocystis pneumonia**
> Cotrimoxazole is the drug of choice, given for treatment and prophylaxis of *Pneumocystis* pneumonia in patients with HIV.

Fusariosis

Fusariosis denotes the group of infections caused by pathogenic *Fusarium* species. *Fusarium* species are soil and plant saprophytes found worldwide. Important species infecting humans are *F. solani*, *F. oxysporum* and *F. verticillioides*.
- **Pathogenesis:** They rarely cause human infections.
  - In immunocompetent individuals, they cause keratitis in contact lens wearers and onychomycosis.
  - In immunocompromised patients—they are angioinvasive and cause pulmonary and sinus infection.

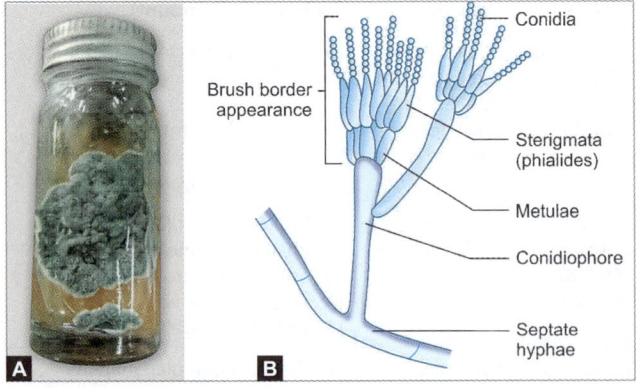

Figs. 58.13A and B: *Penicillium* species: **A.** Colonies on SDA; **B.** Schematic diagram.
Source: **A.** Department of Microbiology, Pondicherry Institute of Medical Sciences, Puducherry (*with permission*).

CHAPTER 58 ❖ Medical Mycology

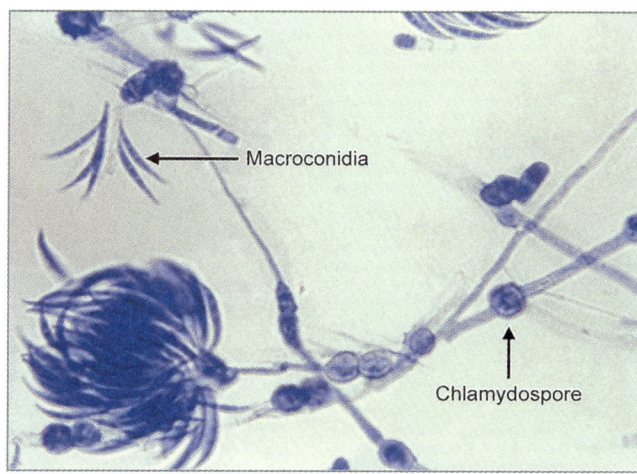

Fig. 58.14: *Fusarium* species (LPCB mount).
Source: Public Health Image Library, ID#: 17970/Centers for Disease Control and Prevention (CDC), Atlanta (*with permission*).

❖ **Laboratory diagnosis:**
- *Fusarium* is a filamentous fungus, grows rapidly on SDA at 25°C and produces woolly to cottony, flat, spreading white to pink colonies.
- LPCB mount of the colony reveals hyaline septate hyphae bearing round microconidia, sickle-shaped large macroconidia and chlamydospores **(Fig. 58.14)**.

❖ **Treatment:** Liposomal amphotericin B, voriconazole or posaconazole are recommended.

■ MYCOTOXICOSES

Mycotic poisoning can be classified into two varieties:
1. **Mycotoxicosis:** Refers to the disease produced following consumption of food contaminated by toxins liberated by certain fungi.
2. **Mycetism:** Refers to the toxic effects produced by eating poisonous fleshy fungi; usually different types of mushrooms.

EXPECTED QUESTIONS

I. Write short notes on:
1. Laboratory diagnosis of dermatophytosis
2. Laboratory diagnosis of candidiasis
3. Laboratory diagnosis of aspergillosis
4. Cryptococcal meningitis
5. Mucormycosis
6. Mycetoma

II. Multiple Choice Questions (MCQs):
1. **All are yeast or yeast-like fungi, *except*:**
   a. Candida
   b. Trichosporon
   c. Cryptococcus
   d. Trichophyton

2. **All are systemic mycoses, *except*:**
   a. Histoplasmosis
   b. Blastomycosis
   c. Dermatophytosis
   d. Coccidioidomycosis

3. **Asteroid bodies are seen in:**
   a. Sporothrix
   b. Rhinosporidium
   c. Candida
   d. Aspergillus

4. **Germ tube test is positive for:**
   a. Candida auris
   b. Candida parapsilosis
   c. Candida albicans
   d. Cryptococcus

Answers
1. d   2. c   3. a   4. c

Applied Microbiology

SECTION 8

SECTION OUTLINE

59. Bloodstream Infections
60. Meningitis
61. Urinary Tract Infection
62. Diarrheal Diseases
63. Respiratory Tract Infections
64. Miscellaneous Infective Syndromes
65. Specimen Collection and Transport

Bloodstream Infections

CHAPTER 59

CHAPTER PREVIEW
- Introduction
- Etiological Agents of BSI
- Types of Bloodstream Infections
- Clinical Manifestations
- Laboratory Diagnosis
- Fever of Unknown Origin

INTRODUCTION

Bloodstream infections (BSI) refer to the presence of microorganisms in blood, which constitute one of the most serious situations among infectious diseases; as they are a threat to every organ in the body. Therefore, timely detection of the causative agent is one of the most important goals of the microbiology laboratory.

Terminologies

- Bacteremia refers to the presence of bacteria in blood without any multiplication
- Septicemia is a condition in which bacteria circulate and actively multiply in the bloodstream and may produce their products (e.g. toxins) that cause harm to the host
- Similarly, the presence of viruses, parasites, and fungi in the blood can be described as 'viremia', 'parasitemia', and 'fungemia' respectively.

Types of Bacteremia

Bacteremia may be transient, continuous, or intermittent.
1. **Transient bacteremia**: It may occur spontaneously or with minor events such as brushing teeth or chewing food, instrumentation of contaminated mucosal site, and surgery involving a non-sterile site. These bacteria are normally cleared from the blood by the host immune system
2. **Continuous bacteremia:** Here, the organisms are released into the bloodstream at a fairly constant rate. It occurs in conditions such as endocarditis
3. **Intermittent bacteremia:** In most other infections, bacteria are released into blood intermittently; e.g. undrained abscess.

ETIOLOGICAL AGENTS OF BSI

Pathogens of all four major groups of microbes—bacteria, viruses, fungi and parasites can cause bloodstream infections.

Bacterial Etiology

Bacterial agents account for the majority of BSIs. The common agents causing **primary BSI** include typhoidal salmonellae, brucellae, or spirochetes (*Leptospira, Borrelia*), HACEK group of pathogens, viridans streptococci, and Rickettsiae.

However, there are various other bacterial agents which can primarily infect other sites and subsequently spill over to the bloodstream to cause **secondary BSI**. These include:
- Gram-positive cocci—staphylococci, beta-hemolytic streptococci, enterococci, and pneumococci
- Gram-negative cocci—meningococci
- Gram-positive bacilli—*Bacillus anthracis* and *Listeria*
- Gram-negative bacilli—*E. coli, Klebsiella, Enterobacter*, non-fermenters (e.g. *Pseudomonas, Acinetobacter, Burkholderia, Stenotrophomonas*), *Haemophilus, Aeromonas,* etc.
- Anaerobes—*Bacteroides*.

Viral Etiology

Although many viruses do circulate in the peripheral blood at some stage of the disease and have a viremic phase, the primary infection usually occurs in the target organs. There are a few viruses that preferentially infect blood cells, which can be considered as **primary viral agents of BSI** such as HIV, agents of hemorrhagic fever such as dengue, chikungunya, Ebola, Marburg, Lassa, yellow fever, etc.

Parasitic Etiology

The parasites causing bloodstream infections are:
- Parasites that directly infect blood cells such as *Plasmodium* and *Babesia* infecting RBCs
- Parasites that may be found in the bloodstream before they migrate to other tissues or organs; e.g. include tachyzoites of *Toxoplasma gondii,* amastigote forms of *Leishmania,* and trypomastigote forms of *Trypanosoma*

- Parasites that may be present in the lymphatics and come to the bloodstream transiently; e.g. microfilariae of filarial parasites.

Fungal Etiology

Fungemia occurs primarily in immunosuppressed patients, patients with malignancies, patients on chemotherapy, and in those with serious or terminal illness—*Candida* species, agents of systemic mycoses (*Histoplasma*, *Blastomyces*, *Coccidioides,* and *Paracoccidioides)* and *Cryptococcus.*

As bacterial agents are the most common group to cause bloodstream infections, therefore the rest of the discussion in this chapter is largely limited to bacterial agents.

TYPES OF BLOODSTREAM INFECTIONS

There are two major categories of bloodstream infections (BSIs): Intravascular and extravascular.

Intravascular Bloodstream Infections

They originate within the cardiovascular system which includes infection of the heart (endocarditis, myocarditis, and pericarditis) and catheter-related BSI (CRBSI).

Extravascular Bloodstream Infections

Most cases of clinically significant bacteremia are of extravascular origin.
- The organisms multiply at the primary site such as the urinary tract, lungs and then invade to reach the bloodstream
- **Portal of entry:** The most common portals of entry for bacteremia are the genitourinary tract (25%), followed by respiratory tract (20%), abscesses (10%), surgical site wound infections (5%), and biliary tract (5%). In up to 25% of cases, the portal of entry remains uncertain.

CLINICAL MANIFESTATIONS

Bloodstream infections have a bacteremia stage followed by a septicemic stage. The clinical manifestations are evident only in the septicemic stage. In this stage, the bacteria multiply and release their products (e.g. toxins) which travel to various organs affecting their functions. Based on the severity and the extent of organ failure; bloodstream infection can be divided into two stages: sepsis and septic shock.
- **Sepsis:** The common signs and symptoms include:
  - Fever or hypothermia with/without chills and rigors
  - Hyperventilation leads to excess loss of CO_2 and subsequent respiratory alkalosis
  - Skin lesions, change of mental status, and diarrhea.
- **Septic shock:** This is the gravest late-stage complication of septicemia and is manifested as—hypotension, multi-organ failure, etc.

LABORATORY DIAGNOSIS

Diagnosis of bloodstream infection depends on the isolation of the causative agent from the blood by performing a blood culture.

Specimen Collection for Blood Culture

Extreme care should be taken while collecting blood for culture, as there is a high risk of contamination with skin flora.
- **Site:** Blood for culture should always be collected in pairs; from two separate venipuncture and 2 separate skin decontamination process. If a central line is present, then one sample from the central line and one from the venipuncture should be collected
- **Preparation of the site:** To avoid contamination with skin flora, blood should be collected under strict aseptic conditions using sterile disposable syringe **(Fig. 59.1)**
- **Skin decontamination:** Skin should be disinfected by two-step procedure—first, treated with 70% isopropyl alcohol, and then a second antiseptic solution such as povidone-iodine or chlorhexidine should be applied
  - The disinfectants should be applied in a circular motion, starting from the center to the periphery
  - The area should be allowed to air dry before venipuncture.

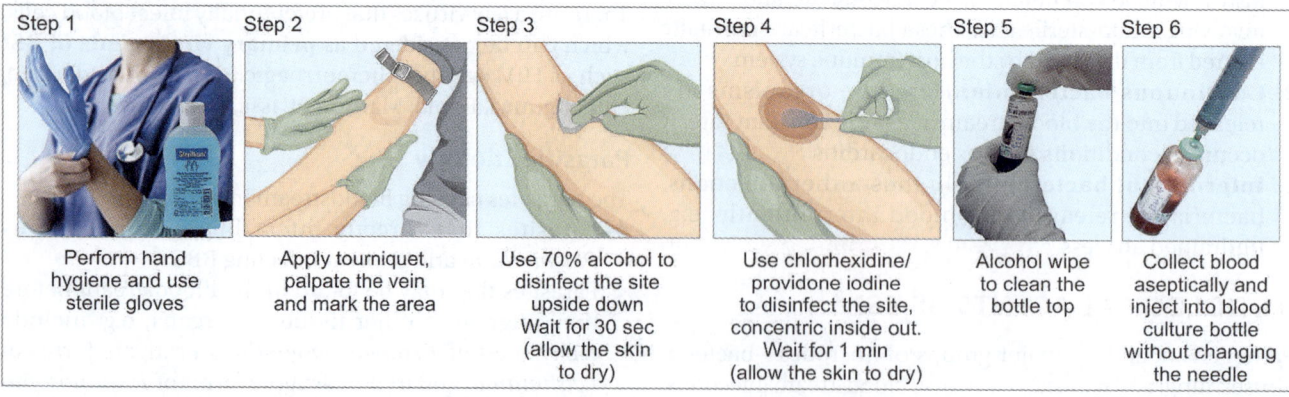

Fig. 59.1: Steps of collection of blood for culture.

- **Timing of collection:** Blood should be collected before starting antimicrobial therapy. If the antimicrobial agent is already started, then the best time for collection is just before the next dose of the antimicrobial agent
- **Blood volume:** A blood specimen is drawn using a sterile syringe and needle. At least **8–10 mL** of blood per bottle for an adult and **1–3 mL** per pediatric bottle is recommended
- **Number of blood cultures:** At least 2–3 blood culture sets (each set consists of two bottles: 1 aerobic and 1 anaerobic) are required to have a good isolation rate. Multiple blood cultures should be collected for endocarditis cases
- **Dispensing:** Collected blood is then directly dispensed into a blood culture bottle at the bedside—either a conventional or automated blood culture **(Figs. 59.2A to C)**.
- **Transport of blood specimen:** The collected blood is gently mixed with the broth and then transported immediately to the laboratory. In case of delay, the blood culture bottle **should never be refrigerated**. It can be kept at 35°C in an incubator (if available) or left at room temperature.

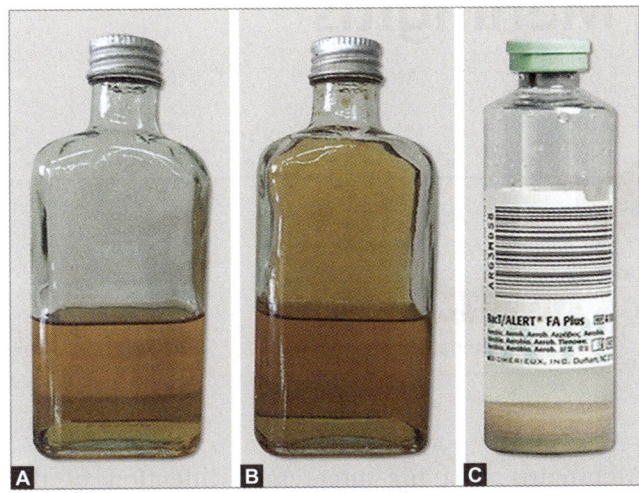

Figs. 59.2A to C: Blood culture bottles: **A.** Monophasic medium (BHI broth); **B.** Biphasic medium (Castaneda's) containing BHI broth and BHI agar slant; **C.** BacT/ALERT bottle.

Source: **A to C.** Department of Microbiology, JIPMER, Puducherry (*with permission*).

FEVER OF UNKNOWN ORIGIN

Fever of unknown origin (FUO) is a very common term used by clinicians to refer to any febrile illness without an initial obvious etiology.

The term FUO is reserved only for prolonged febrile illnesses without an established etiology despite of intensive evaluation and diagnostic testing.

Definition of FUO

The definition of FUO is as follows:
- Fever ≥38.3°C (≥101°F) on at least two occasions
- Duration of illness of ≥3 weeks
- No known immunocompromised state
- The diagnosis that remains uncertain after a thorough history-taking, physical examination, and a set of laboratory investigations.

Etiology of FUO

FUO has both infectious and non-infectious etiology.
- **Infections (36%):** This accounts for the majority of FUO cases. All groups of microbial infections can cause FUO such as mycobacterial infections, typhoid fever, rickettsial infections, etc.
- **Neoplasms (19%):** For example, lymphoma, leukemia, myeloma, renal, colon, and liver cancers, etc.
- **Non-infectious inflammatory diseases (19%):** For example, connective tissue disorders like rheumatoid arthritis, SLE (systemic lupus erythematosus), etc.
- Miscellaneous and undiagnosed causes (26%).

EXPECTED QUESTIONS

I. Write short notes on:
   1. List the etiological agents of bloodstream infection.
   2. List the etiological agents of FUO.
   3. Write in detail about steps involved in blood collection for culture.

Meningitis

CHAPTER 60

CHAPTER PREVIEW
- Acute Bacterial Meningitis
- Acute Viral Meningitis
- Chronic Meningitis

Meningitis is a life-threatening infection of the leptomeninges (arachnoid and pia mater) surrounding the brain and spinal cord, with involvement of the subarachnoid space.

Based on the onset, meningitis can be classified into:
- **Acute meningitis:** Presents as an acute fulminant illness that progresses rapidly in a few hours. It is further divided into acute bacterial (or pyogenic) and acute viral meningitis
- **Chronic meningitis:** Progressively worsens over weeks (>4 weeks).

ACUTE BACTERIAL MENINGITIS

Acute bacterial meningitis (also called as pyogenic meningitis), is an acute purulent infection within the subarachnoid space. It is characterized by elevated polymorphonuclear cells in CSF.

The agents implicated in pyogenic meningitis may vary according to age.
- **Overall:** *Streptococcus pneumoniae* (most common), meningococcus, *Streptococcus agalactiae*, *Listeria*, and *Haemophilus influenzae*
- **Neonates:** The common agents of neonatal meningitis include *Streptococcus agalactiae*, gram-negative bacilli such as *Escherichia coli* and *Klebsiella*, and *Listeria monocytogenes*
- **Elderly (>60 years):** Common agents are *Streptococcus agalactiae* and *Listeria monocytogenes*.

Pathogenesis

The bacteria that cause acute meningitis are transmitted from person-to-person through droplets of respiratory secretions. Organisms may gain access to the meninges by several routes: (i) Hematogenous spread, (ii) direct spread from an infected site (otitis media, sinusitis, etc.) and (iii) via anatomical defects in the CNS as a result of surgery, trauma, etc.

Clinical Manifestations

The incubation period ranges between 2 to 10 days. Patients with meningitis develop various manifestations such as:
- **Important symptoms** include fever, vomiting, intense headache, altered consciousness, etc.
- **Signs of meningism** (meningeal irritation) such as:
    - *Nuchal rigidity* (stiff neck): The neck becomes stiff and resists passive flexion
    - *Kernig's sign:* Severe stiffness of the hamstrings causes an inability to straighten the leg when the hip is flexed to 90°
    - *Brudzinski's sign:* When the neck is passively flexed, results in spontaneous flexion of the hips and knees.
- **In infants:** Babies usually present with fever, irritability, and bulging fontanelle.

Laboratory Diagnosis

CSF is the most ideal specimen for bacterial meningitis. Blood culture is also collected in addition.
- **CSF collection:** CSF is obtained by lumbar puncture under strict aseptic conditions. It is divided into three sterile containers; one each for cell count, biochemical analysis, and bacteriological examination
- **CSF transport:** CSF being the most precious specimen should be examined immediately, and should never be refrigerated as delicate pathogens such as *H. influenzae* may die.

Cytological and Biochemical Analysis

Biochemical analysis and cell count of CSF give a preliminary clue about the type of meningitis **(Table 60.1)**.

In acute bacterial (pyogenic) meningitis:
- CSF usually contains >1,000 leukocytes/μL and predominantly neutrophils (90–95%)
- The total protein content is elevated and the glucose level is diminished or even absent
- CSF pressure is highly elevated.

CHAPTER 60 ❖ Meningitis

Table 60.1: Cytological and biochemical parameters in CSF of normal individuals and in different types of meningitis.

Characteristics	Normal individual	Pyogenic meningitis	Tuberculous meningitis	Viral meningitis
CSF pressure (mm of water)	Normal (50–150)	Highly elevated (>180)	Moderately elevated	Slightly elevated/normal
Total leukocyte count (per mm³)	0–5	100–10,000	10–500	25–500
Predominant cell type	Lymphocytes	Neutrophils	Lymphocytes	Lymphocytes
Glucose (mg%)	40–70	<40 mg/dL (decreased to absent)	20–40 mg/dL (slightly decreased)	Normal
Total proteins (mg%)	15–45	>45 mg/dL (usually >250; markedly increased)	100–500 mg/dL (moderate to markedly increased)	20–80 mg/dL (normal or slightly elevated)

CSF Microscopy (Gram Staining)

Gram staining of CSF may give a preliminary clue about the etiological agent, based on the morphology of the bacteria **(Table 60.2)**. This helps in the early initiation of appropriate empirical antimicrobial therapy.

Direct Antigen Detection

After centrifugation of CSF, the supernatant can be used for antigen detection by latex agglutination test.
- It is available for the detection of capsular antigens of common agents of meningitis such as *S. pneumoniae, N. meningitidis, H. influenzae,* etc.
- Detection of capsular antigens in CSF is more sensitive than CSF microscopy.

Culture

Ideal media for CSF culture are chocolate agar, blood agar, and MacConkey agar.

Table 60.2: Preliminary clue about the etiological agents of pyogenic meningitis based on CSF Gram stain.

Appearance in CSF Gram stain	Suggestive of
Gram-positive diplococci, flame or lanceolate-shaped with clear halo (capsulated) **(Fig. 22.5, Chapter 22)**	*Streptococcus pneumoniae*
Gram-negative diplococci, capsulated, with adjacent sides flattened (lens or half-moon shaped) **(Fig. 23.1, Chapter 23)**	*Neisseria meningitidis*
Pleomorphic gram-negative coccobacilli, capsulated	*Haemophilus influenzae*
Gram-negative bacilli, arranged singly	*Escherichia coli* or others
Gram-positive cocci in short chain	*Streptococcus agalactiae*
Gram-positive short bacilli, often confused with diphtheroids	*Listeria monocytogenes*

- **Culture plates** are incubated at 37°C for 48 hours
- **Identification:** Colonies grown on solid media are processed for identification of the organism either by an automated identification system such as MALDI-TOF or VITEK or by conventional biochemical tests
- **Antimicrobial susceptibility test** should be done to initiate definitive antimicrobial therapy. It is carried out by disk diffusion test or preferably by automated MIC-based methods such as VITEK.

Molecular Methods

Molecular tests are highly sensitive and provide faster results. Multiplex PCR and multiplex real-time PCR can be used for simultaneous detection of common agents of pyogenic meningitis.

TREATMENT — Pyogenic meningitis

Treatment should be initiated as early as possible.
The **empirical therapy** comprises of:
- *Adult:* IV ceftriaxone and vancomycin
- *For neonates:* IV ampicillin plus gentamicin
- IV dexamethasone is added to the regimen to reduce intracranial pressure.

Definitive therapy: After the culture report is available, the empirical therapy is modified based on the organism isolated and its antimicrobial susceptibility pattern.

■ ACUTE VIRAL MENINGITIS

It is caused by a number of viruses, among which enteroviruses account for the majority of cases (>85%). Others include herpesviruses, arboviruses (encephalitis group), HIV, mumps virus, etc.
- The CSF is predominantly lymphocytic
- Although they usually develop meningitis in few days after the infection; many of these viruses progress slower and can also occasionally cause chronic meningitis.

CHRONIC MENINGITIS

Chronic meningitis is defined as the persistence of meningitis that exists for >4 weeks; associated with a persistent inflammatory response in CSF (white blood cell count >5/μL)
- **Etiology:** Caused by both infective etiology **(Table 60.3)** and non-infectious causes such as malignancy, autoimmune diseases, etc.
- **CSF findings:** In chronic meningitis, the CSF is predominantly lymphocytic.

Table 60.3: Agents of chronic meningitis.

Bacterial agents
• Partially treated suppurative meningitis
• *Mycobacterium tuberculosis*
• *Treponema pallidum* (tertiary syphilis)
• *Borrelia burgdorferi* (Lyme disease)

Viral agents: Agents of acute viral meningitis may also present as chronic meningitis, e.g. enteroviruses, herpesviruses, HIV, mumps, etc.
Parasitic agents: *Toxoplasma gondii*, free-living amoebae
Fungal agents: *Cryptococcus neoformans* and *Candida*

Note: Some of these agents may present as a subacute form of meningitis, that progresses over several days to <4 weeks.

EXPECTED QUESTIONS

I. Write essay on:
1. Discuss the etiological agents, pathogenesis and clinical manifestations, and laboratory diagnosis of acute pyogenic meningitis?

II. Multiple Choice Questions (MCQs):
1. Biochemical analysis of pyogenic meningitis reveals all, *except*:
   a. CSF pressure: highly elevated
   b. Total leukocyte count: highly elevated, neutrophilic
   c. Glucose: highly elevated
   d. Total proteins: markedly increased
2. All are the bacterial agents causing meningitis, *except*:
   a. Meningococcus
   b. Gonococcus
   c. *H. influenzae*
   d. Pneumococcus

Answers
1. c 2. b

CHAPTER 61

Urinary Tract Infection

CHAPTER PREVIEW
- Classification
- Predisposing Factors
- Etiology and Pathogenesis
- Clinical Manifestations
- Laboratory Diagnosis
- Treatment

Urinary tract infection (UTI) is defined as a disease caused by microbial invasion of the urinary tract (i.e. kidney, bladder, or urethra). UTI is one of the most common infective syndrome encountered.

Classification
- UTIs may be broadly classified into two types—lower UTI and upper UTI depending on the anatomical sites involved
- Depending upon the source of infection, UTI can be of two types: healthcare-associated (e.g. CAUTI, **Chapter 15** for detail) and community-acquired.

Predisposing Factors
There are a number of factors that predispose to the pathogenesis of UTI.
- **Gender:** UTI more commonly affects females, which is due to—(i) short urethra and (ii) close proximity of urethral meatus to anus; so that there is more chance of migration of bacteria present in perineum into the urinary tract
- **Age:** For females, the incidence of UTI increases with age (10-20% incidence in adult life). Whereas males have a higher risk during infancy and in old age (due to prostate enlargement)
- **Pregnancy:** Anatomical and hormonal changes in pregnancy favor the development of UTIs. Most pregnant women develop asymptomatic bacteriuria
- **Structural and functional abnormality** of the urinary tract may obstruct the urine flow, which can lead to urinary stasis; which predisposes to infection
  - *Structural obstruction:* Renal and ureteric stones, prostate enlargement, etc.
  - *Functional obstruction:* Neurogenic bladder due to spinal cord injury.
- **Catheter:** The presence of an indwelling urinary catheter is the single most important risk factor to develop UTI in hospitalized patients
- **Bacterial virulence** such as the expression of pili helps in bacterial adhesion to uroepithelium.

Etiology
Escherichia coli (uropathogenic *E. coli*) is by far the most common cause of UTIs, accounting for 70% of total cases.
- The endogenous flora such as *E. coli*, *Klebsiella*, *Proteus* and enterococci are the important agents
- In healthcare-associated UTIs, in addition to the above agents, multidrug-resistant *Pseudomonas*, and *Acinetobacter* can also cause UTI.
- In general, viruses, parasites and fungi infrequently infect the urinary tract.

Bacterial pathogens are the major cause of UTI; their pathogenesis, clinical features, laboratory diagnosis and treatment have been discussed in detail in this chapter.

Refer **Table 61.1** for the list of common microorganisms causing UTIs.

Pathogenesis
Bacteria invade the urinary tract mainly by two routes—ascending and descending routes.

Table 61.1: Common microorganisms causing UTIs.	
Bacterial agents	**Other agents**
Gram-negative bacilli: Enterobacteriaceae • ***Escherichia coli:*** Most common (70%) • *Klebsiella pneumoniae* • *Enterobacter* species • *Proteus* species • *Serratia* species **Non-fermenters** • *Pseudomonas aeruginosa* • *Acinetobacter* species	**Fungus:** *Candida albicans* **Parasites:** • *Schistosoma haematobium* • *Trichomonas vaginalis*
Gram-positive cocci: • *Enterococcus* species • *Staphylococcus saprophyticus** • *Staphylococcus aureus* • *Staphylococcus epidermidis* • *Streptococcus agalactiae*	**Viruses:** • BK virus • Adenovirus types–11 and 21

(UTI, Urinary tract infection)
*Common in sexually active females.

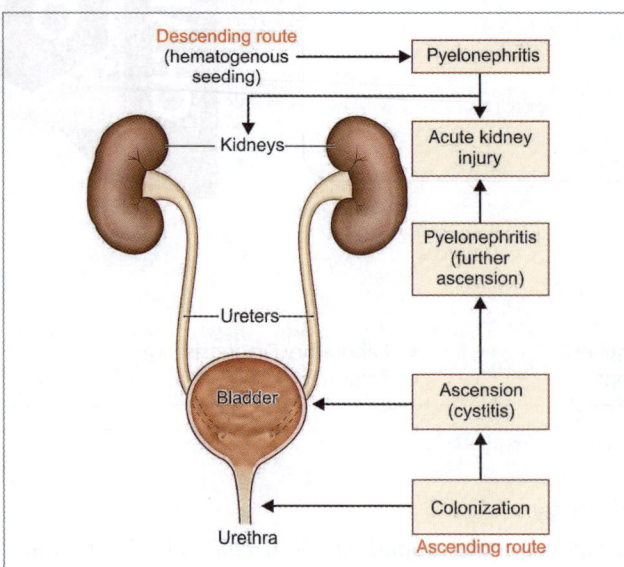

Fig. 61.1: Pathogenesis of urinary tract infection.

Ascending Route

It is the most common route; the enteric endogenous bacteria enter the urinary tract which is facilitated by sexual intercourse, catheterization, etc.
- **Colonization:** Adhesion to the urethral epithelium is the first and the most important step in pathogenesis. A number of virulence factors (e.g. fimbriae) help in adhesion
- **Ascension:** Following colonization, the pathogen ascends through the urethra upwards towards the bladder to cause cystitis
- **Further ascension** through the ureter may occasionally occur if there is vesicoureteral reflux leading to pyelonephritis (infection of renal parenchyma)
- **Acute tubular injury:** If the inflammatory cascade continues, tubular obstruction and damage occurs which may lead to interstitial nephritis.

Descending Route

This refers to the invasion of organisms to renal parenchyma from other organs through the hematogenous route, causing pyelonephritis. This accounts for 5% of total UTIs. Common agents include—*S. aureus*, *Salmonella*, *M. tuberculosis*, and *Leptospira*.

Clinical Manifestations

UTIs may be presented in various forms:
- **Lower UTI:** Asymptomatic bacteriuria, cystitis, urethritis, acute urethral syndrome
- **Upper UTI:** Pyelonephritis.

Lower UTI

Asymptomatic Bacteriuria

It refers to the isolation of a significant count of bacteria in an appropriately collected urine specimen, obtained from a person without symptoms of UTI. It is more common in females and its incidence increases with age.
- **Asymptomatic UTI** is clinically significant in a certain group of people such as pregnant women, people undergoing prostatic surgery, or any urologic procedure where bleeding is anticipated. Therefore, in this group, routine screening and treatment for asymptomatic UTI is highly recommended
- In contrast, **asymptomatic UTI** is not clinically significant in non-pregnant, pre-menopausal women, old age, catheterized patients, or patients with spinal injury. In such cases, neither screening nor treatment of asymptomatic UTI is needed.

Cystitis (Infection of the Bladder)

It is characterized by localized symptoms such as: Dysuria (pain while micturition), frequency, urgency, and suprapubic tenderness (over the bladder area). Urine becomes cloudy, with a bad odor, and in some cases grossly bloody (hematuria).

Acute Urethral Syndrome

This is another form of lower UTI seen in young sexually active females, characterized by:
- Presence of classical symptoms of lower UTI as described for cystitis
- Bacterial count is often low (10^2 to 10^5 CFU/mL)
- Pyuria (pus in urine) is present
- **Agents:** Mostly due to the usual agents of UTI, a few cases may be caused by gonococcus, *Chlamydia*, herpes simplex virus, etc.

Upper UTI (Pyelonephritis)

Pyelonephritis refers to inflammation of kidney parenchyma, calyces, and the renal pelvis, i.e. the part of the ureter present inside the kidney.
- Associated with systemic manifestations such as—fever, flank pain, vomiting
- Lower urinary tract symptoms such as frequency, urgency, and dysuria may also be present.

Laboratory Diagnosis

Specimen Collection

Urine should be collected in a wide mouth screw-capped sterile container by various methods.
- **Clean-voided midstream urine:** It is the most common specimen for UTI; collected after properly cleaning the urethral meatus or glans

CHAPTER 61 ◆ Urinary Tract Infection

- **Suprapubic aspiration** of urine from the bladder: It is the most ideal specimen. It is recommended for patients in coma or infants
- **In catheterized patients,** urine should be collected from the catheter tube (after clamping distally and disinfecting); but not from the urobag.

Transport

The urine sample should be processed immediately. If a delay is expected for more than 1–2 hours, then it can be stored in the refrigerator.

Direct Examination

The screening tests done are as follows:
- **Wet mount examination:** It is done to demonstrate the pus cells in urine. Pyuria of >8 pus cells/mm³ is taken as significant
- **Leukocyte esterase test:** It is a rapid and cheaper method that detects leukocyte esterases secreted by pus cells present in urine.

Culture

- **Culture media:** Urine sample should be inoculated onto CLED agar (cysteine lactose electrolyte deficient agar) or a combination of MacConkey agar and blood agar. CLED agar is preferred in laboratories with higher sample load
- **Kass concept of significant bacteriuria:** This is based on the fact that, though the normal urine is sterile it may get contaminated during voiding, with normal urethral flora. However, the bacterial count in contaminated urine would be lower than that caused by an infection

> **Significant bacteriuria**
> - A count of ≥10^5 **colony forming units (CFU)/mL** of urine is considered as significant—indicates infection (referred to as 'significant bacteriuria')
> - **Count between 10^4 to 10^5 CFU/mL** indicates doubtful significance; should be clinically correlated

Contd...

Contd...

> - **Low count of <10^4** CFU/mL is due to the presence of commensal bacteria (due to contamination during voiding) and is of no significance. However, low counts can be significant in the following conditions:
>   ➢ Patient on antibiotic treatment
>   ➢ Pyelonephritis and acute urethral syndrome
>   ➢ Sample taken by suprapubic aspiration.

- **Quantitative culture:** This is done to count the number of colonies. Each colony on the plate corresponds to one bacterium in the urine sample. Quantitation is done by:
    - A semi-quantitative method such as a standardized loop technique
    - A quantitative method such as the pour plate method.
- **Colony appearance**: It depends upon the organism grown. For example, lactose fermenters such as *E. coli* and *Klebsiella* produce pink colonies on MacConkey agar and yellow colonies on CLED agar; whereas non-lactose fermenters such as *Proteus, Pseudomonas* and *Acinetobacter* produce pale colonies
- **Identification**: The colonies grown are identified either by conventional biochemical tests or automated identification systems such as MALDI-TOF or VITEK
- **AST:** Antimicrobial susceptibility test is essential to guide the appropriate treatment. It is performed conventionally by disk diffusion test (on Mueller-Hinton agar) or by automated MIC-based methods such as VITEK.

TREATMENT — Urinary tract infections

Treatment should be based on the AST report. Quinolones (e.g. norfloxacin), nitrofurantoin, cephalosporins, and aminoglycosides are among the preferred drugs.

Higher antibiotics such as carbapenem (e.g. meropenem), β-lactam/β-lactamase inhibitor combinations (e.g. piperacillin-tazobactam), or fosfomycin are used for the treatment of healthcare-associated UTIs caused by multidrug-resistant gram-negative bacilli.

EXPECTED QUESTIONS

I. **Write an essay on:**
1. Discuss the etiological agents, pathogenesis, clinical manifestations, and laboratory diagnosis of UTI.

II. **Multiple Choice Questions (MCQs):**
1. Which culture medium is preferred for processing of urine specimens?
    a. TCBS agar   b. CLED agar
    c. Chocolate agar   d. XLD agar

2. Which of the following is the most common etiological agent of UTI?
    a. *Escherichia coli*
    b. *Klebsiella*
    c. *Proteus*
    d. *Enterobacter*

Answers
1. b   2. a

CHAPTER 62

Diarrheal Diseases

CHAPTER PREVIEW
- Types of Diarrheal Diseases
- Pathogenesis
- Laboratory Diagnosis

■ DIARRHEAL DISEASES

The diarrheal diseases are one of the leading cause of illness globally; cause significant morbidity and mortality.

There are various clinical types of diarrheal diseases; caused by a wide variety of infectious agents including bacteria, viruses, and parasites **(Table 62.1)**.

Diarrhea

Diarrhea is defined as passage of three or more loose or liquid stools per day, in excess than the usual habit for that person.
- ❖ Acute diarrhea usually lasts for <14 days; most often caused by viral agents, followed by bacterial or parasitic agents
- ❖ Common microbial agents causing diarrhea and the mechanisms involved are summarized in **Table 62.1**.

Dysentery

Dysentery is characterized by diarrhea with increased blood and mucus, often associated with fever, abdominal pain, and tenesmus (feeling of constant need to pass stools, despite an empty colon) **(Table 62.1)**.

Traveler's Diarrhea

Traveler's diarrhea is the most common travel-related infectious illness.
- ❖ **Epidemiology:** Occurs in about 20–50% of people traveling from temperate industrialized countries to tropical regions of Asia, Africa, etc.

Table 62.1: Infectious agents of acute diarrhea and the underlying mechanism.

Mechanism	Examples of pathogens involved	

Non-inflammatory	**Bacteria** (mostly enterotoxin mediated):
	• *Vibrio cholerae*
	• Diarrheagenic *Escherichia coli*:
	   ➢ Enteropathogenic *E. coli*
	   ➢ Enterotoxigenic *E. coli*
	   ➢ Enteroaggregative *E. coli*
	• *Clostridium perfringens*
	• *Bacillus cereus*
	• *Staphylococcus aureus*
	Viruses: Rotavirus, norovirus, adenoviruses—40, 41, caliciviruses and astrovirus
		Parasites (protozoa):
		• *Giardia duodenalis*
		• *Cryptosporidium parvum*
		• *Cyclospora cayetanensis*
		• *Cystoisospora belli*
		Parasites (helminths):
		• *Ascaris*, hookworm
		• *Strongyloides, Trichinella*
		• *Taenia saginata, T. solium*
		• *Hymenolepis nana*
		• *Fasciolopsis buski*

Inflammatory	**Predominantly dysentery:**
	• *Shigella* species
	• *Campylobacter jejuni*
	• Diarrheagenic *Escherichia coli*:
	   ➢ Enterohemorrhagic *E. coli*
	   ➢ Enteroinvasive *E. coli*
	• *Vibrio parahaemolyticus*
	Predominantly inflammatory diarrhea:
	• Non-typhoidal salmonellae
	• *Yersinia enterocolitica*
		Parasite (predominantly dysentery):
		• *Entamoeba histolytica*
		• *Balantidium coli*
		• *Trichuris trichiura*
		• *Schistosoma mansoni*
		• *Schistosoma japonicum*

Penetrating	*Salmonella typhi* (enteric fever)	

- **Microbial agents:** Overall, enterotoxigenic *Escherichia coli* is the most common agent, followed by enteroaggregative *E. coli*, *Campylobacter* and *Shigella*
- **Clinical presentation:** Most cases begin within the first 3–5 days; characterized by a sudden onset of abdominal cramps, anorexia, and watery diarrhea.

Persistent and Chronic Diarrhea

Diarrhea that lasts for ≥14 days (usually 2–4 weeks) is considered persistent. Chronic diarrhea usually lasts for >4 weeks. May result from infections due to various organisms.
- Parasites such as *Cryptosporidium, Cyclospora, Entamoeba histolytica, Giardia*
- Bacteria: *Campylobacter, Clostridioides difficile.*

Gastroenteritis

Gastroenteritis or infectious diarrhea may be defined as inflammation of the mucous membrane of the stomach and intestine resulting in combination of diarrhea, vomiting and pain abdomen with or without mucus or blood in stool, fever or dehydration.

Food Poisoning

Food poisoning refers to an illness acquired through consumption of food or drink contaminated either with microorganisms, or their toxins. The agents of food poisoning have different incubation periods.

Microbial agents of food poisoning

1–6 h incubation period: Food contaminated with preformed toxins, which directly act following intake:
- *Staphylococcus aureus* (enterotoxin)
- *Bacillus cereus* (emetic toxin)

8–16 h incubation period: Food contaminated with organisms which release toxin in the intestine:
- *Clostridium perfringens*
- *Bacillus cereus* (diarrheal toxin)

>16 h incubation period: Food contaminated with organisms which release toxin in the intestine or by other mechanisms:
- *Vibrio cholerae*
- Enterotoxigenic *E. coli*
- Enterohemorrhagic *E. coli*
- Non-typhoidal salmonellae and *Shigella* species

Pathogenic Mechanisms of Diarrhea

Enteric pathogens have developed a variety of strategies to overcome host defenses.

Inoculum Size

Enteric pathogens differ from each other in their infective dose to initiate the infection. For example:
- *Shigella*: 10–100 bacilli
- *Vibrio cholerae:* 10^5–10^8 bacilli
- *Salmonella*: 10^3–10^5 bacilli.

Adherence

Adherence to intestinal mucosa helps the organism to compete with the normal bowel flora and there by colonizing the intestinal mucosa.

Toxin Production

Enteric organisms can produce variety of toxins, which are implicated in pathogenesis of diarrhea. These include:
- *Vibrio cholerae:* Cholera toxin
- *Diarrheagenic E. coli:* Heat labile, heat stable and verocytotoxin
- *Shigella:* Shiga toxin, enterotoxin
- *Clostridioides difficile:* Toxin A and B
- Neurotoxins: *S. aureus* enterotoxin, *Bacillus cereus* toxin, *Clostridium botulinum* toxin.

Invasion

In addition to production of toxins, bacterial invasion is another mechanism by which destruction of intestinal mucosal cells takes place resulting in dysentery.

Predisposing Factors

Alterations of the host defense mechanisms can promote the diarrheal diseases.
- **Suppression of the normal flora:** Leads to loss of protective effect of intestinal normal flora
- **Neutralization of gastric acidity:** Promote the acid labile pathogens (e.g. *V. cholerae*)
- **Inhibition of intestinal motility:** Interfere with the clearance of bacteria from the small intestine
- **Age:** Children (<5 years) are more likely to contract most of the diarrheal diseases (e.g. rotavirus) than adults
- **Location:** Closed and semi-closed communities, including daycare centers, schools, residential facilities, and cruise ships are among the important settings for outbreaks of diarrheal diseases
- **Antibiotic-associated:** Patients on prolonged antibiotic course are more likely to develop *C. difficile* infection leading to diarrhea (*refer* **Chapter 26**)
- **Impaired host immunity:** Immunocompromised hosts (e.g. AIDS) are at a higher risk of developing diarrhea.

Laboratory Diagnosis of Diarrheal Diseases

Specimen Collection

Fecal specimen (containing mucus flakes) is collected in a sterile screw capped wide mouthed container. In carriers, a rectal swab may be collected.
- Specimens should be transported to the laboratory within 1 hour
- If a delay of longer than 1 hour is anticipated, the fecal specimen should be collected in transport media like Cary-Blair medium, or alkaline peptone water (if cholera is suspected).

Macroscopy

The following macroscopic appearances are noted:
* Color of the specimen
* Consistency—formed, semi-formed or liquid
* Presence of blood (suggestive of dysentery), mucus or pus (suggestive of inflammatory diarrhea)
* Presence of adult parasitic forms, e.g. *Enterobius*, *Ascaris*, or *Taenia* segments.

Microscopy

* **Wet mount preparation** in saline or iodine is done for detection of pus cells, RBCs and detection of parasitic cysts, trophozoites, eggs or larvae
* **Hanging drop preparation:** To demonstrate darting motility of *Vibrio cholerae*
* **Gram-stained smear:** Not routinely done because of presence of normal flora
* **Modified acid-fast staining** can be carried out for the detection of oocysts of *Cryptosporidium, Cyclospora* and *Cystoisospora*
* **Electron microscopy** of stool specimen: For the detection of viruses, e.g. rotavirus, astrovirus, etc.

Bacterial Culture

* **Culture media:** Fecal specimen should be inoculated onto the following media:
  - *Enrichment broth:* Selenite F broth and alkaline peptone water
  - *Selective medium:* MacConkey agar, DCA (deoxycholate citrate agar), XLD (xylose lysine deoxycholate) agar and TCBS (thiosulfate citrate bile salt sucrose) agar.

* **Identification** of the enteric pathogens is made by performing either conventional biochemical tests or automated identification systems. Then serotyping is performed with specific group or type specific antisera
* **Antimicrobial susceptibility test:** It is done to choose appropriate drug for treatment.

Tissue Culture

This is carried out for the detection of enteric viruses and also for some diarrheagenic *E. coli*.

Antigen Detection

Various test formats are available to detect microbial antigens in stool.
* ELISA is available for detection of rotavirus antigen in stool
* Immunochromatographic test (e.g. **triage parasite panel**) is available for simultaneous detection of *E. histolytica, Giardia* and *Cryptosporidium* in stool
* Rapid test is available to detect *C. difficile* antigens (glutamate dehydrogenase and toxin A/B) in stool.

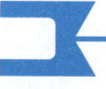

TREATMENT	Diarrhea

Treatment depends up on the severity.
☐ Fluid therapy is the main stay of treatment
☐ Anti-motility agents and adsorbents may be considered in moderate-to-severe diarrhea
☐ Antibiotic therapy is required only for severe diarrhea:
 ➢ Ciprofloxacin or levofloxacin
 ➢ Azithromycin for *Campylobacter*
 ➢ Metronidazole or vancomycin (for *C. difficile*).

EXPECTED QUESTIONS

I. **Write essay on:**
  1. Discuss the etiological agents, pathogenesis, clinical manifestations and laboratory diagnosis of diarrhea.

II. **Write short notes on:**
  1. Dysentery
  2. Traveler's diarrhea
  3. Food poisoning

III. **Multiple Choice Questions (MCQs):**
  1. Which is most common cause of traveler's diarrhea?
     a. *Shigella*   b. ETEC
     c. *V. cholerae*   d. EHEC

  2. Which of the following is the most common etiological agent of acute diarrhea?
     a. Rotavirus
     b. *Shigella*
     c. *V. cholerae*
     d. *Salmonella*

  3. All of the following are predisposing factors for developing diarrhea, *except*:
     a. Suppression of the normal flora
     b. Neutralization of gastric acidity
     c. Inhibition of intestinal motility
     d. Common in adults

Answers
1. b   2. a   3. d

Respiratory Tract Infections

CHAPTER 63

CHAPTER PREVIEW
- Upper Respiratory Tract Infections
- Lower Respiratory Tract Infections

INTRODUCTION

The respiratory tract is divided into two segments, the upper and the lower respiratory tract.
- The upper respiratory tract (URT) includes the nasal cavity, paranasal sinuses, pharynx (throat), epiglottis, and larynx
- The lower respiratory tract (LRT) comprises of trachea, and bronchi, which are divided into bronchioles and lungs, with the surrounding pleura.

UPPER RESPIRATORY TRACT INFECTIONS

The various URT infections (URTI) are pharyngitis and tonsillitis, laryngitis, acute laryngotracheobronchitis (croup), epiglottitis, parapharyngeal infections, infections of the nasal cavity and sinuses.

Pharyngitis and Tonsillitis

Pharyngitis (or sore throat) refers to the inflammation of the pharynx. It commonly affects children, where it presents along with tonsillitis (inflamed tonsils).
- **Agents:** Viral agents are the most common cause, followed by bacterial agents
  - Viral agents: Influenza, parainfluenza viruses, coronaviruses (e.g. COVID-19), adenoviruses, etc.
  - Bacterial agents: *Streptococcus pyogenes, Corynebacterium diphtheriae,* etc.
- **Clinical manifestations** include throat pain, difficulty in swallowing, erythematous (red) and swollen pharynx/tonsil, inflammatory exudate over the pharynx, and rarely membrane over the tonsils (e.g. diphtheria).

Laryngitis

Laryngitis (inflammation of the larynx) has an abrupt onset. The patient presents with hoarseness of the voice. Common causative agents are influenza and parainfluenza viruses, adenoviruses, coronaviruses, etc.

Acute Laryngotracheobronchitis (Croup)

Croup is a more serious disease characterized by fever, inspiratory stridor. It occurs as the infection extends downward from the larynx to involve the trachea or even the bronchi. It is caused by parainfluenza viruses.

Epiglottitis

Epiglottitis is an infection of the epiglottis. It can lead to respiratory obstruction. Children are commonly infected. It is caused by *Haemophilus influenzae* type b.

Parapharyngeal Infections

- **Peritonsillar abscess (or quinsy):** It is a deep neck infection that occurs as a complication of tonsillitis. It usually affects children. The common organisms implicated are *S. pyogenes, S. aureus,* etc.
- **Ludwig's angina:** It is a form of diffuse cellulitis of the mandibular space on the floor of the mouth. This infection most commonly arises from an adjacent dental infection. Often it is polymicrobial infection.

Infections of Nasal Cavity and Sinuses

- **Rhinitis (or common cold):** Rhinoviruses are the most common cause
- **Atrophic rhinitis:** It is caused by *Klebsiella ozaenae,* characterized by chronic foul-smelling mucopurulent nasal discharge
- **Rhinoscleroma:** It is chronic, granulomatous hypertrophy of the nose, caused by *Klebsiella rhinoscleromatis*
- **Sinusitis (i.e. inflammation of the paranasal sinuses):** The common agents are *S. pneumoniae* and *H. influenzae*. Patient usually presents with

frontal headache, loss of smell, nasal congestion, and postnasal drip.

Laboratory Diagnosis of URTI
Specimen Collection and Transport
- **A throat swab** (oropharyngeal swab) containing fibrous exudates is the ideal specimen for pharyngitis. It should be collected by vigorous rubbing of a sterile swab over the posterior pharynx and both the tonsillar pillars. Two swabs may be collected, one for direct smear and the other for culture
- **Specimens** other than throat swabs include:
  - In suspected diphtheria, a portion of the pseudomembrane may be obtained
  - The nasopharyngeal swab is preferred for *B. pertussis* or viruses like influenza or coronavirus. It is collected by inserting a flexible swab through the nose into the posterior nasopharynx and then rotating for 5 seconds.
- **Types of swabs:** Dacron or Rayon swabs are suitable for collecting most URT microorganisms. Flocked swabs are preferable. Cotton swabs can be used for *S. pyogenes*, but are not suitable for viruses
- **Transport:** For isolation of most URT bacterial pathogens, swabs should be processed within 4 hours. However, for molecular diagnosis (bacteria or viruses), the specimens can be stored at 4°C and can be processed late.

Diagnostic Methods
- **Direct smear:** Gram staining is not useful for most of the URTI. Albert stain may be performed when diphtheria is suspected
- **Culture:** Specimens may be inoculated onto blood agar and chocolate agar
- **Molecular methods** such as real-time PCR is the gold standard method for the detection of respiratory viruses such as influenza or coronaviruses and others
- **Antigen detection tests** may be useful for the detection of certain URT pathogens such as SARS CoV-2 from nasopharyngeal swabs.

■ ORAL CAVITY INFECTIONS
Common infections of the oral cavity include:
- **Stomatitis:** It is caused by the herpes simplex virus (HSV); characterized by multiple painful tiny vesicular lesions on the oral mucosa and in the oropharynx
- **Oral thrush:** It is characterized by whitish patches of exudate on the buccal mucosa. It is caused by *Candida* spp., especially in HIV-infected individuals
- **Dental infections** such as root canal infections, dental abscesses, periodontal abscesses, etc., are most commonly caused by anaerobic bacteria and viridans streptococci present in the oral cavity
- **Salivary gland infections** such as parotitis; most often caused by mumps virus or by *Staphylococcus aureus*
- **Vincent's angina:** It is an acute necrotizing ulcerative gingivitis, caused by *Borrelia vincentii* and an anaerobe *Fusobacterium fusiformis*. They are found as normal flora in the mouth.

■ LOWER RESPIRATORY TRACT INFECTIONS
Various lower respiratory tract infections (LRTI) include the infections affecting the bronchus, bronchioles, lungs, and pleura.
- **Bronchitis and bronchiolitis:** It is inflammation of the bronchial tree and bronchioles respectively. Most commonly caused by respiratory syncytial virus (RSV), influenza, and coronavirus and rarely by *Mycoplasma pneumoniae*. It is characterized by expiratory wheeze, tachypnea, nasal flaring, retractions, and irritability
- **Whooping cough:** Caused by *Bordetella pertussis*, characterized by paroxysmal cough—repetitive violent spasmodic coughs, within a single expiration which ends with an audible sound or whoop
- **Pneumonia:** Refers to inflammation of lungs, i.e. either alveoli or interstitium space (discussed below)
- **Tuberculosis:** Caused by *Mycobacterium tuberculosis* (discussed in **Chapter 27**)
- **Fungal lung disease:** It is most often caused by *Pneumocystis jirovecii*
- **Parasitic lung disease:** Agents include *Paragonimus westermani* or larvae of nematodes like *Ascaris*
- **Lung abscess:** Abscess formation in the lung parenchyma, either primary (due to anaerobic bacteria) or secondary to low immunity
- **Pleural effusion:** Presence of an excess quantity of fluid in the pleural space. It could be due to secondary to bacterial pneumonia or tuberculous pleuritic or viral pleural effusion.

Pneumonia
Pneumonia refers to inflammation of the lungs. Pneumonia is classified into two groups:
1. **Lobar or typical pneumonia:** It involves infection of the lung parenchyma and its alveoli. It is characterized by consolidation and productive cough with purulent sputum. It is mostly caused by pyogenic organisms such as: *Streptococcus pneumoniae, Haemophilus influenzae, Staphylococcus aureus, E. coli, Klebsiella, Pseudomonas, Acinetobacter*, etc.
2. **Interstitial or atypical pneumonia** occurs in the interstitial space of the lungs. It is caused by:

- Bacteria such as *Mycoplasma, Chlamydia, Legionella* species, etc.
- Viruses such as influenza, coronaviruses, respiratory syncytial virus, parainfluenza, etc.
- Fungal agents causing pneumonia.

In lieu of epidemiological point of view, pneumonia can also be classified into:

Community-acquired: Patients acquire the infection in the community. Common agents are pneumococcus, *Mycoplasma pneumoniae, H. influenzae, Chlamydia pneumoniae*, and viral pneumonia.

Healthcare-associated: This is more frequently observed in patients on mechanical ventilation, called as **ventilator-associated pneumonia (VAP)**. It is caused by the **multidrug-resistant** pathogens found in the hospital environment such as *Pseudomonas, Acinetobacter, Escherichia coli, Klebsiella pneumoniae* and MRSA (methicillin-resistant *S. aureus*).

Clinical Features

Common clinical features of pneumonia include: Fever with chills and/or sweats, tachycardia, increased respiratory rate, dyspnea (shortness of breath), pleuritic chest pain (in case of pleural effusion) and cough.

Laboratory Diagnosis of LRTI

Specimen Collection

Important specimens for LRTI include sputum, induced sputum, tracheal aspirate, bronchoalveolar lavage (BAL), protected specimen brush (PSB), lung aspirate, and pleural fluid.

Microscopy

- ❖ **Gram staining** of the sputum specimens is done to determine the specimen quality (pus cells are >25 and epithelial cells are <10 per low power field) and also to detect organisms:
  - Gram-positive cocci, pair, lanceolate shaped—suggestive of pneumococcus
  - Pleomorphic gram-negative coccobacilli—suggestive of *Haemophilus influenzae*
- ❖ **Acid-fast staining** of sputum by Ziehl-Neelsen technique is performed to demonstrate the acid-fast bacilli, e.g. *M. tuberculosis*
- ❖ **GMS stain** (Gomori methenamine silver stain) is used to demonstrate *Pneumocystis jirovecii*.

Culture

Specimens should be collected before antibiotic therapy for better yield of organisms.

- ❖ **Bacterial culture** is performed by using media such as blood agar, chocolate agar, and MacConkey agar
- ❖ **For *M. tuberculosis*:** Lowenstein-Jensen medium or automated MGIT (mycobacteria growth indicator tube) may be used
- ❖ **For fungal pathogen isolation:** Sabouraud dextrose agar is used.

Serology (Antibody Detection)

Antibody detection tests by methods such as ELISA can be used for the diagnosis of atypical pneumonia pathogens such as *Mycoplasma, Chlamydia*, and viruses.

Antigen Detection Tests

Various antigen detection methods available include: (i) Enzyme immunoassay (to detect *Legionella pneumophila* antigens in urine) and (ii) Direct fluorescent antibody tests (for influenza virus, respiratory syncytial virus, and *B. pertussis*).

Molecular Test

Molecular methods such as multiplex PCR assays, real-time PCR are available for detection of the agents of pneumonia.

EXPECTED QUESTIONS

I. **Write short notes on:**
   1. Laboratory diagnosis of pharyngitis.
   2. Laboratory diagnosis of pneumonia.

II. **Multiple Choice Questions (MCQs):**
   1. All cause lobar pneumonia, *except*:
      a. *S. pneumoniae*
      b. *H. influenzae*
      c. *B. pertussis*
      d. *Klebsiella*
   2. Interstitial pneumonia is caused by all, *except*:
      a. Mycoplasma
      b. Chlamydia
      c. Legionella
      d. Pneumococci

Answers
1. c   2. d

Miscellaneous Infective Syndromes

CHAPTER 64

CHAPTER PREVIEW
- Skin and Soft Tissue Infections
- Sexually Transmitted Infections
- Congenital Infections
- Eye Infections
- Ear Infections

SKIN AND SOFT TISSUE INFECTIONS

Skin and soft tissue infections (SSTIs) can arise from invasion of organism through skin or from organisms that reach the skin from blood as a part of systemic infection.
- Skin comprises of epidermis, dermis and subcutaneous tissues. Hair follicles and sweat glands originate in the subcutaneous tissues
- Infection can involve any of these layers of skin **(Table 64.1)**.

Clinical Types of SSTIs

Skin infections can be subdivided into primary and secondary lesions:
- **Primary lesion:** An area of tissue with impaired structure/function due to damage by trauma or disease
- **Secondary lesion:** A lesion arising as a consequence of any primary infection.

Agents implicated in surgical site infections and burn wound infections are listed in **Tables 64.2 and 64.3** respectively.

Laboratory Diagnosis

Specimen Collection

Appropriate specimens include:
- Pus from the wound collected by sterile swab
- Pus from abscess collected by incision and drainage, or needle aspiration
- Vesicle or bulla fluid, collected by needle aspiration or sterile swab
- Subcutaneous infections: Sample collected from the base of the lesion or biopsy of the deep tissues
- Skin scrapings, plucked hair or nail clippings in suspected fungal infections.

Microscopy

- Gram staining of the specimen may demonstrate the morphology of the causative organisms
- KOH mount is done for suspected fungal infections (e.g. dermatophyte)
- Tzanck smear of the vesicle fluid suspected of herpes simplex or varicella virus infections.

Culture

- For the culture of aerobic bacteria, specimens are inoculated onto blood agar and MacConkey agar and incubated overnight at 37°C
- **For culture of atypical *Mycobacterium*:** Lowenstein-Jensen medium may be used
- **For dermatophytes:** Sabouraud's dextrose agar is used
- **For anaerobic organisms:** Robertson's cooked meat broth and BHIS (brain heart infusion agar with supplements) should be used. The plates should be incubated anaerobically.

Quantitative Culture

As the degree of bacterial contamination of the wound, is directly related to the chance of development of wound sepsis, hence quantitative culture may be performed to determine the number of colony forming units/gram of the tissue collected from the wound.

Identification

Accurate identification of the causative agent is done based on colony morphology, culture smear, and biochemical reactions or automated identification systems.

CHAPTER 64 ◆ Miscellaneous Infective Syndromes

Table 64.1: Infective skin manifestations and their common causative agents.

Skin lesions	Description	Common etiological agents
Macule	Flat, non-palpable discoloration of skin (≤5 mm size) If size exceeds 5 mm, is called as patch	Dermatophytes, viral rashes (e.g. enterovirus)
Papule	Elevated palpable solid lesion, usually ≤5 mm in size	Molluscum contagiosum, scabies (*Sarcoptes scabiei*), warts (Human Papilloma virus)
Nodule	Elevated palpable solid lesion, usually >5 mm in size	*Corynebacterium diphtheriae*, post kala-azar dermal leishmaniasis, *nocardia* species, etc.
Vesicle	Fluid-filled lesions with a diameter ≤5 mm	Herpes simplex virus, varicella-zoster virus
Bulla	Fluid-filled lesions with a diameter >5 mm	Herpes simplex virus, *Staphylococcus aureus*
Pustule	A fluid-filled vesicle containing pus and is ≤5 mm	*Staphylococcus aureus*
Abscess	A fluid-filled lesion containing pus and is >5 mm	*Streptococcus pyogenes*
Secondary lesions		
Scale	Excess dead epidermal layer	Dermatophytes
Ulcer	A lesion with loss of epidermis and dermis	*Mycobacterium leprae* (leprosy), *Mycobacterium ulcerans* (Buruli ulcer), *T. pallidum* (hard chancre)
Impetigo	Erythematous lesions which may be bullous or non-bullous with exudates and golden-yellow crusts	Non-bullous: *Streptococcus pyogenes* Bullous: *Staphylococcus aureus*
Cellulitis	Diffuse spreading infection involving deep layers of dermis Ill-defined flat red, painful lesions	*Streptococcus pyogenes* *Staphylococcus aureus*
Hair follicle infections		
Folliculitis	Superficial infection of single hair follicle, presents as pustule	*Staphylococcus aureus*
Furuncle	Deeper infections of the hair follicles, presents as abscess, spread deeply into dermis and subcutaneous tissues	
Carbuncle	Represents the coalescence of a number of furuncles	
Infection of fascia and muscles		
Necrotizing fasciitis	Rapidly spreading infection of fascia	*Streptococcus pyogenes* *Staphylococcus aureus*
Pyomyositis	Pus formation in the muscle layer	*Staphylococcus aureus* *Streptococcus pyogenes*
Myonecrosis	Extensive necrosis of the muscle layer with gangrene formation	Clostridial myonecrosis Other anaerobic infections

Table 64.2: Agents causing surgical site wound infection.

Bacterial agents	Fungi
For most clean wounds: • *Staphylococcus aureus* • Coagulase-negative staphylococci • *Enterococcus*	*Candida albicans*
If bowel integrity is compromised: • Gram-negative flora like *E. coli* and • Anaerobic organisms like *Bacteroides*, *Prevotella*, etc.	

Antimicrobial Susceptibility Test
It helps in initiation of appropriate therapy.

Table 64.3: Agents causing burn wound infections.

Bacteria	Fungi
Staphylococcus aureus (may be MRSA) *Pseudomonas aeruginosa* Coagulase-negative staphylococci (e.g. *S. epidermidis*)	*Candida albicans*

(MRSA, methicillin resistant *Staphylococcus aureus*)

TREATMENT — SSTIs

Skin and soft tissue infections are treated by both surgically (incision and drainage or surgical debridement) and medically (antibiotics).

SEXUALLY TRANSMITTED INFECTIONS

The sexually transmitted infections (STIs) are a group of communicable diseases which are transmitted by sexual contact.

Causative agents of STIs may be classified into two groups:
1. Agents causing local manifestations such as:
   - Genital ulcers
   - Urethral discharge
   - Vaginal discharge
   - Genital warts
   - Pelvic inflammatory diseases.
2. Agents transmitted by sexual route, producing only systemic manifestations and do not cause local manifestations (e.g. HIV).

The microorganisms causing STIs are listed in **Table 64.4** and the important features of STIs producing genital ulcers are compared in **Table 64.5**.

Table 64.4: Causative agents of sexually transmitted infections (STIs).

Agents causing local manifestations		
Genital ulcers		
	Syphilis	*Treponema pallidum*
	Herpes genitalis	Herpes simplex viruses
	Chancroid	*Haemophilus ducreyi*
	Lymphogranuloma venereum	*Chlamydia trachomatis*
	Donovanosis	*Klebsiella granulomatis*
Urethral discharge		
	Gonorrhea	*Neisseria gonorrhoeae*
	Non-gonococcal urethritis (NGU)	• *Chlamydia trachomatis* (D-K) • *Ureaplasma urealyticum* • *Mycoplasma genitalium* • *Mycoplasma hominis* • Herpes simplex virus • *Candida albicans* • *Trichomonas vaginalis*
Vaginal discharge		
	Vulvovaginal candidiasis	*Candida albicans* Non-albicans *Candida* species
	Bacterial vaginosis	*Gardnerella vaginalis*
	Trichomonal vaginitis	*Trichomonas vaginalis*
Genital warts		
	Condyloma acuminata	Human papilloma viruses
Agents causing systemic manifestations		
	Pelvic inflammatory diseases (PID)	*Neisseria gonorrhoeae* *Chlamydia trachomatis*
	No genital lesions but only systemic manifestations	HIV Hepatitis B virus (HBV) Hepatitis C virus (HCV)

Laboratory Diagnosis of STIs

Specimen Collection
- Discharge from the infected area such as vaginal or urethral discharge are collected in a sterile container
- **Sterile swabs may be used to collect the discharge** (if scanty): Charcoal impregnated swabs are used for suspected gonococcal infection
- Fluid from the vesicles (genital herpes).

Microscopy
- **Wet mount examination:** It is carried out for the vaginal discharge:
   - In trichomoniasis: Pus cells along with motile trophozoites are seen
   - In candidiasis: Yeast cells along with pseudohyphae are seen.
- **Gram-stained smear** of the discharge or the swab is useful for:
   - Bacterial vaginosis—clue cells are seen, which are vaginal epithelial cells studded with gram variable pleomorphic coccobacilli: suggestive of *Gardnerella vaginalis*
   - In gonorrhea—intracellular kidney-shaped diplococci are seen
   - In candidiasis—gram-positive budding yeast cells along with pseudohyphae are seen.
- **Giemsa stain** is done for:
   - *Klebsiella granulomatis* to detect the presence of Donovan's bodies (macrophage filled with bipolar stained bacilli)
   - *Chlamydia trachomatis* inclusion bodies.
- **Dark field microscopy** and silver impregnation methods—in syphilis, reveals characteristic spirally coiled bacilli.

Culture
Specimens are inoculated onto the appropriate culture media or cell line for the isolation of the causative organism.
- Thayer-Martin medium—for *N. gonorrhoeae*
- McCoy cell line—for *Chlamydia trachomatis*
- Sabouraud's dextrose agar (SDA)—for *Candida* species
- Cell lines such as Vero cells, monkey kidney cell line for herpes simplex virus.

Serology
Serological tests such as venereal disease research laboratory (VDRL) or rapid plasma reagin (RPR) test can be performed for the diagnosis of syphilis.

Molecular Test
Multiplex PCR and real-time PCR have been developed for simultaneous detection of pathogens causing STIs.

CHAPTER 64 ◆ Miscellaneous Infective Syndromes

Table 64.5: Comparison of sexually transmitted infections (STIs) producing genital ulcer.

Feature	Syphilis	Herpes	Chancroid	LGV	Donovanosis
Incubation period	9–90 days	2–7 days	1–14 days	3 days–6 weeks	1–4 weeks (up to 6 months)
Genital ulcer	Painless, indurated, single	Multiple, painful	Painful, soft usually multiple	Painless, firm single lesion	Painless, single/multiple, beefy-red ulcer
Lymphadenopathy	Painless, firm, bilateral	Painful, firm, often bilateral	Painful, soft, marked swelling leads to bubo formation	Painful and soft, unilateral	Absent (pseudobubo may be present due to subcutaneous swelling)

(LGV, lymphogranuloma venereum)

> **TREATMENT** — Urethritis
>
> Combination of ceftriaxone + azithromycin is the recommended regimen. Ceftriaxone will act against gonococcus and azithromycin will treat *C. trachomatis*; as these are the common causative agents of urethritis. Treatment to both the sexual partners is needed.

■ CONGENITAL INFECTIONS

Vertical transmission refers to the spread of infections from mother-to-baby. These infections may occur by transplacental route (congenital infection), during delivery, or after delivery.

Congenital Infection

A congenital infection is an infection that crosses the placenta to infect the fetus. They often lead to defects in fetal development or even death.

TORCH is an acronym used for some common congenital infections. These are:
- **T**oxoplasmosis
- **O**ther infections (congenital syphilis, hepatitis B, Coxsackie virus, Epstein-Barr virus, varicella-zoster virus, *Plasmodium falciparum* and human parvovirus)
- **R**ubella
- **C**ytomegalovirus (CMV)
- **H**erpes simplex virus.

Perinatal Infections (During Delivery)

Perinatal infections occur while the baby moves through an infected birth canal. These infections are usually caused by the agents of STIs. These also include the infections transmitted through contamination with fecal matter during delivery. Common examples of agents causing perinatal infections include:
- Cytomegalovirus
- *Neisseria gonorrhoeae*
- *Chlamydia* species
- Herpes simplex virus
- Human papilloma virus (genital warts)
- Group B streptococci.

Postnatal Infections (After Delivery)

These infections spread from mother to baby following delivery, usually during breastfeeding. Some examples of postnatal infections are: CMV, HIV and group B streptococci.

■ EYE INFECTIONS

In general, ocular infections are grouped into:
- **Infections involving external structures of the eyes:** such as eyelid (blepharitis), conjunctiva (conjunctivitis), cornea (keratitis) and sclera (scleritis)
- **Infections involving internal structures:** Retina (retinitis), uvea (uveitis) and aqueous humor or vitreous humor (endophthalmitis).

The list of the organisms causing various ocular infections is given in **Table 64.6**.

Table 64.6: Ocular infections and their causative agents.

Infections	Organisms
Blepharitis (Infection of eyelids)	*Staphylococcus aureus*
Conjunctivitis (Infection of conjunctiva)	• *Haemophilus influenzae* • *Staphylococcus aureus* • *Chlamydia trachomatis* • *Neisseria gonorrhoeae* • Adenovirus, Herpes simplex virus
Keratitis (Infection of cornea)	• *Staphylococcus aureus* • *Streptococcus pneumoniae* • *Fusarium, Candida* • *Acanthamoeba*
Scleritis (Infection of sclera)	*Staphylococcus aureus*
Chorioretinitis and uveitis (Infection of choroid, retina, and uvea)	• *Mycobacterium tuberculosis* • *Treponema pallidum* • Cytomegalovirus • *Toxoplasma gondii*
Endophthalmitis (Infection of aqueous humor or vitreous humor)	• *Staphylococcus aureus* • *Streptococcus pneumoniae* • *Pseudomonas aeruginosa* • Other gram-negative bacilli • Herpes simplex virus, *Candida*

Table 64.7: Organisms causing ear infections.	
Otitis externa: Infection of external ears	**Otitis media: Middle ear infections**
Acute otitis externa • *Staphylococcus aureus* (most common) • *Streptococcus pyogenes* • *Pseudomonas* (malignant otitis externa) • Other gram-negative bacilli • *Aspergillus* species • *Candida* species	**Acute otitis media** • *Streptococcus pneumoniae*: Most common (33%, in children) • *Haemophilus influenzae* type b (second most common) • *Moraxella catarrhalis* • *Streptococcus pyogenes* • Respiratory syncytial virus • Influenza virus
Chronic otitis externa • Anaerobes (most common) • *Pseudomonas*	**Chronic otitis media** Anaerobes (most common)

■ EAR INFECTIONS

Common ear infections are **(Table 64.7)**.
❖ **Otitis externa:** Inflammation, irritation, or infection of the outer ear and ear canal
  ■ Also called as swimmer's ear—swimming in contaminated water is one of the reasons of contracting swimmer's ear
  ■ Symptoms—itchy ear canal, Inflammation of ear canal's skin and pus formation in ear canal and earache that is aggravated when the ear lobe is pulled.
❖ **Otitis media:** Infections of middle ear; characterized by earache and ear discharge
  ■ It often begins with an infection that causes a sore throat, cold or respiratory problem and eventually spread to the middle ear
  ■ Symptoms include: Intense earache, headache, fever and nausea and leaking of discharge from ear following rupture of the tympanic membrane.

EXPECTED QUESTIONS

I. **Write short notes on:**
  1. TORCH infections.
  2. Laboratory diagnosis of skin and soft tissue infections.
  3. Laboratory diagnosis of sexually transmitted infections.

II. **Multiple Choice Questions (MCQs):**
  1. Which of the following sexually transmitted infection produces painful genital ulcers and painful lymph nodes?
     a. Syphilis
     b. Chancroid
     c. LGV
     d. Donovanosis
  2. The agent of malignant otitis externa is:
     a. *Staphylococcus aureus*
     b. *Pseudomonas aeruginosa*
     c. *Streptococcus pyogenes*
     d. *Candida albicans*
  3. Not a common cause of surgical site infection is:
     a. *Staphylococcus epidermidis*
     b. *Pseudomonas aeruginosa*
     c. *Acinetobacter* species
     d. *Burkholderia pseudomallei*

Answers
1. b   2. b   3. d

Specimen Collection and Transport

CHAPTER 65

CHAPTER PREVIEW
- Specimen Collection
- Specimen Transport

SPECIMEN COLLECTION

Specimen Collection
A young patient with history of high grade fever with chills for two days, presents to the out patient department. Upon detailed clinical examination, clinician decides to admit him and requests for his blood and urine culture and susceptibility testing. After two days of hospitalization he develops diarrhea with two episodes of vomiting. His stool specimen was collected and sent for culture. Discuss the method of collection of the following specimens for culture.
- Blood for blood culture
- Urine specimen for microscopy and culture
- Stool specimen for microscopy and culture

Explanation
The specimen collection has been explained in the following chapters
- Blood collection for culture: *Refer* **Chapter 59**
- Urine specimen collection for microscopy and culture: Explained subsequently in this chapter
- Stool specimen collection for microscopy and culture: Explained subsequently in this chapter.

Specimen collection depends upon the type of underlying infections. *Refer* **Table 3.2.1 of Chapter 3.2** for details regarding various specimens collected in different clinical conditions.

General Principles
The following general principles should be followed while collecting the specimen:
- **Standard precautions** should be followed while collecting and handling all specimens (**Chapter 15** for details)
- Whenever possible, culture specimens should be collected prior to administration of any antimicrobial agents
- **Contamination** with indigenous flora should be avoided
- Tissue, aspirate and body fluids are superior to wound swabs
- **Container:** Specimens should be collected in sterile, tightly sealed, leak proof, wide-mouth, screw-capped containers
- **Labeling:** All specimens must be appropriately labeled with patient identity details.
- **Rejection:** Specimens grossly contaminated or improperly labeled may be rejected (see highlight box below)
- If **anaerobic culture** is requested, proper anaerobic collection containers with media should be used
- Specimen should not be sent in container containing **formalin** for microbiological culture analysis.

Specimen Rejection Criteria
Microbiology samples that do not meet the *appropriate sample* and the *test request requirements* need to be rejected, so as to prevent inaccurate data and to ensure the safety of patients and laboratory personnel. Reasons for sample rejection may include the following:
- Improperly labeled or unlabeled sample
- Incomplete patient information on the sample and/or on the requisition form
- Suboptimal sample, i.e., leaking urine and/or stool containers, insufficient quantity
- Sample delayed in transit more than the accepted limit.

SPECIMEN COLLECTION FOR BACTERIAL INFECTIONS

Blood Specimen
In clinical microbiology laboratories, blood collection is indicated either for blood culture or for serological tests.

Collection of Blood Specimen for Culture
Blood culture is regarded as one of the most important culture investigation performed by clinical microbiology laboratory. As there is a high risk of contamination with skin flora, sterile aseptic precautions must be taken for

collection and skin is disinfected with two agents—70% alcohol followed by chlorhexidine. It is discussed in detail in **Chapter 59**.

Collection of Blood Specimen for Serology

Collection of blood specimen for serological (e.g., virology or immunology) diagnostic tests is similar to as done for culture; except that skin disinfection is performed by only one agent i.e., 70% isopropyl alcohol. This is because contamination with skin flora is not an issue while performing these investigations.

- The blood sample is collected in clean sterile tubes (Vacutainers, **Fig. 65.1B**)
- Tube is filled three-fourths full and then allowed to stand at room temperature for a few hours to allow a solid clot to form and retract
- Then the tube is centrifuged, serum is separated, placed in another clean tube, which can be used for further diagnostic testing.

CSF and Other Sterile Body Fluids

CSF and other sterile body fluids should be collected before the starting of antimicrobial therapy, in sterile screw capped container, under adequate aseptic precautions.

- **CSF:** It is collected by lumbar puncture at interspace L3-L4, or L4-L5. The site is first disinfected with antiseptics similar to that used for blood culture. After collection, CSF is then divided into three sterile tubes (2 mL each) for three diagnostic laboratories
    - Biochemistry (for total protein and glucose)
    - Bacteriology (culture and susceptibility, Gram staining, antigen detection)
    - Cytology (for cell count).
- **Body fluids from other sterile sites** such as ascitic fluid, pleural fluid, peritoneal fluid, and synovial fluid specimens are collected by percutaneous aspiration under aseptic precautions with syringe and needle
- **Body fluid specimens** can also be inoculated at bedside directly on to BacT/ALERT bottles for culture. In these case, a portion of the specimen should be aliquoted separately for Gram stain
- **Transport:** Specimens should be transported immediately (within 15 min) to the laboratory; If any delay is expected, body fluid specimens can be stored at 37°C (in incubator) or at room temperature; *but never refrigerated*, as delicate pathogens such as *H. influenzae*, pneumococci or meningococci may die.

Sterile Universal Specimen Container (Fig. 65.1A)

These are designed for collecting biological specimens, including urine, stool, sputum, peritoneal exudate, joint fluid, biopsy specimen, sterile body fluids and aspirates for microbiological culture and susceptibility testing. It is very convenient for sample collection at the bed side. These containers should have the following specifications:

- They should be sterile, leak-proof, wide mouthed and screw capped
- Each container should bear the name of the patient, from whom the specimen was collected and his hospital register number
- Specimen type and date and time of collection
- A completely filled investigation requisition form should always accompany the specimen indicating the investigation requested along with the probable clinical diagnosis and current antibiotic therapy

Fecal Specimens

A small quantity of semisolid/solid stool or one third of the container in case of liquid stool specimen is collected in a wide mouthed, sterile screw capped, leak proof container (**Fig. 65.1A**); preferably prior to initiation of antibiotics.

- **Rectal swabs** may be collected in case of asymptomatic carriers
- **Transport:** Sample should be immediately transported to the laboratory. In case of delay, suitable transport media may be employed such as Cary-Blair medium or Venkatraman-Ramakrishnan (VR) medium.

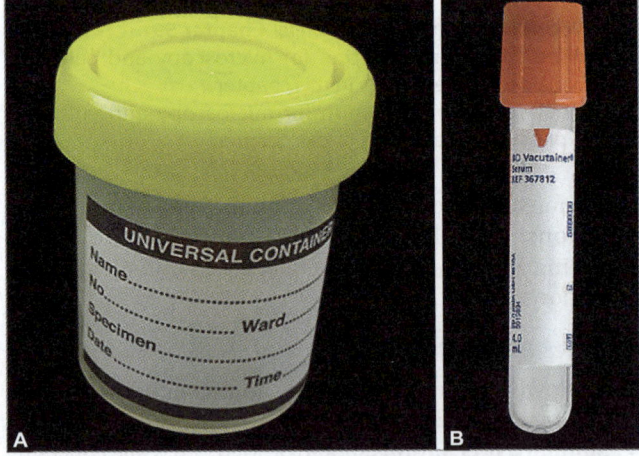

Figs. 65.1A and B: A. Sterile universal container; **B.** Blood collection Vacutainer tube.

Respiratory Specimens

Respiratory specimens are categorized into two groups.
- Upper respiratory tract specimens such as throat swab, nasopharyngeal swabs, bits of membrane from tonsil
- Lower respiratory tract specimens such as sputum, endotracheal aspirate (ETA) and bronchoalveolar lavage (BAL), protected specimen brush (PSB) and lung biopsy.

Sputum

Sputum cultures are indicated to identify the pathogens causing pneumonia.
- Sputum specimen that results following a deep cough is preferable and is collected in a sterile screw capped, wide-mouthed, leak proof container **(Fig. 65.1A)**. Patient should be instructed to place the rim of the container under the lower lip to catch entire expectorated mucopurulent sputum
- **Early morning sputum** samples should be obtained as they contain pooled overnight secretions, as they may contain increased concentration of pathogens
- **For suspected tuberculosis**
  - **Two sputum** specimens are collected- spot and early morning. Sputum collection booths should be located away from other people, outside in an open well ventilated space
  - **Gastric aspirate** may be collected for infants in suspected case of tuberculosis. Early morning specimen is ideal before eating/getting up. Transport time should be <15 minutes.
- Collected specimen has to be transported to the laboratory as soon as possible (within two hours); as delicate pathogens may otherwise die, if there is a delay.

ETA, BAL, PSB and Lung Biopsy Specimens

Collection of endotracheal aspirate (ETA), bronchoalveolar lavage (BAL), protected specimen brush (PSB) and lung biopsy specimens is technically demanding and requires specialized techniques. These specimens should be transported immediately to the laboratory and cultured within one hour of collection.

Throat Swab

Throat swab samples for bacterial culture is collected by depressing the tongue with a tongue depressor. The oropharyngeal swab is rubbed on the back of the throat, over the tonsils, and in any other area where there is redness or pus. Whenever possible, a portion of pseudomembrane may be collected.

Nasopharyngeal Secretions

Nasopharyngeal specimens are the best specimens which may be obtained by:

- **Nasopharyngeal aspiration** (best method): Collected by inserting flexible swab through nose into posterior nasopharynx and rotating for 5 seconds; specimen of choice for *Bordetella pertussis*
- **Per-nasal swab**: Collected by using a sterile swab on a flexible wire.

Note: For culture in a suspected case of pertussis, alginate swabs are the best followed by dacron swabs. Cotton swabs are not satisfactory. It is recommended to collect six swabs, at 1–2 days intervals to achieve maximum yield.

Exudate Specimens

Wound swabs (sterile cotton swab, **Fig. 65.2**) are recommended to identify the etiological agents causing deep-seated wound infection.
- Wound swabs are ideally collected prior to starting of antibiotic therapy and only for clinically infected wounds or that fail to heal even after a long period
- **For closed wounds** disinfect with 70% alcohol or 2% chlorhexidine followed by 10% povidone-iodine. Remove iodine with alcohol just prior to specimen collection
- **Open wounds** are first debrided and then thoroughly rinsed with sterile saline prior to collection
- Preferably sample the **viable tissue** and not the superficial debris
- A portion of the sample also must be placed in Robertson's Cooked Meat (RCM) medium, if anaerobic culture is indicated
- For collection of pus in the form of **abscess**, aspirate the deepest portion of the lesion with a syringe and needle
- **For burn wound** swab collection, consider sampling different areas of the burn, as organisms may not be evenly distributed in a burn wound
- **Aspirates and tissue specimens** should be delivered to the laboratory for further processing within 30 minutes of collection for best recovery. Tissue specimens must be kept moist to preserve viability of organisms
- **For anaerobic culture,** aspirates or tissue specimens are recommended. Specimen which are not suitable include swab, urine, sputum etc.
- **Discharging sinus:** In case of actinomycetoma, **granules** present in the discharge are collected in sterile gauze or loop by pressing the sinuses from the periphery to express them out.

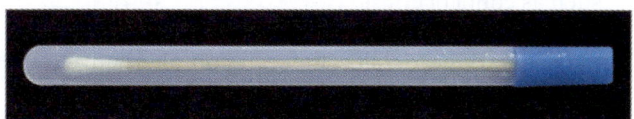

Fig. 65.2: Sterile cotton swab.

Urine Specimen

It is extremely important to collect the urine specimens carefully to avoid the contamination with normal urethral flora. The various type of collection of urine specimen for culture has been described below.

- **Midstream clean catch urine:** It is the most common type of urine specimen collected for culture. After properly cleaning the urethral meatus or glans with soap and water, urine specimen is collected in a sterile, wide mouthed, screw capped, leak proof container by voiding the first portion (which is likely to be contaminated with normal urethral flora) **(Fig. 65.1A)**
- **Indwelling catheter:** Urine specimen should be collected from the catheter tubing (after clamping and disinfecting a portion of the catheter tubing with alcohol), by inserting a sterile syringe and needle directly into the catheter tubing. Urine *must not be* collected from the drainage bag
- **Suprapubic aspiration:** It is the **most ideal** urine specimen, as it avoids the risk of contamination with urethral flora
  - However it is invasive and therefore is recommended only for patients in coma or infants
  - The skin above the bladder is disinfected and then urine is collected needle aspiration above the symphysis pubis through the abdominal wall into the full bladder.
- **Transport:** Urine specimen must be transported to the microbiology laboratory as soon as possible and should be processed immediately. If delay is expected for more than two hours, then it can be stored in refrigerator or stored by adding boric acid or glycerol for maximum 24 hours before plating.

Genital Specimens

Common genital specimens include urethral discharge for urethritis and exudate from genital ulcers.

Urethral Discharge

Urethral swab in men and cervical swab in women are the preferred specimens. Vaginal swab is not satisfactory.
- **Method:** The urethral meatus is cleaned with gauze soaked in saline. The purulent discharge is expressed out by pressing at the base of the penis and collected directly on to slides or swabs
- **Swab:** Dacron or rayon swabs are preferred, as cotton and alginate swabs are inhibitory to many urethral pathogens such as gonococci
- **In chronic urethritis:** As discharge is minimal, prostatic massage is done to collect the secretion; alternatively, the morning drop of secretion may also be collected
- **Transport Media:** Specimens should be transported immediately. If not possible, then charcoal containing Stuart's or Amies transport medium can be used.

Exudate from Genital Ulcers

Surface of the genital ulcer is cleaned with saline, gentle pressure is applied at the base of the lesion, and a drop of exudate is collected on a slide.

Endometrial specimens: Collected by surgical biopsy or trans-cervical aspirate via sheathed catheter.

Other Specimens

- **Ocular specimens:** They are precious specimens, should be transported to laboratory within 15 min. Bedside inoculation onto blood agar may be considered if delay is unavoidable
  - **Conjunctival swab:** Swabs should be pre-moistened with sterile saline and samples should be collected from both the eyes
  - **Corneal scrapings:** Clinicians should instill local anesthetics before collection
  - **Aqueous or vitreous fluid** for endophthalmitis cases.
- **Ear specimens:**
  - **External ear:** Specimen is collected by firmly rotating the swab into the outer ear **(Fig. 65.2)**
  - **Inner ear specimens:** If ear drum is intact, material behind the drum is aspirated with syringe; if ear drum is ruptured, swab is used to collect material from the inner ear. Ear canal should be cleaned with mild soap solution before aspiration.

SPECIMEN TRANSPORT AND STORAGE BEFORE PROCESSING

Specimen Transport

The specimens should reach the laboratory for further processing as soon as possible after the collection. If required appropriate transport media should be used.

For most of the specimens, transport time should not exceed **two hours**. However, there are some exceptions.
- Specimens such as CSF and body fluids, ocular specimens, tissue specimens, suprapubic aspirate and bone specimen should be **transported immediately** (<15 minutes)
- **Urine (midstream)** added with preservative (boric acid) is acceptable up to 24 hours, otherwise should be transported within 2 hours
- **Stool culture:** Stool specimen should be transported within 1 hour, but with transport media such as Cary-Blair medium or Venkatraman-Ramakrishnan (VR) medium, is acceptable up to 24 hours
- **Rectal swabs**—up to 24 hours is acceptable
- **For anaerobic culture:** Specimens should be put into Robertson's cooked meat broth or any specialized anaerobic transport system and transported immediately to the laboratory.

Specimen Storage before Processing

Most specimens can be stored **at room temperature** immediately after receipt, for **up to 24 hours**. However, there are some exceptions.
- **Blood cultures**—should be incubated at 37°C immediately upon receipt
- **Sterile body fluids, bone, vitreous fluid, suprapubic aspirate**—should be immediately plated upon receipt and incubated at 37°C
- **Corneal scraping**—should be immediately plated at bed-side on to blood agar and chocolate agar
- **Stool culture**—stool specimen for culture can be stored up to 72 hours at 4°C
- **Urine** (mid-stream and from the catheter), **lower respiratory** tract specimen, **gastric biopsy** (for *Helicobacter pylori*)—can be stored up to 24 hours at 4°C.

Prioritizing the Specimen for Processing

Certain precious specimens such as CSF and sterile body fluids, ocular specimens, tissue specimens, suprapubic aspirate and bone specimen should be processed immediately as soon as received, not more than 15 min delay. Similarly, blood culture bottles should be immediately incubated upon receipt.

SPECIMEN COLLECTION FOR VIRAL INFECTIONS

Specimen collection has to be done early in the patient's illness as possible, as viruses can be recovered only for a few days after the onset of illness. The following steps should be kept in mind during specimen collection:

Appropriate time: Specimens should be collected as soon as possible, preferably within 3 days after onset of symptoms.
- From the correct site **(Table 65.1)**
- In the correct method of collection
- In adequate volume **(Fig. 65.3)**
- In suitable containers (sterile and chemical free)—e.g., viral transport media
- Transport in correct temperature: Specimen to be kept at 4°C for 3–5 days, after which the sample should be kept at –70°C **(Fig. 65.3)**
- Correctly labeled (patient details and specimen details).

Specimen Collection for COVID-19

Combined oropharyngeal and nasopharyngeal swab is recommended (NP/OP swab) for the diagnosis of COVID-19. Same specimen collection method is followed for detection of other respiratory viruses from nasopharyngeal swab by real-time RCR technique. Refer highlight box for details.

Table 65.1: Various types of viral infections and specimen of choice.

Systemic infections	Specimens to be collected
Respiratory infections	• Swabs (nasal, throat, nasopharyngeal) • Bronchoalveolar lavage, nasal washings • Aspirates (nasal or sinus), serum
Viral encephalitis	• Cerebrospinal fluid • Throat washings • Tissue by brain biopsy (postmortem) • Stool and serum
Viral gastroenteritis	Stool and serum
Exanthematous infections	• Vesicle aspirate • Skin scrapping • Skin biopsy
Poliomyelitis	• Stool and rectal swabs • Serum
Sexually-transmitted infections	Serum
Teratogenic viruses	Serum
Conjunctivitis	Conjunctival swab
Vector-borne diseases	Serum

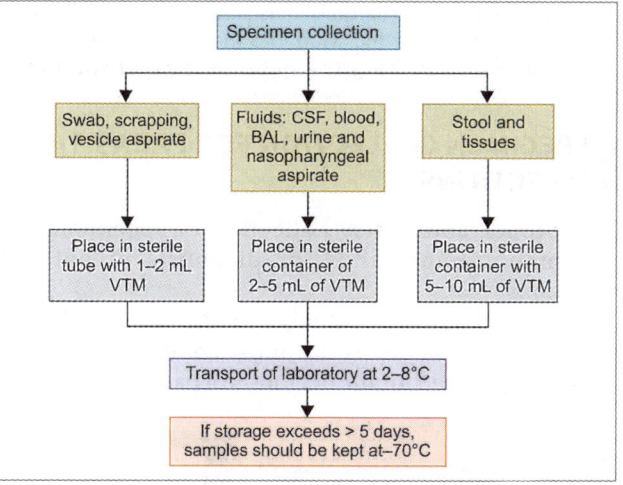

Fig. 65.3: Process of specimen collection and transport for viral infections.
(VTM, viral transport medium; CSF, cerebrospinal fluid; BAL, bronchoalveolar lavage)

> **Specimen collection for COVID-19**
> Combined oropharyngeal and nasopharyngeal swab is recommended (NP/OP swab)—first take the oropharyngeal sample; then using the same swab take nasopharyngeal sample.
> ❑ Dacron or polyester flocked swabs are used, dipped in viral transport media (VTM) after collection **(Fig. 65.4)**
> ❑ Explain the procedure to the patient

Contd...

Contd...

Oropharyngeal swab (e.g., throat swab)
- Tilt patient's head back slightly to improve the view of the throat. Ask the patient to say Ah
- Place a tongue depressor over the anterior 1/3 to anterior 1/2 of the tongue and depress the tongue gently
- Do not press the tongue depressor firmly
- Collect specimen by gently swiping the tip of the swab over tonsillar pillars and posterior pharyngeal wall

Nasopharyngeal swab
- Tilt the patient's head back slightly, so that the nasal passages become more accessible
- Ask the patient to close his eyes to lessen the mild discomfort of the procedure
- Insert the swab into the nostril, and direct it posteriorly. The swab should be passed keeping it close to the nasal septum
- Keep the swab just above the floor of the nasal passage and parallel to the palate. It should not be directed laterally away from the septum or superiorly away from the floor
- You will feel resistance when you reach the nasopharynx
- Once you reach the nasopharynx, leave the swab in place for several seconds to absorb secretions; then rotate the swab several times before removing it

Break of the stem of both the swabs (oropharyngeal and nasopharyngeal) at the groove as shown below (red circle, **Fig. 65.4**), and place the swab into the tube containing the VTM **without touching the outer surface of the tube**.

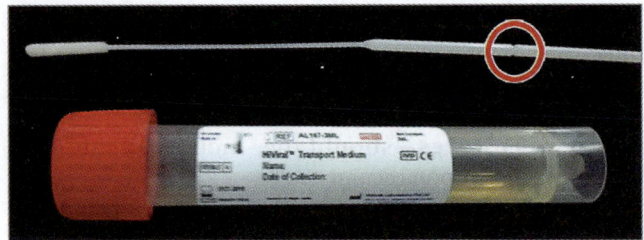

Fig. 65.4: Viral transport medium and swab.
Source: Department of Microbiology, JIPMER, Puducherry (*with permission*).

Refer **Chapter 47** for details on stool specimen collection for stool microscopy and for other diagnostic techniques

- Blood examination is useful in the diagnosis of infection caused by blood parasites, such as *Plasmodium*, *Leishmania* and *Wuchereria bancrofti*. Blood collection technique has been already discussed under specimen collection for bacterial infections. Peripheral smear preparation (thick and thin) and examination has been discussed in detail in **Chapter 51**.

SPECIMEN COLLECTION FOR PARASITIC INFECTIONS

The proper and timely collection of specimen is of paramount importance for diagnosis of parasitic infections.
- As many parasites inhabit in the intestinal tract, stool examination is the most common diagnostic technique used for the diagnosis of parasitic infections.

SPECIMEN COLLECTION FOR FUNGAL INFECTIONS

Specimen collection for diagnosis of fungal infection depends on the site of infection such as skin scraping, hair, nail, sputum, etc.
- Skin, hair and nail are collected for superficial fungal infections
- For systemic mycoses, blood sample is collected
- Cerebrospinal fluid (CSF) is collected for cryptococcal meningitis.

Details on specimen collection for various fungal infections are discussed in **Chapter 58**.

 EXPECTED QUESTIONS

I. Write short notes on:
1. Sterile universal specimen container.
2. Specimen transport for bacterial infections.
3. Specimen collection and transport for viral infections.

Annexures

ANNEXURE OUTLINE

1. Laboratory-acquired Infections and Laboratory Safety
2. Quality Control in Microbiology
3. Practical Microbiology

Annexures

Laboratory-acquired Infections and Laboratory Safety

ANNEXURE 1

■ LABORATORY-ACQUIRED INFECTIONS

Laboratory-acquired infections (LAIs) are defined as all infections acquired through laboratory or laboratory-related activities, regardless of whether they are symptomatic or asymptomatic.

LAIs result from occupational exposure to infectious agents. The most common routes of exposure and accidental inoculation are the following:
- Inhalation (aerosols)
- Percutaneous inoculation (needle and syringe, cuts or abrasions from contaminated items)
- Contact between mucous membranes and contaminated materials (hands or surfaces)
- Ingestion (aspiration through a pipette, smoking, or eating).

The risk-based classification of potential organisms responsible for LAIs is summarized in **Table A1.1**.

■ LABORATORY SAFETY

Safety in a microbiology laboratory is crucial in preventing infections and handling potentially hazardous materials and equipment. General safety protocols to be followed are as follows:

Table A1.1: Risk-based classification of agents causing laboratory-acquired infections.

Group	Definition	Bacteria	Virus	Fungi	Parasite
Group-1	Biological agents that are unlikely to cause human disease	Non-pathogenic organisms	–	–	–
Group-2	Biological agents that can cause human disease and may be a hazard to workers; but are unlikely to spread to the community; effective treatment or prophylaxis is usually available	• *Bacillus* species (**except** *B. anthracis*) • *Clostridium* species • *Corynebacterium diphtheriae* • Enterobacterales • *Staphylococcus* • *Streptococcus* • *Mycobacterium* (**except** *M. tuberculosis*)	• Adenovirus • Calicivirus • Herpesvirus • Influenza virus	• *Cryptococcus* • *Candida* • Dermatophytes • *Aspergillus*	All clinically important parasites

Group-3	Biological agents that can cause severe human disease and are a serious hazard to workers. They may spread to the community; but effective treatment or prophylaxis is usually available	• *B. anthracis*
		• *Brucella* species
		• *Coxiella burnetii*
		• *Francisella tularensis*
		• *M. tuberculosis*
			• Prion
			• LCM virus (Lymphocytic choriomeningitis)
			• Hantavirus
			• SARS-CoV 1 and 2
			• Encephalitis virus such as:
			  ➢ St Louis
			  ➢ Japanese
			  ➢ West Nile
			  ➢ Western equine
				–	–

Group-4	Same as group 3 except that effective treatment or prophylaxis is usually not available	–	• Lassa virus • Ebola virus • Marburg virus • Herpesvirus simiae	–	–

- **Practice safety**: Before starting the work, laboratory personnel should understand the risks of handling microorganisms, chemicals, and equipment
- Always wear appropriate **personal protective equipment (PPE)** such as a lab coat, gloves, mask, goggles, etc., to protect against infectious agents
- **Regularly sterilize and disinfect** the workbench, equipment, and different tools used for processing clinical specimens to minimize the risk of acquiring the infection
- **Handle sharps with caution** to prevent accidental injuries. Follow the guidelines for post-exposure prophylaxis if there is a needle stick injury (*refer* **Chapter 18** for details)
- **Proper disposal of biomedical wastes** as per the standard guidelines (*refer* **Chapter 17** for details)
- **Adhere to the safety protocols:** In case of any emergency be familiar with emergency protocols (eye wash station, blood spill management, first aid kits, fire extinguishers, etc.)
- **Eating and drinking** are strictly prohibited in the laboratory facility area
- **Strict adherence to hand hygiene protocols:** Wash hands thoroughly with soap and water before and after handling the clinical specimens
- **Prompt reporting of accidents** such as chemical spills, exposures, fire accidents, and electrical fire accidents to the safety officer.

Quality Control in Microbiology

ANNEXURE 2

Microbiological investigations play an important role in the diagnosis of infectious diseases and in deciding on selecting appropriate antimicrobial agents for patient care. It is, therefore, essential that the test reports are relevant, reliable, rapid, and interpreted correctly.

QUALITY ASSURANCE (QA)

According to the World Health Organization (WHO), quality assurance has been defined as the total process whereby the quality of laboratory reports can be guaranteed whenever the test is performed.

- ❖ It denotes delivery of the right result, on the right specimen, by the right method, at the right time, by the right interpretation, and at the right price
- ❖ QA has to be dealt in three phases:
  1. Pre-analytical stage—involves sample collection, labeling of the specimen, transportation, etc.
  2. Analytical stage—involves performing the test in actual
  3. Post-analytical—involves reporting and interpretation of the test results.

QA also encompasses monitoring and quality assessment (described later). The components of the quality assurance program are given in the highlight box below.

> **Components of quality assurance**
> - Personnel with adequate competence
> - Proper specimen collection, storage and transport
> - Use of precise and accurate techniques
> - Appropriate processing of test results
> - Good quality equipment and reagents
> - Methods of detecting errors and corrective steps
> - Preventive maintenance of equipment
> - Continual staff training
> - Documentation and timely feedback.

Quality Control (QC)

The term QC covers that part of QA, which refers to the institution of appropriate checks during the performance of tests and verification of test results; that is the analytical phase of QA. QC must cover all aspects of every procedure within the department.

- ❖ All materials, procedures, and equipment must be adequately controlled
- ❖ However, it is mainly restricted to quality control of stains, media, reagents, antibiotic disks, etc. It is not synonymous with quality assurance.

Standard Operating Procedures (SOPs)

Every laboratory must maintain its SOPs. SOP is a laboratory bench manual, which describes the stepwise process and technique of performing a routine or repetitive activity in the laboratory. The laboratory staff refer to the SOPs while performing the tests.

- ❖ **Objectives:** SOPs help in maintaining uniformity while performing the laboratory tests, regardless of who is performing the test. It is also helpful in training the new staff
- ❖ **Preparation of SOPs**: SOPs must be prepared by a qualified laboratory officer in a language clearly understood by users. Each SOP must be given a title and identification number with version and date. It should be signed by an authorized signatory
- ❖ **Review:** It should be reviewed at least annually or whenever the procedure is changed. SOPs should include only those tests which are currently in use
- ❖ The SOP should include requirements for pre-analytic, analytic, and post-analytic phases, keeping the quality issue in view.

Effective QA detects errors early, even before they could lead to incorrect test results. Laboratory personnel need to be aware of the errors that can occur during sample collection (pre-analytical stage), performing the tests (analytical stage), and reporting and interpreting the test results (post-analytical). For factors influencing quality (**Table A2.1**).

Quality Indicators

Quality must be measurable if it has to be managed. It is said that 'If you can't measure it, you can't improve it'.

Table A2.1: Factors influencing quality.

Pre-analytical	Analytical	Post-analytical
Right investigation	Equipment reliability	Accurate recording
Right sample	Reagents stability, integrity, and efficiency	Biological reference intervals
Right collection	Adequate calibration	Age and sex-related variations
Right technique	Correct interpretation	Turnaround time
Right laboratory	Procedural reliability using SOP	Availability of guidance
Right background milieu	Proficiency of personnel	Authorized release of results
Right transportation	Right technique for available reagents	Archiving of specimen
Right quantity	Internal quality control	Transcribing results from worksheet to report forms
Right labeling	External quality assessment	

Source: Adapted from World Health Organization.

- Quality indicators (QI) help the health laboratory to define and measure the progress
- The measurement of quality indicators leads to early detection of system failure, which includes all three stages—pre-analytic, analytic and post-analytic; so that corrective actions can be taken promptly **(Table A2.2)**.

Assessment of Quality

Monitoring is a vital component of a quality system. The main objectives of monitoring are: (i) to confirm consistency, (ii) to identify opportunities for improvement, and (iii) to assess the impact of changes in procedures.

The periodic and retrospective assessment of quality can be undertaken by an independent external agency or internally by a designated staff on behalf of the laboratory management. Assessment is of two types as follows:
- **Material driven:** Internal quality assessment and external quality assessment scheme (EQAS)
- **Man-driven:** Internal audit and external audit (described later).

External Quality Assessment Scheme (EQAS)

External quality assessment schemes vary as per the test method and number of participating laboratories.
- It should include testing for major pathogens; should not be too complicated, costly, or time-consuming
- They are considered a powerful tool to monitor laboratory performance, identify errors, for interlaboratory comparability and reliability of future testing, stimulate staff motivation, assure clients that test results are reliable, and promote high standards of good laboratory practices
- Participation in EQA schemes should always be considered as additional to internal QC. It is conducted by an independent agency, ensures interlaboratory comparability, and improves the performance of participating laboratories
- A scoring system is used in EQAS to stimulate performance and enhance inter laboratory concordance. Participants need to be told whether their test results are in consensus and any corrective action to be taken.

Internal Quality Assessment (IQA)

IQA is similar to EQAS, except that the material preparation, distribution, evaluation, and result assessment are done internally.
- Its main objective is to release reliable results on a day-to-day basis. It is a continuous, concurrent process, which is performed by laboratory staff

Table A2.2: Examples of quality indicators.

Pre-analytic indicators	Analytic indicators	Post-analytic indicators
• Incomplete requisitions • Phlebotomy efficiency • Specimen acceptability/rejection rates • Accuracy of sample accessioning • Specimen transport time	• Internal and external control failures • Performance in external quality assessment scheme (EQAS) • Frequency of unscheduled service and repairs of equipment • On-time performance—calibration and maintenance of equipment • Vendor evaluation (supplier performance) • Inventory—emergency orders, outdating • Misinterpretation of results • Availability of back-up services	• Compliance to turnaround time (TAT) • Errors/incomplete test reports • Availability of archived samples
		Other Quality Indicators
		• Number and type of laboratory accidents • Training and competency evaluation of personnel • Document problems discovered—outdated, incomplete, incorrect • Customer feedback and complaints—physicians, other healthcare staff, patients • Numbers and types of non-conformances • Physician satisfaction with report format and content

Source: Adapted from World Health Organization.

- Each laboratory should have an internal quality assessment scheme that can be carried out by regular use of certified reference material, split sampling, replicate testing, retesting of retained items, and correlation of results
- If the discrepancies are observed, they are recorded and analyzed by a senior professional in discussion with the designated quality manager, and possible corrective and preventive actions are taken.

Assurance

When both IQA and EQAS are in place, a laboratory can assert a level of assurance. QA can be simply stated as the sum of quality control, internal quality assessment, and external quality assessment.

Quality Audit

A quality audit is defined as a planned and documented activity performed by written procedures and checklists to verify the examination and evaluation of applicable elements of a quality assurance program have been developed, documented, and implemented.

There are two types of audits—**internal** and **external**.

Internal Audits

They are performed by laboratory staff to inspect their system and are done by members who are trained in audit techniques. The internal audit allows a better understanding of the day-to-day work and, through the review process, allows one to make better decisions and provides a mechanism for continual quality improvement (CQI).

External Audits

External audits can be of two types.

Second Party External Audits

They are normally supplier audits performed to ensure that goods supplied are of the required standard. They are needed if there is a change of suppliers *or* on a planned basis for regular suppliers.

Third Party External Audits

They are also called **accreditation** and are normally performed by regulatory/statutory bodies; can be voluntary or mandatory. Accreditation is an approved procedure by which an authorized body or regulatory authorities accord formal recognition to a laboratory to undertake specific tasks, provided that predefined standards are met by the laboratory. Standards for laboratory accreditation have been developed by the **International Organization for Standardization (ISO)**. For example, ISO 15189:2022 specifies requirements for quality and competence in medical laboratories.

Practical Microbiology

ANNEXURE 3

Exercises included in the practical assessment and chapter (including page no.) in which these topics are discussed are enlisted in **Table A3.1**.

Table A3.1: Exercises included in the practical assessment and chapter (including page no.) in which these topics are discussed.		
Practical topics	**Chapters**	**Page numbers**
1. Gram staining	3.2	21
2. Acid-fast staining	3.2	22–23
3. Albert staining	3.2	23
4. Hanging drop preparation for motility testing	3.2	23
5. Specimen collection	3.2, 65	19, 365–370
6. Processing of specimens	3.2	27–29
7. Bacterial identification	3.2	30–33
➤ *Staphylococcus aureus*	21	150–152
➤ *Streptococcus* (*S. pyogenes* and *S. agalactiae*)	22	154–156
➤ *Enterococcus*	22	157
➤ *Corynebacterium diphtheriae*	24	162–163
➤ *Mycobacterium tuberculosis*	27	173–174
➤ *Escherichia coli*	29	182
➤ *Klebsiella pneumoniae*	29	183
➤ *Proteus mirabilis*	29	187
➤ *Shigella*	29	186–187
➤ *Salmonella* (*S.* Typhi, *S.* Paratyphi A and *S.* Paratyphi B)	29	184–186
➤ *Vibrio cholerae*	30	190
➤ *Pseudomonas aeruginosa*	31	193
➤ *Acinetobacter baumannii*	31	193–194
8. Antimicrobial susceptibility testing	3.2	33–35
9. Serological tests		
➤ Widal test	8, 29	73, 185–186
➤ VDRL test	8, 34	72, 204
➤ ELISA	8	75–77
➤ Rapid tests	8	79–80
10. Stool examination for parasites (including concentration techniques)	47	268–270
11. Peripheral blood smear examination	47, 51, 56	270, 288–290, 318
12. Lactophenol cotton blue (LPCB) mount for fungi	58	331
13. Fungal identification		
➤ *Candida albicans*	58	337
➤ *Cryptococcus neoformans*	58	338
➤ *Aspergillus*	58	339–340
➤ *Rhizopus* and *Mucor*	58	338–339

Index

Page numbers followed by *f* refer to figure and *t* refer to table.

A

ABO antigens, distribution of 104*t*
ABO blood group 104
    compatibility 97
    system 104
Abscess 346, 367
    brain 171, 179
    liver 274, 276
    lung 358
    peritonsillar 357
Acanthamoeba species 273, 277, 277*f*
Accidents, prompt reporting of 374
Acid
    labile 246
    production 32
Acid-fast
    bacilli 22*f*, 173, 359
    filamentous branching bacilli 179*f*
    organisms 23*t*
    parasites 23
Acid-fast stain 21, 176, 295*f*, 359
    modified 179, 179*f*, 356
    slit skin smear 176*f*
Acidic butt 32
Acinetobacter 32, 56, 192-194, 194*f*, 345, 351, 353, 358, 359
    baumannii 45, 109, 192, 193
    treatment for 194
Acquired immunity 60, 60*t*
    types of 60
Acquired immunodeficiency syndrome 248
    diagnosis of 250*t*
Acquired resistance, development of 47*f*
Acriflavine 180
Actinomadura 178
    madurae 333
Actinomyces 178
    naeslundii 178
    odontolyticus 178
Actinomycetes 178
Actinomycetoma 179, 334, 334*f*, 335
Actinomycosis 178, 178*f*
Actionomycetoma 179
Active immunity, artificial 61
Acute encephalitis syndrome 239
Acute respiratory distress syndrome 234
Acute retroviral syndrome 249
Acute urethral syndrome 352
Acyclovir 223
Adenolymphangitis, acute 317
Adenovirus 101, 214, 224, 225*f*, 260, 261, 357
Adhesion 49, 274
Adult diphtheria toxoid 102
Adult worm 270, 297, 301, 310*f*, 314
Aedes 316-318, 321, 323*t*
    aegypti 236, 237, 238, 240
    albopictus 237
Aerial disinfection 124, 127
Aerophobia 242
Aerosol transmission 234
Aerotolerant anaerobes 168

Aesculin 180
African eye worm 319
African sleeping sickness 285
Agar 4, 24
    dilution 34
    plate technique 313
Agents
    classification of 119*t*
    reducing 29
Agglutination reaction 66, 73, 74
Aggregatibacter species 197
Aging 96
Air
    bacteriology of 139
    fear of 242
    filtration of 123
    particle counters 142
    quality of 141
    sampler method 142*f*
Airborne precautions 116
Air-flow rooms, negative 222
Albendazole 271, 301, 309, 311, 314, 318, 320
Albert's stain 23, 161*f*, 162
Alcohol 125, 128
Aldehyde 124
Algid malaria 288
Alginate coat 192
Alkaline
    butt 32
    slant 32
All trematodes
    except schistosomes, life cycle of 303
    life cycle of 304*f*
Allantoic sac 217
Allergic bronchopulmonary aspergillosis 339
Allergic disease 339
Allergy 91, 92
Alloantigens 63
Allograft 97
Alpha-herpesviruses 219
Alternaria 335
Alum 64
Amantadine 229
Amastigote 282, 282*f*, 283
Amblyomma species 325, 325*f*
Amies medium 159
Amikacin plus cotrimoxazole 335
Aminoglycoside modifying enzymes 48
Aminoglycosides 46
Aminopenicillins 46
Amniotic sac 217
Amoeba 267, 273
    free-living 8*f*, 273, 277
    nonpathogenic 276
Amoebiasis 271, 276
    invasive 274
Amoebic antigen 275
Amoebic dysentery 274, 276
Amoebic keratitis 277
Amoebic liver abscess 270, 273, 274, 276
Amoebic stool 274
Amoxicillin-clavulanate 45, 201

Amphitrichous 14*f*
Amphotericin B 271, 332, 336, 338, 340
Ampicillin 45, 171, 180, 196
Amsel's criteria 202
Anaerobes
    facultative 17
    non-sporing 168, 171
Anaerobic culture 19, 20, 365, 367, 368
    media 26
    methods 29
Anaerobic glove box 29, 168
Anaerobic organisms 22, 360
Anaerobic work station 29
Anaerobiosis, indicator of 29
Anaphylactic reactions 300
Anaphylaxis, localized 92
Anchovy sauce pus 274
Ancylostoma 312, 313, 315
    brasiliensis 315
    caninum 315
    ceylanicum 315
    duodenale 312
Anemia 287
Angiostrongylus cantonensis 315
Angiotensin-converting enzyme-2 234
Animal anatomical waste 133
Animal inoculation 162, 216, 293
Animalia minuta 3
Anopheles 318
    barbirostris 319
    mosquito 286, 321, 323*t*
Anorexia 228
Anoxomat anaerobic system 29*f*
Anoxomat system 168
Anthracoid bacilli 165, 167
Anthrax 165, 166
    toxin 165
Antibacterial spectra 145
Antibiogram 38, 145
Antibiotic 163, 331, 355
    broad-spectrum 336
    ineffective 145
    misuse, stoppage of 152
    use 171
Antibody 63, 64, 71, 86, 93, 256
    blocking 74
    circulating 97
    excess 186
    function of 65*f*
    general structure of 64*f*
    markers 256
    secreting 88
    structure of 64
    surge 61
    titer 73, 186
Antibody detection 74, 176, 199, 204, 209, 210, 221, 222, 229, 230, 232, 238, 242, 245, 250, 254, 276, 279, 293, 295, 299, 301, 305, 306, 311, 318, 332, 359
    assay 71, 234
    latex agglutination test for 74
    methods 319

Index

serology for 206
specific 208
tests 270
screening 250
Antibody-dependent
cell-mediated cytotoxicity 88
cellular cytotoxicity 91, 93
enhancement 237
Antibody-mediated immune
effector functions of 89
response 86, 88
Anti-Epstein-Barr virus antibodies 223
Antifolates 47
Antigen 63, 71, 72, 185, 250, 289
administration, route of 64
binding 65
biological classes of 64
chemical nature of 63
doses of 64
host relationship 63
markers 256
production of 43
release of sequestered 94
role of 66
size of 63
soluble 72
somatic 187
tumor-associated transplantation 98
tumor-specific transplantation 97
variation 227
Antigen detection 74, 79, 186, 190, 209, 222, 230, 276, 280, 284, 288, 299, 305, 306, 318, 332, 338, 339, 356
assay 71, 234
direct 349
from stool 279, 295, 298
tests 271, 359
Antigen-antibody reaction 71, 72
general properties of 71
types of 72, 72t
Antigenic detection 210
Antigenic drift 228t
Antigenic peptides 84
Antigenic shift 228t
Antigenic types 244
Antigenicity 63
Antiglobulin test 74
Anti-hepatitis
A virus 254
B
precore antibody 256
surface antibody 256
Antimicrobial agent 45, 46t, 47
broad-spectrum 52
rational use of 144
Antimicrobial resistance 45, 143
mechanism of 48
Antimicrobial stewardship 143
program 117, 143
team 143
Antimicrobial susceptibility test 33, 144, 151, 155-157, 182, 186, 187, 190, 193, 196, 349, 353, 356, 361
interpretation of 35
methods, classification of 33
Antiparasitic agent 299, 301
Antiparasitic drugs 271

Anti-rabies prophylaxis 243t
Antiretroviral therapy 137, 253
Antiseptics 118, 125, 128
Antiviral agents 257
direct-acting 258
Antiviral drugs 215, 221, 234
Apicomplexa 267
Appendix 82
Appetite, loss of 237
Aquatic plant 303
Aqueous humor, infection of 363
Arabinitol 337
Arachnoid 348
Arboviruses 214, 216, 262, 236
prevalent 237t
Argasid tick 325
Artemisinin derivatives 271
Arthralgia, severe 238
Arthritis 238, 258
Arthropod 322
acting 322t
classification of 321t
control of 325
vector 236
Arthropod-borne viruses 236
Arthus reaction 93
Ascariasis 271, 311
Ascaris 56, 270, 310, 358
lumbricoides 310
eggs of 311f
life cycle of 311f
Ascoli's thermoprecipitation test 166
Ascorbic acid 168
Asepsis 118
Aseptate hyaline hyphae 338
Asexual cycle 292
Asexual spores, types of 329
Aspergillosis 336, 339
Aspergillus 330, 332, 339, 339t, 340f
flavus 339, 340f
fumigatus 339, 340f
nidulans 333
niger 339
Aspirin 221
Asthma 92, 209, 339
Astrovirus 260, 261, 356
Atherosclerosis 209
Atopic dermatitis 92
Atovaquone plus azithromycin 291
Atrophic rhinitis 357
Audits, types of 377
Auraminephenol solution 173
Autofluorescence 9
Autograft 96
Autoimmune
diseases 95, 95t
hemolytic anemia 95
Autoimmunity 94, 96
mechanisms of 94
Autoinfection 268, 294, 313, 314
Automated antimicrobial susceptibility tests 35
Automated blood culture
systems 185
techniques 26
Autonomic dysfunction 242
Avian flu 228

Avidin-biotin system, use of 77
Azithromycin 200, 209
Azoles 336

B

B cell 60, 82, 83, 86, 89
activation of 89
defects 96
differentiation of 89, 89f
lymphoid follicles 82
proliferation of 89
receptor 65
B lymphocytes 82, 83
Babesia 270, 286, 291
infecting 345
Baby hamster kidney 242
Bachman intradermal test 320
Bacillocid extra 124
Bacillus 16, 17, 40, 165, 167
anthracis 14, 50, 165, 166, 345
gram stain of 166f
atrophaeus 167
spores of 122, 123
Calmette-Guerin 102
cereus 167
isolation of 170
pumilus 124
stearothermophilus 167
Bacitracin susceptibility test 31
Bacteremia 154, 156, 171, 192, 345
continuous 345
intermittent 345
primary 184
secondary 184
transient 345
types of 345
Bacteria 5t, 6, 11, 15, 40, 105, 139, 354, 361, 373
classification of 12t
discovered 4
factors affecting growth of 17, 18
gene transfer in 40
imparts toxigenicity to 42
medically important 11, 11t
miscellaneous 11
morphology of 11, 12f
opsonization of 90f
physiology of 11, 16
shape of 11
used for common 25t
vector into 43
Bacterial adhesion 15
Bacterial agents 345, 350, 351, 357, 361
Bacterial capsule 64
Bacterial cell
anatomy 12
division 16
structure of 12f
wall 12
Bacterial chromosome 42
Bacterial conjugation 42f
Bacterial count 16
Bacterial culture 356, 359
Bacterial endotoxins 50t
Bacterial etiology 345
Bacterial exotoxins 50t
Bacterial flagellar arrangement, types of 14f

Index

Bacterial genetics 40
Bacterial growth
    and nutrition 16
    curve 16, 17*f*, 17*t*
Bacterial identification, automated systems for 32
Bacterial infections 19
    anaerobic 11
    diagnosis of 19
    laboratory diagnosis of 19
    mode of transmission of 49*t*
    secondary 221, 230, 300
    specimen collection for 365
Bacterial meningitis, acute 348
Bacterial motility 15
Bacterial opportunistic infections 249
Bacterial pathogenesis 49
Bacterial spore 15, 15*f*
Bacterial taxonomy 11
Bacterial vaginosis, treatment of 202
Bacterial virulence 14, 351
Bacterial vitamins 16
Bacteriological incubator 28, 29*f*
Bacteriology, general 11, 19, 40, 52
Bacteriophage 224-226
    morphology of 226*f*
    uses of 226
Bacteriuria
    asymptomatic 351, 352
    significant 353
Bacteroides 26, 171, 345
    fragilis 52, 171
Balamuthia 273, 277
    cysts of 277
    mandrillaris 277
Balantidium coli 296
    morphology of 296*f*
Bamboo stick appearance 166, 166*f*
Banana-shaped gametocyte 290*f*
Bancroftian filariasis 316
Barbour-Stoenner-Kelly medium 205
Barrel-shaped arthrospores 336
Bartonella 208
    bacilliformis 208
Basal media, uses of 24
Basophils 84
Bedrails 125
Bedside tables 125
Benznidazole 285
Beta-D-glucan assay 332
Beta-herpesviruses 219
Beta-lactamases 182
Bifidobacterium 171
Bile duct carcinoma 307
Bilharziasis 306
Binary fission 16
Biochemical identification 30, 151, 155, 182
Biochemical tests 162, 193
Biofilm 119
    formation 50
Biological control methods 326
Biological oxygen demand incubators 331
Biological safety cabinet 28*f*
Biological transmission 321
Biomarkers-guided therapy 144
Biomedical waste 130
    disposal of 124
    hazards with 130
    proper disposal of 374
    segregation of 133*f*
    treatment facility 132, 133
Biomedical waste management 130, 235
    monitoring of 134
    Rule 131, 131*t*
    steps of 132
Biopsy 176
    urease test 201
Biosafety cabinet 28
Biosynthesis 214
Biphasic medium 26
Bipolaris 335
Bird seed agar 331
Bivalent vaccine 224
BK virus 224
Blackfly 319, 322
Blackwater fever 288
Bladder 351
    carcinoma 306
    infection of 352
Blastocystis hominis 296
Blastomyces 346
    dermatitidis 330, 335, 336
Blastomycosis 336
Blepharitis 363
Blood
    collection vacutainer tube 366*f*
    concentration of 270
    donors, screening of 215
    flukes 303, 305
    spillage of 116
    transfusion 249
    volume 347
Blood agar 24, 24*f*, 141, 154, 162, 166, 185, 193, 331
    hemolysis on 30, 30*f*
    proteus on 187*f*
    vibrio cholerae on 191*f*
Blood culture 20, 184, 198, 369
    bottles 347*f*
    media 25, 26
    number of 347
    positivity 185
    specimen collection for 346
    steps of collection of 346*f*
Blood group 74
    distribution of 104
    for blood transfusion, selection of 104
Blood smear, thick 173, 288, 288*f*
    examination of 270
Blood specimen 365
    for culture, collection of 365
    for serology, collection of 366
    transport of 347
Blood spill
    kit 116*f*
    large 126
    management 116, 134
Blood-borne virus 136
Bloodstream infection 110, 182, 345, 346
    diagnosis of 346
    etiological agents of 345
    types of 346
Blood-sucking
    arthropods 236
    insects 201
Body clothing, protective 114
Body fluid 116, 366
    specimens 366
    potentially infectious 135
Body lice 324, 324*f*
Bone marrow 81, 97, 198, 215, 271, 282, 335
    aspiration 283
    culture 198
    dysfunction 283
    transplant units 141
Bone, abscess of 179
Bordetella 196
    pertussis 197, 358, 367
Borrelia 203, 205, 345
    burgdorferi 205
    species 205
    vincentii 358
Bothria 301
Botulinum
    antitoxin 103, 170
    toxin 42, 170
Botulism
    diagnosis of 170
    infant 170
    treatment of 170
Bowie-Dick test 121
Bradyzoites 293
Brain 84
    biopsy 242*f*
Brain heart infusion 184
    agar 179, 331
    broth 26*f*
Brevundimonas diminuta 124
Brick-red pigment 340
Bright-field microscope 7*f*
Brill-Zinsser disease 207
Bronchial asthma, severe 339
Bronchiolitis 358
Bronchitis 358
Bronchoalveolar lavage 367, 369
Brood capsule 300
Broth dilution 34
Brown-Brenn modification 178
Brucella 31, 196, 198, 226
    melitensis 198
    species 198
Brucellosis 74, 198
Brudzinski's sign 348
Brugia 319
    malayi 270, 308, 316, 318
    timori 316, 319
Brugian filariasis 316
Brush border appearance 340
Buccal mucosa 230*f*
Budding 329
Bunyaviridae 237
Burkholderia 345
    cepacia 192, 194
    pseudomallei 192, 194
    species 194
Burkitt's lymphoma 288
Burn wound swab collection 367
Bystander activation 95

C

Calabar swelling 319
Calcofluor white stain 330
Campylobacter 29, 200, 200*f*, 355

jejuni 200
   species 200
Cancers, diagnosis of 98*t*
Candida 110, 329, 330, 336, 350
   albicans 109, 336, 337, 337*f*
   infecting humans 336
   species 336, 337, 346, 358
Candidiasis 336, 337, 337*f*
Candle jar 29*f*
Capnophilic bacteria 29
Capsid 213
Capsule 14
Carbapenems 46
Carbon dioxide 18
Cardiac surgeries 115
Cardiobacterium hominis 197
Carpet culture 28
Cartridge-based nucleic acid amplification test 174
Cary-Blair medium 366
Cascade reaction 67
Case-fatality rate 231
Casoni's test 271, 301
Caspofungin 332
Castaneda's biphasic blood culture medium 198*f*
Cat's feces 293
Catalase test 31, 31*f*
Catheter 351
   indwelling 368
Catheterized patients 353
C-carbohydrate antigens 153
CD molecules 82
CD4 T cells 249
Ceftazidime 180
Ceftriaxone 144, 160, 196
Cell 81, 88
   antigen-presenting 83, 84, 87
   clue 202
   culture, viral growth in 217
   cytotoxic 88
   dendritic 59, 81, 84, 84*f*, 86
   endothelial 215
   epithelial 81
   follicular dendritic 84, 89
   granulocytic 84
   inflammatory 179
   lines, types of 217
   lymphoid 81, 82
   mast 59, 65, 84, 92
   membrane 13
   memory 61, 83, 88, 89
   microglial 84
   parent 329
   sperm 84
   stem 97
   surface adhesins 149
   tumor 87
   virus-infected 87
Cell wall
   appendages 12, 14
   deficient forms 15
   theory 21
Cell-mediated
   immune response 86, 87
   immunity 175
Cellophane tape 310*f*
Cell-to-cell interaction 81

Cellular anergy 94
Cellular fraction 99
   vaccine 100
Cellular immunodeficiency 96
Central lymphoid organs 81
Central nervous system
   complications 230
   infections 220
   manifestations 203
   spread to 241
Central sterile supply department 118
Centrifugal spread 242
Centroblasts 89
Centrocytes 89
   differentiation of 89
Cephalosporin 45, 171
   third-generation 159, 160, 191
Cercarial dermatitis 305
Cerebellum 241
Cerebral malaria 288
Cerebrospinal fluid 271, 330, 366, 369, 370
   antibodies 72, 204
   collection 348
   examination 158
   gram staining of 349
   microscopy 349
   smear 159*f*
   third portion of 159
   transport 348
Cervix, carcinoma of 224
Cestode 267, 297
   adult worm of 297*f*
   life cycle of 297, 298*t*
Chagas' disease 285
Chancroid 197
Chandler's index 312
Charcot-Leyden crystals 276, 311
Chemical control 326
Chemical disinfection 133
   tests for 128
Chemical indicator 29
Chemical sterilant 122
Chemical wastes, hazards from 130
Chemiluminescence immunoassay 78
   advantages of 79
Chemiluminescence system 78*f*
Chemoprophylaxis 291
Chemotherapy 96
Chick Martin test 128
Chickenpox 55, 116, 221
   rashes of 222*f*
   vaccine 99
Chiggerosis 208
Chiggers 208
Chikungunya 238, 239, 345
   virus 236
Childhood flaccid paralysis 244
Childhood immunization program 170
Chilomastix mesnili 281, 281*f*
Chip-based nucleic acid amplification techniques 174
Chlamydia 75, 87, 207, 208, 352, 359
   pneumoniae 209, 359
   psittaci 208
   species 363
   trachomatis 208, 362
Chlamydospore 337*f*
Chloramphenicol 46, 196, 331

Chlorhexidine
   gluconate 126, 129
   hand wash 111
Chlorine 125, 126, 129
Chloroquine 271
   resistance 290
Chocolate agar 24*f*, 25, 196
Cholera 189, 190
   red reaction 190
   resembling 295
   toxin 42, 189
   vaccine 99, 190
Cholesterol 329
Chorioallantoic membrane 217
Chorioretinitis 363
Choroid, infection of 363
Christie-Atkins-Munch-Petersen test 30, 154, 155
CHROMagar *Candida* medium 331
Chromoblastomycosis 335
Chromogenic technique 141
Chromosome 40
Chronic disease 258
Chyluria 317
Cicatricial skin lesions 221
Cirrhosis 258
Citrate
   test 193
   utilization test 31, 32*f*
Citrobacter 31, 181, 184
Cladosporium 335
Cleaning agents 127
   chemicals 127
   detergents 127
   enzymatic cleaners 127
   proteolytic cleaners 127
   types of 127
Clean-voided midstream urine 352
Clindamycin 171
Cloning 43
   vector 226
Clonorchis 304, 306
   eggs of 307
   sinensis 306
Clostridia 168
Clostridial enteric infections 168
Clostridial wound infections 168
Clostridioides difficile 168, 170, 355
Clostridium 16, 165, 168
   botulinum 50, 168, 170
   species 168
   tetani 50, 100, 168, 169
Clostridium difficile 170
   diarrhea 109
   infection 116
Clostridium perfringens 140, 168
   gram-stained smear of 169*f*
Coagulase test 151, 151*f*
Coagulase-negative staphylococci 149, 150, 152
Coal tar, distillation of 125
Coccidioides 346
   immitis 330, 335, 336
Coccidioidomycosis 336
Cockroach 322
Co-infection 258
Cold agglutination test 74
Cold chain 101

Index

Colicin typing 187
Coliform
    bacilli 181
    bacteria 140
Colistin 144
Colloidal gold 79
Colonic mucosa 275
Colony appearance 353
Colony morphology 30
Colpitis macularis 280
Coma 242
Combined immunization 218
Combined immunodeficiencies 96
Common pili 15
Common sterilization agents 128*t*
Common sterilization disinfectants 128*t*
Communicable disease 175
Community acquired
    pneumonia 209
        interstitial 210
Complement deficiency diseases 69, 69*t*
Complement fixation test 75
Complement pathways 59, 68*f*
Complement proteins 60
Composting 134
Concentration techniques 269, 279
Condenser 7
Condylomata lata 203
Confirmatory tests 250
Congenital rubella syndrome 232
Congenital varicella syndrome 221
Conjugation, role of 43
Conjunctiva 230
    infection of 363
Conjunctival swab 368
Conjunctivitis 208, 363, 369
Conventional biochemical tests 190, 201
Conventional blood culture 26, 184
Coombs
    antiglobulin test 74
    test 74
Coproantigen 275, 279
Core polysaccharide 13
Corkscrew motility 203
Corn meal agar 331
Cornea, infection of 363
Corneal scraping 20, 271, 368, 369
Coronavirus disease-2019 (COVID-19) 55, 214, 233, 234, 357
    diagnosis of 369
    home isolation 234
    hospitalization 234
    prevention of 235
    situation 234
    specimen collection for 369
    symptomatic management 234
    vaccines 235
Cortex 81, 82
Corynebacteria 161
Corynebacterium 161, 162
    diphtheriae 23, 42, 50, 73, 100, 161, 161*f*, 357
    jeikeium 164
    minutissimum 164
    pseudotuberculosis 164
    ulcerans 164
    urealyticum 164
    xerosis 23

Cotrimoxazole 194, 271, 293
Coughs, containment of 229
Covaxin 235
Cover slip 269
Covishield 99, 235
Coxiella 50
    burnetii 208
Coxsackie 244
Coxsackievirus 216, 244, 246
Crab 303, 322
    lice 324
Crayfish 303, 322
C-reactive protein 60, 144
Creamy white colonies 336
Crepitus 168
Cresol 128
Critical device 120
Crushed ping-pong balls 340
Cryoglobulinemia, mixed 258
Cryptococcal capsular antigen 332
Cryptococcal meningitis 330, 336-338, 370
Cryptococcosis 338
    type of 338
Cryptococcus 330, 346
    neoformans 329, 330, 337, 338*f*, 350
Cryptosporidiosis 296
Cryptosporidium 23, 139, 269-271, 292, 294, 294*f*, 294*t*, 295, 355, 356
    parvum 268, 275, 295*f*
Culex
    bites 317
    mosquito 239, 321, 323*t*
    quinquefasciatus 317
    tritaeniorhynchus 239
    vishnui 239
Culicoides, bite of 319
Culture 206
    condition 331
    identification 30, 331
    techniques 271
Culture media 24, 162, 331, 353
    constituents of 24
    conventional 24
    types of 24
Culture smear 30, 155, 166, 182, 187, 190, 193, 198
    microscopy 150
Cup-like depressions 261
Curvularia 335
Cutaneous anthrax 165
Cutaneous candidiasis 337
Cutaneous filariasis 319
Cutaneous forms 282
Cutaneous larva migrans 314, 315
    causes of 315
Cutaneous leishmaniasis 282, 284
Cycloheximide 331
Cyclops 320, 322, 325
Cyclospora 23, 139, 269, 270, 292, 294, 294*f*, 294*t*, 295, 355, 356
    cayetanensis 294, 295*f*
    cycle of 294
Cyclosporiasis 296
Cyst 270, 273, 274, 275*f*, 276, 277*f*, 278, 279, 281, 281*f*
    mature 273
    pressure effect of enlarging 300
    quadrinucleated 275

    wall 300
Cysteine 168
    lactose electrolyte-deficient agar 25, 26*f*, 27
Cysticercosis 297-299
Cystitis 352
Cystoisospora 23, 269, 270, 292, 294, 294*f*, 294*t*, 295, 356
    belli 294, 295*f*
    cycle of 294
Cystoisosporiasis 296
Cystoscopes 128
Cytoadherence 288
Cytokine 60, 81, 85
    classes of 85
    functions of 85
    storm 234
Cytological analysis 348
Cytolysis, complement-mediated 90*f*
Cytomegalovirus 222, 363
    infections 222
Cytopathic effect 217
Cytopathology 220
Cytoplasm 12
Cytoplasmic matrix 14
Cytoplasmic tails 85
Cytostomal fibrils 281
Cytostome 281
Cytotoxic
    drug waste, disposal of 133
    factors 88*f*
    necrotizing factor 181
    T lymphocyte 86, 87
    waste, hazards from 130

D

Dead bacilli 176
Deep burial 133
Deer fly 322
Dehydration, severe 190
Dengue 237, 238, 345
    antigen 77
    fever 237
    hemorrhagic fever 237
    infection 237
    shock syndrome 238
    vaccine 238
    virus 215, 236
Dental caries 53
Deoxycholate citrate agar 25, 27, 356
Deoxyribonucleic acid
    vaccine 100
    virus 99, 224, 255
        vaccine 99
Depth filters 123
Dermatolymphangitis 317
Dermatophyte 330, 332, 333, 334*f*, 360
Dermatophytosis 332, 333
    types of 333*t*
Dettol 125, 128
Diabetes mellitus 336
Diabetic ketoacidosis 338
Dialysis water 139, 141
Diamond's media 280
Diarrhea 181, 230, 354, 356
    chronic 355
    fatty 278
    infantile 225

Index

infectious agents of acute 354*t*
inflammatory 200, 356
pathogenic mechanisms of 355
persistent 355
profuse 295
Diarrheal diseases 20, 354, 355
Diarrheal stool 126
Diarrheal toxin 167
Dientamoeba fragilis 281
Diethylcarbamazine 318
Dilution tests 34
Dimorphic fungus 335
Diphtheria 161, 163, 357
    antitoxin 103
    bacilli 162
    incidence of 163
    pathogenesis of 161
    toxin 42, 73, 161
    vaccine 163
Diphtheroids 161, 163, 163*f*
Diphyllobothrium
    latum 298, 301
        egg of 302*f*
    species 297, 302
Direct agglutination test 73
Direct disk diffusion test 33
Direct smear 150*f*, 193, 358
    microscopy 150, 154, 162, 182
Direct wet mount 268
    examination 270
Discarding jars, disinfectant in 129
Disease
    causation, epidemiological determinants of 55, 55*t*
    germ theory of 4
Disinfectant 119, 125
    factors influencing efficacy of 119
    high-level 118-120, 124
    intermediate-level 118, 119, 125
    level of 118*t*
    low-level 118-120, 126
    surface 126, 128
    test efficacy of 128
    type of 118
Disinfection 118, 127
Disk diffusion
    method 33
    test, interpretation of 34*t*
Disposable
    gowns 115
    needles 135
Disposal after use 135
Dizziness 231
Doffing 115
Donning 114, 115
Donovani amastigotes 284*f*
Doxycycline 194, 199, 209
Dracunculiasis 320, 320*f*
Dracunculus 309
    medinensis 308, 316, 320
Drinking water
    contaminated with enteric pathogens 139
    disinfection of 126
    supply, classification of quality of 141*t*
Drowsiness 231
Drug
    allergy 92
    newer 143
    resistance 174
        transferrable 47, 48, 48*t*, 266
    susceptibility test 174
Drum stick appearance 169
Dry heat sterilizer 123, 123*f*
Dumb rabies 242
Duodenal aspirate 271
Duodenal capsule 280*f*
Duodenal contents 268
Duodenal sampling 279
Duodenal ulcer 201
Durham's tube 140
Dysentery 200, 354

E

Ear
    external 368
    infections 20, 192, 364
    specimens 368
Early intestinal
    manifestations 184
    phase 313
Early morning sputum 367
Eaton's agent 209
Ebola 261, 345
    river 261
    virus 115, 262*f*
        disease 261
Eccentric scolex 299*f*
Echinococcus 297
    granulosus 297, 298, 300
        eggs 300
        life cycle of 300*f*
Ectoparasites 267, 321
Ectothrix 332
Eczema
    allergic 92
    herpeticum 220
Eczematous lesion 220
Edema, transient local 317
Effector cell 61, 87-89
    function 82
    nonspecific 87
    specific 87
Effluent treatment plan 133
Efflux pumps 48
Egg
    counting methods 270
    inoculation 217
Ehrlichia 208
Eijkman test 140
Eikenella corrodens 197
Electrical field 122
Electrical heater 120
Electroencephalogram, abnormal 263
Electrolyte replacement 200
Electron microscope 9, 9*t*
    applications of 10
Elek's gel precipitation test 73, 162, 163*f*
Elephantiasis 317, 317*f*
Embryonated egg 217*f*
Emetic toxin 167
Eminent microbiologists 4*f*
Emmons modification 331
Empirical therapy 144
Empyema 171
Encapsulation 133
Encephalitis 215, 221, 231, 292
    group 236
    stage, acute 239
Encystation 274
Endemic hemoptysis 307
Endemic index 312
Endemic typhus 207
Endocarditis 53, 339, 346
    infective 192
Endogenous source 109
Endometrial specimens 368
Endoparasites 267
Endophthalmitis 339, 363
Endoscopes 128
Endothrix 50, 332
    detection 141
Endotracheal aspirate, collection of 367
Endotracheal intubation 110, 234
Enriched media 24
Enrichment broth 25
Entamoeba 273
    coli 273, 276, 276*f*, 276*t*
    dispar 274-276
    histolytica 139, 273-275, 275*f*, 276, 276*t*, 295, 355
    life cycle of 273*f*
Enteric fever 184, 186
    clinical manifestations of 184
Enteric flora, passage of 314
Enterobacter
    infections, treatment of 184
    species 31, 48, 109, 181, 183, 345
Enterobacterales 181
Enterobacteriaceae 351
Enterobiasis 310
Enterobius 308, 309
    vermicularis 268, 309, 310*f*
    egg of 309*f*
Enterobius
    eggs of 310
    life cycle of 309*f*
Enterococcus 153, 154, 154*t*, 157
    faecalis 46
    faecium 109
Enteromonas hominis 281
Enterotest 279
Enterotoxins 181
Enteroviruses 215, 244, 350
Env gene 248
Envelope 214, 219
Environmental cleaning 116, 127
Enzymatic inactivation 48
Enzyme 49, 75, 192
    detection 337
    extracellular 149
    immunoassay 79
Enzyme-antibody complex 77
Enzyme-linked fluorescence assay 77, 216
Enzyme-linked immunosorbent assay 75, 76*f*, 77, 216, 238, 261, 275, 279, 307
    advantages of 77
    applications of 77
    capture 293
    direct 76
    disadvantages of 77
    indirect 76
    modification of 77
    principle of 75
    procedure of 75

sandwich 76, 77f
    types of 76
Eosinophilia 311
Eosinophils 65, 84, 88
Epidemic relapsing fever 324
Epidemic typhus 207, 324
Epidermodysplasia verruciformis 224
Epidermophyton
    floccosum 334f
    species 332
Epiglottitis 357
Epitope 63
Epsilometer 34, 34f
Epstein-Barr virus 219, 222, 262
    infections 223
        diagnosis of 223
Equipment
    entero-test 280f
    external surfaces of 125
    patient dedicated 116
Erythema
    infectiosum 224
    migrans 205
    multiforme 220
Erythrocytic schizogony 286
Erythromycin 163, 200, 209
Escherichia coli 14, 16, 17, 25, 31, 46, 48, 52, 69,
    109, 144, 181, 183, 348, 351, 358, 359
    biochemical reactions of 182f
    diffusely adherent 182
    enteroaggregative 182
    enterohemorrhagic 182
    enteroinvasive 181
    enteropathogenic 181
    enterotoxigenic 181
    meropenem for 144
Esophageal candidiasis 337
Esophagus 224
Espundia 284
E-test 34, 34f
Ethylene oxide 121
    sterilizer 121, 122, 122f, 128
Eukaryotes 3t
Eukaryotic cells, unicellular 267
Eumycetoma 333, 334, 334f
Exogenous
    antigens 86
    sources 109
Exotoxins 50, 50t
Extrahepatic complications 256
Extrahepatic manifestations 258
Extraintestinal amoebiasis 273
Extrapulmonary tuberculosis 172
Extravascular bloodstream infections 346
Extravascular lysis 105
Eye 335
    external structures of 363
    fundoscopy of 299
    infections 20, 192, 363
    protective 115
Eyelids, infection of 363

■ F

Face wear 115
Facial paralysis 221
Facial spasms 170f

Facultative intracellular bacteria 50
Falciparum malaria 288, 290
    complications of 288
Family Caliciviridae 261
Family Streptococcaceae, classification of 153f
Fascia, infection of 361
Fasciitis, necrotizing 154
Fasciola 304, 306
    hepatica 303, 306, 306f
Fasciolopsis 304
    buski 303, 306, *306f*
        adult worm of 303f
Fastidious gram-negative bacilli 196
Fat, malabsorption of 278
Fatty acid, unsaturated 168
Faucial diphtheria 162
Febrile blisters 220
Febrile episodes, recurrent 205
Febrile neutropenia 336
Febrile paroxysm 287
Fecal carriers 184
Fecal specimens 366
Feces 128
    examination of 268
Feco-oral route 273
Feline cycle 293
Fernandez reaction 176
Fertility 40
Fertilization 287
Fertilized eggs 311, 311f
Fetal immunity 65
Fever 230, 242, 245, 283, 346
    high-grade 206, 228, 317
Fever of unknown origin 347
Field's stain 270
Filamentous bacteria 334
Filarial dance sign 318
Filarial fever 317
Filarial nematodes 316, 316t
Filariasis 271, 317, 317f
Filariform larva 312, 314, 316
Filoviruses 261
Filtration methods 123f
Fimbriae 15, 49, 352
Fimbrial antigen 181
First aid 136, 136t
Fish tapeworm 301
Flaccid paralysis 244
Flagella 14, 64
    detection of 15
Flagellates 267
Flask-shaped ulcers 274
Flaviviridae 237
Flavivirus 239
Flea 267, 324
Flea-borne 207
Fletcher's semisolid medium 206
Flies 321
Floppy child syndrome 170
Flora
    normal 53t
        microbiology of 52
        suppression of 355
    role of normal 52
Flotation techniques 269
Fluconazole 332
Flucytosine 338

Fluid 200
    loss, mild 190
Flukes 267
Flu-like self-limited illness, milder 201
Flu-like symptoms, mild 228
Fluorescence
    measurement of 79
    microscope 9, 9f
Fluorescent dye, microbes coated with 9
Fluorescent staining 173
Fluoroquinolones 47, 171, 191
Folic acid synthesis inhibitors 47
Folinic acid 293
Fonsecaea 335
Food
    bacteriology of 139
    poisoning 150, 355
    processing 142
    sampling 142
    sources, common 179
    surveillance 142
Food-borne
    botulism 170
    pathogens, number of 142
Forchheimer spots 232
Foreign antigens 63
Formaldehyde 124
Formalin 268, 365
Fosfomycin 46
F-plasmids 40
Fragilis 281
Fragment A 162
Framing antimicrobial policy 143
Francisella tularensis 201
Freshwater snail 304
Fried egg
    appearance 210
    colonies 332
Frothy pale offensive stool 268
Frozen vaccines 101
Fundoscopy 299
Fungal agents 350
Fungal disease 330
    classification of 330t
    clinical classification of 330
Fungal etiology 346
Fungal hyphae 330f
Fungal identification 331
Fungal infection 330
    diagnosis of 370
    laboratory diagnosis of 330
    specimen collection for 370
    treatment of 332
Fungal lung disease 358
Fungal opportunistic infections 249
Fungal pathogen isolation 359
Fungus 6, 351, 361, 373
    classification of 329
    microscopic appearance of 331
    morphological forms of 329f
Funiculitis, chronic 317
Fusariosis 340
Fusarium 341
    oxysporum 340
    solani 340
    species 340, 341f
    verticillioides 340

Fusion 249
Fusobacterium 171
   fusiformis 358

G

Gabbet's method 23
Gabbet's methylene 23
Gag gene 248
Galactomannan antigen 332
Gambusia fish, use of 326
Gamete 286
   female 293
   male 293
Gametocytes 286, 289, 293
Gametogony 286
Gamma-herpesviruses 219
Gardner and Venkatraman classification 189
Gardnerella vaginalis 23, 202
Gas
   gangrene 168, 169
   plasma 122
   production 32
GasPak
   anaerobic system 30*f*
   system 168
Gastric acidity, neutralization of 355
Gastric aspirate 367
Gastric biopsy 20, 369
Gastric flu 261
Gastric mucosa, colonization of 200
Gastric ulcers 201
Gastroenteritis 214, 355
   agents of 261
Gastrointestinal tract 52
Gastrointestinal tuberculosis 172
Gel electrophoresis 36, 79
Gelatin stab agar 166
Gene
   targets 234
   therapy 43
   transfer
      artificial methods 43
      horizontal 40
Genetic
   engineering 43
   factor 63
   makeup 56
Genital chlamydiasis 208
Genital flagellates 278
Genital herpes 362
Genital lesions 220
Genital mucosa 224
Genital specimens 368
Genital ulcer 203, 362
   producing 363*t*
Genital warts 362, 363
Genitourinary tract 52, 346
Genitourinary tuberculosis 172
Genotypic methods 39
Gentamicin 180, 188
Genus specific tests 206
Geobacillus stearothermophilus 16, 17, 128, 167
   spores 121-123
German measles 232
Germinal center 82
Giant-cell
   multi-nucleated 221*f*, 230*f*
   pneumonitis 230

Giardia 295, 355
   intestinalis 268
   lamblia 139, 275, 278, 279, 279*f*
      life cycle of 278, 278*f*
Giardiasis 280
Giemsa 280
   stain 205, 270, 362
      blood smear 291*f*
Global Polio Eradication Initiative 245
Glomerulonephritis 258
Glossina 323
Glove 112
   donning, steps of 113*f*
   removal
      indications for 113
      steps of 113*f*
   use 112, 113*t*
      indications for 113
Glucose 168
   only fermenters 32
Glutaraldehyde 124, 128
Glutathione 168
Glycopeptides 46
Glycoprotein 85, 248
   G 241
Glycylglycines 46
Gomori's methenamine silver stain 359
Gomori's stained smear 178*f*, 179
Gonococcal infection, disseminated 159
Gonococcus 158, 160*f*
Gonorrhoea 159
Gown donning, steps of 115*f*
Gown removal, steps of 115*f*
Graft rejection
   acute 97
   chronic 97
   prevention of 97
   types of 97, 97*t*
Graft-versus-host reaction 87, 97
Gram stain 11, 16, 21, 156, 157, 159, 162, 165, 166, 169, 179, 180, 183, 188, 190, 190*f*, 193, 330, 338, 349
   interpretation of 21
   principle of 21, 21*f*
   procedure of 21*f*
   property 12, 12*f*
   uses of 22
Gram-negative
   bacilli 11, 12, 30, 185, 196, 201, 351
   bacteria, hospital antibiogram of 145*t*
   cell wall 13, 13*f*, 13*t*
   cocci 11, 12
   diplococci 159*f*, 160*f*
   spiral rods 200*f*
Gram-positive
   filamentous bacilli 178*f*
   bacilli 11, 12, 163*f*
   cocci 11, 12, 30, 351
   cell wall 13, 13*f*, 13*t*
Gram-stain 178, 197*f*, 198
   smear 356, 362
Granules 367
   histopathology of 179
Granuloma formation 93
Granulomatous reaction 334
Graves' disease 93, 95
Griffith experiment 40
   demonstrating transformation 41*f*
Griseofulvin 332

Ground-glass chromatin 220
Growth retardation 311
Guillain-Barre syndrome 210
Guinea
   pig 162
   worm disease 320

H

H agglutination 185*f*
H antibody 185
H antigen 73, 181
H1N1 flu 228
HACEK group 197
Haemaphysalis species 325
Haemophilus 40, 196, 345
   aegyptius 196
   ducreyi 196, 197
   influenzae 14, 16, 25, 50, 99, 196, 348, 349, 357-359
      B 163
      satellitism of 197*f*
   parainfluenzae 196
   species 196, 197
Hair follicle 360
   infections 361
Halogens 125
Halophilic *Vibrios* 189, 191
Hand hygiene 111, 112
   before gloves use 112
   methods, types of 111
   moments for 111*f*
   product 127
   protocols 374
Hand rub 111, 125, 128, 129
   advantage 111
   indications 111
   steps of 111, 112*f*
Hand scrub, surgical 111
Hand wash 111, 116, 129
   after glove use 112
   steps of 111, 112*f*
Hanging drop
   method 23*f*, 190
   preparation 23
Hanging groin 319
Hanging mask syndrome 114
Hansen's bacillus 172, 175
Hantavirus 262
   pulmonary syndrome 262
Hapten 63
Harada-Mori filter paper tube method 313
Hard tick 291, 322, 325
   female 325*f*
Hashimoto's thyroiditis 95
Hassall's corpuscles 81
Hay fever 92
Head
   cover 115
   louse 324, 324*f*
Health-care worker 135, 136, 138
Healthcare-associated infection 54, 109
   factors affecting 109
   prevention of 110
   surveillance 117
   types, major 110
Heart 154
Heat fixation 20, 22
Heat labile 66
Heat-sensitive critical items 128

Index

Heavy larva load 314
Hecht's pneumonia 230
Hela cell line 217
Helical symmetry 213
Helicobacter 29
   pylori 31, 79, 200
      diagnosis of 201
Helminthic infections 66
Helminths 267, 267*t*, 354
Helper T cells 83, 84, 87
   differentiation of 87
Helper T lymphocyte 87
Hemagglutination
   inhibition test 75
   test 74
Hemagglutinin 227
Hematuria 352
Hemoflagellates 282
Hemolysis 30
   complete 153
   partial 153
Hemolytic reactions, acute 105
Hemorrhagic cystitis 225
Hemorrhagic fever
   agents of 345
   risk of 237
Hendra virus 231
Hepadnavirus 214
Hepatic complications 256
Hepatic flukes 303, 306
Hepatitis
   acute 255, 258, 259
   chronic 256, 258
   fulminant 259
   immunoreactive 256
   virus 215, 224, 254, 254*t*
Hepatitis A 255
   vaccine 99
   virus 139, 254
      antigen detection 254
      particles, detection of 254
Hepatitis B 66, 77, 79, 101, 102, 134, 163, 214, 218, 254, 255, 257
   core
      antibody 256
      antigen 256
   immunoglobulin 103, 138, 257
   infection 257*f*
   laboratory diagnosis of 256
   post-exposure prophylaxis for 138*t*
   surface antigen 76*f*, 77, 100, 138, 256
   vaccine 99, 257
   virus 109, 135, 224, 254, 255, 255*f*, 262
      antigens 256
      infection 216, 255
      vaccination 135
Hepatitis C 79, 134, 258
   virus 109, 135, 254, 257, 262
      infection 258
Hepatitis D 259
   virus 254, 258
Hepatitis E 259
   virus 139, 259
   infections 259
Hepatorenal hemorrhagic syndrome 206
Herd immunity 62
Herpes gladiatorum 220
Herpes simplex virus 219, 219*f*, 352, 363

infections 221
Herpesvirus 214, 219, 350
   replication of 219
Herpetic whitlow 220
Heteroantigens 63
Heterophile
   agglutination tests 74
   antigen 63
Hide porter's disease 165
High-efficiency particulate air filters 123
Hiss's serum sugar media 162
Histocompatibility antigens 84
Histocompatibility complex, major 84, 86, 87
Histopathological stain 330, 334, 336
Histoplasma 346
   capsulatum 330, 335
Histoplasmosis 335
Hookworm 270, 308, 312
   eggs of 313, 313*f*
   infections 313
   life cycle of 312*f*
Hormone 77, 98
Horn cells, anterior 244
Hortaea werneckii 332
Hospital antibiogram 145
Hospital environment 109
Hospital infection control 3, 107
   committee 117
Hospital information system 143
Hospital organisms 109
Hospital waste, disposal of 130
Host cell
   entry 234
   receptors 60
Host immune cells 59
Host immunity, impaired 355
Hot air oven 123*f*
Housefly 321, 322, 322*f*
Human acquire infection 306
Human anatomical waste 133
Human cycle 286, 292, 317
Human diploid cell vaccine 218
Human fungal infections 332
Human herpesvirus-8 223, 262
Human host, normal flora of 52*t*
Human immunodeficiency virus 79, 96, 109, 134, 248, 350
   diagnosis of 250*t*, 251, 252, 252*f*
   disease, acute 249
   genome 248
   infection 253
      specific tests for 250
      symptomatic 249
   prognosis of 251
   RNA detection 252
   serotyping 248
   structure of 248*f*
   testing 136
Human immunoglobulin 255
Human intestine 301
   development in 273
Human leukocyte antigens 84
Human lice 324
Human lysozyme 290
Human oncogenic viruses 262*t*
Human papillomavirus 262, 363
   vaccine 99, 100
Human parainfluenza viruses 230

Human prion diseases 263
Human rabies, prevention of 242
Human T cell lymphotropic virus 262
Human tissues 154
Humidity, relative 119
Humoral immune responses 87
Humoral immunity 175
Humoral immunodeficiency 96
Hutchinson's teeth 203
Hyaluronic acid 153
Hyaluronidase 153
Hybridizes 38
Hydatid cyst 300, 301*f*
   microscopy of 301*f*
Hydatid disease 271, 301
Hydatid fluid 300
   microscopy 301
Hydatid sand 300
Hydrocele 317
Hydroclaving 133
Hydrogen peroxide 124, 128
Hydrophobia 242
Hygiene 56
Hymenolepis
   nana 268, 269, 297, 298, 301
      egg of 302*f*
   species 297
Hyperinfection syndrome 314
Hyperpigmentation 283
Hypersensitivity
   detection of 92
   mechanism of 91
   reaction 91, 92*f*, 93
   types of 91*t*
Hyphae 329
Hypnozoites 286
Hypochlorite 125, 126
Hyposensitization 92
Hypothermia 346

I

Icosahedral symmetry 213
Illnesses, types of 205
Immune
   cells, development of 81
   response 61, 86, 91
   status 109
   stimulation 52
Immune system 85
   cells of 81, 83
   components of 81
   comprises 81
   structure of 81*t*
Immunity 13, 59
   active 61, 62*t*
   local 61
   low 335
   natural 61
   types of 61
Immunization
   active 217, 257
   schedule 99
Immunoassays, conventional 72
Immunochromatographic test 79, 216, 275
Immunocompetent host 293
Immunodeficiency
   diseases 96, 99
      classification of primary 96*t*

Index

disorders 94, 96
    secondary 96
Immunodiagnostic methods 270
Immunoelectrophoresis 72
Immunofluorescence 9
    antibody, indirect 208
    assay 78, 78f
    test, direct 198, 229
Immunogen 63
Immunogenicity 63
Immunoglobulin 101, 64, 218
    A 66
    administration 99
    class 65, 65t
    D 66
    E 66
    functions of 65
    G 65
    M 65
Immunohematology 104
Immunological complication 105
Immunological memory 61
Immunological methods 250, 251, 332
Immunological reactivity 63, 63
Immunological tolerance 63, 94
Immunology 3, 57, 366
Immunoprophylaxis 99, 101, 103t, 217
Immunosorbent 75
    agglutination assay 293
Immunosuppression 96
Immunosuppressive therapy 97
Impetigo 255
Impregnation methods 21
In vitro test 162, 163
Indirect agglutination test 74
Indole
    negative 31
    positive 31
    test 31, 31f
Infection 54, 96, 182, 347
    abdominal 182
    abortive 245
    acute 65
    anaerobic 20
    asymptomatic 258
    chlamydial 209
    chronic 313
    community-associated 54
    congenital 363
    control 183, 194
        measures 152, 157, 159, 163, 175, 221, 222
        practice 139
    cutaneous 177
    dental 358
    disseminated 177
    exanthematous 369
    genital 20
    human 179
    inapparent 245
    intravascular bloodstream 346
    parapharyngeal 357
    perinatal 363
    postnatal 363
    prevention and control 235
    primary 219, 238, 324
    recurrent 220
    reservoir of 256
    risk of contracting 135

secondary 238
sequence of 237
source of 109, 221
spread of 338
subcutaneous 360
surgical site 110
systemic 369
toxin-mediated 150
types of 20t
Infectious agents, variety of 354
Infectious diseases 77
    epidemiology of 54
Infectious mononucleosis 74, 222
Infectious plastic waste 131
Infectious sharps, hazards from 130
Infectious waste
    hazards from 130
    pathogens in 130
Infective dose 49, 55
Infective syndromes, miscellaneous 360
Inflamed tonsils 357
Inflammatory response 59, 69
Influenza 75, 229
    B viruses 227
    epidemiological surveillance for 228
    illness, development of 234
    severe 228
    surveillance 228, 229
Influenza vaccine 217, 229
    cell culture-based inactivated 229
    recombinant 229
Influenza virus 214, 215, 227, 227f, 228, 247, 357, 359
    evolution of pandemic 228f
Inguinal lymph nodes 197
Inhibit cell wall synthesis 46
Innate immunity 59, 60t, 88
Inner ear specimens 368
Interferon 217
    alfa plus ribavirin 258
Interleukin 82, 85
Internal audits 377
Internal quality assessment 376
Interstitial pneumonia 209, 358
Intestinal amoebae 273
Intestinal amoebiasis 274
    laboratory diagnosis of 274
Intestinal anthrax 165
Intestinal cestodes 297
Intestinal coccidian
    infections 296
    parasites 292, 294
Intestinal complications 274, 311
Intestinal flagellates 278, 281
Intestinal fluke 303, 306
Intestinal motility, inhibition of 355
Intestinal nematodes 267, 308
Intestinal phase 310, 311
Intestinal taeniasis 297, 298, 298f
Intestine 313
    large 273
Intracellular antigens 83, 86
Intracellular bacteria 50t
Intracytoplasmic inclusions 14
Intradermal skin tests 271
Intravascular organisms 66
Intrinsic resistance 35, 45
Invasive tests 201
Iodine 21, 125

mount 268, 269, 269f, 275f
tincture of 125
Iodophor 125
Ionizing radiation 124
Iris diaphragm 7
Iron
    deficiency 336
    hematoxylin stain 276f
Isoantibody, natural 104
Isoantigens 63
Isograft 96
Isolation 116, 162
    room 229
Isonicotinic acid hydrazide 47
Isopropyl alcohol 366
Itch
    ground 313, 315
    mite 322, 324, 324f
    severe 324
Itraconazole 333, 335, 336
Ivermectin 314, 318
Ixodid tick 325

J

Japanese B encephalitis 236, 239
    diagnosis of 239
    vaccine 99
JC virus 224
Jeryl Lynn strain 231
Joint
    pain 258
    swelling 238
Jumping genes 43

K

Kala-azar 282
    elimination 284
    vector of 323
Kaposi's sarcoma 223
Katayama fever 305
Kelsey-Maurer test 128
Kelsey-Sykes test 128
Keratitis 339, 363
Keratoconjunctivitis 126
Kernig's sign 348
Kidney 154, 351
    abscess of 179
    parenchyma, inflammation of 352
Killed influenza vaccine 99
Killed injectable polio vaccine 218
Killed vaccine 61, 99, 100, 100t
    injectable 191
Killed viral vaccines 218
Killed whole-cell vaccine 190
Kingella kingae 197
Kinyoun's cold acid-fast staining 173
Kinyoun's method 23, 179
Kirby-Bauer disk diffusion 33, 34f
Klebsiella 56, 181, 183, 345, 348, 353, 358
    granulomatis 183
    ozaenae 183
    pneumoniae 14, 31, 45, 109, 183, 183f, 359
    rhinoscleromatis 183, 357
    species 48, 183, 183f
Koch's postulates 4
Koplik's spots 230, 230f
Korthof's medium 206

Index

Kovac's reagent 31
Kupffer cells 84
Kyasanur forest disease virus 236, 239

L

L form 15
Labile toxin 181
Laboratory coats 114
Laboratory safety 373
Laboratory-acquired infections 373, 373*t*
Lactophenol cotton blue 331
Lactose
    fermenters 181
    non-fermenting colonies 194, 194*f*
Lag phase 16
Langhans giant cells 175
Larva 297, 302
    currens 314, 315
    migrans 315
        etiology of 315*t*
    migrating 313, 314
Laryngitis 357
Laryngotracheobronchitis, acute 357
Larynx 224
    inflammation of 357
Lash's cysteine hydrolysate serum media 280
Lassa 345
Late intestinal phase 313
Latent syphilis 203
Latent tuberculosis infection 174
Latex agglutination test 14
Lattice hypothesis 71
Laundry management 235
Lawn culture 28
Lectin pathway 69
Legionella 201, 359
    pneumophila 109, 359
Leishman's stain 270
Leishman-Donovan bodies 283
Leishmania 267, 270, 271, 282, 282*f*, 284, 345, 370
    braziliensis complex 284
    chagasi 284
    donovani 282
        life cycle of 283*f*
    mexicana complex 284
    tropica complex 284
Leishmaniasis 271, 282, 283*f*
Leishmanin test 284
Lepra bacilli 175
Lepromatous leprosy 175*t*
Lepromin test 175, 176
Leprosy 54, 175, 176
    elimination 176
Leptomeninges 348
Leptospira 203, 345, 352
    interrogans 205, 206*f*
Leptospirosis 35, 79, 206
Lesion 225
    benign 224
    cutaneous 220
    edge of 176
    primary 360
    secondary 360, 361
Lethal parasitic disease 288
Leukemia 96
Leukocyte esterase test 353
Leukocytosis, moderate 276
Levaditi stain 203
Levofloxacin 194
L-form 209
Lid 120
Life-threatening systemic infections 149
Light microscope 9*t*
Light-emitting diode 173
Limb hypoplasia 221
Lincosamides 46
Line probe assay 38, 174
Lip, vesicular lesions on 220*f*
Lipo-oligosaccharide 159
Lipopeptides 47
Lipopolysaccharide 13, 64
Liposomal amphotericin B 284, 341
Lipoteichoic acid 153
Lipschutz body 220
Liquid
    culture 28
    filtration of 124
    media concept 4
    waste, pre-treatment of 126
Listeria 345, 348
    monocytogenes 179, 348
Listeriosis, neonatal 180
Lithium chloride 180
Little animalcules 4
Live attenuated influenza vaccine 99, 229
Live bacilli 176
Live oral polio vaccine 61
Live vaccination 61
Live vaccines 100, 100*t*, 218
Liver 215, 271, 282, 335
    aspirate 271
    biopsy 283
    flukes, life cycle of 306
    pus, microscopy of 276
LJ media, culture on 177
Loa loa 270, 308, 316, 319
Lobar pneumonia 358
Lockjaw spasms 170*f*
Loeffler's serum slope 25, 27, 162, 162*f*
Loeffler's syndrome 311
Lophotrichous 14*f*
Louse 322, 324, 324*f*
Louse-borne 207
Low infective dose 55
Lowenstein-Jensen medium 25, 25*f*, 174*f*, 179, 335, 359
Lower respiratory tract 357, 369
    infections 358
        laboratory diagnosis of 359
Ludwig's angina 357
Lugol's iodine 268
Luminescence 78
Lumpy jaw 178
Lung 277
    biopsy specimens 367
    fluke 303, 307
Lutzomyia 282
Lyme disease 205
Lymph node 82, 271
    aspiration 271, 283
    biopsy 271
    infection 177
Lymphadenopathy 203, 232, 249, 283
Lymphatic filariasis 271, 316, 316*t*, 317, 318
Lymphatic inflammation 317
Lymphoblasts 82, 83
types of 82
Lymphogranuloma venereum 208, 363
Lymphoid follicles 82, 89, 89*f*
Lymphoid lineage 83
Lymphoid organs 81, 82, 89
    peripheral 81, 82
Lymphoid tissue
    group of 82
    mucosa-associated 82
Lymphokines 85
Lymphoma 96
Lysogenic conversion 42, 226
Lysogenic cycle 41, 226
Lysol 128
Lysosomal enzymes 83
Lytic cycle 41, 225

M

M protein 154
M'Fadyean capsule stain 14
MacConkey
    agar 25, 26*f*, 150, 183*f*, 185, 185*f*, 190, 193, 194, 194*f*, 359
    broth 142
    purple broth 140*f*
Macroconidia 333
Macrolides 46
Macrophage 81, 83, 83*f*, 88, 93, 175
    activated 84, 93
    activating response 172
Madura foot 333
Maduramycosis 333
Madurella
    grisea 333
    mycetomatis 333
Magnesium ribonucleate theory 22
Malaise 242, 245
Malaria 271, 290
    benign 287
    chronic complications of 288
    epidemiology of 288
    recrudescence of 286
    relapse of 286
    severe 290
Malaria parasite 271, 286
    life cycle of 287*f*
    morphological forms of 289*f*
    speciation of 289
Malassezia furfur 332
Malignancy 223
Malnutrition 96, 311
Man, development in 278, 300
Mannitol 180, 337
Mannose binding lectins 68
Mansonella 270
    species 308, 316, 319
Mansonia 318, 321
Mantle area 82
Marburg 345
Mask
    donning, steps of 114*f*
    front of 114
    removal, steps of 114*f*
Matted hair 166
McCoy cell line 220, 362
McCrady table 141
McFadyean's reaction 166, 166*f*
Mcintosh and Filde's anaerobic jar 29*f*

Index

Measles 55, 103, 116, 231
   vaccine 99, 231
   virus 230
      infection 61
Meatballs appearance 332
Mebendazole 271, 309, 311, 320
Mechanical vector 322
Medical entomology 321
Medical microbiology 3
Medical mycology 329
Medical products, number of 124
Medulla 81, 82
Medusa head appearance 166
Megaloblastic anemia 302
Membrane attack complex 69, 90
   formation of 67, 67*f*
Membrane filter 123, 123*f*
   method 141
Memory
   B cells 82, 83
   present 60
Meningitis 20, 156, 182, 215, 221, 348
   acute 348
   agents of chronic 350*t*
   chronic 348-350
   types of 349*t*
Meningococcal
   infection, pathogenesis of 158
   vaccine 99
Meningococcus 158
Meropenem 194, 353
Mesophiles 17
Mesosomes 14
Metabolic defects 41
Metacercaria larva 303
Metachromatic granules 161
Metallic body implants 132
Metallic iron 168
Metastatic spread 149
Methanol fixation 20
Methicillin resistant *Staphylococcus aureus* 47, 48, 152, 361
Methylcholanthrene 98
Metronidazole 171, 271
Mickey mouse 336
Microaerophilic bacteria 17, 29
Microbial agents 355
Microbial antigens, extracellular 86
Microbial exposure, requires prior 60
Microbial flora, normal 52
Microbial typing 38
Microbiological tests 201
Microbiological waste 133
Microbiology
   general 1
   laboratory, support from 143
   quality control in 375
Micrococcus 149
Microconidia 333
Microfilaremia, asymptomatic 317
Microfilaria 316-318
   detection of 318, 319
Micrometry, principle of 7*f*
Microorganisms 5*t*
   classification of 3
   discovery of 5
Microscopic agglutination test 74, 206
Microsporum
   canis 334*f*
   species 332
Microwave 124, 133
Micturition, pain while 352
Middle ear infections 364
Middle east respiratory syndrome coronavirus 233
Milk, pasteurization of 4
Miltefosine 284
Minimum inhibitory concentration-guided therapy 144
MiniVIDAS system 77*f*
Minocycline 194
Mites 267, 324
Mitsuda reaction 176
Mobile genetic elements 43
Mobiluncus 171
Moistened sterile swabs 142
Molecular diagnosis 159, 275, 276, 293, 295, 313
Molecular method 36, 174, 186, 190, 199, 216, 222, 224, 225, 271, 280, 284, 290, 318, 332, 349
Molecular mimicry 95, 154
Molecular test 143, 229, 232, 359, 362
Molluscum
   bodies 225
   contagiosum virus 225
Monkeypox virus 225
Monobactam 46
Monoclonal antibody 66
Monocytes 88
Monokines 85
Monophasic medium 26
Monotrichous 14*f*
Monozygotic twins 96
Monsur's gelatin taurocholate tellurite agar 190
Montenegro test 271, 284
Morganella 181, 187
Morphological classification 329
Morula 208
Mosquito 321, 322
   aedes 236
   anopheles 236
   bites 317
   body of 321
   breeding 319
   culex 236
   cycle 286, 317
   larvae of 326
Motile bacilli 200
Motility 182, 193, 269, 279
   darting 190
   differential 180
   gliding 209
   testing 30, 190
   types of 15, 15*t*
Mouse footpad cultivation 176
Mucocutaneous histoplasmosis 335
Mucoid bloody stool 268
Mucor 330, 338, 339
Mucormycosis 338
Mucosal candidiasis 336
Mucosal immunity 66
   mediates 90
Mucosal transmission 249
Mueller-Hinton agar 33, 193, 353
Multibacillary leprosy 175
Multi-disinfectant resistance 192
Multidrug resistance 192
Multiple drugs 182
Multiple tube method 140, 140*f*
Multiplex polymerase chain reaction 216
Mumps 55, 350
   prevention of 231
   salivary gland for 215
   vaccine 99
   virus 231
Munch-Peterson test 155
Mupirocin 46
Musca domestica 321
Muscle
   abscess of 179
   biopsy 320
   encystment 320
   infection of 361
   tissue 271
Muscular cysticercosis 299
Musculoskeletal infections 150
Mutation 40
Mutational drug resistance 47, 48, 48*t*
Mutational resistance 47
Myalgia 228, 320
Myasthenia gravis 93, 95
Mycelium 329
Mycetism 341
Mycetoma 333, 335
Mycobacteria 172
   growth indicator tube 174
Mycobacterium
   atypical 360
   leprae 4, 16, 23, 50, 172, 175, 176*f*, 361
   tuberculosis 16, 17, 22, 23, 47, 172, 174, 352, 358, 359
Mycolic acid synthesis inhibitors 47
Mycology 327, 329
Mycoplasma 207, 209, 359
   antibodies 74
   colonies 210*f*
   infections 75
   pneumonia 35, 74, 209, 358, 359
Mycoses, superficial 330, 332
Mycotic poisoning 341
Mycotoxicosis 341
Myeloma, multiple 96
Myocarditis 346
Myxovirus 213, 214, 227, 232

N

N95 respirator 114, 175
Naegleria 273, 277
   fowleri 277
Nagler's reaction 75
Naïve lymphocytes 82
Nasal cavity
   and sinuses, infections of 357
   infections of 357
Nasal specimens 176
Nasopharyngeal aspiration 367
Nasopharyngeal swab 370
Nasopharynx 52
National AIDS Control Organization 132, 137, 251, 252
National Immunization Program 239
National Immunization Schedule 101, 102*t*, 245, 261
National Institute of Health 275

Index

National TB Elimination Programme 175
National Vector Borne Disease Control
　　Programme 284, 288
Native valves 192
Natural killer cell 59, 65, 83, 86, 88, 96
Nausea 237
Necator 313
　　americanus 312, 315
Needle
　　recapping of 136*f*
　　type of 135
Needle stick injury 135
　　prevention of 135
　　transmitted infections 109
Negri body 242, 242*f*
Neisseria 25, 40, 158
　　gonorrhoeae 158*t*, 159, 363
　　meningitidis 50, 82, 158, 158*t*, 349
Nemathelminths 267
Nematodes 308
　　developmental stages of 308*f*
Neonatal herpes 220
Neoplasia 249, 249*t*
　　malignant 224
Neoplasms 347
Nerve
　　cells, latency in 219
　　lesion 175
Neuraminidase 227
Neurocysticercosis 299, 299*f*
Neurologic manifestations 184, 210
Neurologic phase, acute 242
Neuron degeneration 245
Neuropathological diagnosis 263
Neurotoxins 355
Neurotropic viruses 215
Neutralization test 75
Neutrophils 60, 84, 88
Never recap needles 135
Newer techniques 75
Newer vaccine 100
Nichols strain 204
Nicotinamide adenine dinucleotide 196
Niger seed agar 331
Nigrosin stains 330
Nikshay 175
Nipah virus 115, 231
　　transmission of 231
Nitazoxanide 296
Nitrocellulose membrane 79
Nitrofuran 47
Nitrofurantoin 45
Nitroimidazoles 47
Nocardia 23, 178, 179, 333
Nocardiosis 179
Nodules resembling leprosy 283
Non-bile stained eggs 269
Non-chromogens 177
Non-coronavirus disease-2019 vaccines 235
Non-critical instruments, smaller 125
Non-critical surfaces, disinfection of 125
Non-fermenting gram-negative bacilli 192
Nonhalophilic vibrios 189
Non-hazardous solid waste 130
Nonimmunological complications 105
Non-infectious inflammatory diseases 347
Noninvasive tests 201

Non-ionizing radiation 124
Non-lactose fermenters 181
Non-microbiological parameters 142
Nonparalytic poliomyelitis 245
Non-plastic infectious waste 124
Non-treponemal test 204, 205
Nontuberculous mycobacteria 176, 177*t*
　　classification of 176
Non-typhoidal salmonellae 184
Nonvenereal treponema species 205
Norfloxacin 353
Normal resident flora 60
Norovirus 139
Norwalk virus 260, 261
Nose specimen 162
Nosocomial candidiasis 336
Nosocomial wound infection 110
NS1 antigen detection 238
Nuchal rigidity 348
Nuclear antigen 223
Nucleic acid 213
　　amplification
　　　　techniques 36
　　　　tests 209
　　probes 38
　　　　types of 38
　　synthesis inhibitors 47
　　type of 213
Nucleocapsid 219, 248
Nucleoid 14
Nucleoprotein 227, 241
　　antigens 241
　　N gene 231, 232
Nutrient agar 24, 24*f*, 150, 166, 193, 193*f*
Nutrient broth 24
Nutritional status 56

O

O agglutination 185*f*
O antibodies 185
O antigen 181
O blood group 104
Objective lens 7
Obligate aerobes 17
Obligate anaerobes 17, 29, 168
Obligate intracellular 50
Obstructive pulmonary disease, chronic 209, 339
Obstructive uropathies 306
Occult filariasis 317
Ocular cysticercosis 299
Ocular filariasis 316
Ocular infections 225, 363*t*
Ocular larva migrans 315
Ocular lens 7
Ocular lesions 220
Ocular micrometer 6
Ocular specimens 368
Ofloxacin 209
Oil immersion fields 173
Oliguria 190
Omicron detection 234
Onchocerca volvulus 308, 316, 319
Onchocercoma 319
Oncofetal antigens 98
Oncofetal proteins 98

Oncogenic viruses 262
Onychomycosis 337*f*, 339
Oocyst 287, 292, 294, 295
　　sporulated 294, 294*f*
　　types of 294
Ookinete 287
Operation theatre 141
　　disinfection of 127
Ophthalmia neonatorum 159
Opisthorchis 304, 306
　　eggs of 307
　　viverrini 306
Opportunistic coccidian parasites 292
Opportunistic mycoses 330, 336
Opsonin 65
Oral cavity 52
　　infections 358
Oral cholera vaccines 190
Oral doxycycline 205, 206
Oral fluconazole therapy 338
Oral live attenuated vaccines 191
Oral macrolides 200
Oral polio vaccine 99, 246*t*
Oral terbinafine 333
Oral thrush 336, 337*f*, 358
Oral vancomycin 171
Oral-cervicofacial actinomycosis 178
Oral-facial mucosal lesions 220
Organic matter 119
Organism
　　causing ear infections 364*t*
　　load 119
　　nature of 119
　　pathogenicity 55
Oriental sore 284
Orientia
　　tsutsugamushi 207
Oropharyngeal candidiasis 336
Oropharyngeal swab 358, 370
Orthomyxoviruses 227, 229
Ortho-phthalaldehyde 124, 128
Osteolytic bone lesions 338
Otitis externa 364
Otitis media 364
Otomycosis 339
Outer membrane 13
　　protein 159
Oviparous 308
Ovoviviparous 308
Oxazolidinones 46
Oxidase test 31, 31*f*
Oxygen 17
　　absorption of 29

P

P24 antigen, detection of 250-252
PALCAM agar 180
Palisade arrangement 164
Panencephalitis, subacute sclerosing 230
Papilloma 224
Papillomaviruses 224
Papovaviruses 214
Papular-purpuric gloves 224
Paracoccidioides 346
　　brasiliensis 330, 335, 336
Paracoccidioidomycosis 336

Index

Paracortical area 82
Paragonimus 304, 307
    life cycle of 307
    westermani 303, 306f, 307, 358
Paralytic disease 245
Paralytic poliomyelitis 245
    vaccine-associated 245, 246
Paralytic rabies 242
Paramyxoviruses 227, 229
Paranasal sinuses, inflammation of 357
Parasite 6, 139, 267, 345, 351, 354, 373
    lactate dehydrogenase 271
    life cycle of 267
    sequestration of 288
Parasitic agents 350
Parasitic cysts 268
Parasitic diseases
    laboratory diagnosis of 268
    treatment of 271
Parasitic etiology 345
Parasitic infections
    diagnosis of 268
    specimen collection for 370
Parasitic lung disease 358
Parasitic opportunistic infections 249
Parasitology 265
Paratyphi 184
Paromomycin 271, 284
Paroxysms, stimulation of 198
Parvoviruses 214, 224
Passive agglutination test 74, 74f
Passive immunity 61, 62t, 66
    artificial 61
Passive immunization 218
Pasteurella 201
    multocida 201
Pasteurization 126
Patent ductus arteriosus 232
Pathogenic bacteria, metabolism of 18
Patient movement 116
Paucibacillary leprosy 175
Paul-Bunnell test 63, 74
Pediculus humanus
    capitis 324
    corporis 324
Pelvic inflammatory disease 171, 362
Penetration air filters 123
Penicillin 92, 163, 205
    G 201
    resistance 156
Penicillinase resistant-penicillins 46
Penicilliosis 339
Penicillium 330
    marneffei 330, 339, 340
    species 339, 340f
Penicillosis 336
Pentamidine 271
Pentatrichomonas hominis 281
Pentavalent
    antimonials 284
    vaccine 102
Peplomeres 214
Pepper appearance 338
Peptic ulcer disease 201
Peptidoglycan layer 13, 149
Peptone water 24, 24f
Peptostreptococcus 171
Peracetic acid 124, 128
Percutaneous injury 135

Percutaneous transmission 249
Perianal pruritus 309
Perianal skin samples, microscopy of 310
Perianal swabs 268
Pericarditis 346
Periodic acid Schiff stain 275, 330
Peripheral blood smear 285, 319
    examination 285, 285f, 288
    types of 288
Periplasmic space 13
Peritonitis 53
Peritrichous 14f
Permanent stain 274
    smear 269
Per-nasal swab 367
Pernicious malaria 288
Personal protective equipment 111, 113f, 133, 374
    cap 113f
    coverall 113f
    disposable gown 113f
    face shield 113f
    gloves 113f
    goggles 113f
    gum boot 113f
    heavy duty gloves 113f
    linen gown 113f
    N95 respirator 113f
    plastic apron 113f
    shoe cover 113f
    shoes 113f
    surgical mask 113f
Pertussis toxin, tracheal cytotoxin, adhesins 197
Pertussis vaccine 99
Peyer's patches 82, 244
pH 18
    local 119
    theory 21
Phaeohyphomycosis 335
Phaeoid fungi 335
Phage, life cycles of 41
Phagocytes 59
Phagocytosis 65, 83
    disorders of 96
    opsonization of 90f
Pharmaceutical waste 130
Pharyngitis 154, 209, 357
Pharyngoconjunctival fever 225
Phenol coefficient test 128
Phenolic 125
    compounds 128
Phenotypic methods 38
Phenotypic skewing 94
Phenylpyruvic acid test 187
Phialophora 335
Phlebotomus 282
    argentipes 282, 323
    longipes 284
    sergenti 284
Photochromogens 177
Phylum Arthropoda 321, 321t
Physical control methods 325
Physical destruction 53
Pia mater 348
Picornaviruses 214, 244
Piedraia hortae 332
Pigment 150, 192
    production 177

Pili 15, 49, 159, 181
Pilot wheel appearance 336
Pinworm 309
Piperacillin 353
Pistia plants, removal of 319
Placenta, cross 65
Plague 187
    vaccine 99
Plaque inhibition test 75
Plasma
    membrane 13
    pyrolysis 133
    regain, rapid 35, 73, 204
    sterilization 122, 128
Plasma cell 66, 83, 88, 89
    antibody-producing 83
    pneumonia 340
Plasma sterilizer 122f
    uses of 122
Plasmids 14, 40
    functions of 40
    transfer of 226
Plasmodium 87, 270, 286, 289, 321, 345, 370
    falciparum 286, 288, 290f
    malariae 286
    ovale 286
        infections 286
    vivax 286
Plastic
    aprons 114
    bags 132
    infectious waste 124
Platelets 84
Platyhelminths 267
Plerocercoid larva 302
Pleura 357
Pleural effusion 358
Pleural fluid 173
Pleuropneumonia-like organisms 209
Pneumococcal conjugate vaccine 102, 157
Pneumococcal vaccine 99
Pneumococci, properties of 156f
Pneumococcus 153, 154t, 156
Pneumocystis 87
    jirovecii 340, 359
        pneumonia 336
    pneumonia 340
Pneumonia 194, 225, 234, 339, 358
    atypical 209, 210, 358
    infant 208
    primary atypical 209
    severe 234
    typical 358
    ventilator-associated 110, 359
Pneumonic plague 187
Pol gene 248
Polio vaccine, injectable 99, 246t
Poliomyelitis 244, 245f, 369
Poliovirus 215, 244, 244f
    strains, vaccine-derived 245
    vaccine-derived 244-246
Polyclonal B cell activation 95
Polyclonal lymphocyte activation 95
Polymerase chain reaction 36, 216, 332
    applications of 36
    disadvantages of 37
    modifications of 37
    nested multiplex 275
    principle of 36

Index

Polymicrobial infection 357
Polymorphonuclear leukocytes 84
Polymyxin 45, 47, 180
Polyomaviruses 224
Porphyromonas 171
Posaconazole 341
Positive germ tube test 337*f*
Post-exposure management 136
    steps of 136, 136*t*
Post-herpetic neuralgia 222
Post-kala-azar dermal leishmaniasis 282, 283
Postnatal rubella infection 232
Post-streptococcal glomerulonephritis 95
Post-traumatic patients 193
Posture, abnormal 169
Postzone 71*f*
    phenomenon 72
Potassium
    hydroxide preparation 330
    tellurite agar 25, 27, 162, 162*f*
Potency, high 50
Povidone iodine 125, 129
Poxvirus 214, 224, 225
Practical microbiology 378
Praziquantel 306
Precipitation reaction 72
Precyst 273
Predominantly dysentery 354
Predominantly inflammatory diarrhea 354
Pre-erythrocytic schizogony 286
Pregnancy 100
Pressure chamber 120
Prevotella 171
Prion disease 262, 263*t*
    mechanism of 263
Probiotics 53
Procalcitonin 144, 145, 77
Prodromal phase 242
Proglottids 298
Prokaryotes 3*t*
Promastigote 282, 282*f*, 284
Prophylaxis 163
    against malaria 290
    post-exposure 103, 136, 137*t*, 163, 215, 218, 222, 231, 243
    pre-exposure 243
Propionibacterium 171
Proteeae 181
    A 74, 80, 149
        conjugate 80
        detection 151
    coagulation 60
    extracellular surface 157
    production of 43
    synthesis inhibition 46
Proteus 181, 187, 353
    mirabilis 31
    species 31, 45
    swarming 24
Protozoa 105, 267, 267*t*, 354
    miscellaneous 267
Providencia 181, 187
Provirus 249
Prozone 71*f*
    phenomenon 71, 74
Pruritic rashes 319
Pseudallescheria boydii 333
Pseudohyphae 329
Pseudomembranous colitis 170

Pseudomonas 17, 31, 32, 40, 48, 56, 50, 69, 110, 192, 194, 345, 353, 358, 359
    aeruginosa 45, 46, 109, 140, 192, 193, 193*f*
    infection 193
Psychrophiles 17
Pthirus pubis 324
Pubic lice 324, 324*f*
Pulmonary anthrax 165
Pulmonary aspergillosis 339
Pulmonary cryptococcosis 338
Pulmonary edema 288
Pulmonary eosinophilia, tropical 317
Pulmonary histoplasmosis 335
Pulmonary infection 177, 336
Pulmonary phase 310
Pulmonary symptoms 314
Pulmonary tuberculosis 20, 172
Pulp, white 82
Pulse polio immunization 245
Pus
    cells 280
        numerous 156
    containing sulfur granules 179
Pustule, malignant 165, 165*f*
Pyelonephritis 352
Pyocyanin 192
Pyogenic meningitis 348, 349
    causes 158
    etiological agents of 349*t*
Pyorubin 192
Pyoverdin 192

Q

Q fever 208
Quadrivalent vaccine 224
Quality assurance, components of 375
Quality audit 377
Quality control 375
Quality indicators 375, 376*t*
Quantitative buffy coat 270
    capillary tube 290*f*
    examination 289
Quantitative culture 353, 360
Quaternary ammonium compound 126, 129
Quellung reaction 14, 156
Quinsy 357

R

Rabid dogs, bite of 241
Rabies 66, 215, 218, 242
    antigen detection 242
    encephalitic 242
    furious 242
    immunoglobulin 61, 103, 243
    prevention of 242
    vaccine 99, 243
    virus 214, 215, 241, 241*f*
Radiation 124
Radioactive waste, hazards from 130
Radiologic examination 276
Ramsay Hunt syndrome 221
Rapid antibody detection tests 186
Rash 184, 221, 232, 324
Rat flea 321, 322, 324
    male 323*f*
Rat-bite fever 201, 202
    agents of 202

Reaction
    localized 93
    manifestations of 92
Real-time polymerase chain reaction 38, 38*f*, 216, 276
Recombinant DNA technology 43
Rectal swabs 20, 366, 368
Red blood cell 82, 104, 276
    antibody in 104
    size, parasitized 289
Red pulp 82
Reduviid bug 322
Re-emerging disease 238
Relapse 286
Relapsing fever 205
Remdesivir 234
Remittent fever 184
Renal parenchyma, infection of 352
Renal stones 351
Renal syndrome 262
Reoviridae 237
Replication, primary site of 214
Respirator 114
    negative pressure seal of 114
    positive pressure seal of 114
Respiratory contact 246
Respiratory diphtheria 162
Respiratory diseases 227
Respiratory droplets 234
    inhalation of 228
Respiratory infections 225, 369
Respiratory protection 112
Respiratory secretions 215
Respiratory specimens 367
Respiratory support 234
Respiratory syncytial virus 229, 231, 358
Respiratory tract 52, 230
    infections 233, 357
Respiratory viruses 261
Restriction enzyme, treatment with 43
Retina, infection of 363
Retroviruses 214
Reverse passive agglutination test 74
Reverse passive hemagglutination assay 74
Reverse transcriptase polymerase chain reaction 216, 230, 231, 234, 239
Revised National Tuberculosis Control Programme 175
Reye's syndrome 221
Rhabditiform larva 314*f*
Rhabdoviridae 237
Rhabdoviruses 213
Rh-antigen 104
Rh-blood group
    antigen 104
    system 104
Rheumatoid arthritis 95, 96
Rhinitis 357
    allergic 92
Rhinocerebral mucormycosis 338
Rhinoscleroma 357
Rhinosporidiosis 335
Rhinosporidium seeberi 335
Rhinovirus 244, 246, 247
Rhizoids 339
Rhizopus 330, 338, 338*f*
Ribavirin 231
Ribonucleic acid
    hepatitis viruses 214

synthesis inhibitors 47
vaccine 99, 100
virus 214, 233
    miscellaneous 260
Ribosomes 14
    aggregates of 245
Rice starch agar 331
Rice-water stool 190
Rickettsia 75, 87, 207
    akari 207
    conorii 207
    genera related to 208
    members of 207
    prowazekii 207
    rickettsii 207
    typhi 207
Rickettsial infections 35, 208
Rickettsialpox 207
Rideal and Walker test 128
Rifampicin 199
Rifamycins 47
Ring forms 289
Ring worm infections 333*f*
Ringer's solution 142
Ringworm infections, types of 332
Rituximab 223
River blindness 319
Robertson's cooked meat 170
    broth 26
    medium 26*f*
Rocky mountain spotted fever 207
Rodent-borne viral infections 262
Romana's sign 285
Romanowsky stains 270
Rose Gardner's disease 335
Rose spots 184
Rose-Waaler test 96
Rotavirus 102, 214, 139, 260, 261*f*, 355, 356
    diarrhea 260
    from stool 10
    isolation of 260
    vaccine 99, 102
Roundworm 310
Rubella 55, 103, 232
    vaccine 99, 232
    virus 227

S

S gene 101
Sabin-Feldman dye test 75, 293
Sabouraud's dextrose agar 179, 331, 362
Safe blood transfusion practices 104
Saline mount 268, 269, 269*f*
Saliva, shed in 242
Salivary gland infections 358
Salmonella 25, 31, 39, 46, 55, 69, 87, 128, 139, 181, 184, 185*f*, 352
    from sewage, isolation of 186
    typhi 73, 185, 226
Salt appearance 338
Sandfly 283, 322, 322*f*
    diseases transmitted by 323
Sapovirus 260, 261
Sarcoidosis 339
Sarcoptes scabei 324, 324*f*
Satellitism 196
Saturated salt solution 269

Savlon 129
Scabies 267, 325
    crusted 324
Scalded skin syndrome 150
Schaeffer-Fulton stain 16
Schistosoma 303, 306
    adult worm of 303*f*
    eggs 303, 305*f*
    haematobium 305, 305*f*, 306
    japonicum 305, 305*f*
    mansoni 305, 305*f*
Schistosomes 304, 305
    life cycle of 304, 304*f*
Schistosomiasis 305, 306
Schizogony 286
Schizonts 286, 289
Schneider's Drosophila insect medium 284
Sclera, infection of 363
Scleritis 363
Sclerosis, multiple 95
Scotochromogens 177
Scrotum, hydrocele of 317*f*
Scrub typhus 207
Seasonal flu 228
Sedimentation techniques 269
Seizure 299
Self-antigen, sequestration of 94
Semi-critical device 120
Semipermeable membrane 13
Semisolid medium 24
Sensitization phase 91, 93
Sepsis 346
Septic
    arthritis 210
    shock 346
Septicemia 165, 345
Septicemic plague 187
Sequencing 234
Serological tests 71, 260
Serology 35, 155, 204, 209, 232, 275, 359, 362
Serotyping 187, 225
Serovar specific test 206
Serpiginous tracks 313
Serratia 187
    marcescens 124, 187
Serum
    amyloid 60
    antibody 104, 230, 259
        detection 185, 238, 261, 284
    anti-diphtheritic 163
    antigen 261
    immunoglobulin A 66
    inactivated 66
    sickness 93
Severe acute respiratory syndrome coronavirus disease 233, 233*f*
Sex pili 15
Sexual cycle 293
Sexual mode 249
Sexual practices 56
Sexual spores, types of 329
Sexual transmission 255
Sexually active females 351
Sexually transmitted infection 197, 280, 362, 363*t*, 369
    causative agents of 362*t*
    laboratory diagnosis of 362
Shanghai fever 192

Sharp injury 135
Sharp pit 133
Sheather's sugar floatation technique 270, 295
Sheep, development in 300
Shepherd's crook 281
Shigella 25, 31, 39, 46, 50, 139, 181, 186, 355
    dysenteriae 186
    identification of 187
Shigellosis, treatment of 187
Shingles 221
Shock, risk of 237
Shoe cover 115
Sieve impactor 141
Silver 79
    impregnation method 204*f*
    staining 203
Simulium
    bite of 319
    species 322
Single hand scoop technique 136*f*
Sinus 357
    discharging 367
Sinusitis 357
Skeletal tuberculosis 172
Skin 52, 230, 271
    abscess of 179
    contact, direct 255
    decontamination 346
    flora 366
    infection 20, 149, 193, 360, 361
        superficial 154
        types of 360
    lesions 175, 203, 338, 346, 361
    manifestations, infective 361*t*
    rashes 203
    scrapping 325
    specimen 162
    test 301
Skin-to-skin contact 324
Skirrow's media, growth on 200*f*
Sleeping sickness 285
Slide agglutination 73
    test 73*f*, 185
Slide coagulase test 151
Slide culture technique 331*f*
Slide flocculation test 72
Slit sampler method 141
Slit skin smear 176
Slow virus 263*t*
    disease 262, 263
    infections 262
Small blood spill 126
Small intestine 273
Small medical items, disinfection of 125
Smallpox 55
    virus 225
Smear microscopy 176
Smear preparation 22
Sneezes, containment of 229
Socks syndrome 224
Sodium hypochlorite 126, 129, 235
Soft tick 322, 325
Soft-tissue
    infection 20, 149, 154, 193, 360, 361
    types of 360
Solid waste 134
Somatic cestodes 297

Index

Somatic nematodes 267, 308
Sore throat 154
Spaghetti appearance 332
Sparganosis 302
    diagnosis of 302
Sparganum larva 302
Spaulding's classification of medical devices 120, 120*t*
Species identification 193
Specimen 162, 169, 177-179, 234, 368
    exudate 367
    inoculation of 27
    number of 310
    preparation 10
    quality of 22
    rejection criteria 365
    storage before processing 20, 368, 369
    transport 19, 198, 368
    types 27*t*
Specimen collection 19, 158, 159, 165, 197, 242, 246, 268, 330, 333, 334, 352, 355, 359, 360, 362, 365
    and transport 358, 365
    process of 369*f*
Spermatheca 324
Spermatozoa 94
Spherules 335
Spike protein 101, 234
Spill management 135
    steps of 116
Spirillum minus 202
Spirochetes 203
Spirometra species 302
Spleen 82, 215, 282, 335
Splenic aspirate 271
Splenic aspiration 283
Splenomegaly 287
Sporangia, large 335
Spores 166
    demonstration of 16
Sporicidal agents 16
Sporogony 287
Sporothrix schenckii 330, 335, 335*f*
Sporotrichosis 335
Sporozoites 287, 292
Sputnik V vaccine 235
Sputum 271, 367
    microscopy 307
    smear
        grading of 173
        Zn staining of 173*f*
    specimen 22
Stains 242, 289
    differential 21
    simple 20
    special 21
    techniques 20
Standard agglutination test 74
Standard operating procedures 375
Staphylococcal
    abscess 50, 150*f*
    folliculitis 150*f*
Staphylococcus 31, 69, 149
    aureus 17, 30, 37, 46, 48, 50, 74, 95, 109, 149, 150*t*, 151, 151*f*, 196, 226, 352, 358
Steam jacket 120
Steam sterilizer 120, 121, 121*f*, 128

components of 120
    types of 121
    uses of 120
Steatorrhea 278
Stenotrophomonas 345
    maltophilia 192, 194
Sterilant 119, 120
    factors influencing efficacy of 119
    level of 118*t*
    test efficacy of 128
Sterile
    body fluids 366
    cotton swab 367*f*
    swabs 362
    universal specimen container 366, 366*f*
Sterilization 118, 121
    agents of 119
    conditions 120
    control 121, 122, 124
    cycle 121
    practice 118
    techniques 4
Sterilizers
    biological indicator 128
    chemical indicator 128
    physical indicator 128
    tests for 128
Stiff neck 348
Stomatitis 358
Stool
    antigen detection 275
    concentration 274
        techniques 295
    consistency 268
    culture 20, 185, 275, 313, 314, 368, 369
    examination 278, 295, 298, 311
    macroscopy 274, 305, 306, 313, 314
    saline mount of 309*f*
    sample container for 268*f*
    wet mount examination of 269*f*
Stool specimen 245
    demonstrating oocysts 295*f*
    normal constituents of 269
    parasite in 270*t*
Stormy clot reaction 169
Streak culture method 28, 28*f*
Streptobacillus moniliformis 202
Streptococcal infections 50
Streptococci 154*t*
Streptococcus 31, 39, 40, 69, 153
    agalactiae 155, 169, 348
    pneumoniae 48, 50, 69, 82, 154, 156, 348, 349, 358
    pyogenes 49, 50, 153, 155, 155*f*, 357
Streptodornase 153
Streptogramins 46
Streptokinase 153
Streptomyces 178
Streptomycin 188, 199
Strict hand hygiene 229
String test 190, 191*f*
Stroke culture 28
Strongyloides 270, 308, 309
    life cycle of 312*f*
    stercoralis 268, 313, 314*f*, 315
Strongyloidiasis 271, 314
    complications of 314*t*
    disseminated 314

Subcutaneous cysticercosis 299
Subcutaneous granulomatous disease 335
Subcutaneous mycoses 330, 333
Subcutaneous tissues 302
Substrate-chromogen system 75, 77
Sugar fermentation test 162
Sulbactam 45
Sulfonamides 92
Sulfur granules 178
Sun-rays appearance 179
Superantigens 64
Super-infection 258
Supplemental antibody detection tests 250
Suprapubic aspiration 353, 368
Surface disinfection 127
Surgical mask 113
    and respirators 112, 123
Surveillance, surface 142
Swabs, types of 358
Swarming growth 170
Swimmer's ear 192
Swimmer's itch 305
Swimming pool granuloma 177
Sympathetic dysfunction 242
Syngeneic graft 96
Synthesize vitamin 52
Syphilis 72, 79, 203, 205
    congenital 203
    diagnosis of congenital 205
    late 203
    primary 203
    secondary 203
Systematic bacteriology 147
Systemic anaphylaxis 92
Systemic autoimmune diseases 95
Systemic lupus erythematosus 95
Systemic mycoses 330, 335
Systemic reaction 93

■ T

T cell 60, 81, 82, 86, 91
    anergy, breakdown of 94
    area 82
    cytotoxic 83, 86
    defects 96
    development 83
    maturation of 81
    receptor 86, 87
    regulatory 94
    types of 83
T lymphocytes 82, 83
Tachyzoite 292
    comma-shaped 293
    transform into 292
Taenia 270
    infection 268
    life cycle of 297
    species 298
Taenia saginata 297, 298
    egg of 299*f*
    life cycle of 298*f*
Taenia solium 268, 297, 298, 298*f*, 299
    causing cysticercosis, life cycle of 299
    egg of 299*f*
Tapeworm 267, 299
Target cell 88
    lysis 69, 87, 88

Index

Tazobactam 353
Tbilisi phage typing 226
T_C cells 88
    activation of 86f, 87
    differentiation of 86f
T-dependent antigens 64
T_{DTH} cells 91, 93
Tegument 219
Teichoic acid 13, 149
Tertian malaria, malignant 288
Test band 79
Test dots 80
Tetanospasmin 169
Tetanus 66, 102
    immune globulin 103
    neonatal 54
    toxoid vaccine 170
Tetracycline 45, 46, 191, 209
Tetramethyl benzidine 75
T_H cell 91
    activation of 87, 87f
    effector 87
Thermocycler machine 36f
Thermophiles 17
Thin blood smear 288, 288f
Thioglycollate broth 26f
Thiosulfate-citrate-bile-salt sucrose agar 25, 27, 190, 191f
Threadworm 309
Throat swab 358, 367, 370
Thumb print appearance 198
Thymocytes 81
Thymus 81
    transplants 97
Ticks 267, 325
T-independent antigens 64
Tinea
    barbae 333, 333f
    corporis 333, 333f
    cruris 333
    faciei 333, 333f
    nigra 332
    pedis 333, 333f
    unguium 333
    versicolor 332
Tissue
    cestodes 297
    culture 10, 217, 246, 293, 356
    cyst 292
        containing bradyzoites 293f
    damaging response 172
    enzymes, antigen to 63
    injury 49
    nematodes 308, 316
    specimens 367
Titer 71, 185
    protective 163
TLD regimen 253
Tocilizumab 234
Togaviridae 237
Tongue, vesicular lesions on 220f
Tonsillitis 357
Tonsils 82
Toxic shock syndrome 150, 154
Toxigenicity test 170

Toxin 49, 50, 149, 181, 192, 345
    antitoxin neutralization test 75
    code for 226
    coregulated pilus 189
    demonstration 162, 170
    phage coded 42
    production 355
    treatment of 101
Toxocara canis 315
Toxoid 163
    vaccine 99, 100
Toxoplasma 75
    gondii 292, 293f, 345
        life cycle of 292f
    infection 293, 294
Toxoplasmosis 293
Trachea 357
Tracheobronchitis 210
Trachoma 208
Transduction
    role of 41
    types of 41
Transfusion 109
    reactions 105
Transfusion-transmitted infections 105
Transplant
    classification of 96
    immunology 96
Transposons, types of 43
Traveler's diarrhea 354
Treg cells, loss of 94
Trematode 267, 303
    infections 305
    life cycle of 304t
Trench fever 324
Treponema 203
    pallidum 4, 18, 72, 75, 203, 205
        direct microscopy of 204f
        specific antigen 204
Treponemal tests 204
Triage parasite panel 271, 356
Tribe proteeae 187
Trichinella spiralis 308, 316, 320
Trichomonas 271
Trichomonas
    tenax 281
    vaginalis 280
        trophozoite of 280f
Trichomoniasis 280
    diagnostic modalities for 280
Trichophyton
    mentagrophytes 334f
    species 332
Trichosporon beigelii 332
Trichuris 56, 270, 308
    life cycle of 309f
    trichiura 309
    egg of 309f
Triple sugar iron test 31, 32f, 193
Triple-drug regimen 201
Trombiculid mite 322, 324, 324f
Trophozoite 270, 273, 275, 275f, 276, 276f, 277, 277f, 278, 279, 279f, 280, 281, 281f, 286
Tropism 215
Trypanosoma 270, 282, 285, 345

    cruzi 285, 285f
Trypanosoma brucei 285
    gambiense 285
    rhodesiense 285
    trypomastigote forms of 285f
Tsetse fly 322, 323, 323f
Tube agglutination 73
Tube coagulase test 151, 151f
Tubercle bacilli 9f
Tuberculoid leprosy 175t
Tuberculosis 174, 339, 358
    infection, diagnosis of latent 174
    suspected 367
Tuberculous
    lymphadenitis 172
    meningitis 172
    skin lesions 172
Tularemia 201
Tumor
    antigens 83, 98
    immunology 94, 97
    markers 98t
Turbidimetric method 141
Tyndallization 126
Typhi 184
Typhoid
    fever 73
        vaccines for 186
    vaccine 99
Typhoidal salmonella 184
Typhus fever 63, 74
Tzanck cell 220, 221f
Tzanck preparation 220
Tzanck smear 221f, 360

U

Ultraviolet
    light 98
    radiation 126
Unfertilized eggs 311, 311f
Upper respiratory tract 357
    infections 357
        laboratory diagnosis of 358
Upper urinary tract infection 352
Urea hydrolysis test 31, 32f
Urease test 193, 198
    rapid 201
Ureteric stones 351
Urethra 351
Urethral discharge 362, 368
Urethral exudates, gram staining of 159
Urethritis 363, 368
Urinary carriers 184
Urinary tract 351
    functional abnormality of 351
    structural abnormality of 351
Urinary tract infection 20, 53, 150, 181, 192, 351, 351t, 353
    asymptomatic 352
    catheter with 110
    lower 352
    pathogenesis of 352f
    symptoms of 352
Urine 20, 271, 368, 369

Index

culture 185
microscopy 306
midstream clean catch 368
specimen 368
Urogenital disease 306
Urogenital mycoplasmas 210
Uvea, infection of 363
Uveitis 363
post-traumatic 94

V

Vaccine
commonly used 99t
inactivated 99, 100
nine valent 224
production of 43
subunit 99, 100, 218
vial monitor 101
stages of 101f, 101t
Vagina 52
Vaginal discharge 362
pH of 202
Vaginal mucosa, strawberry appearance of 280
Vaginal secretion depicting clue cell, wet mount of 202f
Vancomycin resistant enterococci 47, 48, 157
Varicella-zoster
immunoglobulin 103, 222
virus 221
treatment of 222
Variola 225
Vector control strategies 291
Vector-borne diseases 369
Veillonella 171
Venereal disease research laboratory 72
slide 204f
test 204, 204f
Venezuelan equine encephalitis viruses 236
Venkatraman-Ramakrishnan medium 366
Vernier caliper 34f
Vero cell line 217
Verocytotoxin 42
Vi antigen vaccine 186
Viable plate count 142
Viable tissue 367
Vibrio
alginolyticus 191
cholerae 14, 25, 39, 50, 55, 139, 189, 190, 190f, 191f, 226, 355
classification of 189
parahaemolyticus 191
species 191
vulnificus 191
Vincent's angina 358
Viral agents 345, 350, 357
Viral antibody, detection of 216
Viral antigen 83
detection of 216, 220, 260
Viral culture 234
Viral deoxyribonucleic acid 256
Viral diseases 217
diagnosis of 75
laboratory diagnosis of 215
treatment of 217
Viral encephalitis 369
Viral etiology 260, 345
Viral gastroenteritis 260, 369
Viral growth 225
Viral infections
manifestations of 215
pathogenesis of 214
specimen collection for 369
transport for 369f
types of 369t
Viral isolation 220, 230
Viral load 249
monitoring 251
Viral meningitis, acute 349
Viral neutralization 69
test 75
Viral opportunistic infections 249
Viral pneumonia 359
Viral protein 244, 227
Viral replication 214
Viral ribonucleic acid 227
detection 251
Viral transport medium 369
and swab 229f, 370f
Viral vaccines 217
Viral vector vaccine 99, 101
Viremia 215
Viridans streptococci 154, 155, 156f
Virology 211, 366
general 213
Virulence factors 13, 149, 153, 158, 159, 161, 165, 181
Virulence pathogenesis 165
Virulent cycle 41, 225
Virus 105, 139, 351, 354, 373
causing gastroenteritis 260t
direct demonstration of 216
direct detection of 260
entry 249
fixed 241
isolation of 216, 222, 229, 232, 242, 245, 246
mode of transmission of 215t
morphology of 213
parainfluenza 229, 230, 357
ribonucleic acid detection 242
shape of 214
size of 214
spread of 215
street 241
teratogenic 369
Visceral larva migrans 315
causes of 315
Visceral leishmaniasis 282, 284
epidemiology of 282
prevention of 284
Visceral organs 302
Vitamin B$_{12}$ 52
supplement 302
VITEK 2 automated system 33, 33f
Vitreous fluid 368
Vitreous humor 363
Vivax malaria 290
Viviparous 308
Vomiting 237
Voriconazole 332, 341
Vulvovaginitis 280, 336

W

Warts 224
Waste
disposal of 131
general 134
generated 130
in hospitals 130
management hierarchy 131
produced antagonizes 52
receptacles 132
segregation in hospitals 132
sharps including metal sharps 132
Waste-to-energy 134
Water
bacteriology of 139
contaminated with healthcare, test of 141
fleas 325
recent fecal contamination of 140
sample, collection and transport of 140
sampling methods 140f
supply, quality of 141
surveillance 139
Waterborne pathogens 139
Water-lily sign 301
Wayson staining 188
Weil's disease 206
Weil-Felix
reaction 74
test 208
Welsh regimen 335
West-Nile
encephalitis 236, 239
fever 239
virus 239
Wet mount
examination 353
preparation 187
Whiff test 202
Whooping cough 197, 358
Widal test 73, 185, 185f, 186, 186f
Wild polioviruses 244
Wilson and Blair media 186
bismuth sulphite 185
Winter vomiting disease 261
Wool sorter's disease 165
Worm load, mild-to-moderate 314
Wound 182
botulism 170
care, local 243
clean 110, 361
closed 367
open 367
Wound infection
agents causing burn 361t
agents causing surgical site 361t
cause of 201
Wuchereria bancrofti 270, 308, 316-318, 321, 370
life cycle of 317f
microfilaria of 318f, 319f

X

X. astia 324
Xenodiagnoses 285
Xenograft 97
Xenopsylla cheopis 207, 322, 324
Xylose lysine deoxycholate 25, 27, 356

Y

Yeast 22, 329
   dried 128
   like fungi 330, 332
Yellow fever 240, 345
   17D vaccine 99, 240
   vaccine 217
Yersinia 181
   enterocolitica 188
   pestis 187, 321
   pseudotuberculosis 188
   species 187, 188
Yersiniosis 188
Yolk sac inoculation 217

Z

Ziehl-Neelsen stain 173
   microscopy by 177
   modified 16
Ziehl-Neelsen technique 22, 23, 359
Zika
   fever 240
   syndrome, congenital 240
   virus 240
Zinc 336
   sulphate 270
Zoonotic 236
   tetrad 208
Zoster 221
   ophthalmicus 221
   rashes of 222*f*
Zygomycosis 336, 338, 339
Zygote 287